PAIN MANAGEMENT AND SEDATION

PAIN MANAGEMENT AND SEDATION

Emergency Department Management

Edited by

Sharon E. Mace, MD, FACEP, FAAP
Associate Professor
Department of Emergency Medicine
Ohio State University School of Medicine
Faculty, Cleveland Clinic/MetroHealth Emergency
   Medicine Residency Program
Director, Pediatric Education/Quality Improvement
Director, Observation Unit
The Cleveland Clinic Foundation
Cleveland, Ohio

James Ducharme, MD, CM, FRCP
Professor
Department of Emergency Medicine
Dalhousie University
Clinical Director
Department of Emergency Medicine
Atlantic Health Sciences Corporation
Saint John, New Brunswick, Canada

Michael F. Murphy, MD
Professor and Chair
Department of Anesthesiology
Dalhousie University
Attending Emergency Physician
Queen Elizabeth II Health Sciences Center
Halifax, Nova Scotia, Canada

McGraw-Hill
Medical Publishing Division

New York   Chicago   San Francisco   Lisbon
London   Madrid   Mexico City
Milan   New Delhi   San Juan   Seoul
Singapore   Sydney   Toronto

Pain Management and Sedation: Emergency Department Management

Copyright © 2006 by The McGraw-Hill Companies, Inc. All rights reserved. Printed in the United States of America. Except as permitted under the United States Copyright Act of 1976, no part of this publication may be reproduced or distributed in any form or by any means, or stored in a data base or retrieval system, without the prior written permission of the publisher.

1 2 3 4 5 6 7 8 9 0   DOC/DOC   0 9 8 7 6 5

ISBN: 0-07-144202-2

This book was set in Times by International Typesetting and Composition.
The editors were Marc Strauss and Robert Pancotti.
The production supervisor was Catherine Saggese.
Project management was provided by International Typesetting and Composition.
The cover designer was Aimee Nordin.
The indexer was Susan G. Hunter.
RR Donnelley was printer and binder.

This book is printed on acid-free paper.

Library of Congress Cataloging-in-Publication Data
Pain management and sedation : emergency department management / edited by Sharon E.
   Mace, James Ducharme, Michael F. Murphy.
      p. ; cm.
   Includes bibliographical references and index.
   ISBN 0-07-144202-2 (alk. paper)
   1. Pain—Treatment. 2. Analgesia. 3. Anesthesia. 4. Sedatives. 5. Emergency medicine. I.
Mace, Sharon E. II. Ducharme, James. III. Murphy, Michael F.
   [DNLM: 1. Pain—drug therapy. 2. Analgesics—therapeutic use. 3. Emergency Service,
Hospital—organization & administration. 4. Emergency Treatment—methods. WL 704
P146575 2006]
RB127.P332342 2006
615′.78—dc22
                                                                    2005049138

To my family, especially my parents, and my friends for their love and encouragement.

Sharon E. Mace

To my father, who could not rely on his physicians to treat his pain in the final years of his life. May we serve our patients better than this.

James Ducharme

Time is a fixed commodity. In my case, the time that I spend writing and editing books diminishes the time that I have to spend with my family, time I'll never get back. At times, we both resent it. I dedicate this effort to my wife Debbi, my sons Teddy and Ryan, and my daughter Amanda. No work like this is possible without the dedication, toil, and expertise of others. I recognize the efforts of my fellow editors, Sharon and Jim, and the authors, who gave selflessly of their time to make us better at what we do and to take better care of people.

Michael F. Murphy

CONTENTS

SECTION IX   The Future: What's to Come

CONTRIBUTORS

Eric Anderson, MD, MBA, FACEP [5]
Faculty, Cleveland Clinic/MetroHealth
Emergency Medicine Residency Program
Associate Director of Operations
Department of Emergency Medicine
The Cleveland Clinic Foundation
Cleveland, Ohio

Scott Bailey, MD [45]
Resident Physician
Emergency Medicine Residency Program
University of California at Los Angeles/Olive View
Los Angeles, California

Ashley E. Booth, MD [7]
Clinical Instructor, Healthcare Policy Fellow
Department of Emergency Medicine
University of Florida Health Science Center–Jacksonville
Jacksonville, Florida

Lance Brown, MD, MPH, FACEP [50]
Chief, Division of Pediatric Emergency Medicine
Associate Professor of Emergency Medicine and Pediatrics
Loma Linda University Medical Center and
    Children's Hospital
Loma Linda, California

William H. Cordell, MD [36]
Adjunct Clinical Professor in Emergency Medicine
Department of Emergency Medicine
Indiana University School of Medicine
Senior Clinical Research Physician
Eli Lilly & Company
Indianapolis, Indiana

Ann M. Dietrich, MD, FAAP, FACEP [35]
Associate Professor of Pediatrics
Ohio State University of Medicine and Public Health
Attending Physician, Section of Emergency Medicine
Children's Hospital
Columbus, Ohio

James Ducharme, MD, CM, FRCP [30,33,34,39,51]
Professor
Department of Emergency Medicine
Dalhousie University
Clinical Director
Department of Emergency Medicine
Atlantic Health Sciences Corporation
Saint John, New Brunswick, Canada

Pamela Dyne, MD [45]
Associate Professor of Clinical Medicine
David Geffen School of Medicine
University of California at Los Angeles
Residency Program Director
Emergency Medicine Residency Program
University of California at Los Angeles/Olive View
Codirector
University of California at Los Angeles/
    Olive View–University of California at
    Los Angeles Combined Emergency Medicine/
    Internal Medicine Residency Program
Sylmar, California

Jonathan Glauser, MD, FACEP [4]
Clinical Assistant Professor
Department of Medicine
Case Western Reserve University
Attending Staff
Department of Emergency Medicine
The Cleveland Clinic Foundation
Cleveland, Ohio

Steven A. Godwin, MD, FACEP [7]
Assistant Professor
Director of Medical Education
Residency Director
Department of Emergency Medicine
University of Florida Health Science
    Center–Jacksonville
Jacksonville, Florida

Ran D. Goldman, MD [49]
Pediatric Research in Emergency Therapeutics
  (PRETx) Program
Division of Pediatric Emergency Medicine
The Hospital for Sick Children
Department of Pediatrics
University of Toronto
Toronto, Ontario, Canada

Kathleen Hogan, RN, CEN [9]
Nurse Manager
Department of Emergency Medicine
Hospital of the University of Pennsylvania
Philadelphia, Pennsylvania
Our Lady of Lourdes Medical Center
Camden, New Jersey

Orlando Hung, MD [27]
Staff Anesthesiologist
Queen Elizabeth II Health Sciences Center
Professor
Departments of Anesthesiology, Pharmacology,
  and Surgery
Director of Research
Department of Anesthesia
Dalhousie University
Halifax, Nova Scotia, Canada

Fredric M. Hustey, MD [44]
Staff Physician
Department of Emergency Medicine
The Cleveland Clinic Foundation
Assistant Professor
The Cleveland Clinic Lerner College of Medicine
Case Western Reserve University
Cleveland, Ohio

Grant D. Innes, MD, FRCP(C) [31]
Department of Emergency Medicine
Providence Health Care and St. Paul's Hospital
Vancouver, British Columbia, Canada

Sandra H. Johnson, JD, LLM [6]
Tenet Chair in Health Law and Ethics
Center for Health Law Studies of the School of Law
  and Center for Health Care Ethics
Professor of Law in Internal Medicine
School of Medicine
Saint Louis University
St. Louis, Missouri

Anne-Maree Kelly, MD, MClinEd, FACEM [10,38]
Professor and Director, Department of
  Emergency Medicine
Western Hospital
Melbourne, Australia
Director, Joseph Epstein Centre for Emergency
  Medicine Research
Melbourne, Australia
Department of Medicine
The University of Melbourne
Melbourne, Australia

Marc Leder, MD [35]
Clinical Associate Professor of Pediatrics
Ohio State University of Medicine and
  Public Health
Attending Physician
Section of Emergency Medicine
Children's Hospital
Columbus, Ohio

Jacques S. Lee, MD, MSc, DABEM, FRCPC [11,45]
Assistant Professor, Department of Medicine
University of Toronto
Director, Emergency Medicine Research Program
Sunnybrook and Women's College Health
  Sciences Center
Associate Researcher, Clinical Epidemiology Unit
Sunnybrook Research Institute
Scholarly Activities Coordinator
University of Toronto
Royal College Training Program in Emergency Medicine
Toronto, Ontario, Canada

Sharon E. Mace, MD, FACEP, FAAP [1-3,12,15,17-22,26,37,43,47,48]
Associate Professor
Department of Emergency Medicine
Ohio State University School of Medicine
Faculty, Cleveland Clinic/MetroHealth Emergency
  Medicine Residency Program
Director, Pediatric Education/Quality Improvement
Director, Observation Unit
The Cleveland Clinic Foundation
Cleveland, Ohio

Lilit Minasyan, MD, MS [50]
Fellow, Pediatric Emergency Medicine
Loma Linda University Medical Center and
  Children's Hospital
Loma Linda, California

Michael F. Murphy, MD [1,7,8,16,23,24,25,27,28,48]
Professor and Chair
Department of Anesthesiology
Dalhousie University
Attending Emergency Physician
Queen Elizabeth II Health Sciences Center
Halifax, Nova Scotia, Canada

L. Connor Nickels, MD [40]
Department of Emergency Medicine
Orlando Regional Medical Center
Orlando, Florida

Blake O'Brien, MD [40]
Department of Emergency Medicine
Orlando Regional Medical Center
Orlando, Florida

Tammie E. Quest, MD [46]
Assistant Professor
Department of Emergency Medicine
Emory University School of Medicine
Atlanta, Georgia

George A. Ralls, MD, FACEP [40]
Medical Director
Orange County Emergency Medical
    Services System
Orange County, Florida
Attending Emergency Physician
Department of Emergency Medicine
Orlando Regional Medical Center
Orlando, Florida

Alex L. Rogovik, PhD, MD [49]
Pediatric Research in Emergency Therapeutics
    (PRETx) Program
Division of Pediatric Emergency Medicine
The Hospital for Sick Children
Department of Pediatrics
University of Toronto
Toronto, Ontario, Canada

Alfred D. Sacchetti, MD, FACEP [9, 42]
Assistant Clinical Professor of Emergency Medicine
Thomas Jefferson University
Philadelphia, Pennsylvania
Chief of Emergency Medicine
Our Lady of Lourdes Medical Center
Camden, New Jersey

Sandra M. Schneider, MD, FACEP [32]
Professor and Chair
Department of Emergency Medicine
University of Rochester
Rochester, New York

Ghazala Q. Sharieff, MD, FACEP, FAAEM, FAAP [41]
Director of Pediatric Emergency Medicine
California Emergency Physicians (CEP)
Associate Clinical Professor
Children's Hospital and Health Center
University of California at San Diego
San Diego, California

Salvatore Silvestri, MD, FACEP [40]
Medical Director
Orange County Emergency Medical Services System
Orange County, Florida
Assistant Residency Director
Department of Emergency Medicine
Orlando Regional Medical Center
Orlando, Florida
Clinical Assistant Professor
Department of Emergency Medicine
University of Florida College of Medicine
Gainesville, Florida

James I. Syrett, MD [32]
Senior Instructor
Department of Emergency Medicine
University of Rochester
Rochester, New York

Knox H. Todd, MD, MPH [13, 29]
Director, Pain and Emergency Medicine Initiative
Adjunct Associate Professor
Rollins School of Public Health
Atlanta, Georgia

Thomas F. Turco, PharmD [42]
Director of Pharmacy
Our Lady of Lourdes Medical Center
Camden, New Jersey

Michael A. Turturro, MD, FACEP [14]
Clinical Associate Professor of Emergency Medicine
University of Pittsburgh School of Medicine
Vice Chair and Director of Academic Affairs
Department of Emergency Medicine
The Mercy Hospital of Pittsburgh
Pittsburgh, Pennsylvania

Ron M. Walls, MD [28]
Chairman, Department of Emergency Medicine
Brigham and Women's Hospital
Associate Professor of Medicine
Division of Emergency Medicine
Harvard Medical School
Boston, Massachusetts

John Ward, MD, FRCP(C) [31]
Department of Emergency Medicine
Providence Health Care and St. Paul's Hospital
Vancouver, British Columbia, Canada

Bernie Whitaker, RN, BapplSci(AdvNur), MNst, PhD [10]
Lecturer in Nursing
School of Nursing
University of Ballarat
Ballarat, Victoria, Australia

Robert J. Zalenski, MD [46]
Director of Clinical Research
Professor, Emergency Medicine
Wayne State University
Detroit, Michigan

"SAY IT AIN'T SO, SAY IT AIN'T SO." This saying arises from the fact that Shoeless Joe Jackson took a $5000 bribe and might have been involved in deliberately guiding his team, the Chicago White Sox, to lose the 1919 World Series. More shocking than Shoeless Joe's action is the reality that patients have needlessly suffered pain and anxiety while in the care of competent health care providers.

Over half of the approximately 120 million patients presenting to emergency departments each year in the United States have pain as part of their chief complaint.[1] Prompt, titrated, and effective analgesia should be a high priority for basic humane concerns and for positive physiologic benefits including decreased myocardial oxygen consumption, decreased sympathetic outflow, decreased carbon dioxide production, and unaltered immune function and coagulability. Furthermore, due to central nervous system plasticity, unrelieved acute pain may occasionally progress to chronic pain.

Oligoanalgesia remains the silent epidemic.[2] In 1973, Marks and Sachar noted that undertreatment of medical patients in pain with opioid analgesics was more the rule than the exception.[3] During the past three decades, this observation has been repeated in all specialties and medical settings examined. The reason why oligoanalgesia has existed throughout the world is open to speculation.

Since postoperative pain is the commonest type of acute pain that exists in hospitals, many of our pain management patterns have evolved from academic surgeons. In Zachary Cope's text *The Early Diagnosis of the Acute Abdomen*, his well-meaning statement has haunted us for decades: "If morphine be administered, it is possible to die happy in the belief that he is on the road to recovery, and in some cases the medical attendant may for a time be induced to share the same delusive hope."[4] This philosophy dated from a time before modern diagnostic techniques. Studies now indicate that titrated opioid analgesia can be safely administered without obscuring or delaying the diagnosis of acute abdominal pain. The latest author of

this text, William Silen, has a dramatically different opinion: "The cruel practice of withholding analgesics is to be condemned, but I suspect that it will take many generations to eliminate it because the rule has become so firmly ingrained in the minds of physicians."[5]

Education can be instrumental in eliminating oligoanesthesia. The textbook *Pain Management in Emergency Medicine* was published in 1988.[6] In 1992, the U.S. Department of Health and Human Services published the clinical practice guideline "Acute Pain Management in Adults: Operative Procedures."[7] The American College of Emergency Physicians (ACEP) has clinical policies on the treatment of abdominal pain and procedural sedation.[8] In 2005, this textbook *Pain Management and Sedation: Emergency Department Management* is being published. Such information should promote knowledge about safe and effective pain management and procedural sedation, advance the clinical practice of emergency medicine, and improve patient care.

Providing relief from pain and anxiety can never be an excuse for an unsafe procedure. First "do no harm" but then "do some good." We must provide the scientific basis for the practice of analgesic techniques. We must be cognizant of the fact that other specialties will often criticize practices that they are unfamiliar with or believe to be unsafe due to habit and antiquated teachings. An example involved a review of the text *Pain Management in Emergency Medicine*, which contained a chapter on ketamine that recommended doses that would now be considered too low.[8] The recommended IM doses were 0.5 mg to 1.0 mg/kg IM and 0.5 mg/kg IV loading dose. The journal *Anesthesia and Analgesia* stated, "The doses suggested in the text would induce a state of general anesthesia in most patients if given as an intravenous bolus. Without ventilatory support, some of these patients could easily suffer hypoxic damage or death."[9] This grossly inaccurate, non-evidence-based assessment points out some critical issues. Many other specialties and physicians are behind the curve in progressive, humane approaches to acute pain management. In many emergency departments, drugs such as fentanyl, ketamine, and etomidate have been prohibited or were obtained only after the rattling of sabers and gnashing of teeth. These misguided actions are by well-intentioned physicians who believe that they are carrying the burden of patient safety. Like our fellow specialists, we are "patient safety" advocates but we must remind our colleagues that patient safety is not incompatible with effective analgesia, anxiolysis, or procedural sedation.

There is no specialty of medicine or surgery that has taken a leadership role in education and research into the humane treatment of acute pain. As a specialty, emergency medicine has the opportunity to become a lighthouse in the sea of human suffering from acute pain. We must be the beacons of information, role modeling, and advocating for safe and effective analgesia. This text can be our ally as we go to war to combat the plight of acute pain.

The editors of this text are to be lauded for compiling 51 chapters that cover the entire gamut of topics pertinent to practicing emergency physicians. Some topics are unique and represent novel additions to our literature. Topics such as the Joint Commission on Accreditation of Healthcare Organizations, preprocedural assessment, and postprocedural sedation assessment present information that is exceedingly important to emergency department directors, including those responsible for establishing policies. The authors represent leading pain researchers and educators in our specialty. All patient populations are represented, including neonates, children, geriatrics, and pregnant women. Nonpharmacologic techniques are also well represented. This text allows ready availability of crucial information that pertains to more than half of our patients. It is ideally suited to be used by emergency medicine residents to become more expert at the pharmacology and practice of analgesia and procedural sedation. This is why it should be part of any emergency department library of reference texts.

This text can help emergency medicine guide the health care system to achieve a new reality that will include the following:

- Prompt and effective analgesia and sedation for all emergency department patients with acute pain states.
- Use of pain scores to guide pain management and continuous quality improvement efforts.

- Prospective studies confirming success in the early, safe, and successful treatment of patients with acute pain.
- Prescriptions for analgesics given to all *appropriate* patients discharged with acute pain states.
- Procedural sedation routinely used for all indicated procedures and following guidelines to ensure safety and patient comfort.
- Evidence-based (contributing to research) use of the analgesic class best suited for the given indication.

When this day comes, we can all imagine ourselves, our loved ones, and our fellow humans en route to an emergency department with the confident expectation that safe, compassionate pain relief is only moments away. "Say it is so, say it is so, please say it is so."

Paul M. Paris, MD
Department of Emergency Medicine
Executive Director
Pittsburgh Emergency Medicine Foundation
Pittsburgh, Pennsylvania

REFERENCES

1. Cordell WH, Keene KK, Giles BK, et al. The high prevalence of pain in emergency medical care. *Am J Emerg Med.* 2002; 20:165–169.
2. Wilson JE, Pendleton JM. Oligoanalgesia in the emergency department. *Am J Emerg Med.* 1989;7:620–623.
3. Marks RM, Sachar EJ. Undertreatment of medical inpatients with narcotic analgesics. *Ann Intern Med.* 1973;78:173–181.
4. Cope Z. *The Early Diagnosis of the Acute Abdomen.* New York: Oxford University Press; 1921.
5. Silen W. *Cope's Early Diagnosis of the Acute Abdomen.* 21st ed. New York: Oxford University Press; 2004.
6. Paris PM, Stewart RD. *Pain Management in Emergency Medicine.* Norwalk, CT: Appleton & Lange; 1988.
7. Acute Pain Management Guideline Panel. *Acute Pain Management in Adults: Operative Procedures. Quick Reference Guide for Clinicians.* AHCPR Pub. No 92-0019. Rockville, MD: Agency for Health Care Policy and Research, Public Health Service, U.S. Department of Health and Human Services.
8. American College of Emergency Physicians. Clinical policy: Critical issues for the initial management and evaluation of patients presenting with a chief complaint of nontraumatic abdominal pain. *Ann Emerg Med.* 2000;36:406–415.
9. Smith KW. *Anesth Analg.* 1990;70:678–679.

PREFACE

THE EDITORS OF THIS BOOK have dedicated much of their careers to the alleviation of the pain and suffering of emergency patients. We have advocated and will continue to advocate for adequate analgesia and procedural sedation in both adults and children. Unfortunately, all too often in the past, severe abdominal pain may have been untreated, a dislocated ankle was relocated without adequate analgesic medication, and small children undergoing procedures were restrained without receiving analgesics. Health care providers, including physicians, were taught that these were safe and appropriate practices within the standard of care. Thankfully, with the growth and maturation of medicine, much has changed.

Emergency medicine, a specialty focused on the care and treatment of the emergency patient, must play a leading role in the provision of adequate analgesia and sedation. Now the issue is not "Should the patient receive analgesia and/or sedation?" but "How do we ensure that our patients receive adequate analgesia and how is procedural sedation administered safely in the emergency department setting?"

Although some groups of patients—children and infants, the elderly, and the cognitively impaired—suffer more from oligoanalgesia than others, all patients can benefit from improved pain management and sedation. Failure to treat pain adequately has both short- and long-term negative consequences. Progress in the treatment of emergency department patients has been made. However, adequate sedation and analgesia must continue to be a priority issue for all who practice the specialty of emergency medicine so that suboptimal analgesia and sedation no longer exist in emergency departments.

Most medical schools fail to provide adequate emphasis on the teaching of pain, analgesia, and sedation. We must ensure that undergraduate and postgraduate professional education, both in residency programs and beyond, stress the importance of the effective management of pain and sedation. Emergency department administrators need to ensure that patients' pain and sedation needs are being met by developing effective departmental policies regarding sedation and analgesia. Emergency medicine organizations, whether local, national, or international, must make adequate pain management and sedation an ongoing priority. We must maintain our role as patient advocates.

The purpose of this text is to deal with issues of analgesia and procedural sedation as they relate to emergency medicine. Furthermore, much of the information in this textbook is not readily available elsewhere. Some of the chapters, such as those on nerve blocks and specific sedative agents, are detailed enough to serve as a "how to" manual. The authors' intent was to provide a concise, practical overview of analgesia and sedation in emergency medicine practice. We have attempted to highlight the risks and benefits contingent on the use of potent medications and techniques and have recommended safe procedures by which they might be employed. As with the use of any therapeutic agent or medical procedure, practitioners are advised to use their own knowledge and skills in order to employ the techniques and therapeutic agents in a safe and prudent manner.

We hope that emergency physicians will find this textbook a useful addition to their libraries, a valuable resource in their clinical practice, and a tool for training their students and residents. Furthermore, any discussion engendered by this textbook should promote education and research in analgesia and procedural sedation. May all our patients benefit.

Terminology

Opioids, opiates, or narcotics are terms that have been used to describe a class of drugs that have effects related to binding to opioid receptors. Because these terms have been used interchangeably for years, it is difficult to change old habits. The editors have endeavored to incorporate the preferred usage (e.g., opioids) throughout this textbook. However, there may be instances where the older terminology is used. Eventually, time and consistent usage of the term opioids will prevail.

PAIN MANAGEMENT AND SEDATION

1

The History of Procedural Sedation

Michael F. Murphy
Sharon E. Mace

EARLY HISTORY

The history of medicine and the human condition is inextricably entwined with pain, and our attempts to escape it.

The alleviation of pain and suffering is fundamental to the practice of medicine, perhaps even more so when painful procedures must be performed. Before the discovery and introduction of diethyl ether in the late 1840s, pain was considered an inevitable consequence of surgery. Prior to that time, combinations of opium (opioid) and ethanol (sedative hypnotic) were commonly used to blunt the pain inflicted during such procedures, though with the advent of general anesthesia such concoctions faded in importance. In fact, it really was not until the 1970s that the concept of procedural sedation (PS) and analgesia was resurrected.

The 1970s

Driven by constraints placed on it by the public's demand for less painful and anxiety-provoking dentistry, and malpractice carrier restrictions on general anesthesia for routine dental procedures, it was the dental profession that sought out alternative techniques. Thus, by the mid-1970s, the concept of *conscious sedation* was borne of necessity.[1–6] In fact, a monograph totally concerned with the practice of conscious sedation was published in 1974.[1] At its earliest stages it consisted of varying amounts of:

- Hypnosis, to address the psychologic aspects of fear and suffering.
- Analgesia, typically nitrous oxide.

- Local anesthesia.
- Anxiolysis employing oral agents such as chloral hydrate and barbiturates.

The goal was a state of consciousness characterized by the patient's indifference to and cooperation with the procedure, without pain, anxiety, fear, or the loss of protective reflexes.

Dental practitioners pioneered many of the concepts of safety in providing conscious sedation to dental patients. They were the first to explore and report on the use of oxygenation monitoring during sedation.[7,8]

The 1980s

By the mid to late 1980s, the adoption of this terminology and practice was widespread in medicine and dentistry:

- Anesthesia providers employed it to facilitate investigational studies, as an adjunct to regional anesthesia and for minor surgery (e.g., D&C, epilepsy surgery, and laparoscopy).[9–12]
- Gastroenterologists for endoscopy.[13,14]
- Podiatrists for minor surgery.[15]
- Ophthalmologists for cataract surgery.[16]
- Radiologists and anesthesiologists for pediatric cardiac catheterization.[17]
- Cardiologists for cardioversion.[18]

The subject of conscious sedation was probably first introduced to emergency medicine by the American Academy of Pediatrics in 1985.[19] A sign of the importance of sedation in all aspects of medicine and dentistry is its early publication in the emergency medicine literature.[20] Bennett and Stewart elaborated the concept beyond pediatrics in the late 1980s touting conscious sedation as an alternative to general anesthesia, and a procedure appropriate to emergency medicine practice.[21] They also were probably the first to introduce the term *dissociative sedation* to refer to the state induced by subdissociative doses of ketamine. By 1990, "Conscious Sedation and

Analgesia" had become an annual presentation at the American College of Emergency Physicians Scientific Assembly.

Issues that would frame the discussion regarding sedation in the 1990s began to appear in the literature throughout the 1980s:

- The concept, the importance, and components of the presedation evaluation.[22,23]
- Safety:
    - A general discussion of risks and benefits.[24,25]
    - The types of medications and their relative risks.[26–30]
    - Depth of sedation.[26,29]
    - Monitoring: What to monitor, how to monitor it, and by whom,[30–40] including an early discussion of the use of end-tidal carbon dioxide monitoring[35,36] and an initial red flag regarding the unpredictable occurrence of hypoxemia and apnea in patients receiving midazolam and fentanyl.[37]
- Education programs in the United States and internationally to train dental practitioners specifically in sedation.[41–47]
- Legal issues, followed immediately by legislation, regulations, and credentialing.[48–52]
- Early guidelines by organizations and societies.[19,53–56]

There are early references to the turf battles that are about to emerge in the 1990s and crystallize in the early part of the twenty-first century!

The 1990s

By the 1990s, the use of sedation to facilitate the performance of procedures had expanded widely. The literature of the late 1980s paved the way for the explosion of publications seen in the 1990s. The number of publications regarding sedation had grown geometrically from 27 between 1970 and 1980 to 183 between 1981 and 1990, to 1936 between 1991 and 2000.

The 1990s was the decade to explore medication options, craft standards and guidelines, and hone the terminology.

Medications

Virtually all combinations and permutations of medications, and routes and methods of administration were explored and evaluated for efficacy and safety in a variety of venues:

- Opioids, sedative hypnotics, dissociative agents, neuroleptic agents, local anesthetic agents, anesthetic gases and vapors, and others.

- Administered orally, intramuscularly, rectally, topically, or by inhalation.
- By bolus dose or titrated.
- In the field, the emergency department, radiology suites (magnetic resonance imaging [MRI], computed tomography [CT], and others), cardiac catheterization suite, endoscopy suite, pediatric dental chair, outpatient pediatric ear, nose, and throat (ENT) and ophthalmology clinic, pulmonary function lab, electroencephalogram (EEG) facility, plastic surgery clinic, lithotripsy suite, and so forth.

Standards and Guidelines

Standards and guidelines serve to systematize the process of sedation, define parameters within which sedation ought to occur, and clarify documentation expectations. At least 10 American professional organizations and 6 English-speaking foreign countries crafted and published guidelines, standards, or policies related to PS between 1991 and 2000:

- Gastroenterology: The American Society for Gastrointestinal Endoscopy (1995) and the Society of Gastroenterology Nurses and Associates (1997, 1999, 2000).[57–62]
- Plastic surgery: Plastic Surgery Nurses (1992) and the American Society of Plastic and Reconstructive Surgeons (1999).[63,64]
- Emergency medicine: The American College of Emergency Physicians produced two documents, one on pediatric sedation (1997) and the other on the broader clinical topic of sedation in the emergency department (ED) (1998) and the Emergency Nurses Association (1992). The Canadian Association of Emergency Physicians also produced ED sedation guidelines (1999).[65–68]
- Critical care: The Critical Care Nurses (1997).[69]
- General nursing: The American Nurses Association (1992).[70]
- Operating room (OR) nurses: The Association of Operating Room Nurses (1993, 1997).[71,72]
- Anesthesia: The American Society of Anesthesiologists.[73]
- Harvard Medical School: Guidelines for Non-Anesthesiologists (1994).[74]

- Dental Surgeons and Dentists in Australia and New Zealand (1992).[75]
- Dentists in the United Kingdom (1991, 1992).[76,77]
- South Africa: Separate Documents from Anesthetists (1992), the Medical Association (1997), and the Dentists (1999).[78–80]

Terminology

Coming out of the 1990s is clarity of terminology with respect to sedation end points, and more importantly how patient safety is optimized:

- The qualifications of the individuals that will administer PS and how they are to be trained and credentialed.
- Clear end points for sedation (light and moderate).
- Monitoring to be employed.
- Documentation to be kept.
- Quality oversight expected.

The most important advance on which the other items rely is clarity of terminology. The term conscious sedation meant different things to different people. To some it meant light sedation, to others moderated sedation; dissociative sedation really had no home and for many, deep sedation was inseparable from general anesthesia.[73,81–83]

The term *procedural sedation and analgesia* was adopted as a general term. The following terms were introduced into the lexicon awaiting even clearer definition after the turn of the century:

- Light sedation/minimal sedation/anxiolysis
- Moderate sedation
- Deep sedation
- General anesthesia

CURRENT TERMINOLOGY

In 1974, Ramsay proposed an eight-point sedation scale that has subsequently been validated for the assessment of sedation in the intensive care unit (ICU).[84] This scale has recently been modified to correlate with the Joint Commission on Accreditation of Healthcare Organizations (JCAHO) sedation definitions.[85] Table 1-1 presents this information in a clear and concise manner.

Table 1-1. Ramsay Sedation Scale Modified to Correlate with JCAHO Definitions of Minimal Sedation, Moderate Sedation, Deep Sedation, and General Anesthesia

Score	Modified Ramsay Sedation Scale Score Definition	JCAHO Sedation Definition
1	Awake and alert, minimal or no cognitive impairment	Minimal sedation (anxiolysis) is a drug-induced state during which patients respond normally to verbal commands. Although cognitive function and coordination may be impaired, ventilatory and cardiovascular functions are unaffected.
2	Awake but tranquil, purposeful responses to verbal commands at conversational level	Moderate sedation/analgesia: A drug-induced depression of consciousness during which patients respond purposefully to verbal commands, either alone or accompanied by light tactile stimulation. No interventions are required to maintain a patent airway and spontaneous ventilation is adequate. Cardiovascular function is usually maintained.
3	Appears asleep, purposeful responses to verbal commands at conversational level	
4	Appears asleep, purposeful responses to commands but at a louder than usual conversational level, requiring light glabellar tap, or both	

(Continued)

Table 1-1. Ramsay Sedation Scale Modified to Correlate with JCAHO Definitions of Minimal Sedation, Moderate Sedation, Deep Sedation, and General Anesthesia (*Continued*)

Score	Modified Ramsay Sedation Scale Score Definition	JCAHO Sedation Definition
5	Asleep, sluggish purposeful responses only to loud verbal commands, strong glabellar tap, or both	Deep sedation/analgesia is a drug-induced depression of consciousness during which patients cannot be easily aroused but respond purposefully following repeated or painful stimulation. The ability to independently maintain ventilatory function may be impaired. Patients may require assistance in maintaining a patent airway, and spontaneous ventilation may be inadequate. Cardiovascular function is usually maintained.
6	Asleep, sluggish purposeful responses only to painful stimuli	
7	Asleep, sluggish withdrawal to painful stimuli only (no purposeful responses)	
8	Unresponsive to external stimuli, including pain	General anesthesia is a drug-induced loss of consciousness during which patients are not arousable, even by painful stimulation. The ability to independently maintain ventilatory function is often impaired. Patients often require assistance in maintaining a patent airway, and positive pressure ventilation may be required because of depressed spontaneous ventilation or drug-induced depression of neuromuscular function. Cardiovascular function may be impaired.

Note: Because sedation is a continuum, it is not always possible to predict how an individual patient will respond. Hence, practitioners intending to produce a given level of sedation should be able to rescue patients whose level of sedation becomes deeper than initially intended. Individuals administering moderate sedation/analgesia (conscious sedation) should be able to rescue patients who enter a state of deep sedation/analgesia, while those administering deep sedation/analgesia should be able to rescue patients who enter a state of general anesthesia.

REFERENCES

1. Bennett CR. *Conscious Sedation in Dental Practice.* St. Louis, MO: Mosby; 1974.
2. Weiner AA. Patient management through conscious sedation. *J Mass Dent Soc.* 1975;24:227–230.
3. Bennett CR. Conscious-sedation as an alternative to general anesthesia. *N Y State Dent J.* 1976;42:351–358.
4. Laskin DM. Conscious sedation or general anesthesia? *Anesth Prog.* 1977;24:146.
5. Bennett CR. Conscious sedation in dentistry (I). *Quintessence Int.* 1978;9:131–134.
6. Bennett CR. Conscious sedation in dentistry (II). *Quintessence Int.* 1978;9:73–76.
7. Cheek JA. Arterial O_2 concentrations during conscious sedation. *J Oral Surg.* 1979;37:781.
8. Kraut RA. Continuous transcutaneous O_2 and CO_2 monitoring during conscious sedation for oral surgery. *J Oral Maxillofac Surg.* 1985;43:489–492.
9. Trop D. Conscious-sedation analgesia during the neurosurgical treatment of epilepsies—practice at the Montreal Neurological Institute. *Int Anesthesiol Clin.* 1986;24:175–184.
10. Archer DP, McKenna JM, Morin L, et al. Conscious-sedation analgesia during craniotomy for intractable epilepsy: a review of 354 consecutive cases. *Can J Anaesth.* 1988;35:338–344.
11. Shane SM, Speedie LJ, Rao L, et al. Conscious sedation for minor gynecologic surgery in the ambulatory patient. A pilot study. *Anesth Prog.* 1987;34:211–214.
12. Beilin B, Vatashsky E, Aronson HB. Conscious sedation for laparoscopy. *Isr J Med Sci.* 1986;22:346–349.
13. Brouillette DE, Leventhal R, Kumar S, et al. Midazolam versus diazepam for combined esophogastroduodenoscopy and colonoscopy. *Dig Dis Sci.* 1989;34:1265–1271.
14. Wilcox CM, Forsmark CE, Cello JP. Utility of droperidol for conscious sedation in gastrointestinal endoscopic procedures. *Gastrointest Endosc.* 1990;36:112–115.

15. Harris WC Jr, Alpert WJ, Gill JJ, et al. Nitrous oxide and valium use in podiatric surgery for production of conscious-sedation. *J Am Podiatry Assoc.* 1982;72:505–510.

16. Shane SM. Conscious sedation and behavioral modification with local standby anesthesia for ophthalmologic surgery. *Ophthalmic Surg.* 1982;13:50–52.

17. Meretoja OA, Rautiainen P. Alfentanil and fentanyl sedation in infants and small children during cardiac catheterization. *Can J Anaesth.* 1990;37:624–628.

18. Khan AH, Malhotra R. Midazolam as intravenous sedative for electrocardioversion. *Chest.* 1989;95:1068–1071.

19. Guidelines for the elective use of conscious sedation, deep sedation, and general anesthesia in pediatric patients. Committee on Drugs. Section on anesthesiology. *Pediatrics.* 1985;76:317–321.

20. Hawk W, Crockett RK, Ochsenschlager DW, et al. Conscious sedation of the pediatric patient for suturing: a survey. *Pediatr Emerg Care.* 1990;6:84–88.

21. Bennett CR, Stewart RD. Ketamine. In: Paris PM, Stewart RD, eds. *Pain Management in Emergency Medicine.* Norwalk, CT: Appleton & Lange; 1988:295–310.

22. Ash MR, Ford ML. Evaluation for conscious sedation using physical examination techniques. *Gen Dent.* 1986;34:272–274.

23. Yagiela JA. Preoperative assessment of patients for conscious sedation and general anesthesia. *Anesth Prog.* 1986;33:178–181.

24. Conscious sedation. Benefits and risks. *J Am Dent Assoc.* 1984;109:546–557.

25. Lofstrom B. Risk evaluation and patient assessment in sedation. *Acta Anaesthesiol Scand Suppl.* 1988;88:17–20.

26. Allen GD. Cardiorespiratory effects of conscious sedation. *SAAD Dig.* 1980;4:181–186.

27. Giovannitti JA, Henteleff HB, Bennett CR. Cardiorespiratory effects of meperidine, diazepam, and methohexital conscious sedation. *J Oral Maxillofac Surg.* 1982;40:92–95.

28. O'Connor KW, Jones S. Oxygen desaturation is common and clinically underappreciated during elective endoscopic procedures. *Gastrointest Endosc.* 1990;36(suppl 3):S2–S4.

29. Bennett CR. Management of adverse drug reactions in conscious-sedation. *Dent Clin North Am.* 1984;28:509–528.

30. Weaver JM. Intraoperative management during conscious sedation and general anesthesia: patient monitoring and emergency treatment. *Anesth Prog.* 1986;33:181–184.

31. Giglio JA, Campbell RL. The dental assistant's role in monitoring conscious sedation and general anesthesia. *Dent Assist.* 1985;54:17–18.

32. A.D.S.A. guidelines of intra-operative monitoring of patients undergoing conscious sedation, deep sedation and general anesthesia. *J Conn State Dent Assoc.* 1988;62:210–211.

33. Rodrigo MR, Rosenquist JB. Effect of conscious sedation with midazolam on oxygen saturation. *J Oral Maxillofac Surg.* 1988;46:746–750.

34. Fleischer D. Monitoring the patient receiving conscious sedation for gastrointestinal endoscopy: issues and guidelines. *Gastrointest Endosc.* 1989;35:262–266.

35. Iwasaki J, Vann WF Jr, Dilley DC, et al. An investigation of capnography and pulse oximetry as monitors of pediatric patients sedated for dental treatment. *Pediatr Dent.* 1989;11:111–117.

36. Ackerman WE, Phero JC, Reaume D. End tidal carbon dioxide and respiratory rate measurement during conscious sedation through a nasal cannula. *Anesth Prog.* 1990;37:199–200.

37. Bailey PL, Pace NL, Ashburn MA, et al. Frequent hypoxemia and apnea after sedation with midazolam and fentanyl. *Anesthesiology.* 1990;73:826–830.

38. Benjamin SB. Overview of monitoring in endoscopy. *Scand J Gastroenterol Suppl.* 1990;179:28–30.

39. Bell GD. Monitoring—the gastroenterologist's view. *Scand J Gastroenterol Suppl.* 1990;179:18–23.

40. Cousins MJ. Monitoring—the anaesthetist's view. *Scand J Gastroenterol Suppl.* 1990;179:12–17.

41. Jacobsohn PH. General anesthesia and conscious sedation in dentistry: current concepts, educational requirements and safety. *J Wis Dent Assoc.* 1984;60:19–21.

42. Reed MJ, Requa-Clark B, Shultz RE. Undergraduate education in the use of intravenous conscious sedation for dentistry. *J Dent Educ.* 1989;53:273–276.

43. Malamed SF. The role of the dental school in teaching conscious sedation. *J Dent Educ.* 1989;53:271–272.

44. Stacy G, Sheridan P, McDonald D. Conscious sedation courses. The University of Sydney. *Dent Anaesth Sedat.* 1984;13:45–48.

45. Sykes P. Teaching of sedation and anesthesia in the United Kingdom. *Anesth Prog.* 1989;36:215–216.

46. Barclay JK. Current status of education in anesthesia and sedation in New Zealand, 1988. *Anesth Prog.* 1989;36:214–215.

47. Matsuura H. Current status of education in anesthesia and sedation in Japan. *Anesth Prog.* 1989;36:212–213.

48. Reyes-Guerra A Jr. Concerns related to sedation, local and general anesthesia, with special reference to the Protopappas case. *Anesth Prog.* 1989;36:279–280.

49. Berry RM. Legal considerations in the administration of conscious sedation, deep sedation, and general anesthesia in dentistry. *Anesth Prog.* 1986;33:201–202.

50. Permit will be required to administer general anesthesia, conscious sedation and nitrous oxide/oxygen analgesia. *Pa Dent J (Harrisb).* 1988;55:22–23.

51. General anesthesia and conscious sedation. Regulations for Kentucky dentists. *Ky Dent J.* 1988;40:22–23.

52. Feldsott AF. The new regulations on conscious sedation. *N Y State Dent J.* 1989;55:8–10.

53. Guidelines for the elective use of conscious sedation, deep sedation, and general anesthesia in pediatric patients. *ASDC J Dent Child.* 1986;53:21–22.

54. Creedon RL. Guidelines for the elective use of conscious sedation, deep sedation, and general anesthesia in pediatric patients. *Anesth Prog.* 1986;33:189–190.

55. Smith RG. Conscious sedation: is it dentistry or medicine? *Dentistry.* 1988;8:9–11.

56. Peskin RM. The use of conscious sedation and general anesthesia in dentistry. *N Y State Dent J*. 1988;54:4.

57. Sedation and monitoring of patients undergoing gastrointestinal endoscopic procedures. American Society for Gastrointestinal Endoscopy. *Gastrointest Endosc*. 1995;42:626–629.

58. Guidelines for nursing care of the patient receiving sedation and analgesia in the gastrointestinal endoscopy setting. Society of Gastroenterology Nurses and Associates, Inc. *Gastroenterol Nurs*. 1997;20(suppl):1–6.

59. Guidelines for documentation in the gastrointestinal endoscopy setting. Society of Gastroenterology Nurses and Associates, Inc. *Gastroenterol Nurs*. 1999;22:69–97.

60. Sedation and analgesia. Society of Gastroenterology Nurses and Associates. *Gastroenterol Nurs*. 1999;22:29–30.

61. Society of Gastroenterology Nurses and Associates, Inc. Sedation and analgesia. *Gastroenterol Nurs*. 2000;23:281–282.

62. Society of Gastroenterology Nurses and Associates. SGNA guidelines for nursing care of the patient receiving sedation and analgesia in the gastrointestinal endoscopy setting. *Gastroenterol Nurs*. 2000;23:125–129.

63. Position statement on the role of the registered nurse (RN) in the management of patients receiving IV conscious sedation for short-term therapeutic, diagnostic, or surgical procedures. *Plast Surg Nurs*. 1992;12:31.

64. Iverson RE. Sedation and analgesia in ambulatory settings. American Society of Plastic and Reconstructive Surgeons. Task Force on Sedation and Analgesia in Ambulatory Settings. *Plast Reconstr Surg*. 1999;104:1559–1564.

65. Neff JA. Patient care guidelines. Conscious sedation. *J Emerg Nurs*. 1992;18:170–173.

66. Use of pediatric sedation and analgesia. American College of Emergency Physicians. *Ann Emerg Med*. 1997;29:834–835.

67. Clinical policy for procedural sedation and analgesia in the emergency department. American College of Emergency Physicians. *Ann Emerg Med*. 1998;31:663–677.

68. Innes G, Murphy M, Nijssen-Jordan C, et al. Procedural sedation and analgesia in the emergency department. Canadian Consensus Guidelines. *J Emerg Med*. 1999;17:145–156.

69. Polomano RC, Soulen MC, McDaniel CE. Sedation and analgesia for oncological patients undergoing interventional radiologic procedures. *Crit Care Nurs Clin North Am*. 1997;9:335–353.

70. ANA position statements. The role of the registered nurse in the management of patients receiving IV conscious sedation for short-term therapeutic, diagnostic, or surgical procedures. *SCI Nurs*. 1992;9:55–56.

71. Recommended practices. Monitoring the patient receiving i.v. conscious sedation. Association of Operating Room Nurses. *AORN J*. 1993;57:978–983.

72. Recommended practices for managing the patient receiving conscious sedation/analgesia. Association of Operating Room Nurses. *AORN J*. 1997;65:129–134.

73. Practice guidelines for sedation and analgesia by non-anesthesiologists. A report by the American Society of Anesthesiologists Task Force on Sedation and Analgesia by Non-Anesthesiologists. *Anesthesiology*. 1996;84:459–471.

74. Holzman RS, Cullen DJ, Eichhorn JH, et al. Guidelines for sedation by nonanesthesiologists during diagnostic and therapeutic procedures. The Risk Management Committee of the Department of Anaesthesia of Harvard Medical School. *J Clin Anesth*. 1994;6:265–276.

75. RACDS and ANZCA policy on sedation for dental procedures. *Aust Dent J*. 1992;37:234–236.

76. James DW. General anaesthesia, sedation and resuscitation in dentistry. *Br Dent J*. 1991;171:345–347.

77. General Dental Council. Professional conduct and fitness to practice. *Br Dent Surg Assist*. 1992;51:4.

78. James MF. Sedation and safety: South African Society of Anaesthetist. *S Afr Med J*. 1992;81:394–395.

79. Pinkney-Atkinson VJ. Conscious sedation clinical guideline. Conscious Sedation Working Group, Medical Association of South Africa. *S Afr Med J*. 1997;87:484–492.

80. General Dental Council. GDC new guidelines for sedation. *SAAD Dig*. 1999;16:17–19.

81. Murphy MF. Sedation. *Ann Emerg Med*. 1996;27:461–463.

82. Green SM, Krauss B. Procedural sedation terminology: moving beyond "Conscious Sedation." *Ann Emerg Med* 2002;39:433–435.

83. Cote CJ. Conscious sedation: time for this oxymoron to go away! *J Pediatr*. 2001;139:15–17.

84. Ramsay M, Savage T, Simpson B, et al. Controlled sedation with alphaxalone-alphadolone. *BMJ*. 1974;2:656–659.

85. Gill M, Green SM, Krauss B. A study of the bispectral index monitor during procedural sedation and analgesia in the emergency department. *Ann Emerg Med* 2003;41:234–241

2

Pain Management and Procedural Sedation: Definitions and Clinical Applications

Sharon E. Mace
Michael F. Murphy

HIGH YIELD FACTS

- Pain is the number one reason for seeking health care and is the chief complaint in up to 70% of emergency department (ED) visits.

- Oligoanesthesia is the inadequate treatment of pain.

- Patients at higher risk for oligoanesthesia are children, especially infants, the elderly, pregnant patients, those with special health care needs, minorities, and chronic pain (vs. acute pain) patients.

- Pain has a physiologic basis while the expression of pain is modified by cognitive, behavioral, and sociocultural dimensions.

- Failure to adequately treat pain can have a negative impact: ↑ difficulty treating subsequent episodes of pain, ↑ risk of chronic pain, ↑ complications, poorer clinical outcomes, ↑ costs.

- Procedural sedation is a continuum from minimal sedation, moderate sedation, deep sedation, to general anesthesia.

- Select the desired state for procedural sedation, the most appropriate medication by the safest route.

- Evaluate the patient's "physiologic reserve," titrate medications to a central nervous system (CNS) end point with appropriate monitoring by an individual who is not performing the procedure.

- Pain management and procedural sedation are an essential component of emergency medicine practice.

PAIN MANAGEMENT

Overview

Pain is the number one reason given for seeking health care, representing the chief complaint in up to 70% of all visits to an emergency department (ED).[1] Unfortunately, the under-treatment of pain—oligoanalgesia—has been a common occurrence not only in the ED but throughout medicine.[2–5] Oligoanalgesia may be more frequent in certain patient populations, including patients at the extremes of age, pregnant patients, patients with special health care needs, members of minority ethnic groups, and chronic pain (vs. acute pain) patients.[6–21] Hopefully, this tendency for oligoanesthesia will become a trend of the past. There are encouraging signs that adequate treatment of pain and sedation are becoming commonplace and the norm for both emergency medicine and medicine in general.[22–26]

Definitions

Pain has been defined by the International Association for the Study of Pain as "an unpleasant sensory and emotional experience associated with actual or potential tissue damage, or described in terms of such damage."[27] This definition reflects the subjective nature and multifaceted experience of pain. The patient's response to pain, the physician's response to the patient in pain, as well as the patient-physician interactions, all occur in a specific setting that is affected by multiple interconnected parameters. The *induction* of pain has a physiologic basis with nociceptive and sensory components.[28] The *sensation* of pain is much more complex, being modified by cognitive, affective, and sociocultural dimensions[29] as well as the patient's past experiences (including treatment or lack of treatment) with pain.[30–43] Indeed, pain is a very complex entity, which we are only beginning to understand.

  The physician will encounter patients with many different types of pain. Acute and chronic pain are defined by duration. Acute pain implies recent onset of pain that lasts a few days to several weeks. Chronic pain has previously been defined as pain lasting for more than 3–6 months. Another more useful definition for chronic pain is pain that lasts longer than the usual expected time period for tissue healing. Recurrent pain, a subset of chronic pain, may allow a patient to be relatively symptom-free between painful episodes. Examples of disorders with recurrent episodes of pain include migraine headaches, inflammatory bowel disease, or sickle cell disease.

Most patients with chronic pain will have acute exacerbations of the painful condition. This is similar to a patient with chronic obstructive pulmonary disease (COPD). Patients with COPD or chronic pain have an underlying baseline dysfunction for which they are maintained on various medications as part of a management regimen. An event occurs which worsens their chronic condition and precipitates the need for further medication therapy. The physician may feel more comfortable treating the COPD patient with an acute exacerbation than the chronic pain patient with a flare-up of his pain. This is unfortunate, for the undertreated chronic pain patient who deserves care as much as the COPD patient often develops abnormal behavior in an attempt to obtain that care. Patients whose pain is inadequately treated may appear to be inappropriately "drug seeking," or have pseudoaddiction.[44–46] They may become fixated on obtaining analgesics and resort to deception and illegal drug use as a means to achieve pain relief.

Pseudoaddiction should be differentiated from addiction. There is a consensus statement from the American Academy of Pain Medicine, the American Pain Society, and the American Society of Addiction Medicine that deals with "Definitions related to the use of opioids for the treatment of pain."[44] They define addiction as a primary, chronic, neurobiologic disease with genetic, psychosocial, and environmental factors influencing its development and manifestations. It is characterized by behaviors that include one or more of the following: impaired control over drug use, compulsive use, continued use despite harm, and craving. Addicted patients will demonstrate even greater behavior disorders if prescribed opioids whereas the abnormal behavior of pseudo-addicted patients returns to normal once their pain is properly treated.

Two other important definitions from this document are physical dependence and tolerance. Physical dependence is a state of adaptation that often includes tolerance. It is manifested by a drug-class-specific withdrawal syndrome that can be produced by abrupt cessation, rapid dose reduction, decreasing blood level of the drug, and/or administration of an antagonist. Tolerance is a state of adaptation in which exposure to a drug induces changes that result in a diminution of one or more of the drug's effects over time. It is well accepted that as part of having chronic pain treated with opioids, patients will develop dependence. This should be no greater a concern than expecting a diabetic to become dependent on insulin. Physicians treating chronic pain need to be vigilant for signs of addiction, not dependence.

Pathophysiology of Acute and Chronic Pain

Acute pain generally is a response to tissue injury and resolves when the acute injury heals. Acute pain is part of an adaptive response that occurs in conjunction with protective reflexes. Examples of such protective reflexes include the purposeful withdrawal of an extremity from danger or muscle spasms that immobilize a limb. Acute pain is often accompanied by obvious signs of physical suffering and indicators of a hyperactive sympathetic nervous system. Although acute pain is an adaptive response of the body to an acute threat, evidence suggests that occasionally such responses may be counterproductive or even harmful. Such maladaptive actions can result in increased myocardial oxygen consumption, decreased immune responses, hypercoagulable status, and atelectasis.

In contrast to acute pain, there is no adaptive function with chronic pain, and obvious signs of pathology, such as activation of the autonomic nervous system, are few or nonexistent. Furthermore, patients with chronic pain may have "adapted" to their situation and often lack the behaviors usually manifest in patients with acute pain. This relative paucity of physiologic indicators and distinctive behavioral patterns in chronic pain patients often misleads the health care provider into assessing the patient's pain as minimal or nonexistent, thereby undertreating the patient's pain.[45,46]

Anatomy and Pathophysiology of Acute Nociceptive and Neuropathic Pain

Pain receptors or nociceptors are the free nerve endings that convert various stimuli (mechanical, chemical, or thermal) into electrical activity thereby initiating an impulse.[28] Chemical mediators such as prostaglandins, leukotrienes, platelet-activating factor, substance P, serotonin, and bradykinin may be involved in the process. The chemical mediators may sensitize the receptors to stimuli and/or be involved in the conduction of stimuli.

The nociceptor or pain receptor is part of a sensory neuron located in the periphery within a given skin dermatone. The sensory neuron consists of this receptor and a cell body located in the dorsal root ganglia. Fibers from the dorsal root ganglion link to the dorsal horn of the spinal cord and transmit cephalad via the ascending spinal cord tracts to the brain. The sensation of pain can also be modulated by the brain via descending tracts in the spinal cord (see also Chap. 30).

Nociceptive and neuropathic pain results from two different physiologic mechanisms. Noxious stimuli such as trauma or inflammation activate the peripheral nociceptors. In general, pain resulting from activation of superficial structures such as the skin or subcutaneous tissues is well localized and sharp. Activation of nociceptors in deeper structures (for example, tendons, bones, or joints) tends to be achy or crampy and diffuse or radiating. Pain due to activation of visceral nociceptors in internal organs is perceived as deep aching and poorly localized. Nociceptors in internal organs can be activated by inflammation, ischemia, or distention as occurs with cholecystitis, pancreatitis, ulcers, ischemic bowel disease, or acute urinary retention.

Neuropathic pain is classically described as a burning, tingling, searing, or shooting pain. Neuropathic pain is due to abnormal signal processing in the nervous system either centrally or peripherally. Examples of neuropathic pain include the complex regional pain syndrome (see Chap. 37), shingles (herpes zoster), all the various mono/polyneuropathies (diabetic, alcoholic), phantom limb pain (deafferentation), and the central pain states associated with multiple sclerosis or after a stroke.

Barriers to the Treatment of Pain

Several of the barriers to the treatment of pain can be related to concerns regarding the use of opioids. Physicians may be fearful that they will be subject to increased surveillance and even punishment or sanctions if they prescribe or administer excessive amounts.[47–49] This latter fear appears to be unfounded (see Chap. 6). Appropriate prescribing of opioids for patients in pain does not violate any regulation or law, although failure to adequately treat pain may subject the physician to malpractice claims, Emergency Medical Treatment and Active Labor Act (EMTALA) violations, and other regulatory infractions.

Health care providers (and patients as well) may fear addiction and/or adverse effects from opioid use. We need to recognize that the prescription of opioids for acute pain, or for a limited time for chronic pain very rarely leads to addiction. Health care providers may also have a fear of being duped by patients who seek opioids for illegal or nonmedical use. Each case should be evaluated on its own merit, but rates of malingering are lower than 2% in patients complaining of pain even in urban centers. Coadministration of other analgesics, such as acetaminophen or nonsteroidal anti-inflammatory drugs (NSAIDs), may help decrease the required opioid dose needed for analgesia.

A lack of education on pain management and procedural sedation has been cited as a barrier to the adequate treatment of pain.[50] Pain, as a specific topic, is not included in the core content of emergency medicine.[51] Likewise, there is a lack of formal teaching/training in pain management in our medical schools and residencies. Recent literature (including this textbook) is an attempt to address this knowledge deficiency.

A lack of health care provider accountability for substandard care has been cited as an obstacle; however, with the new Joint Commission on Accreditation of Healthcare Organizations (JCAHO) recommendations and other regulations/standards this may no longer be applicable.[52]

Further, several recent clinical policies or statements have emphasized the importance of adequate sedation and analgesia in the ED, and even in prehospital care.[53–61]

Other barriers to effective pain management may be more complex.[29] In our medical training, we are taught to deal with diseases and pathology ahead of symptoms expecting that by treating the pathology the symptoms will resolve. This may not be possible with many of our patients experiencing pain.

Patients may be unable or reluctant to report pain; however, even in preverbal children/infants, nonverbal (illiterate, speak another language) adults, cognitively impaired adults, or special needs children, pain scales and other methods for addressing a patient's pain can be used (see Chaps. 11, 12, 43). Patients may fail to report their pain for various reasons: fear, an attempt to please a parent/family member/health care providers, and cultural/social/religious issues.[29]

Health care providers and families may have difficulty quantifying or assessing the abstract concept called pain.[62] We can quantify anemia by a hematocrit or hypoxemia by pulse oxygen saturation, but there is no objective test (laboratory, radiographic, or other) for pain. The use of pain scales to quantify and measure pain helps overcome this barrier and emphasizes the importance of quantifying and assessing pain (both before and after therapeutic measures).

Why Treat Pain?

In addition to the obvious moral, ethical, and legal/regulatory reasons to treat pain adequately and expeditiously (see Chap. 6), failure to properly treat may make it much more difficult to treat future pain and may increase the likelihood of developing chronic pain.[30,36,46,63,64]

Failure to treat pain adequately may affect later responses and behaviors to pain. Negative experiences with painful procedures may cause an individual to delay or even avoid seeking medical care, creating delays in diagnosis and treatment with worse (and more costly) outcomes.[46] Inadequate pain therapy may lead to increased pain thresholds making it more difficult to treat later episodes of pain as well as negatively impacting later behavioral responses, and predisposing the patient to chronic pain.

There is evidence that inadequate analgesia and/or sedation leads to worse clinical outcomes and more complications (whether in an intensive care unit or for postoperative patients).[2,65,66] A possible pathophysiologic mechanism for the negative effects of inadequate analgesia/sedation may be an excess of stress hormones causing catabolism, immunosuppression, and hemodynamic instability.[65]

Management of Pain

Pain management can include both pharmacologic and non-pharmacologic methods. The use of one of these modalities does not exclude the other. Similarly, a combination of pharmacologic agents, for example, hydro-codone plus aceta-minophen, may be appropriate in a given patient. No one analgesic (or sedative) or modality is appropriate for every patient in every clinical situation so the physician should be familiar with a variety of therapeutic options (see Chaps. 4, 17–23, 48–50)

What should be our approach to managing pain? First, we must acknowledge that all individuals can experience pain irrespective of our ability to communicate with that individual. All ages and types of patients can experience pain, from the premature infant to the cognitively impaired elderly, the special needs child, the psychiatric or behavioral patient, and the patient unable to articulate their pain for whatever reason (illiteracy, different language, and so forth).

Next, we must recognize and be able to assess pain. We should be aware that health care professionals in general (not just physicians) and even families (for example, parents) tend to underestimate a patient's pain.[9,62] Patient self-report is judged to be the most accurate assessment of pain severity. We need to accept and rely on (with perhaps only a few exceptions) what the patient tells us. Furthermore, we should reassess a patient's pain after treatment as we would verify any other medical condition after a therapeutic intervention.

We should also allow the patient and/or family to be involved in their care as part of family-centered care. Patients may decide not to accept certain therapeutic options including analgesics for various reasons (for example, social, cultural, religious, or ethical). We can give input or advice but should respect their decisions.

Finally, our therapy should be timely. Inordinate delays for pain therapy are unacceptable. Protocols for the early administration of appropriate analgesics should be developed. This may involve triage protocols for nursing to administer analgesics or even emergency medical services personnel as part of the prehospital management (see Chap. 40)

ED policies and procedures can be developed to foster safe and effective analgesia in a timely fashion to ED patients in pain and distress. The need for and importance of pain management has been cited in policy statements and informational papers by various professional organizations including the American College of Emergency Physicians, the American Academy of Pediatrics, the Canadian Association of Emergency Physicians, the American Pain Society, the Canadian Paediatric Society, and the National Association of EMS Physicians.[53–60]

PROCEDURAL SEDATION

Emergency medicine serves as a health care safety net for a community. As such, it must ensure quality and compassionate patient care, and advocate for the patient in the realm of pain management and procedural sedation. These facets of care are integral to the practice of emergency medicine. With procedural sedation, even more than with pain, one must be keenly aware of the balance between benefit and harm.

The Lexicon of Procedural Sedation: Defining the Terms

The terminology of sedation has undergone considerable evolution over the years as described in Chapter 1. Different medical and dental specialties have used imprecise and at times confusing terms to describe what is being done. It is essential that the lexicon be firmly established and agreed upon in order to assure unambiguous communication across specialty lines and among practitioners of the same specialty. This is particularly important to investigators as they attempt to make "apples-to-apples" comparisons, and to the readers of such studies for the same reason.

The consciousness continuum spans cognition from "awake and alert" to "death." The continuum is arbitrarily punctuated by points defined as closely as possible by the clinical appearance of the patient. As it currently stands:

1. Minimal sedation (anxiolysis) is a drug-induced state during which patients respond normally to verbal commands. Although cognitive function and coordination may be impaired, ventilatory and cardiovascular functions are unaffected.

2. Moderate sedation/analgesia is a drug-induced depression of consciousness during which patients respond purposefully to verbal commands, either alone or accompanied by light tactile stimulation. No interventions are required to maintain a patent airway and spontaneous ventilation is adequate. Cardiovascular function is usually maintained.

3. Deep sedation/analgesia is a drug-induced depression of consciousness during which patients cannot be easily aroused but respond purposefully following repeated or painful stimulation. The ability to independently maintain ventilatory function may be impaired. Patients may require assistance in maintaining a patent airway and spontaneous ventilation may be inadequate. Cardiovascular function is usually maintained.

4. General anesthesia is a drug-induced loss of consciousness during which patients are not arousable, even by painful stimulation. The ability to independently maintain ventilatory function is often impaired. Patients often require assistance in maintaining a patent airway, and positive pressure ventilation may be required because of depressed spontaneous ventilation or drug-induced depression of neuromuscular function. Cardiovascular function may be impaired.

General anesthesia may be subdivided into *stages* and *planes* as classically described for inhalational induction and maintenance:

a. Stage 1: Light sleep
b. Stage 2: Excitement
c. Stage 3: Surgical anesthesia; further divided into four planes depending on vital function stability and response to stimulation; Plane 3 is generally considered to be *surgical anesthesia*
d. Stage 4: Death

General anesthesia is composed of three subcomponents:

a. Hypnosis (sleep)
b. Analgesia
c. Muscle relaxation

Some agents (e.g., volatile anesthetic agents) produce all three to varying degrees. Typically, total intravenous anesthesia (TIVA) requires the administration of a hypnotic (e.g., propofol), an analgesic (e.g., fentanyl), and a neuromuscular blocking drug (e.g., rocuronium) depending on the requirements of the procedure. Employing the best features of both together is called *balanced anesthesia*. Procedural sedation and analgesia employing both sedative hypnotic agents and analgesics is similar.

The Consciousness Continuum

It is generally agreed that an individual administering procedural analgesia and sedation ought to be capable of managing one level beyond the level desired on the consciousness continuum. For example, if one is attempting to produce moderate sedation, one ought to be competent to manage the physiologic concomitants of deep sedation and if one is attempting to produce deep sedation, competency in managing general anesthesia is expected. Having said that, it is well known that individuals have varying, and at times unpredictable, responses to the medications employed to produce procedural sedation and analgesia.

Sedation, Analgesia, and Dissociation

Sedation and analgesia, for the most part, are separate issues. Sedative hypnotics do not possess analgesic activity, and in fact, may be antianalgesic. The apparatus of pain transmission is not interrupted by even very deep levels of sedative hypnotic hypnosis leading to "wind-up" and postprocedure pain transmission facilitation.

Parenteral analgesic agents ordinarily employed in procedural sedation and analgesia possess varying degrees of sedating side effects (e.g., morphine and sufentanil) that may be useful in managing individual patients. However, employing an opioid as the primary agent to achieve sedation is rather like attempting to insert a round peg in a square hole; it can be done, but it is a poor fit and often at the expense of ventilatory drive.

Ketamine is a unique agent that in a dose-dependent fashion produces sedation, analgesia, and hypnosis, followed by dissociation. The dissociated state is unique in that patients do not respond to surgical stimuli (i.e., appear as though they are under general anesthesia), but maintain and protect their airway, maintain ventilation and hemodynamics, and muscle tone (catalepsy), provided the dose of ketamine is reasonable. In a *quantitative* sense they are much like patients in the moderate sedation/analgesia category. Although qualitatively and cognitively these patients fit the general anesthesia definition, from a safety perspective they conform to the moderate sedation/analgesia definition. This state has a unique name: *dissociative sedation*.

Clinical Approach

The best advice is to know precisely how deeply sedated this patient will need to be to accomplish what is required in a manner acceptable to the patient. Further, consider the reserve of the patient and whether or not it is sufficient to withstand the effects of the medications that are contemplated balanced against the stimulation to be inflicted by the procedure (see Chap. 8). Consider the aspiration risk, particularly if a deeply sedated or general anesthetic state may supervene. In the final analysis, one must be confident that sedation and analgesia can be safely and effectively undertaken in a manner that is acceptable to the patient and that referral for general anesthesia is unnecessary.

In summary, select the *desired state*, select the *most appropriate medications* to get the patient there, and administer them by the *safest route*. Take into account whether or not the procedure will inflict pain. The following are common end points in an ED setting:

- Minimal sedation (e.g., child requiring suturing of a minor laceration): oral (PO) (or alternative routes of sedative administration) and/or topical anesthetics is acceptable. Parenteral (intramuscular [IM] or intravenous [IV]) administration of sedatives/ analgesics may also be acceptable (see Chaps. 43, 47).
- Moderate sedation for nonpainful procedures (e.g., computed tomography [CT] and magnetic resonance imaging [MRI] scanning): IV titration using *titratable drugs* is safest, with the probable exception of ketamine.
- Moderate sedation and analgesia for painful procedures: Select a titratable opioid (e.g., fentanyl) and titrate it IV to establish an acceptable level of analgesia, then use a titratable sedative hypnotic to titrate the patient to the moderate sedation end point. In the author's experience, avoiding the practice of alternating small doses of sedative hypnotic agents with small doses of opioids reduces the risk of sudden and unpredictable apnea. Alternatively, employ ketamine IV, PO, or IM.

The use of single large, bolus doses of any class of medication (sedative hypnotic, opioid, and ketamine) by any route (IV, PO, IM, subcutaneous [SC], PR, IN) is inherently more dangerous (respiratory and cardiovascular depression) than a measured IV titration to a defined end point. Some agents have a broader safety profile (ketamine) than others (midazolam, propofol, and thiopental) and some are intermediate in risk (pentobarbital and chloral hydrate).

Titratable drugs are safer and preferable for IV titration to a moderate sedation end point. These drugs have a rapid onset, rapid offset, and a clearly identifiable effect on a dose-by-dose basis (e.g., fentanyl, propofol, and ketamine-propofol combinations). They permit one to adjust both the dose and dosage interval in a safe and effective manner. Medications such as diazepam are difficult to titrate and midazolam is of intermediate ease, possessing as much as a 2-minute delay to peak effect profile.

Remember to evaluate the physiologic reserve of the patient. For the most part, one will be titrating to a *CNS end point*, i.e., degree of sedation and adequacy of analgesia. However, some patients will be too sick or unstable (e.g., hypotensive patient with ventricular tachycardia and decompensated COPD patient) to use the CNS end point and titration will be against ventilatory (e.g., hypoxia and hypercarbia) or cardiovascular (e.g., hypotension) end points. In the very ill, one will use only an amnestic (e.g., small dose of midazolam) to obtund memory as higher doses may lead to further decompensation.

Administration of the drugs and monitoring of the patient should *not* be undertaken by the same individual performing the procedure if sedation beyond anxiolysis is induced.

Monitoring Standards

The intensity of the monitoring is governed mostly by the extent to which the medications employed are anticipated to affect the vital organ functions of the particular patient, though it must take into account the specific medications to be used and the depth of sedation contemplated.

Minimal sedation: For these patients direct observation by a suitably trained and experienced health care provider (e.g., nurse) and pulse oximetry (if the patient will tolerate it) is generally sufficient.

Moderate sedation: Continuous pulse oximetry, cardiac monitoring, and blood pressure determination every 3–5 minutes. In the near future it is likely that continuous end-tidal carbon dioxide monitoring will become the standard of care for moderate sedation.

Intravenous Access

IV access is generally considered to be unnecessary in patients receiving minimal sedation unless the condition of the patient suggests that resuscitation or reversal medications may be rapidly needed (e.g., severe COPD, concomitant CNS depressants such as ethanol).

Patients receiving moderate sedation for nonpainful procedures will usually have an IV in place unless they are children receiving PO or IM sedation (or alternate routes of sedative administration) for nonpainful procedures. Though, strictly speaking it is not required, it ought to be carefully considered (see Chaps. 43, 47)

Patients receiving moderate sedation and analgesia must have IV access. The exception is patients undergoing dissociative sedation where IV access is generally considered unnecessary, particularly if a single-dose PO or IM methodology is employed, unless a risk factor for laryngospasm (e.g., mild upper respiratory infection [URI]) or cardiovascular decompensation (very young) exists. (see Chap. 20)

REFERENCES

1. Cordell WH, Keene KK, Giles BK, et al. The high prevalence of pain in emergency medical care. *Am J Emerg Med.* 2002;20:165–169.
2. Drayer RA, Henderson J, Reidenberg M. Barriers to better pain control in hospitalized patients. *J Pain Symptom Manage.* 1999;17:434–440.
3. Wilson J, Pendelton J. Oligoanalgesia in the emergency department. *Am J Emerg Med.* 1989;7:620–623.
4. Rupp T, Delaney KA. Inadequate analgesia in emergency medicine. *Ann Emerg Med.* 2004;43:494–503.
5. Tcherny-Lessenot S, Karwoski-Soulie F, Lamarche-Vadel A, et al. Management and relief of pain in an emergency department from an adult patients' perspective. *J Pain Symptom Manage.* 2003;25:539–546.
6. Maurice SC, O'Donnell JJ, Beattie TF. Emergency analgesia in the paediatric population. Part I: Current practice and perspectives. *Emerg Med J.* 2002;19:4–7.
7. Purcell-Jones G, Dormon F, Sumner E. Pediatric anesthetists' perception of neonatal and infant pain. *Pain.* 1988;33:181–187.
8. Broome ME, Richtsmeier A, Maikler V, et al. Pediatric pain practices: a national survey of health professionals. *J Pain Symptom Manage.* 1996;11:312–320.
9. Romsing J. Assessment of nurses' judgment for analgesic requirements of postoperative pain. *J Clin Pharm Ther.* 1996;21:159–163.
10. Goddard JM, Pickup SE. Postoperative pain in children. *Anesthesia.* 1996;51:588–590.
11. DeLima J, Lloyd-Thomas AR, Howard RF, et al. Infant and neonatal pain; anaesthetists' perceptions and prescribing patterns. *Br Med J.* 1996;313:787.
12. Porter FL, Wolf CM, Gold J, et al. Pain and pain management in newborn infants: a survey of physicians and nurses. *Pediatrics.* 1997;100:626–632.
13. Selbst SM, Clark M. Analgesic use in the emergency department. *Ann Emerg Med.* 1990;19(9):1010–1013.
14. Friedland LR, Kulick RM. Emergency department analgesic use in pediatric trauma victims with fractures. *Ann Emerg Med.* 1994;23(2):203–207.
15. Brown JC, Klein EJ, Lewis CW, et al. Emergency department analgesia for fracture pain. *Ann Emerg Med.* 2003;42(2):197–205.
16. Jones JS, Johnson K, McNinch M. Age as a risk factor for inadequate emergency department analgesia. *Am J Emerg Med.* 1996;14(2):157–160.
17. Spedding RL, Harley D, Dunn FJ, et al. Who gives pain relief to children? *J Accid Emerg Med.* 1999;16:26–34.
18. Todd KH, Deaton C, D'Adamo AP, et al. Ethnicity and analgesia practice. *Ann Emerg Med.* 2000;35:11–16.
19. Todd KH, Samaroo N, Hoffman JR. Ethnicity as a risk factor for inadequate emergency department analgesia. *JAMA.* 1993;269:1537–1539.
20. Green CR, Anderson KO, Baker TA, et al. The unequal burden of pain: confronting racial and ethnic disparities in pain. *Pain Med.* 2003;4:277–294.
21. Bonham VL. Race, ethnicity, and the disparities in pain treatment. *J Law Med Ethics.* 2001;29:52–68.
22. Todd KH. Emergency medicine and pain: a topography of influence. *Ann Emerg Med.* 2004;43:504–506.
23. Goldman RD, Balasubramanian S, Wales P, et al. Sedation and analgesia for incarcerated inguinal hernia in the pediatric emergency department. *J Pain.* 2005;117.
24. Pace S, Burke TF. Intravenous morphine for early pain relief in patients with acute abdominal pain. *Acad Emerg Med.* 1996;3:1086–1092.
25. Kim MK, Strait RT, Sato TT, et al. A randomized clinical trial of analgesia in children with acute abdominal pain. *Acad Emerg Med.* 2002;9:281–287.
26. LoVecchio F, Oster N, Sturmann K, et al. The use of analgesics in patients with acute abdominal pain. *J Emerg Med.* 1997;15:775–779.
27. Merkey H, Bogduk N, eds. *Classification of Chronic Pain.* 2nd ed. Seattle, WA: IASP Press; 1994.
28. Paris PM, Stewart R. Pain management. In: Rosen P, Barkin R, Danzl DF, et al, eds. *Emergency Medicine Concepts and Clinical Practice.* St. Louis, MO: Mosby; 1998:276–300.
29. Ducharme J. Whose pain is it anyway? Managing pain in the emergency department. *Emerg Med.* 2001;18:271–273.
30. Jabbur SJ, Saadé NE. From electrical wiring to plastic neurons: evolving approaches to the study of pain. *Pain.* 1999; Suppl 6:S87–S92.
31. Gordon SM, Dionne RA, Brahim J, et al. Blockade of peripheral neuronal barrage reduces postoperative pain. *Pain.* 1997;70:209–215.
32. Bowsher D. The effects of preemptive treatment of postherpetic neuralgia with amitriptyline: a randomized, double-blind, placebo-controlled trial. *J Pain Symptom Manage.* 1997;13:327–331.
33. Bowsher D. Acute herpes zoster and postherpetic neuralgia: effects of acyclovir and outcome of treatment with amitriptyline. *Br J Gen Pract.* 1992;42:244–246.
34. Bach S, Noreng MF, Tjellden NU. Phantom limb pain in amputees during the first 12 months following limb amputation, after preoperative lumbar epidural blockade. *Pain.* 1988;33:297–301.
35. Dworkin RH, Boon RJ, Griffin DR, et al. Postherpetic neuralgia: impact of famciclovir, age, rash severity, and acute pain in herpes zoster patients. *J Infect Dis.* 1988;178(Suppl 1):S76–S80.
36. Weisman SJ, Bernstein B, Schecter NL. Consequences of inadequate analgesia during painful procedures in children. *Arch Pediatr Adolesc Med.* 1998;152:147–149.
37. Johnston CC, Stevens BJ. Experience in a neonatal intensive care unit affects pain response. *Pediatrics.* 1996;98(5):925–930.
38. Taddio A, Ipp M, et al. Effect of neonatal circumcision on pain responses during vaccination in boys. *Lancet.* 1995;345:291–292.
39. Johnston CC, Stevens BJ, Franck LS, et al. Factors explaining lack of response to heel-stick in preterm infant. *JOGNN.* 1999;28:587–594.

40. Grunau RVE, Whitfield MF, Petrie JH, et al. Early pain experience, child and family factors, as precursors of somatization: a prospective study of extremely premature and full term children. *Pain.* 1994;56:353–359.

41. Oberlander TF, Grunau RV, Whitfield MF. Behavioral responses in formed extremely low-birthweight infants at 4 months corrected age. *Pediatrics.* 2000;105:E6–E18.

42. Grunau RV, Whitfield MF, Petrie JH. Pain sensitivity and temperament in extremely low-birth-weight premature toddlers with preterm and full-term controls. *Pain.* 1994; 58:341.

43. Grunau RE, Whitfield MF, Petric JH. Children's judgment about pain at age 8 years: do extremely low birthweight (≤1000 g) children differ from full birthweight peers? *J Child Psychol Psychiatry.* 1998;39:587–594.

44. American Society of Addiction Medicine. Definitions related to the use of opioids for the treatment of pain. Consensus document from the American Academy of Pain Medicine, the American Pain Society, and the American Society of Addiction Medicine, February 2001. Available at *http://www.asam.org.* Accessed February 12, 2005.

45. Todd KH. Pain management in the emergency department. American College of Emergency Physicians CME Monograph. Dallas, TX: American College of Emergency Physicians; 2004:4.

46. Ducharme J. Acute pain and pain control: state of the art. *Ann Emerg Med.* 2000;35:592–603.

47. Johnson SH, ed. Symposium: appropriate management of pain: addressing the clinical, legal, and regulatory barriers. *J Law Med Ethics.* 1996;24:285. Available in full text at *http://aslme.org/research/painjournals.php*

48. Johnson SH, ed. Symposium: the undertreatment of pain: legal, regulatory, and research perspectives and solutions. *J Law Med Ethics.* 2001;29:11. Available in full text at *http://aslme.org/research/painjournals.php*

49. Johnson SH, ed. Symposium: improving the treatment for pain: legal, regulatory, and research perspectives. *J Law Med Ethics.* 2003;31:15. Available in full text at *http://aslme.org/research/painjournals.php*

50. Jones JB. Assessment of pain management skills in emergency medicine residents: the role of a pain education program. *J Emerg Med.* 1999;17:349–354.

51. Hockberger RS, Binder LS, Graver MA, et al, for the American College of Emergency Physicians Core Content Task F, II. The model of the clinical practice of emergency medicine. *Ann Emerg Med.* 2001;37(6):745–770.

52. Joint Commission for the Accreditation of Healthcare Organizations. Background on the development of the Joint Commission standards on pain management. Available at *http://www.jcaho.org/news+room/health+care+issues/pain.htm.* Accessed July 21, 2004.

53. ACEP. American College of Emergency Physicians. Clinical policy for procedural sedation and analgesia in the emergency department. *Ann Emerg Med.* 1998;31:663–677.

54. Zempsky WT, Cravero JP, Committee on Pediatric Emergency Medicine and Section on Anesthesiology and Pain Medicine. Relief of pain and anxiety in pediatric patients in emergency medical systems. *Pediatrics.* 2004; 114(5):1348–1356.

55. Mace SE, Barata IA, Cravero JP, et al. Clinical policy: evidence–based approach to pharmacologic agents used in pediatric sedation and analgesia in the emergency department. *Ann Emerg Med.* 2004;44:342–377.

56. American Academy of Pediatrics and Canadian Paediatric Society. Prevention and management of pain and stress in the neonate. *Pediatrics.* 2000;105(2):454–461.

57. American College of Emergency Physicians Clinical Policy. Procedural Sedation. Approved October 20, 2004 by ACEP Board of Directors, for publication. *Ann Emerg Med.* 2005.

58. Ducharme J.: Emergency pain management: a Canadian Association of Emergency Physicians (CAEP) consensus document. *J Emerg Med.* 1994;12:855–866.

59. American Academy of Pediatrics and American Pain Society. The assessment and management of acute pain in infants, children, and adolescents. *Pediatrics.* 2001;108(3): 793–797.

60. Alonso-Serra HM, Wesley K, for the National Association of EMS Physicians Standards and Clinical Practices Committee. Prehospital pain management. *Prehosp Emerg Care.* 2003;7:482–488.

61. American College of Emergency Physicians. *Pain Management in the Emergency Department* [policy statement]. Approved March 2004. Available at *www.acep.org/1,33678,0.html.* Accessed February 12, 2005.

62. Chambers CT, Reid GJ, Craig KD, et al. Agreement between child and parent reports of pain. *Clin J Pain.* 1998;14: 336–342.

63. Katz J. Perioperative predictors of long-term pain following surgery. In: Jensen T, Turner J, Weisenfeld-Hallin Z, eds. *Proceedings of the 8th World Congress on Pain.* Vol 8. Seattle, WA: IASP Press; 1997.

64. Kalso E. Prevention of chronicity. In: Jensen T, Turner J, Weisenfeld-Hallin Z, eds. *Proceedings of the 8th World Congress on Pain.* Vol 8. Seattle, WA: IASP Press; 1997.

65. Bursch B, Zelter LK. Pediatric pain management. In: Behrman RE, Kliegman RM, Jenson HB, eds. *Nelson Textbook of Pediatrics.* Philadelphia, PA: W.B. Saunders; 2004: 358–366.

66. Anand KJS, McIntosh N, Lagercrantz H, et al. Analgesia and sedation in preterm neonate requiring ventilatory support. *Arch. Pediatr Adolesc Med.* 1999;153:331–338.

3

Procedural Sedation in the Emergency Department

Regulations as Promulgated by the Joint Commission on Accreditation of Healthcare Organizations and Establishment of Procedural Sedation Policy within the Emergency Department

Jonathan Glauser
Sharon E. Mace

HIGH YIELD FACTS

- Joint Commission on Accreditation of Healthcare Organizations (JCAHO) standards address sedation and anesthesia for operative and other procedures.
- Each hospital must develop protocols for patient sedation.
- The four levels of sedation are minimal sedation (anxiolysis), moderate sedation/ analgesia (*conscious sedation*), deep sedation/analgesia, and general anesthesia with sedation being a continuum.
- Patient assessment is done prior to and after the sedation or anesthesia.
- Monitoring of the patient is done during the procedure or anesthesia and during the recovery period.
- Monitoring includes assessment of the patient's oxygenation, ventilation, and circulation.
- Prior to discharge, the patient's vital signs should be in the patient's normal range, and the mental status, verbal skills, and muscular control status should be at presedation state.

OVERVIEW

The appropriate management of pain and anxiety in the emergency department (ED) is an important component of emergency care in all age groups. Administering medications for analgesia and sedation can facilitate interventional procedures and minimize patient pain and suffering. The use of such medicines, procedural sedation, is an integral part of the practice of emergency medicine. Procedural sedation is performed regularly by other nonanesthesiologists, including gastroenterologists, radiologists, and cardiologists.[1]

For successful and safe procedural sedation, appropriate drugs and dosages must be chosen and administered in the proper setting on appropriate patients. Patient evaluation should be performed before, during, and after their use.

The Joint Commission on Accreditation of Healthcare Organizations (JCAHO) recognizes that operative or other procedures and the administration of sedation or anesthesia often occur simultaneously. Sedation or anesthesia may be administered for noninvasive procedures as well. Specifically cited by the JCAHO are hyperbaric treatment, computed tomography (CT), or magnetic resonance imaging (MRI).[1] Their standards therefore address both operative or other procedures, as well as the administration of moderate or deep sedation or anesthesia. The American Society of Anesthesia formally approved definitions of General Anesthesia and Levels of Sedation/Analgesia on October 13, 1999.[2]

For JCAHO, standards for sedation and anesthesia care apply when patients receive, for any purpose or by any route, either of the following:

1. General, spinal, or other major regional sedation and anesthesia.
2. Sedation with or without analgesia that, in the manner used, may be reasonably expected to result in the loss of protective reflexes. For ED purposes, the modified Ramsey score is frequently used to define depth of sedation (Table 3-1).

It is understood by JCAHO that sedation is a continuum and that individual patient response to sedation may be unpredictable. Therefore, each hospital is expected to develop specific and appropriate protocols for the care of patients receiving sedation. Such protocols address the following[1]:

1. Sufficient qualified individuals are present to perform the procedure and to monitor the patient throughout administration and recovery.

Table 3-1. Modified Ramsay Score
for Procedural Sedation

1 = Anxious
2 = Awake, tranquil
3 = Drowsy, responds easily to verbal commands
4 = Asleep, brisk response to tactile or loud auditory stimulus
5 = Asleep, minimal response to tactile or loud auditory stimulus
6 = Asleep, no response

2. Appropriate equipment for care and resuscitation is available.

3. There is appropriate monitoring of vital signs, specifically heart rate, respiratory rate, and oxygenation.

4. Documentation of care.

5. Monitoring of outcomes.

Four levels of sedation are specifically defined and described in tabular form (Table 3-2).[2]

Minimal sedation (anxiolysis) is a drug-induced state during which patients respond normally to verbal commands. Although cognitive function and coordination may be impaired, ventilatory and cardiovascular functions are unaffected.

Moderate sedation/analgesia (conscious sedation) is a drug-induced depression of consciousness during which patients respond purposefully to verbal commands, either alone or accompanied by light tactile stimulation. No interventions are required to maintain a patent airway and spontaneous ventilation is adequate. Cardiovascular function is usually maintained.

Deep sedation/analgesia is a drug-induced depression of consciousness during which patients cannot be easily aroused but respond purposefully following repeated or painful stimulation. The ability to independently maintain ventilatory function may be impaired. Patients may require assistance in maintaining a patent airway and spontaneous ventilation may be inadequate. Cardiovascular function is usually maintained.

General anesthesia is a drug-induced loss of consciousness during which patients are not arousable, even by painful stimulation. The ability to independently maintain ventilatory function is often impaired. Patients often require assistance in maintaining a patent airway, and positive pressure ventilation may be required because of depressed spontaneous ventilation or drug-induced depression of neuromuscular function. Cardiovascular function may be impaired.

Because sedation is a continuum, it is not always possible to predict how an individual patient will respond. Hence, practitioners intending to produce a given level of sedation should be able to rescue patients whose level of

Table 3-2. Definition of General Anesthesia and Levels of Sedation/Analgesia

	Minimal Sedation (Anxiolysis)	Moderate Sedation/ Analgesia (Conscious Sedation)	Deep Sedation/ Analgesia	General Anesthesia
Responsiveness	Normal response to verbal stimulation	Purposeful response to verbal or tactile stimulation	Purposeful response following repeated or painful stimulation	Unarousable even with painful stimulus
Airway	Unaffected	No intervention required	Intervention may be required	Intervention often required
Spontaneous ventilation	Unaffected	Adequate	May be inadequate	Frequently inadequate
Cardiovascular function	Unaffected	Usually maintained	Usually maintained	May be impaired

Note: Approved by House of Delegates of the American Society of Anesthesiology on October 13, 1999.

sedation becomes deeper than initially intended. Individuals administering moderate sedation/analgesia (conscious sedation) should be able to rescue patients who enter a state of deep sedation/analgesia, while those administering deep sedation/analgesia should be able to rescue patients who enter a state of general anesthesia.

- Monitored anesthesia care does not describe the continuum of depth of sedation. Rather it describes "a specific anesthesia service in which an anesthesiologist has been requested to participate in the care of a patient undergoing a diagnostic or therapeutic procedure."
- Reflex withdrawal from a painful stimulus is *not* considered a purposeful response.
- Rescue of patients from a deeper level of sedation than intended should be interpreted as an intervention by a practitioner proficient in airway management and with advanced life support skills. All efforts at this point by the qualified practitioner should be directed to returning the patient to the originally intended level of sedation. It is not appropriate to continue the procedure and maintain the patient at an unintended level of sedation.

Specific standards listed by JCAHO are enumerated as PC.13.20, PC.13.30, and PC.13.40, and are discussed in turn.

Standard PC.13.20 addresses when operative or other procedures and/or the administration of moderate or deep sedation or anesthesia are planned. Since it is not always possible to predict how an individual patient will respond, qualified individuals are trained in professional standards and techniques to manage patients in case of a potential harmful event.[1]

Elements enumerated for performance of PC.13.20 include the following:

1. Sufficient numbers of qualified staff are available to evaluate the patient, perform the procedure, monitor, and recover the patient.
2. Individuals administering moderate or deep sedation and anesthesia are qualified and have the appropriate credentials to manage patients at whatever level of sedation or anesthesia is achieved, either intentionally or unintentionally. In this case, the JCAHO provides details as to the minimum competency-based education, training, and experience expected.
3. A registered nurse supervises perioperative nursing care.

4. Appropriate equipment to monitor the patient's physiologic status is available.
5. Appropriate equipment to administer intravenous fluids and drugs, including blood and blood components, is available as needed.
6. Resuscitation capabilities are available.

Qualified: The individuals providing moderate or deep sedation and anesthesia have at a minimum had competency-based education, training, and experience in the following:

1. Evaluating patients before moderate or deep sedation and anesthesia.
2. Performing moderate or deep sedation and anesthesia including rescuing patients who slip into a deeper than the desired level of sedation or analgesia. This includes the following:
   a. Moderate sedation—are qualified to rescue patients from deep sedation and are competent to manage a comprised airway and to provide adequate oxygenation and ventilation.
   b. Deep sedation—are qualified to rescue patients from general anesthesia and are competent to manage an unstable cardiovascular system as well as a comprised airway and inadequate oxygenation and ventilation.

Also, before operative or other procedures or the administration of moderate or deep sedation or anesthesia, the following steps are taken:

1. Patient acuity is assessed to plan for the appropriate level of postprocedure care.
2. Preprocedural education, treatments, and services are provided according to the plan for cure, treatment, and services.
3. The site, procedure, and patient are accurately identified and clearly communicated, using active communication techniques during a final verification process, such as "time out," prior to the start of any surgical or invasive procedure.
4. A presedation or preanesthesia assessment is conducted. Tables 3-3 to 3-5 give a suggested ED assessment, centering on elements of history, physical, and airway.
5. Before sedating or anesthetizing a patient, a LIP (licensed individual practitioner) with appropriate clinical privileges plans or concurs with the planned anesthesia.
6. The patient is reevaluated immediately before moderate or deep sedation and anesthesia induction.

Table 3-3. Relevant History and Physical Examination

1. Patient age
2. History of abnormalities of major organ systems, including heart, lungs, kidneys, or airway (e.g., sleep apnea, snoring, and stridor)
3. Pregnancy test only in women who are unable to ensure (based on history) that they are not pregnant
4. Current medications
5. History of any allergies or any adverse or allergic drug reactions with anesthesia or sedation/analgesia
6. History of prior sedation/analgesia including adequacy of pain control for those procedures
7. History of tobacco, alcohol, or substance use or abuse
8. Vital signs (weight, heart rate, blood pressure, and respiratory rate)
9. Cardiopulmonary examination
10. Airway examination (see Table 3-4)
11. Laboratory evaluation based on the patient's medial condition and the effect the results of such evaluation will have on the plan for procedural sedation/analgesia

Table 3-4. Preprocedural Examination of the Airway

Indicators of potential problematic airway
Decreased mouth opening
Micrognathia
Retrognathia
Significant malocclusion
Dentures
Macroglossia
Nonvisible uvula
Decreased neck flexibility
Advanced rheumatoid arthritis
Dysmorphic facial features
  Pierre Robin syndrome
  Trisomy 21
<3 cm hyoid-mental distance (adult)
Tracheal deviation

PATIENT SELECTION

The emergency physician determines whether a patient is appropriate for procedural sedation. This determination is based on the intended procedure, the patient's medical status as defined by the history and physical, and by the level of sedation/analgesia required to complete the procedure. Recent food intake is not a contraindication for administering procedural sedation and analgesia, but should be considered in choosing the depth of sedation. The American Society of Anesthesiologists (ASA) recommends fasting 6 hours for solids and 2 hours for liquids,[3] but the literature to date does not show a change in outcomes or adverse events with fasting for procedural sedation.[4,5] Ranitidine and metoclopramide can be given 30–60 minutes prior to sedation to increase gastric pH and reduce gastric volume.[6] NPO guidelines by age are summarized in Table 3-6, but are not mandated by JCAHO.

Table 3-5. Presedation Assessment on the Day of the Procedure

Documentation of any changes in history and physical
Time and nature of last oral intake
Vital signs, including heart rate, blood pressure, respiratory rate, and temperature
Baseline ambulation status
Patient or legal guardian must be informed about the risks, benefits, and alternatives to the proposed procedural sedation/analgesia

Table 3-6. NPO Status for Children

Children <6 months old
2 hours fast clear liquids
4 hours fast milk, solids

Children 6 months to 3 years
3 hours fast clear liquids
6 hours fast milk, solids

Children >3 months old
3 hours fast clear liquids
6–8 hours fast milk, solids

As part of the procedure ledger, a preprocedure history and physical examination is performed on the patient and documented. Pertinent aspects include medical history, particularly cardiac or pulmonary disease, sleep apnea, renal or hepatic disease, and prior central nervous system (CNS) disease (Table 3-3). Alcohol and tobacco, or illicit drug use, previous problems with sedative or analgesic agents, current medications, allergies, pregnancy status, and last PO intake must be documented. A history of prior sedation/analgesia including the adequacy of pain control for those procedures can be helpful. Along with vital signs and oxygen saturation, the examination may include auscultation of the heart and lungs, and examination of the airway for potential problems (Table 3-4). Baseline ambulation status should be documented.[7]

Pertinent laboratory evaluation and/or radiographs should be considered. Currently, there is no literature to support the need for specific laboratory testing before procedural sedation and analgesia. Laboratory testing should be driven by the patient's comorbid status.[8]

Finally, discussion with the patient or legal guardian to obtain informed consent includes the risks, benefits, and alternatives to sedation, as well as the planned procedure (Table 3-5). Written and verbal postprocedure and sedation discharge instructions are reviewed with the patient and/or responsible adult prior to the procedure.[6,9,10] Documentation and appropriate signatures are obtained before any medication is administered. The patient must have a responsible adult with whom to be discharged once the procedure is finished.[7]

Obtaining and preparing the appropriate equipment for sedation and managing the airway is paramount prior to beginning the procedure. A nurse or respiratory therapist dedicated to sedation, and skilled in the use of airways, bag and mask, monitors, and pharmacology of sedatives and analgesics should be at the patient's bedside throughout the procedure and recovery period. Oxygen delivery equipment (bag-valve mask, nasal cannula, and/or facemask) must be available at the bedside. Age-appropriate resuscitation equipment, including oxygen, intubation equipment, suction, emergency cart, and defibrillator, likewise, are immediately available at all times.[11]

A respiratory therapist, if available at the particular institution, should be notified of all conscious sedation procedures and ensure availability of all necessary airway and oxygen equipment at the bedside. The therapist provides an additional set of hands for assistance with any needed airway management. Capnometry has been recommended for patients with the potential for decreased hypoxic ventilatory drive,[12] but is not mandated by JCAHO.

Standard PC.13.30 states that patients are monitored during the procedure and/or administration of moderate or deep sedation or anesthesia. Elements of performance for PC.13.30 include the following:

1. Appropriate methods are used to continuously monitor oxygenation, ventilation, and circulation during procedures that may affect the patient's physiologic status.

2. The procedure and/or the administration of moderate or deep sedation or anesthesia for each patient are documented in the medical record.[1]

Certain specifics as to how the monitoring should be accomplished do not appear in JCAHO regulations. For example, the use of pulse oximetry to detect hypoxemia, electrocardiogram (ECG) for cardiac monitoring, and blood pressure monitoring are traditionally recommended, while other modalities such as end-tidal CO_2 for capnography are not mandated.

Standard PC.13.40 states that patients are monitored immediately after the procedure and/or administration of moderate or deep sedation or anesthesia. The elements of performance for PC.13.40 are the following[1]:

1. The patient's status is assessed on arrival in the recovery area.

2. Each patient's physiologic status, mental status, and pain level are monitored.

3. Monitoring is at a level consistent with the potential effect of the procedure and/or sedation or anesthesia.

4. Patients are discharged from the recovery area and the hospital by a qualified LIP or according to rigorously applied criteria approved by the clinical leaders.

5. Patients who have received anesthesia in the outpatient setting are discharged in the company of a responsible, designated adult. Table 3-7 contains suggested discharge criteria from the ED.

Table 3-7. Postsedation and Analgesia Discharge Criteria

Return to baseline verbal skills
Can understand and follow directions
Can verbalize, including correct diction

Return to baseline muscular control function
If an infant, can sit unattended
If a child or adult, can walk unassisted

Return to baseline mental status
Patient or responsible person with patient can understand procedural sedation and/or analgesia ED discharge instructions
Transportation home can be arranged

Table 3-8. Adverse Events as a Result of Sedation and Analgesia

---

Death
Cardiopulmonary arrest
Airway compromise during procedural sedation
Prolonged sedation
New neurologic deficit
Significant hypoxemia (saturation <90% for 1 minute in
    otherwise healthy patient
Aspiration
Significant hypotension
Significant bradycardia
Significant tachycardia
Admissions to the hospital as a direct result of intravenous
    conscious sedation

ADVERSE EVENTS REPORTING MANDATES BY JCAHO

Standard PI.2.20, element #8 specifies that an analysis is performed for adverse events or patterns of adverse events during moderate or deep sedation and anesthesia use.[1] Table 3-8 lists potential adverse events as a result of sedation. Table 3-9 lists a suggested quality assurance pathway for an ED.

DOCUMENTATION IN THE MEDICAL RECORD

The final mention of sedation and anesthesia in the JCAHO manual pertains to documentation of operative or other procedures, and the use of moderate or deep sedation or anesthesia. Specifically, Standard IM.6.30 applies to operative or other invasive and noninvasive procedures that place the patient at risk. The focus of JCAHO is on procedures and is not meant to include use of medications that place patients at risk.[1] Elements of performance for IM.6.30 include the following:

1. The history and physical examination, the results of any indicated diagnostic tests, as well as a provisional diagnosis are recorded before the operative procedure by the LIP responsible for the patient.

2. An operative progress note is entered into the medical record immediately after the procedure.

3. Operative reports dictated or written immediately after a procedure record the name of the primary surgeon and assistants, findings, procedures performed and description of the procedure, estimated blood loss, as indicated, specimens removed, and postoperative diagnosis.

4. The completed operative report is authenticated by the surgeon and made available in the medical record as soon as possible after the procedure.

5. Postoperative documentation records the patient's vital signs and level of consciousness; medications (including

Table 3-9. Model Quality Assurance Pathway

Each procedural area should identify an individual responsible for adverse event reporting and follow-up.
Each procedural area should determine a system for assuring compliance with documentation requirements.
Monthly summary reports should be made to the quality management authority or equivalent. Among specific events
    to be reported include the following:
    Total number of sedation cases per month per physician and whether the cases were moderate or deep sedation.
    Recovery phase >3 hours.
    Admissions as a direct result of procedural sedation.
    Emergency resuscitation of any type (drugs, airway, or cardiopulmonary support) initiated due to procedural
        sedation.
    Procedure cancellation due to adverse events related to sedation/analgesia.
    Any prolonged airway intervention.
    For moderate sedation cases any need to rescue the patient from slipping into deep sedation.
    For deep sedation cases any need to rescue the patient from slipping into general anesthesia.
The monthly reports should be reviewed by the hospital quality management board and the quality review officer of
    the department from which the report originated.

---

intravenous fluids) and blood and blood components administered, if applicable; and any unusual events or complications, including blood transfusion reactions and the management of those events.

6. Postoperative documentation records the patient's discharge from the postsedation or postanesthesia care area by the responsible LIP or according to discharge criteria.

7. The use of approved discharge criteria to determine the patient's readiness for discharge is documented in the medical record.

8. Postoperative documentation records the name of the LIP responsible for discharge.

Table 3-7 gives suggested postsedation and analgesia discharge criteria and discharge instructions.

The physician performing the procedure or his or her physician designee should be immediately available for consultation until the patient is discharged. Patients who are still sedated at the end of the procedure or those who received narcotic or benzodiazepene reversal are recovered within the ED prior to discharge home. The duration of all agents used, especially including reversal agents must be taken into consideration before discharging the patient.

To ensure safe recovery, vital signs and level of consciousness are continually assessed until the patient's mental status has returned to baseline and the patient completely awakens from sedation. Recovery should take place in the presence of an individual capable of monitoring patients and recognizing complications. Vital signs are monitored until they are within 20% of the patient's normal range. Assessment for pain, wound drainage, any nausea and vomiting, bladder distention, or compromised neurovascular status should be carried out prior to discharging the patient. No patient should be discharged, or sent to a medically unsupervised setting (x-ray, clinics, and so forth) until the mental status has returned to the presedation state. If the patient is transferred prior to the return to the presedation mental status, a nurse accompanies the patient.

A standard set of discharge criteria help to ensure safe discharge of the patient (Table 3-7). Discharge criteria, including level of consciousness criteria, should be met for at least a 30-minute period prior to the patient's discharge. The patient should be able to ambulate with assistance consistent with age and prior ambulatory status. The postprocedure and sedation discharge instructions are reviewed once again with the patient and/or responsible party prior to the patient's leaving the ED.

CONCLUSION

Procedural sedation enables the emergency physician to perform therapeutic interventions in a safe and humane fashion. Sedation also enables diagnostic testing to be done accurately and in a controlled setting. As with other interventions, proper use of sedative agents requires screening, preparation, and an ongoing quality monitoring process. The JCAHO lists a number of guidelines to be adhered to in order to ensure patient safety.

REFERENCES

1. Hospital Accreditation Standards. Oakbrook Terrace, IL: Joint Commission on Accreditation of Healthcare Organizations; 2004:163–166, 206, 287–288.

2. Definition of General Anesthesia and Levels of Sedation. American Society of Anesthesiology. Approved October 13, 1999. Available at *http://www.asahq.org/publications AndServices/standards/20.htm*

3. American Society of Anesthesiologists. Practice guidelines for sedation and analgesia by non-anesthesiologists. *Anesthesiology*. 1996;84:459–471.

4. American College of Emergency Physicians. Clinical policy for procedural sedation and analgesia in the emergency department. *Ann Emerg Med*. 1998;31:663–677.

5. Innes G, et al. Procedural sedation and analgesia in the emergency department. Canadian consensus guidelines. *J Emerg Med*. 1999;17:145–156.

6. Sacchetti A, Schafermeyer R, Gerardi M, et al. Pediatric analgesia and sedation. *Ann Emerg Med*. 1994;23:237–250.

7. Rose J, Koenig K. Procedural sedation and analgesia. *Crit Decis Emerg Med* 1996;10:9–15.

8. Van Vlymen JM, White PF. Outpatient anesthesia. In: Miller RD, Cucchiara RF, Miller ED Jr, et al, eds. *Anesthesia*. 5th ed, Vol 2. Philadelphia, PA: Churchill Livingstone; 2000: 2213–2240.

9. American College of Emergency Physicians. Use of pediatric sedation and analgesia. *Ann Emerg Med* 1997;29:834–835.

10. American Academy of Pediatrics. Guidelines for monitoring and management of pediatric patients during and after sedation for diagnostic and therapeutic procedures. *Pediatrics* 1992;89:1110–1115.

11. Green SM, Krauss B. Procedural sedation and analgesia. In: Roberts JR, Hedges JR, Chanmugam AS, et al, eds. *Clinical Procedures in Emergency Medicine*. Philadelphia, PA: W.B. Saunders; 2004:596–620.

12. Gross JB, et al. Guidelines for sedation and analgesia by nonanesthesiologists. *Anesthesiology*. 1996;84:459.

4

Documentation and Standard Forms for Use during Procedural Sedation in the Emergency Department

Jonathan Glauser

HIGH YIELD FACTS

- Procedural sedation is an integral part of emergency medicine.
- Procedural sedation is performed on a regular basis by nonanesthesiologists, including radiologists, gastroenterologists, and cardiologists.
- Patient selection for procedural sedation is based on the patient's medical status, the intended procedure, and the level of sedation/analgesia required for completing the procedure.
- The patient's medical status is defined by the history and physical (H&P) examination, which includes written documentation as part of the preprocedural patient assessment.
- Joint Commission on Accreditation of Healthcare Organizations (JCAHO) requires a documented H&P prior to procedural sedation, which for the emergency department (ED) is done on the day of sedation.
- Preprocedural assessment, intraprocedural monitoring, and postprocedural assessment are documented on a standardized form that becomes part of the patient's permanent medical record.

INTRODUCTION

Procedural sedation is an integral part of the practice of emergency medicine and is performed regularly by other nonanesthesiologists, including gastroenterologists,

radiologists, and cardiologists.[1] For successful and safe procedural sedation, appropriate drugs and dosages must be chosen and administered in the proper setting on appropriate patients. Patient evaluation should be performed before, during, and after their use.

In this section, we will provide a pragmatic overview of documentation from an emergency medicine perspective, although these documents and forms are widely applicable across other medical specialties. Forms will concentrate on the procedure itself, on preparation for the procedure, on quality monitoring, and on discharge instructions. Tables and figures are included for purposes of procedural guidelines and as suggestions for protocols in ED assessment and management.

PATIENT SELECTION

The emergency physician determines whether a patient is appropriate for procedural sedation. This determination is based on the intended procedure, the patient's medical status as defined by the H&P, and by the level of sedation/analgesia required to complete the procedure. Recent food intake is not a contraindication for administering procedural sedation and analgesia, but should be considered in choosing the depth of sedation. The American Society of Anesthesiologists (ASA)[2] recommends fasting, 6 hours for solids and 2 hours for liquids,[3] but the literature to date does not show a change in outcomes or adverse events with fasting for procedural sedation.[4,5] Recent literature suggests that even when fasting guidelines are not met or adhered to, adverse events are rare, with emesis in 1.5% of patients and no recorded significant episodes of aspiration in 509 patients who did not meet fasting guidelines.[6] Suggested NPO guidelines by age are summarized in Table 4-1.

In complicated patients or patients with severe systemic disease in which the sedation/analgesia and the complexity of the procedures would reduce the patient's reserve, the physician may find an anesthesiology consult helpful in determining if the ED or operating room is best for the required procedure. Likewise, the physician should use caution with patients who have significant oxygenation or anatomic airway/ventilation abnormalities as noted by history or physical examination (see further). Relative contraindications include hemodynamic instability, respiratory depression, and significant underlying medical problems.

In general, patients with severe systemic disease (ASA III or IV) require consultation with an anesthesiologist. Similarly, infants <3 months of age, premature infants <60 weeks postconceptual weeks of age, and children

Table 4-1. NPO Status for Children

Children <6 months old
2 hours fast clear liquids
4 hours fast milk, solids

Children 6 months to 3 years
3 hours fast clear liquids
6 hours fast milk, solids

Children >3 months old
3 hours fast clear liquids
6–8 hours fast milk, solids

with underlying respiratory airway disease, neurologic conditions, central nervous system (CNS) injury, multiple trauma, or liver/kidney disease are at increased risk for sedation complications and require consultation with an anesthesiologist.[7-9] This chapter applies only to patients classified as ASA I or II (Table 4-2).

DOCUMENTATION OVERVIEW

The attending staff physician is responsible for the performance of residents and of physician extenders under his or her supervision. The procedural sedation record (Fig. 4-1) is to be signed by the ED staff, although collection of data for some sections may be delegated to a nurse/monitor. Physicians may think that they are following sedation guidelines when they are not.[10] The H&P for any procedure requiring sedation must be done within 30 days of that procedure by Joint Commission standards, but in the ED should be done the same day. Pertinent aspects of the medical history should emphasize cardiac or pulmonary disease, sleep apnea, renal or hepatic disease, or prior CNS disease. Alcohol and tobacco, or illicit drug use, previous problems with sedative or analgesic agents, current medications, allergies, pregnancy status (when appropriate), and last PO intake must be documented. A history of prior sedation/analgesia including the adequacy of pain control for those procedures can be helpful. Along with vital signs and oxygen saturation, the examination may include auscultation of the heart and lungs and examination of the airway for potential problems. Baseline ambulation status should be documented.[11]

Pertinent laboratory evaluation and/or radiographs should be considered. Currently, there is no literature to support the need for specific laboratory testing before procedural sedation and analgesia. Laboratory testing should be driven by the patient's comorbid status.

Finally, discussion with the patient or legal guardian to obtain informed consent includes the risks, benefits, and alternatives to sedation, as well as the planned procedure. Written and verbal postprocedure and sedation discharge instructions are reviewed with the patient and/or responsible adult prior to the procedure.[8,12,13] Documentation and appropriate signatures are obtained before any medication is administered.

Table 4-2. American Society of Anesthesiologists Classifications

Class	Patient Status
I	Normally healthy patient. The pathologic process for which the procedure is to be performed is localized and not a systemic disturbance.
II	Mild systemic disease under control (e.g., asthma).
III	Severe systemic disease from any cause.
IV	Severe systemic disease, which is a constant life threat, not always correctable by the operative procedure.
V	Moribund patient who is not expected to survive without the operation.

THE PROCEDURE FORM ITSELF

A suggested form for routine use for sedation in the ED is appended (Fig. 4-1), which also notes that the patient is deemed to be a suitable candidate for sedation in the ED by the ED attending. This form becomes part of the patient's permanent medical record.

Intraprocedural monitoring is documented on a monitoring record throughout the procedure. Cardiorespiratory monitoring should be performed on all patients. This includes, but is not limited to, noninvasive blood pressure, electrocardiogram (ECG) monitoring, pulse oximetry, and vital sign observation. During deep sedation, vital signs are recorded every 5 minutes. For other conscious sedation this should be no less frequent than every 15 minutes for adequate safety.[7]

Evaluation, at a minimum, requires assessment of and recording of vital signs and level of consciousness, before the beginning of the procedure, after administration of sedative/analgesic drugs, at regular intervals during a procedural sedation, and at the end of the procedure.

THE CLEVELAND CLINIC FOUNDATION
PROCEDURAL SEDATION RECORD

Name: _____

CCF ID: _____

D.O.B.: _____

Date: _____/_____/_____   Age: _____

I.D. verified by: _____

PHYSICIAN DOCUMENTATION (Check one)

☐ See H & P dated _____/_____/_____ If H & P completed within 30 days and present on chart, complete shaded areas.

  Anything changed since H & P completed? ☐ No ☐ Yes (explain) _____

☐ H & P below.

Indication for procedure: _____

Procedure: _____ **Verified c̄ pt. by:** _____

HISTORY AND PHYSICAL

Chief complaint: _____

History of present illness: _____

_____
_____
_____
_____
_____

Past medical history PATIENT	NO	YES	EXPLAIN	Current medications MEDICATION NAME	COMMENTS
Hypertension					
Heart disorders					
Lung disorders					
Neuro disorders					
Diabetes					
Kidney disorder					
Bleeding disorder					
ETOH/Substance abuse					
Anes./Sed. complications					
Hx stridor, apnea, snoring					
Hx poor surg. pain mgmt.					
Other				Allergies: ☐ NKA or update composite list	
				Pregnancy/LMP	

Physical examination: BP _____ **P** _____ **R** _____ **Wt.:** _____ **Labs (as applicable)** _____

  Heart: _____   Lung: _____

  Other: _____

Impressions/Plan: _____

_____

  Airway: visualization of uvula: ☐ yes ☐ no   Neck: full range of motion: ☐ yes ☐ no

  Mouth opening ≥ 2 fingerbreadths? ☐ yes ☐ no   Other: _____

Patient candidate for procedural sedation? _____ moderate _____ deep

Informed consent for procedure & sedation:

  Risk, benefits, & alternatives discussed? _____ Pt. agrees to proceed? _____
  (yes or no)   (yes or no)

Physician signature: _____ _____/_____ / Beeper _____
                                        (PRINT NAME)

Fig. 4-1. Sample procedural sedation record.

Nursing assessment:

NPO since: _____

I.D. band check: _____

Dentures   ☐ yes   ☐ no   ☐ N/A

Glasses   ☐ yes   ☐ no   ☐ N/A

Other: _____

Patient education re: procedure   ☐ yes   ☐ no   ☐ N/A

Nursing plan of care initiated: ☐ yes   ☐ no   ☐ N/A

Patient assessment score

	pre	post
Moves 4 extremities voluntarily on command	2	2
Moves 2 extremities voluntarily on command	1	1
Moves 0 extremities voluntarily on command	0	0
Able to breathe deeply & cough freely	2	2
Dyspnea or limited breathing	1	1
Apneic	0	0
Fully awake	2	2
Arousable on calling	1	1
Not responding	0	0
Able to maintain O_2 saturation > 90% on RA	2	2
Needs O_2 to maintain O_2 sat > 90%	1	1
O_2 sat < 90% with O_2	0	0
Able to stand up and walk upright	2	2
Vertigo when erect	1	1
Dizziness when supine	0	0
Non-ambulatory	0	0
TOTAL		

PRE-PROCEDURAL VASCULAR ASSESSMENT ☐ No deferred/not indicated

PALPABLE: 4+= Bounding 3+= normal 2+= decreased 1+= weak 0=absent

Pulses: Pre	F	P	DP	PT	Other
RL					
LL					

Pre-procedure vital signs: Time:_____ BP: _____ P: _____ R: _____ T: _____ O_2 sat _____ Pain rating* _____

Audible time out: Time: _____ Physician: _____ Assistant: _____

Prep: _____

Transportation home verified?   ☐ yes   ☐ no   ☐ N/A

IV site/gauge: _____

_____ Initials _____

	INTAKE		
TIME	SOLUTION - ml's/hr	ABSORBED	CREDIT

		OUTPUT		
TIME	URINE	EBL		

Procedure start time: _____

Procedure finish time: _____

Total fluoroscopy time: _____

Electrosurgical unit # _____ Pad # _____

Pad location _____

Site condition p̄ removal _____

Specimens collected _____

Dressing: _____

TIME	BP	P	R	O_2SAT	LOC**	Pain rating 0-10	MEDS/O_2	NOTES RN/LPN/Tech	INITIALS

Modified ramsay score LOC 1 = Anxious 2 = Awake, tranquil, 3 = Drowsy, responds easily to verbal commands 4 = Asleep, brisk response to tactile or loud auditory stimulus 5 = Asleep, minimal response to tactile or loud auditory stimulus 6 = Asleep, no response
*Pain scale: 0 1 2 3 4 5 6 7 8 9 10 (0 = none 10 = worst)

Fig. 4-1. (*Continued*).

Vital signs (continued):

TIME	BP	P	R	O$_2$SAT	LOC	Pain rating 0-10	MEDS/O$_2$	NOTES	INITIALS
POCT-stickers									

POST-PROCEDURAL VASCULAR ASSESSMENT ☐ No deferred/not indicated
Palpable: 4+= Bounding 3+= normal 2+= decreased 1+= weak 0= absent

Pulses: Pre	F	P	DP	PT	OTHER
RL					
LL					

Physician signature: _____
  (for medication orders)

Print name: _____ Beeper: _____

Discharge care:

  I.V. discontinued: _____

  Condition of I.V. site: _____

Discharge assessment

MET

☐ Patient returned to pre-procedure patient assessment score.
☐ Cardiovascular function and airway patency are satisfactory and stable.
☐ Pulse oximetry > or = to 90% on room air or at pre-procedure baseline.
☐ Patient is able to move within pre-sedation abilities.
☐ Ability to retain oral fluid when appropriate.
☐ Pain adequately controlled, pain rating _____

Patient discharged to:

☐ Hospital unit _____   ☐ Other: _____
☐ Home, in the care of responsible adult _____

Discharge time: _____

Mode of transportation:

☐ gurney ☐ wheelchair ☐ bed ☐ crib ☐ ambulated ☐ stroller

Discharge instructions:

☐ Written and verbal post procedure & sedation discharge instruction giver to patient and/or family with stated understanding
☐ Discharge prescriptions given to patient
☐ Medication use explained to patient with stated understanding

Returned to patient: ☐ Belongings   ☐ Dentures
          ☐ Glasses   ☐ Other _____

TIME	NURSE SIGNATURE	INITIALS	TIME	NURSE SIGNATURE	INITIALS

Fig. 4-1. (*Continued*).

Pulse oximetry is used to continuously and quantitatively assess oxygenation. In general, oxygen saturation should be maintained with oxygen at >95%. In patients with chronic hypoxemia, a reasonable goal is to maintain saturation at or above their baseline.[3,4] Capnography can be used to monitor ventilation.[5,13]

Electrocardiographic monitoring should be considered for use on those patients who have or are at increased risk for cardiac disease. This may include, but is not be limited to, those with a history of congestive heart failure, dysrhythmias, diabetes, coronary artery disease, peripheral vascular disease, age over 50, or >20 pack-year smoking history.[3,14]

In certain circumstances, one of the above monitoring requirements may be temporarily suspended if performance of that requirement would result in interference with the procedure (i.e., computed tomography/magnetic resonance imaging [CT/MRI] scans). The requirement for monitoring heart rate and oxygen saturation by pulse oximetry, however, should never be suspended.

Recall also the need for a "time out" prior to a procedure, at which time the patient's name and hospital number and/or date of birth are verified prior to proceeding.

DISCHARGE FORMS

The patient must have a responsible adult with whom to be discharged once the procedure is finished.[9] A suggested set of discharge guidelines follows (Fig. 4-2). Discharge instructions include general warnings regarding decreased mental acuity following sedation and specific activities to avoid.[15] The patient is warned that the anesthetics used may still be active for 24 hours after the procedure.

Activity is minimized during the day following sedation, progressing to regular activities as tolerated. Instructions to avoid driving cars and operating dangerous machinery or power tools for 24 hours should be given. As examples, instructions can include patients avoiding sewing machines, blenders, as well as heavy equipment. Patients are advised not to drink alcohol or take any other sedatives for 1 day, and not to make important decisions for 1 day following anesthetics. Caution is advised when climbing or descending stairs. Typical diet instructions for an adult entails, clear liquids are best tolerated at first. If the patient has no nausea 6 hours after the procedure, the diet can be advanced as tolerated to solid foods. Suggested criteria for discharge are listed in Table 4-3.

For pediatric patients, a similar but more age-appropriate set of instructions are used. Parents are advised that their children may feel sleepy, and that sleeping, rest, or

Table 4-3. Postsedation and Analgesia Discharge Criteria

Return to baseline verbal skills
Can understand and follow directions
Can verbalize, including correct diction

Return to baseline muscular control function
If an infant, can sit unattended
If a child or adult, can walk unassisted

Return to baseline mental status
Patient or responsible person with patient can understand procedural sedation and/or analgesia ED discharge instructions
Transportation home can be arranged

quiet play (coloring and watching TV) are recommended activities after sedation. The child's diet is likewise started with fluids, and advanced as tolerated to the appropriate diet for the child's age.

Warnings included in discharge instructions request the patient to return or contact their doctor if the patient has persistent vomiting for more than 24 hours, experiences signs of infection such as fever or chills, or if there are any complications from the procedure performed. In children, if the patient has pain unrelieved by acetominophen or other prescribed pain medication, the patient is warned to return.

MONITORING POSTPROCEDURE QUALITY ASSURANCE

Monthly audits should be performed on all patients undergoing procedural sedation. Reports should be generated to the institution's quality assurance office on a quarterly basis, documenting agents used, adverse events, and types of procedures performed by individual staff. Although this book focuses on emergency medicine, other departments performing sedation outside the operative suite must do the same, for example, cardiology, gastroenterology, interventional radiology, and pediatrics . A standard form is appended (Fig. 4-3). Adverse events mandating reporting are listed elsewhere (see Chap. 3).

CONCLUSIONS

Procedural sedation enables the emergency physician to perform therapeutic interventions in a safe and humane fashion. Sedation by nonanesthesiologists has become

Emergency Department
Cleveland Clinic Foundation
9500 Euclid Avenue
Cleveland, OH 44195

GENERAL INFORMATION: You or your child were give medications to induce sleepiness so the doctors could perform a procedure on you with minimal discomfort. The anesthetics, sedatives, or pain-killers which were given to you in the emergency department may still be active for the next 24 hours. You or your child may feel a little drowsy from them.

The medications you or your child received:

_____

_____

_____

INSTRUCTIONS:

Activity

<u>Adult</u>: Rest at home today, progressing to regular activities as tolerated. Do not drive a car, operate dangerous machinery or power tools for 24 hours. This includes sewing machines and blenders, as well as heavy equipment. Do not drink alcohol or take unprescribed medication for 24 hours. Do not make any important decisions. Be careful climbing stairs.

<u>Child</u>: Restrict activity to quiet play, watching TV, coloring. Do not let child play unattended for 24 hours due to possible dizziness or drowsiness. Do not let your child ride bicycles or play on swingsets for the next 24 hours.

You or your child may feel sleepy. It is fine to sleep.

Diet

<u>Adult</u>: Clear liquids are best tolerated at first. If you are not nauseated, you can progress your diet to solid foods as tolerated.

<u>Child</u>: Start with fluids, then advance to appropriate diet for child's age, as tolerated. Fluids are more important for the first 24 hours.

CONTACT YOUR DOCTOR OR RETURN TO THE EMERGENCY DEPARTMENT IF:

1. There is vomiting more than 24 hours.
2. There are signs of infection such as fever or chills.
3. You or your child have pain unrelieved by acetaminophen or other prescribed pain medication.
4. There are any complications from the procedure performed.

Fig. 4-2. Sample set of guidelines for discharge of a patient from an emergency room.

THE CLEVELAND CLINIC FOUNDATION PROCEDURAL SEDATION LOG
(Privileged Quality Management Communication as defined in the Ohio Revised Code 2305.24,2305.25)
UNIT _____ MONTH _____ YEAR _____ PAGE _____ OF _____

DATE	TIME	PATIENT LABEL	PROCEDURE PERFORMED	AGENT USED/ DOSE	DURATION OF SEDATION (TIME)	QM/ADVERSE EVENTS	COMMENTS	PHYSICIAN	RN RRT
					CS:_____ * DS:_____ **				
					CS:_____ * DS:_____ **				
					CS:_____ * DS:_____ **				
					CS:_____ * DS:_____ **				

PLACE THE APPROPRIATE LETTER IN THE QUALITY MONITORING(QM)/ADVERSE EVENTS BOX

(A) NO ADVERSE EVENTS
(B) USE OF REVERSAL AGENT
(C) RECOVERY PHASE > 3 HOURS
(D) ADMISSION TO THE HOSPITAL AS DIRECT RESULT OF PROCEDURAL SEDATION
(E) EMERGENCY RESUSCITATION OF ANY TYPE (medications, airway, cardiopulmonary support)
(F) PROCEDURE CANCELLATION DUE TO ADVERSE EVENTS RELATED TO SEDATION/ANALGESIA
(G) ANY PROLONGED MANUAL INTERVENTION OF THE AIRWAY > 20 MINUTES

*Conscious sedation (CS)/Analgesia: Purposeful response following repeated or painful stimulation; airway intervention may be required; adequate spontaneous ventilation with cardiovascular function usually maintained.
**Deep Sedation (DS)/Analgesia: Purposeful response following repeated or painful stimulation; airway intervention may be required; spontaneous ventilation may be inadequate with cardiovascular unction usually maintained. Note: Reflex withdrawal from a painful stimulus is not considered a purposeful response.

Fig. 4-3. Sample procedural sedation log.

widely accepted; however, documentation of procedures, adherence to discharge guidelines, and a quality assurance program are all mandatory. Recommended forms in this chapter may be modified according to the needs and characteristics of a given institution, but should still retain the essential elements cited.

REFERENCES

1. Holzman R, Cullen D, Eichhorn J, et al. Guidelines for sedation by nonanesthesiologists during diagnostic and therapeutic procedures. *J Clin Anesth*. 1994;6:265–276.
2. American Society of Anesthesiologists. Practice guidelines for pre-operative fasting and the use of pharmacologic agents to reduce the risk of pulmonary aspiration: application to healthy patients undergoing elective procedures. *Anesthesiology*. 1999;50:896–905.
3. American Society of Anesthesiologists. Practice guidelines for sedation and analgesia by non-anesthesiologists. *Anesthesiology*. 1996;84:459–471.
4. American College of Emergency Physicians. Clinical policy for procedural sedation and analgesia in the emergency department. *Ann Emerg Med*. 1998;31:663–677.
5. Innes G, et al. Procedural sedation and analgesia in the emergency department. Canadian consensus guidelines. *J Emerg Med*. 1999;17:145–156.
6. Agrawal D, Manzi SF, Gupta R, et al. Preprocedural fasting state and adverse events in children undergoing procedural sedation and analgesia in a pediatric emergency department. *Ann Emerg Med*. 2003;42(5):647–650.
7. Holzmann R, Cullen D, Eichhorn J, et al. Guidelines for sedation by nonanesthesiologist during diagnostic and therapeutic procedures. *J Clin Anesth*. 1994;6:265–276.
8. American College of Emergency Physicians. Use of pediatric sedation and analgesia. *Ann Emerg Med*. 1997;29:834–835.
9. Ostman PL, White PF. Outpatient anesthesia. In: Miller RD, ed. *Anesthesia*. 4th ed. New York: Churchill Livingstone; 1994:2213–2246.
10. Slomka J, Hoffman-Hogg L, Mion LC, et al. Influence of clinicians' values and perceptions on use of clinical practice guidelines for sedation and neuromuscular blockade in patients receiving mechanical ventilation. *Am J Crit Care*. 2000;9(6):412–418.
11. Rose J, Koenig K. Procedural sedation and analgesia. *Crit Decis Emerg Med*. 1996;10:9–15.
12. Sacchetti A, Schafermeyer R, Gerardi M, et al. Pediatric analgesia and sedation. *Ann Emerg Med*. 1994;23:237–250.
13. American Academy of Pediatrics. Guidelines for monitoring and management of pediatric patients during and after sedation for diagnostic and therapeutic procedures. *Pediatrics*. 1992;89:1110–1115.
14. Practice guidlines for sedation and analgesia by non-anesthesiologists. *Anesthesiology*. 1996;84:459–471.
15. Ward KR, Yealy DM. Systemic analgesia and sedation for procedures. In: Roberts JR, and Hedges JR, eds. *Clinical Procedures in Emergency Medicine*. 3rd ed. Philadelphia, PA: W.B. Saunders; 1998:516–531.

5

Quality Improvement and Risk Management

Eric Anderson

HIGH YIELD FACTS

- Most quality problems are related to flaws in systems or processes, and not personnel.
- Quality improvement is an evolutionary process, not a "quick fix."
- The quality cycle, process control charts, cause and effect diagrams, parieto diagrams, and flow diagrams are used to identify potential problems.
- Risk management's goal is to identify potential problem areas and make interventions before a problem becomes manifest. Steps should be taken, within an institution's capability, to identify and correct problem areas.
- When adverse events occur, be open and honest with the patient and family about what happened and what you have done about it.

INTRODUCTION

The key to quality improvement in emergency department (ED) procedural sedation is a coordinated hospitalwide uniform set of guidelines.[1-4] These guidelines may include definition of terms, presedation evaluation of patients, exclusions, equipment needed in the area of the sedation, qualifications of personnel involved in the sedation, areas where it is acceptable to perform sedation, pharmacologic agents used, intraprocedural patient monitoring, postprocedure recovery period, discharge criteria, and home-going instructions.[5] Appropriate feedback mechanisms to report any complications and education of personnel when complications occur should be part of the quality improvement program.[5,6]

Risk management is essentially applied quality improvement. The essence of risk management is to identify potential problem areas *before* there is an adverse event and correct the potential problem area (procedure) or at least make everyone involved aware that there is the potential for a problem. Risk management also involves medical personnel behavior after there is an adverse event. Steps should be taken to minimize the injury to the patient. The patient and family should be notified of the unexpected adverse event, reasons it occurred, and steps taken to correct the event. Here, frankness and honesty can save the patient frustration and anger and can help to maintain the trust of the patient with the practitioner.

QUALITY IMPROVEMENT

Improvement in patient care is an evolutionary process. Medications and techniques change over time, and the process of assessing the efficacy of the chosen treatment modality should be continuously revised. We have moved from the quality assessment days where bad outcomes were felt to be the result of bad practitioners. Now it is well recognized that 85% of problems are the result of flaws in systems and not in personnel. By continuously observing the system and noting variances in outcomes, practitioners can make adjustments in the system that will result in more uniform outcomes. Continuous quality improvement has evolved from efforts to improve manufacturing systems in order to produce a more consistent product. Continuous quality improvement when applied to health care systems, specifically procedural sedation, should allow for more uniform and predictable outcomes. Treating patients is considerably different from manufacturing; however, the quest to decrease variation and provide uniform outcomes is the same. The quality cycle is a simplified way of illustrating how basic quality improvement should work (Fig. 5-1).[7,8]

Plan for good outcomes. Study the system. Ishakawa (fish bone) diagrams, flowcharts, and parieto analysis and brainstorming are helpful (Figs. 5-2 to 5-4).[7,9] Determine personnel needed, personnel qualifications, physical plant, special equipment, and patient inclusions and exclusions discussed in Chap. 8.[5] Evaluate how patients and equipment are moved in the ED. Get perspectives of all personnel involved in the procedural process: doctors, nurses, respiratory therapist, radiology technicians, and consultants who may do procedures in the ED that require procedural sedation. Educate staff about the need for change and the expected behavior and procedure changes before the changes are implemented.

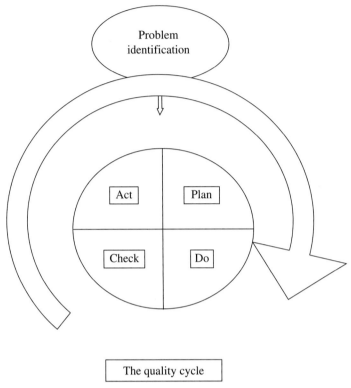

Fig. 5-1. Quality cycle.

Do, implement changes to the system, to move toward the desired result. Small changes initially, unless circumstances demand immediate drastic change. The staff can more easily accept smaller visible changes. Visible changes can be observed by all of the staff, which will then acknowledge that the quality process can have some positive results. Visible improvements motivate the staff to pursue further quality projects. Conflicts and "turf battles" must be resolved at this stage to assure project success. Those resistant to change must be further educated or reassigned to less sensitive duties.

Check to see if implemented changes are having the desired effects: decreased complication rate, decreased sedation time, and increased physician and patient satisfaction with the procedure. Visual analog satisfaction scales of physician and patient satisfaction with the sedation analgesia and procedure ease will help to asses the efficacy of the chosen procedural sedation modalities. Decreasing the complication rate is indicative of increasing patient safety. Patient selection for procedural sedation will be a key determinant in the ultimate complication rate (Chap. 8).

Act to maximize the therapeutic benefit to the patient. Use data to make adjustments for variances in procedures that were exposed in the check part of the cycle. Implement the adjustments and run the plan, do, check, act, cycle again, to reassess for the desired improvements. Remember that without data, there can be no quality improvement.

Development of process control charts can help illustrate how a process evolves over time. An average complication rate is calculated from available data. Upper and lower control limits are developed and subsequent complication rates are charted on a weekly, monthly, or quarterly basis. The general trend should be downward until the maximal amount of quality is obtained from the system in its present condition. At that point, the complication rate will plateau, until there is some new medicine, process, or technology that improves the process to the point where a new quality plateau will be obtained. The degree of variation in outcomes (between doctors, nurses, shifts, and procedures) should decrease as the system becomes more uniform in outcome results.

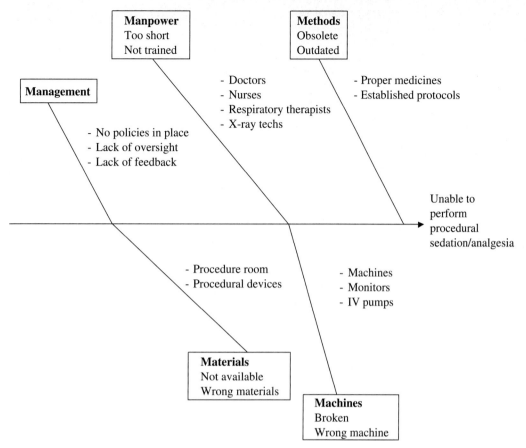

Fig. 5-2. Cause and effect diagram (also known as a Ishikawa or fishbone diagram).

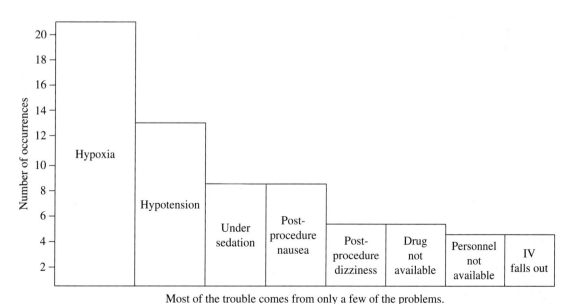

Most of the trouble comes from only a few of the problems.

Fig. 5-3. Parieto diagram (80% of the trouble comes from 20% of the problems).

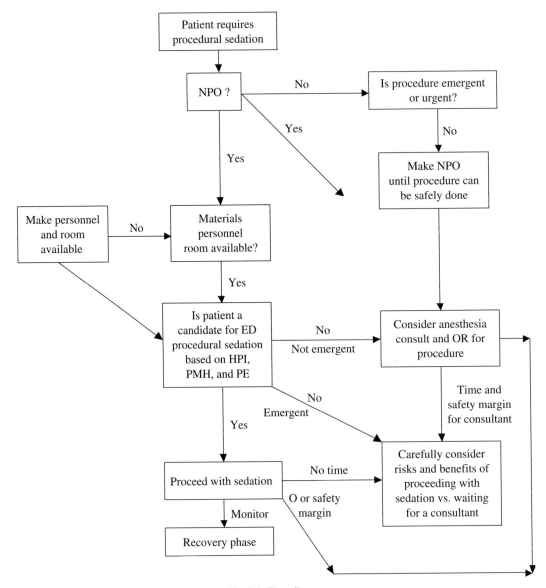

Fig. 5-4. Flow diagram.

RISK MANAGEMENT

Patient safety is paramount in medicine. The Institute of Medicine's 2001 report "To Error is Human: Building a Safer Health System" indicated there were approximately 90,000 deaths in hospitals of the United States due to "medical errors."[10] Routine practices to prevent medical errors, improve patient safety, and decrease the medicolegal risk to the practitioners and institutions involved should be initiated. Selecting patients appropriate for sedation and analgesia for an ED procedure is important. Many complications can be avoided by proper patient selection as outlined in Chapter 8.

Confusion with soundalike drugs like narcan (Nalaxone) and norcuron (Vecuronium) can have devastating results. Soundalike dosages like 15 mg and 50 mg can have similar results when dosing sedative/analgesic drugs.[11] Preventive measures like having the physician write down medications and dosages will decrease confusion at the time of administration. It is recognized that during a sedation procedure, it may be necessary to give verbal orders for medication administration. Verbal confirmation, having the nurse repeat back the medication and dosage is a good double check on what is being administered.[11] Verbal orders should always be given to a specific individual and not just shouted into the air. This will avoid double dosing or meds not being given.[11] Usage of dosage charts and previously established sedation/analgesia protocols will increase the safety and decrease the chance for errors.[11]

When and if errors or unexpected complications or situations occur, it is best to be up front with the family about what happened and the steps taken to correct the problem. This is not the time to place blame on another member of the health care team. The families will be somewhat stressed by the news of a problem and will want information. This is the time to answer family and patient questions. We must also assure that the patient has no further problems because of the event. One of the things families complain the most about is the medical community "clamming up" over concerns about a lawsuit. It is important to deal with patients and families as people, and not as potential adversaries in a lawsuit. This is particularly important since, in the ED, they are still under your care.

SUMMARY

Procedural sedation/analgesia has been found to be both safe and efficacious in a variety of clinical situations. Pediatric use of procedural sedation/analgesia is also safe and efficacious.[12,13] Preestablished procedural sedation protocols help establish measurable quality goals. One of the most common reasons for complications during procedural sedation/analgesia is inadequate monitoring.[14] By following established protocols, preventable complications as well as time and expense of an operating room visit can be avoided.[15] Risks can be anticipated and minimized by proper patient selection, room preparation, and training of personnel for monitoring, recognition, and intervention if complications occur.

REFERENCES

1. Gross JB, Framington CT, Bailey PJ. Practice guidelines for sedation and analgesia by non-anesthesiologists. *Anesthesiology.* 2002;96(1):1004–1017.

2. Innes G, Murphy M, Nijssen-Jordan C, et al. Procedural sedation and analgesia in the emergency department: Canadian consensus guidelines. *J Emerg Med.* 1999;17(1):145–156.

3. Jagoda AS, Campbell M, Karas J, et al. Clinical policy for procedural sedation and analgesia in the emergency department. *Ann Emerg Med.* 1998;31(5):663–677.

4. Sklar DP. Joint commission on accreditation of healthcare organizations requirements for sedation. *Ann Emerg Med.* 1996;27(4):412–413.

5. Cleveland Clinic Foundation. Guidelines for procedural sedation/analgesia. Cleveland, OH: Cleveland Clinic Foundation; 2001:1–10.

6. Zebris J, Maurer W. Quality assurance in the endoscopy suite: sedation and monitoring. *Gastroenterol Clin North Am.* 2004;14:415–429.

7. Othman JE. Quality assurance and continuous quality improvement in sedation analgesia. In: Malviya S, Naughton NN, Tremper KK, eds. *Sedation and Analgesia for Diagnostic and Therapeutic Procedures.* Totowa, NJ: Humana Press; 2003:275–295.

8. Buckley LL. Continuous quality improvement in emergency services: what and why. In: Siegel DM, Crocker PJ, eds. Continuous quality improvement for emergency departments. *Am Coll Emerg Phys.* Dallas, TX; 1994:1–14.

9. Bromley M. A team approach to the quality improvement process. In: Siegel DM, Crocker PJ, eds. Continuous quality improvement for emergency departments. *Am Coll Emerg Phys.* Dallas, TX; 1994:21–31.

10. Institute of Medicine, committee on quality of health care in America. To error is human: building a safer health system. In: Kohn LT, Corrigan JM, Donaldson MS, eds. Washington, DC: National Academy Press; 2000.

11. Sucov A, Wears RL. Reports spotlight medication errors: make changes before tragedy strikes. *ED Manag.* 2000;12 (6 suppl 1–2):61–65.

12. Pitetti RD, Singh S, Pierce MC. Safe and efficacious use of procedural sedation and analgesia by nonanesthesiologists in a pediatric emergency department. *Arch Pediatr Adolesc Med.* 2003;157 (11):1090–1096.

13. Mace SE, Barata IA, Cravero JP, et al. Clinical policy: evidence-based approach to pharmacologic agents used in pediatric sedation and analgesia in the emergency department. *Ann Emerg Med.* 2004;44(4):342–350.

14. Holtzman RS, Cullen DJ, Eichorn JH, et al. guidelines for sedation by nonanesthesiologists during diagnostic and therapeutic procedures. The risk management committee of the department of anaesthesia of Harvard medical school. *J Clin Anesth.* 1994;6:265–276.

15. Koenig KL, Lambe S. A model emergency department systematic sedation record. *Acad Emerg Med.* 1997;4(12):1178–1180.

6

Legal and Ethical Issues in Pain Management and Procedural Sedation in the Emergency Department

Sandra H. Johnson

HIGH YIELD FACTS

- Pain drives most patients to seek care in an emergency department (ED).
- Treatment of pain in medicine generally including emergency medicine (EM) has been inadequate with racial and ethnic disparities but this is changing.
- Obstacles to effective ED pain management include financial, educational, cultural, legal, and regulatory concerns.
- There is an ethical and legal duty to treat pain.
- Litigation concerning negligent treatment for pain has occurred.
- Under the Emergency Medical Treatment and Labor Act (EMTALA), pain assessment should be part of the medical screening examination.
- State and federal regulations on the ED may affect the emergency physician's (EP's) treatment of patients in pain.

CONTEXT AND CHALLENGES

It is pain that drives most patients to seek care in an emergency department (ED).[1] Pain is most commonly, and necessarily, viewed as a symptom that guides the physician to a diagnosis of an underlying pathology. Pain management and pain relief should be a priority in emergency medicine (EM).

Pain associated with an emergency condition might be viewed as a temporary, though serious and intense, experience. Studies on the relationship between chronic pain and acute pain episodes indicate that an experience of unrelieved acute pain can make a person vulnerable to a pattern of chronic pain[2,3] or to a repeat pain episode.[4] Studies have indicated that managing pain postsurgically promotes recovery while persons with untreated pain are more likely to experience complications.[5] A patient's experience with painful procedures could lead the patient to delay or avoid necessary medical diagnosis and treatment of a later episode or a new symptom. In fact, the procedure may be more painful the next time it is employed if analgesia was not addressed in the first instance.[4] For some patients with chronic diseases associated with acute episodes of pain, the sole purpose for the visit is pain relief. Although it is important to rule out other conditions that may be causing this particular pain episode, the treatment of the pain itself is the goal of emergency treatment in these cases.

Research on Pain Management in the ED

In the past, the treatment of pain in medicine generally including EM has revealed a pattern of inadequacy.[5–9] Similarly, in EM and medicine in general, there is evidence of disparities in the treatment of patients for pain based on race and ethnicity.[10–13]

There are some areas that show significant improvement and demonstrate the desire and capacity to aggressively treat pain in EM.[14] Acute abdominal pain is now treated during the course of diagnosis in contrast to the prior practice that viewed such intervention as confounding attempts to diagnosis[15–19]; although some evidence indicates that ED physicians still withhold analgesia for acute abdominal pain,[8] illustrating the difficulties in changing embedded professional knowledge.

Obstacles to Effective Pain Management in the ED

Literature on barriers to effective pain management in other areas of medical practice reveal financial restrictions, educational deficiencies, cultural challenges, and legal and regulatory concerns.[20–23] Some of the reasons for undertreatment of pain in the ED mirror those for medical practice generally. For example, some observers and practitioners have identified deficiencies in the educational programs that prepare emergency physicians (EPs).[8,24] Other reasons for neglect of pain in EM are likely to be distinctive. Most of the causes given for the phenomenon in EM emerge from intuition and experience or are extrapolated from the few existing studies.

Effective pain management begins with recognizing pain. Perceptions of the patient and physician as to the degree of pain experienced or expected are often divergent.[25]

Studies indicate that pain assessment is ordinarily a one-time evaluation in the ED and is not performed, or at least not recorded, at important points after the initial assessment.[1] Pain assessment may be particularly difficult when the patient is unable to communicate.[7]

The EP's priority is diagnosis. There has been a belief that analgesia may impede diagnosis in some cases, and that belief has been an obstacle to pain management in the ED. Patients and physicians share a priority for diagnosis and treatment, and may have high expectations for suffering and low demands for analgesia.[25] Where evidence can be produced to reject that hypothesis, the practice of withholding analgesia can change.

Consideration of the culture of the ED, including the nature of the physician-patient relationship in EM and the type of person who is attracted to the specialty, may reveal other reasons for undertreatment of pain.[26] The professional priority for diagnosis may produce a detachment from the suffering of the patient, and this detachment may increase over time as the ED physician and nurse develop a tolerance for suffering as an immutable and relentless characteristic of their environment.[8,11] The personality of individuals attracted to EM may personally discount the seriousness of pain and discomfort both for themselves and their patients.

EM is acutely aware of its role as providers of care to those persons whom everyone else has forgotten or avoids. Although this self-concept motivates EPs to undertake the care of the abandoned as a part of their professional mission, it also speaks of a differentiation or even alienation from the patients served. EM serves patients who are strangers to the care team, and there is some evidence that patients with whom the physician is familiar receive more effective treatment for pain.[27]

Like other physicians, EPs fear being duped by patients who have no medical need for controlled substances for pain relief.[28] This fear leads to heightened distrust of patients' reports of pain, especially when those patients fall within marginalized groups.[8]

ETHICAL DUTIES TO TREAT FOR PAIN

The relief of pain is an essential prerequisite for almost all other human values, to allow the human being to enjoy relationships, to reflect, and to make choices. Although there may be ethical and medical concerns about particular pain management interventions in particular circumstances, the core ethical obligation to relieve pain is not generally disputed. This duty extends to all individuals.

Barriers to effective pain relief are professional, social, educational, financial, and legal, but embedded in these barriers are ethical challenges. Situations where individuals are denied pain relief because of their health status (for example, because they have sickle cell or because they are chemically dependent) or because of stereotypes about a specific population implicate the ethical commitment to relieve pain.

A lack of education and training is often identified as a barrier to effective pain management both in medical practice, generally, and in EM. Advocates work to change this phenomenon as a matter of policy and systems reform, but the lack of education and training also involves a professional obligation: the duty to continue to learn how to treat patients effectively and carefully throughout the course of the physician's or nurse's career.

The concern that EPs have over individuals who may be lying about their symptoms in order to get medically unnecessary drugs also presents an ethical issue. This challenge is faced by all physicians who treat a large number of patients in pain, but is especially acute in the ED where the physician and the patient are usually strangers to one another. The ethical physician is alert to situations like this, but a serious ethical problem arises when the physician becomes hypervigilant or relies on profiling that gives only a general and often inaccurate picture of the drug-seeking patient with the result that many patients in pain are denied necessary care. When race, socioeconomic status, source of pay for care, and related generalities are used to exclude patients from effective treatment, ethical principles of medical practice are violated.

The individual physician takes responsibility for responding to these obstacles in his or her own practice. For example, the individual EP may not be able to change the curriculum for EM training, but can alter [their] practice in response to new learning.

LEGAL ISSUES IN PAIN MANAGEMENT

Legal issues relating to pain management and procedural sedation in the ED emerge from at least three different areas of law. They are (1) malpractice and general tort liability; (2) the federal Emergency Medical Treatment and Labor Act (EMTALA); and (3) state and federal regulation of medical practice, especially as it relates to the prescription of controlled substances.

Malpractice and General Tort Liability

Malpractice and negligence lawsuits are governed by state law, in contrast to EMTALA claims, which are based on federal legislation. The law governing malpractice and negligence litigation varies among the states, but to be successful in any state, plaintiffs must prove that a physician-patient or hospital-patient relationship existed; that the health care provider breached a duty owed to the plaintiff; that the care provided breached applicable standards and amounted to negligence or malpractice; and that this negligence or malpractice caused the plaintiff's injuries.

The Physician-Patient and Hospital-Patient Relationship

A physician's legal duty toward a patient begins when the physician-patient relationship is established. The contract between physician and patient is voluntary, unless the physician has undertaken contractual obligations that require him or her to treat particular patients. In the context of EM, a contractual obligation to treat patients who come to the ED is typically included or implied in the physician's agreement with the physician group that contracts to provide emergency services for the hospital, or in the EP's employment with the hospital, or in the on-call physician's agreement with the hospital, sometimes as part of staff privileges.[29] In the absence of such an agreement, the duty of the doctor to the patient arises when the relationship actually begins, i.e., when the physician agrees to or actually undertakes the care of the patient. The triggering event may be a consultation with or examination of the patient in such cases.

Substantial litigation has also arisen over the issue of whether the hospital has a duty to a patient who has presented at the ED for treatment. Courts have variably relied on several factors to decide whether a hospital-patient relationship has been established. Some courts have relied solely on the fact that the hospital has held itself out publicly as providing emergency services, while others have required that the patient should have been admitted to the ED or have been physically present in the ED for some amount of time.[30] For claims brought under EMTALA, the federal regulations establish the point at which the hospital's duty to treat the patient arises.

Duty to Treat Pain

Physicians have a well established legal duty to treat pain as part of their medical treatment of a patient.[31,32] The doctor's duty to relieve pain is generally supported by policy statements and standards of professional organizations and by the standards enforced by state licensing boards.[33,34] Joint Commission on Accreditation of Healthcare Organizations (JCAHO) standards on the assessment and treatment of pain in the ED also provide support for a legal duty to treat pain effectively.[35] American College of Emergency Physicians (ACEP) has adopted several policies that assert the importance of treating pain.[18,36] The courts rely on policy statements and practice guidelines promulgated by such organizations to establish a legal duty to which physicians and hospitals are held.

Litigation Concerning Negligent Treatment for Pain

Studies of malpractice lawsuits have concluded repeatedly that patients injured through negligence or malpractice generally do not file suit.[37,38] In considering legal risks, efforts to improve pain management may be viewed pragmatically as a method for avoiding litigation, although this conclusion is largely intuitive.

While undertreatment of pain is commonly viewed as an exacerbating factor in malpractice or negligence lawsuits, neglectful pain treatment alone can also form the basis of a malpractice or negligence claim. In *Bergman v. Eden Medical Center* and *Tomlinson v. Bayberry Care Center*,[39] the surviving family members of two patients in California filed suit against the physicians, hospitals, and nursing homes that treated the patients. In *Bergman*, the jury returned a verdict of $1.5 million, which the court reduced to $250,000. In *Tomlinson*, the defendants (the patient's hospital physician, nursing home physician, hospital, and nursing home) entered into voluntary settlements with the plaintiffs, with undisclosed sums paid to the family.

Bergman and *Tomlinson* illustrate that it is possible for patients to bring suit for inadequate pain management in the absence of other negligence or malpractice, but these were extreme cases. In each case, the patient was in the end stages of terminal cancer, was transferred from hospital to nursing home for the final days or weeks of care, received inadequate medication, and the lawsuits were both brought under the state's elder abuse statute. The diagnosis was clear: the standard interventions for pain management were well accepted but were not provided. Treatment for cancer pain and pain at the end of life are areas of treatment for pain where there are strong medical and legal consensus. There is no concern over addiction or diversion, and the state medical boards have long viewed the use of controlled substances for cancer pain, even over a long time and in large doses, as permissible.[40]

The transfer from hospital to nursing home care in each case caused a discontinuity in care with no discharge orders for pain medication from the hospital physician, in at least one of the cases, despite awareness of the patient's medical condition and prognosis.

A terminally ill patient who has been cared for in a nursing home or at home may be brought to the ED when death is imminent. EPs need to be familiar with current practices and standards for effective treatment of pain at the end of life, and hospitals should have a plan to assure that the ED is well prepared to care for or admit these patients.

EPs encounter cases in which a patient who regularly receives care elsewhere for a chronic illness comes to the ED for treatment for an exacerbation of their condition or for an acute pain episode. These situations present continuity of care challenges, as in *Bergman* and *Tomlinson* in part because the EP is not as familiar with the patient as is the patient's own physician. An even more difficult situation occurs when the ED doctor is convinced that patients are receiving inadequate treatment, for pain or otherwise, from their own physician or the facility in which they reside. In such cases, consultation with the patient's doctor may help, serious and detailed information to the patient directly may allow the patient to take action, or admission to the hospital under the care of another attending physician may allow for more thorough assessment and a change in treatment plan.[41]

Both *Bergman* and *Tomlinson* involved inadequate orders for pain medication on discharge. The EP has to be an expert in transfer and discharge planning and assure that adequate medication and follow-up orders, including those required for pain management postdischarge, are provided for the patient.[4] Ongoing pain assessment in the ED is required for both treatment and discharge. The ACEP policy on procedural sedation requires that continuing or developing pain and discomfort be addressed prior to discharge.[36]

Lawsuits claiming neglected pain as the only basis for legal action face several obstacles. Many states have a cap or limit on the amount of damages that can be awarded for pain and suffering. In some states, damages for pain and suffering do not survive the death of the patient and cannot be awarded to surviving family. It is for this latter reason that the plaintiffs in *Bergman* and *Tomlinson* brought their suits under a state elder abuse statute that provided a private right of action for elderly persons and their surviving family. Under this statute, however, the plaintiffs had to prove that the providers had been reckless and not merely negligent. This is a very difficult burden to meet in medical cases, where professional judgment is so often the core of the issue. The statute provided for the payment of attorneys' fees by the defendants to the plaintiff's attorneys, and these fees amounted to approximately $500,000 in the *Bergman* case.

SPECIFIC AREAS OF LEGAL RISK IN PAIN MANAGEMENT IN THE ED

Informed Consent for Pain Management Interventions

All medical care requires the informed consent of the patient, and medical treatment provided without consent is considered battery. A limited exception to the requirement of informed consent exists in emergency situations. The classic statement of the exception for emergency treatment declares that the exception "comes into play when the patient is unconscious or otherwise incapable of consenting, and harm from a failure to treat is imminent and outweighs any harm threatened by the proposed treatment."[42] The exception ordinarily would include treatment for pain in such circumstances.

The emergency exception is actually quite narrow. It certainly does not give the ED *carte blanche* to treat every ED patient without consent. It only applies where the patient's condition is urgent and the time required for consent would put the patient at serious risk of death or severe injury.[43] In the case of the incapacitated patient, the nurse or doctor should secure the consent of a family member or other surrogate where possible without serious harm to the patient.

In litigation alleging emergency treatment without consent, several courts have concluded that consent for emergency treatment is implied by the patient's coming to the ED.[44] This implied consent does not extend to situations where the physician knows that the patient objects to treatment or particular interventions; however,[45] the notion of implied consent should not be relied on too broadly. Quite frequently, an ED patient will sign a general consent form. Even with general consent, the care provider should continue to inform the patient about his or her treatment, and a more specific consent should be sought for any procedure or medication with serious risks. Procedural sedation presents risks of damage to the central nervous system and depression of cardiac and respiratory functions. ACEP policy states that implied consent may be acceptable where the patient is unable to understand the necessary information due to altered mental status or severe pain and anxiety[36], otherwise separate consent to sedation is recommended.[46]

One of the most serious problems regarding informed consent in the ED is the difficulty in ascertaining whether the patient is incapacitated. The stress and duress of an emergency condition, especially one associated with severe pain, may compromise the ability of the patient to consent, but the patient will not be legally incapacitated. The same judgment call is required for patients whose mental state is impaired by abuse of drugs or alcohol. The key components to informed consent are that the patient is able to understand what options exist as well as the consequences of choosing one over another and is able to evaluate the costs and benefits of these consequences by relating them to a framework of values and priorities.[47]

Doctors should not assume that opioid analgesia will incapacitate the patient and should not withhold all pain medication for this reason.[8] In regard to any medication that may impair judgment, alertness, or physical capacity, including pain medication, the physician must inform the patient clearly and accurately of these limitations prior to discharge. The physician should warn the patient specifically if the medication might interfere with driving or other similar activity and document this warning.[48]

Patients may choose among different options, with differing levels of effectiveness and adverse effects, for treatment of pain. Some patients may forego the most effective pain relief if it will compromise other goals.[4] Physicians and nurses need to educate their patients so that the patient does not make this decision based on inaccurate assumptions about the potential for sedation or addiction.

Legal Significance of ED Policies, Protocols, and Guidelines

Hospitals typically have policies, protocols, clinical pathways, and practice guidelines governing treatment in the ED, including treatment for pain management and procedural sedation. The advantage of establishing written policies is that they can contribute to assuring that care in the ED meets the current standards of practice. Both the adequacy and the violation of written policies will be at issue in malpractice or negligence litigation. Professional standards for treatment of pain in all settings are evolving quickly. It is not enough for policies to adopt customary practice in this situation.

Written department or hospital policies are not helpful if they are violated in practice. In fact, violation of the ED's own written standards creates a strong inference of negligence. Nonconformance with hospital policies is not viewed legally as negligence per se, i.e., the plaintiff must prove that the treatment provided violated the appropriate standards of practice and not just the hospital's own policies. Nonconformance with the hospital's own policies and practices, however, can be very persuasive to a jury and on its own provide the legal basis for liability in a claim brought under EMTALA, as discussed further.

Scope of Practice of Nonphysicians

One of the issues that arises is whether nonphysician health care professionals have the authority to administer the treatment. The question of authority arises in two ways: are the professionals authorized to provide the intervention under hospital policy and are they authorized to do so within their scope of practice under state law? The scope of practice of nonphysician health care professionals varies widely among the states. If professionals exceed their statutory scope of practice, it is likely, absent exculpatory circumstances, that this action will be viewed as negligence per se without further proof of the standard of care[49]; however, some states treat this situation only as evidence, but not conclusory evidence, of negligence.

A related but distinct legal issue arises in the context of procedural sedation and other similar interventions. Although the procedure may be within the scope of practice allowed to professionals under state licensure, they must also be competent by virtue of education, training, and experience in performing the procedure. For example, a physician license is not limited to a particular range of medical practice, but not all physicians are competent to perform procedural sedation. ACEP policy asserts that all EPs should be capable and competent in performing procedural sedation and that anesthesiologists are ordinarily not required.[36]

Inadequate Equipment, Staff, or Training

Generally, the hospital may be held liable if the patient's injuries are caused in whole or in part by deficiencies in the physical facilities—equipment, selection, training, and monitoring of staff, including both employees and physicians with privileges—or policies or procedures that fail to meet current standards of practice. In regard to procedural sedation, violation of standards relating to the equipment and the number and level of staff required for safety[36] will be pursued under theories of direct liability. Direct liability also applies to the physician corporation or partnership that contracts to provide emergency medical services within the hospital.

EMERGENCY MEDICAL TREATMENT AND LABOR ACT

The federal EMTALA requires that a hospital receiving Medicare and operating an ED provide to any individual who "comes to" the ED with a request for aid receive an "appropriate medical screening examination . . . to determine whether or not an emergency medical condition exists." If the hospital determines that the individual has *an emergency medical condition*, the hospital must provide medical treatment to stabilize the condition or, alternatively, arrange for transfer through appropriate means if the patient requests transfer or if the physician (or another authorized person) certifies that the *medical benefits* of transfer outweigh the increased risks of transfer.

Pain Assessment and the Appropriate Medical Screening

The courts have consistently held that the EMTALA requirement for an "appropriate medical screening examination" requires no more than that the hospital screen each and every ED patient in the manner of the hospital's usual policy, custom, and practice.[50,51] The courts have refused to apply general professional standards of care to the screening requirement. With the implementation of the JCAHO standards on pain assessment, each accredited hospital should now include assessment for pain within their usual and customary medical screening examination process, making pain assessment an element of the appropriate medical examination required under EMTALA.

Pain and the Emergency Medical Condition

The statute defines *emergency medical condition* as "a medical condition manifesting itself by acute symptoms of sufficient severity (*including severe pain*) such that the absence of immediate medical attention could reasonably be expected to result in" serious harm to the patient. The statute references severe pain, not as an emergency medical condition itself, but rather as a *symptom* of an emergency medical condition. Despite the explicit reference to pain as a symptom of an emergency medical condition and the likelihood that the hospital's customary medical screening includes a pain assessment, it is not clear that EMTALA requires *treatment* for pain.

Stabilization and the Relief of Pain

The statutory definition seems to anticipate that a patient may have the symptom of severe pain—a manifestation of an emergency medical condition—but not actually have an emergency medical condition. The EMTALA treatment requirement is limited to that treatment required to stabilize the patient. Stabilization is defined as providing "such medical treatment of the condition as may be necessary to assure . . . that no material deterioration *of the condition* is likely to result from or occur during [transfer]." Unless pain will result in a material deterioration of the patient's emergency medical condition, treatment for the pain itself is not required under EMTALA.

Although it cannot be said that EMTALA absolutely requires that the ED have the patient's pain managed prior to discharge or transfer, there is one caveat. Under EMTALA, the adequacy of the medical treatment required to stabilize the patient is measured against professional standards of care, not the hospital's own practices. EMTALA incorporates a malpractice standard in reviewing the adequacy of treatment of emergency patients. As medical practice begins to view interventions to relieve pain as essential to minimally adequate care, the emerging standards may infiltrate EMTALA cases either through the malpractice standard for stabilization or because of new understandings and evidence of what constitutes a *material deterioration* of a patient's emergent condition and how unrelieved pain can result in such deterioration. Where the emergency medical condition is mental or emotional, conditions also within the EMTALA obligation, unrelieved pain may be a cause of material deterioration in the patient's medical condition.

STATE AND FEDERAL REGULATION OF PRESCRIBING PRACTICES

Physicians' fear of regulatory scrutiny and intervention on the part of the Drug Enforcement Administration (DEA), the state bureau of narcotics, or the state licensure board has been identified as a substantial barrier to effective pain relief for patients requiring medications that are listed as controlled substances in the schedules of the Federal Controlled Substances Act (CSA)[52] and its state counterparts. The fear of providing controlled substances to patients with no medical need for the drugs also appears to be a substantial fear among ED physicians.[4,8] It is not clear whether the fear on the part of EPs is related to a fear of legal sanctions or a more culturally embedded concern for being tricked by duplicitous individuals posing as patients.

The public policy concerns underlying the CSA and medical discipline for prescribing practices are the risk of addiction and the diversion of certain medications. The public policy challenge in implementing both the CSA and state standards concerning prescribing is to establish restrictions and penalties for the dangerous or reckless prescriber while encouraging the responsible physician to treat pain aggressively.[53]

Certain areas of pain management have been recognized by the regulators as requiring special attention and support. State medical boards have recognized that individuals with cancer pain or pain associated with terminal illness are not at substantial risk of addiction or diverting their medications and are likely to need large amounts of pain medication over what can be a very long period of time.[53] In contrast, the stereotypical setting that draws regulatory scrutiny is the physician's private office that is treating a high volume of chronic pain patients with less than minimal contact with patients or documentation of history, examination, or treatment plan.

It does not appear that EDs are particular targets for regulatory intervention in regard to prescribing controlled substances for pain relief. The private office of a reckless or criminal doctor can provide a number of patients who are addicted or diverting drugs with large volumes of medication over some amount of time, although it should be clear that no data support the notion that private physician office practices are a major source of diverted drugs. EPs have not been targeted by these agencies generally because of the limited risk of high-volume diversion.

The risk of hypervigilance, when EPs become overly concerned with the risk of providing controlled substances to patients who may not require them for relief of pain, is serious. There is often confusion, for example, between drug-seeking and pain relief-seeking behaviors, and this confusion can penalize particular patient groups, such as sickle cell patients.[13] The EP should engage in reasonable practices to assure that prescriptions for controlled substances meet current standards, such as those offered by the Federation of State Medical Boards[34] but adjusted to the practice of EM.

CONCLUSION

Legal, ethical, and professional standards for medical practice are converging on a common ground to set a priority for the effective treatment of pain. Treatment of pain in the ED is an important part of emergency medical practice. Some studies have identified particular areas of difficulty, and more research will follow. As evidence builds to support both the duty to treat pain and more effective techniques for doing so, EM will need to incorporate these developments into practice.

REFERENCES

1. Eder SC, Sloan EP, Todd K. Documentation of ED patient pain by nurses and physicians. *Am J Emerg Med.* 2003;21: 253–257.
2. Katz J. Perioperative predictors of long-term pain following surgery. In: Jensen T, Turner J, Weisenfeld-Hallin Z, eds. *Proceedings of the 8th World Congress on Pain.* Vol 8. Seattle, WA: IASP Press; 1997.
3. Kalso E. Prevention of chronicity. In Jensen T, Turner J, Weisenfeld-Hallin Z, eds. *Proceedings of the 8th World Congress on Pain.* Vol 8. Seattle, WA: IASP Press; 1997.
4. DuCharme J. Acute pain and pain control: state of the art. *Ann Emerg Med.* 2000;35:592–603.
5. Drayer RA, Henderson J, Reidenberg M. Barriers to better pain control in hospitalized patients. *J Pain Symptom Manage.* 1999;17:434–440.
6. Wilson J, Pendleton J. Oligoanalgesia in the emergency department. *Am J Emerg Med.* 1989;7:620–623.
7. Maurice SC, O'Donnell JJ, Beattie TF. Emergency analgesia in the paediatric population. Part I: Current practice and perspectives. *Emerg Med J.* 2002;19:4–7.
8. Rupp T, Delaney KA. Inadequate analgesia in emergency medicine. *Ann Emerg Med.* 2004;43:494–503.
9. Tcherny-Lessenot S, Karwoski-Soulie F, Lamarche-Vadel A, et al. Management and relief of pain in an emergency department from an adult patients' perspective. *J Pain Symptom Manage.* 2003;25:539–546.
10. Todd KH, Samaroo N, Hoffman JR. Ethnicity as a risk factor for inadequate emergency department analgesia. *JAMA.* 1993;269:1537–1539.
11. Todd KH, Deaton C, D'Adamo AP, et al. Ethnicity and analgesia practice. *Ann Emerg Med.* 2000;35:11–16.
12. Green CR, Anderson KO, Baker TA, et al. The unequal burden of pain: confronting racial and ethnic disparities in pain. *Pain Med.* 2003;4:277–294.
13. Bonham VL. Race, ethnicity, and the disparities in pain treatment. *J Law Med Ethics.* 2001;29:52–68.
14. Todd KH. Emergency medicine and pain: a topography of influence. *Ann Emerg Med.* 2004;43:504–506.
15. Pace S, Burke TF. Intravenous morphine for early pain relief in patients with acute abdominal pain. *Acad Emerg Med.* 1996;3:1086–1092.
16. LoVecchio F, Oster N, Sturmann K, et al. The use of analgesics in patients with acute abdominal pain. *J Emerg Med.* 1997; 15:775–779.
17. Kim MK, Strait RT, Sato TT, et al. A randomized clinical trial of analgesia in children with acute abdominal pain. *Acad Emerg Med.* 2002;9:281–287.
18. American College of Emergency Physicians. Clinical policy: critical issues for the initial evaluation and management of patients presenting with chief complaint of non–traumatic acute abdominal pain. *Ann Emerg Med.* 2000;36:406–415.
19. *Evidence Report/Technology Assessment No. 43, Making Health Care Safer: A Critical Analysis of Patient Safety Practices.* Rockville, MD: AHRQ; 2001:396. AHRQ publications 01-E058.
20. Johnson SH, ed. Symposium: appropriate management of pain: addressing the clinical, legal, and regulatory barriers. *J Law Med Ethics.* 1996;24:285. Available in full text at *http://aslme.org/research/painjournals.php*
21. Johnson SH, ed. Symposium: appropriate management of pain: addressing the clinical, legal, and regulatory barriers. *J Law Med Ethics.* 1996;24:285. Available in full text at *http://aslme.org/research/painjournals.php*

22. Johnson SH, ed. Symposium: the undertreatment of pain: legal, regulatory, and research perspectives and solutions. *J Law Med Ethics.* 2001;29:11. Available in full text at *http://aslme.org/research/painjournals.php*

23. Johnson SH, ed. Symposium: improving the treatment for pain: legal, regulatory, and research perspectives. *J Law Med Ethics* 2003;31:15. Available in full text at *http://aslme. org/research/painjournals.php*

24. Jones JB. Assessment of pain management skills in emergency medicine residents: the role of a pain education program. *J Emerg Med.* 1999;17:349–354.

25. Singer AJ, Richman PB, Kowalska A, et al. Comparison of patient and practitioner assessments from commonly performed emergency department procedures. *Ann Emerg Med.* 1999;33:652–658.

26. Sanders AB. Unique aspects of ethics in emergency medicine. In Iserson KV, Sanders AB, Methieu D, eds. *Ethics in Emergency Medicine.* 2nd ed. Tucson, AZ: Galen Press; 1995:7.

27. Tait RC, Chibnall JT. Physician judgments of chronic pain patients. *Soc Sci Med.* 1997;45:1199–1205.

28. Wilsey B, Fishman S, Rose JS, et al. Pain management in the ED. *Am J Emerg Med.* 2004;22:51–57.

29. *Hiser v. Randolph,* 617 P.2d 774 (Ariz. App. 1980). But see, *Miller v. Martig,* 754 N.E.2d 41 (Ind. App. 2001).

30. *Wilmington General Hospital v. Manlove,* 174 A.2d 135 (Del. 1961); *Davis v. Johns Hopkins Hosp.,* 585 A.2d 841 (Md. App. 1991), *affirmed* 622 A.2d 128 (Md. 1993).

31. Furrow BR. Pain management and provider liability: no more excuses. *J Law Med Ethics.* 2001;29:28–51.

32. Rich BA. Physicians' legal duty to relieve suffering. *West J Med.* 2001;175:151–152.

33. 11 BNA Health Law Reporter 1222.

34. Federation of State Medical Boards. *Model Policy for the Use of Controlled Substances for the Treatment of Pain,* 2004. Available in full text at *http://www.fsmb.org*

35. Joint Commission on Accreditation of Healthcare Organizations. *Accreditation Issues of Emergency Departments.* Oakbrook Terrace, IL: Joint Commission Resources; 2003.

36. American College of Emergency Physicians. Clinical policy for procedural sedation and analgesia in the emergency department. *Ann Emerg Med.* 1998;31:663–677.

37. Brennan TA, Leape LL, Laird MM, et al. Incidence of adverse events and negligence in hospitalized patients: results of the Harvard medical practice study. *New Engl J Med.* 1991;324:370–376.

38. Brennan TA, Leape LL, Laird MM, et al. Incidence of adverse events and negligence in hospitalized patients: results of the Harvard medical practice study. *New Engl J Med.* 1991;324:370–376.

39. Tucker KL. Medico-legal case report and commentary: inadequate pain management in the context of terminal cancer. The case of Lester Tomlinson. *Pain Med.* 2004;5: 214–217.

40. Johnson SH, et al. Commentary on medico-legal case report. *Pain Med.* 2004;5:218–228.

41. Frader J. Referral back to an incompetent primary care provider. In Iserson KV, Sanders AB, Methieu D, eds. *Ethics in Emergency Medicine.* 2nd ed. Tucson, AZ: Galen Press; 1995:276.

42. *Canterbury v. Spence,* 464 F.2d 772 (D.C. App. 1972).

43. *Miller v. Rhode Island Hosp.,* 625 A.2d 778 (R.I. 1993); Shine v. Vega, 709 N.E.2d 58 (Mass. 1999).

44. *Wright v. John Hopkins Health System Corp.,* 728 A.2d 166 (Md. 1999).

45. *Anderson v. St. Francis–St. George Hosp.,* 614 N.E.2d 841 (Ohio App. 1992).

46. Blackburn P, Vissers R. Pharmacology of emergency pain management and conscious sedation. *Emerg Med Clin North Am.* 2000;18:76–101.

47. Iserson KV, Sanders AB, Mathieu D. Autonomy and informed consent. In Iserson KV, Sanders AB, Mathieu D, eds. *Ethics in Emergency Medicine.* 2nd ed. Tucson, AZ: Galen Press; 1995;51.

48. *Burroughs v. Magee,* 118 S.W.3d 323 (Tenn. 2003); *McKenzie v. Hawai'i Permanente Medical Group, Inc.,* 47 P.3d 1209 (Hawaii, 2002).

49. *Central Anesthesia Assoc. v. Worthy,* 325 S.E.2d 819 (Ga. App. 1984).

50. General Accounting Office. *EMTALA Implementation and Enforcement Issues.* GAO–01-747; 2001.

51. Access to health care. In: Furrow B, Greaney T, Johnson S, et al, eds. *Health Law Cases, Materials, and Problems.* 5th ed. St. Paul, MN: Thomson West; 2004:528.

52. 21 U.S.C. s 801 *et seq.*

53. Hoffmann D, Tarzian A. Achieving the right balance in oversight of physician opioid prescribing for pain: the role of the state medical boards. *J Law Med Ethics* 2003; 31:21. Available in full text at *http://aslme.org/research/ painjournals.php.*

7

Policies and Procedure

Ashley E. Booth
Steven A. Godwin

HIGH YIELD FACTS

- Emergency physicians treat a very diverse patient population so policies should encompass the varied patient population.
- When developing guidelines, criteria required by the institution's accrediting organizations such as Joint Commission on Accreditation of Healthcare Organizations (JCAHO) should be considered.
- Physicians performing procedural sedation must be competent in airway management and cardiopulmonary resuscitation.
- A screening history and physical examination must be done and documented prior to the procedural sedation.
- Procedural sedation requires enough personnel to provide continuous monitoring of the patient's cardiopulmonary status during and after the sedation.
- Supportive equipment and medications should be present and readily available at all times during procedural sedation and analgesia (PSA).

INTRODUCTION

Emergency physicians are called to provide oversight in their department for procedural sedation in a very diverse patient population. In an effort to maximize patient safety, emergency physicians should provide departmental guidelines that encompass sedation in patients ranging from those severely injured by trauma to pediatric patients requiring sedation prior to imaging. As with all systems, education of all participants is critical to ensuring successful implementation.

This chapter addresses the policies and procedures that guide pain management and procedural sedation in the emergency department. It should be noted, however, that there is little scientific evidence at this time to support or reject many of the policies that are used in procedural sedation. Many policies concerning pain management and procedural sedation have been developed by consensus and are deemed merely guidelines. Guidelines are not intended as standards of care or absolute requirements.[1–5] It must also be noted that individual hospitals and health care institutions are accredited by their respective accrediting organizations such as Joint Commission on Accreditation of Healthcare Organizations (JCAHO) and specific criteria required by these organizations should be considered when developing policy.[6]

DEFINITIONS

The American College of Emergency Physicians defines procedural sedation as the administration of "sedatives or dissociative agents with or without analgesics to induce a state that allows the patient to tolerate unpleasant procedures while maintaining cardiorespiratory function."[1] Procedural sedation, previously referred to as conscious sedation, is a continuum that ranges from minimal sedation or anxiolysis to general anesthesia.[7] Individuals respond differently to sedative and hypnotic agents and, as a result, it is often difficult to predict exactly where on the continuum each patient will fall following administration of a given sedative or hypnotic. In view of potential complications, physicians performing procedural sedation must be competent in airway management and cardiopulmonary resuscitation.[1,4,6]

GENERAL GUIDELINES

Numerous organizations have developed procedural sedation and analgesia (PSA) policies and guidelines in an effort to provide a framework by which patients can be safely managed.[1–4,6] Due to the diverse nature of the emergency department patient population, no policy addresses all patient care scenarios. It is therefore important that individual departments develop guidelines based on sound and safe medical principles.

Candidates for PSA include any patient, regardless of age, who needs pain control or anxiety management for an emergent condition, interventional procedure, or diagnostic study. However, there are some general principles that should be adopted to aid in determining required medication dosing and depth of sedation. Importantly, individual patients at the extremes of age will react differently to sedative agents, and therefore extra vigilance should be taken when administering sedatives and analgesics to these patients. Patients with underlying medical conditions and those with recent central nervous system depressant use may also react differently to certain sedative/hypnotic agents, mandating caution when treating these patients.[1,2]

Only personnel trained in PSA should provide procedural sedation. The person providing procedural sedation must be skilled in administration of pharmacologic agents, monitoring of patients during and after sedation for desired levels of sedation, as well as recognition and management of complications. They must also be able to effectively titrate medications to achieve the desired level of sedation without oversedation.[6] The American College of Emergency Physicians recommends that "procedural sedation and analgesia in the ED be supervised by an emergency physician or other appropriately trained and credentialed specialist."[1] There is no clear scientific evidence as to the number of personnel needed to safely provide PSA. Enough personnel to provide continuous monitoring of the patient's cardiopulmonary status during and after sedation must be present. JCAHO, the American College of Emergency Physicians, and the American Academy of Pediatrics recommends that at least one support personnel be present to continuously monitor the patient and assist in any supportive or resuscitative measures.[1-3,6]

Supportive equipment and medications should be present and readily available at all times during PSA. Although rare, complications such as an allergic reaction, respiratory arrest, cardiopulmonary arrest, or induction of general anesthesia may occur during PSA. Having medications and equipment available on-site to manage complications reduce morbidity and mortality associated with PSA.[1-5] Supportive equipment includes, but is not limited to, oxygen, suction, and airway management equipment for all age ranges for which PSA is performed. Advanced cardiac life support (ACLS) medications must be present and readily accessible during PSA. Reversal medications such as the opioid antagonist naloxone and the benzodiazepine antagonist flumazenil should also be available if these drug classes are used in the PSA.[1,2,4] Supplemental oxygen is recommended if deep sedation is anticipated during PSA, however, there is no evidence to support its routine use. There is no scientific evidence to support intravenous (IV) access as a requirement for patients undergoing procedural sedation. The choice and route of administration of sedative/hypnotic agents should be based on the individual patient's status and needs as determined by the emergency physician.[1,4]

EVALUATION/MONITORING/DOCUMENTATION

All patients should undergo a screening history and physical examination with attention paid to past medical history and prior anesthetic history, medications, allergies, last meal, vital signs, and assessment of the patient's cardiopulmonary status. Patients should also routinely have their airway assessed for potential difficulties with airway management and intubation prior to initiating PSA. There is a lack of scientific evidence as to the extent of evaluation needed before PSA; however, when potential risks are identified, such as a patient with a recognized difficult airway, the need for the emergent procedure as well as the depth of sedation must be reconsidered. Appropriate backup, such as advanced airway equipment and personnel trained in advanced airway management, should be immediately available.[1-4] At present there is no literature to support routine laboratory or radiologic testing. Laboratory testing should be based on an individual's past medical history and the presence of underlying medical problems.[1,4]

There is no scientific evidence to support preprocedural fasting. The time and nature of a patient's last meal must be taken into account when determining the timing of sedation, the specific drugs used, and the target level of sedation. Nevertheless, sedation/analgesia should never be withheld in an emergent or urgent medical condition based on recent food intake alone. The emergency physician must weigh the risk of pulmonary aspiration versus the benefit of PSA on an individual case basis.[1,3,4,6,8-10]

JCAHO requires that informed consent, whether written or verbal depending on the patient's level of acuity, be obtained when patients are competent to understand the risk, benefits, and alternatives to procedural sedation.[6] Often patients presenting to the emergency department are in extreme pain or have significant anxiety secondary to their medical condition. This may limit their ability to understand the options presented to them and informed consent may not feasible; however, it is recommended that the patient or their legal guardian be informed of the risk and complications of procedural sedation, as well as the benefits and alternatives. It is important to document any discussions concerning patient consent in the patient's medical record if the patient or patient's legal guardian is unable to sign an informed consent.[1,2,4]

Patients undergoing procedural sedation must be monitored by direct visualization at all times during and after procedural sedation. Monitoring must include assessment of the patient's level of consciousness and cardiopulmonary status. This monitoring may include, but is not limited to, blood pressure, respiratory rate, heart rate, oxygen saturation, exhaled carbon dioxide, and continuous cardiac rhythm monitoring. Documentation of the monitored parameters must be recorded at regular intervals during procedural sedation.[1,2,4] Some sources recommend documentation of recorded parameters at least every 5 minutes,[3,6] however, there is no scientific evidence as to how frequently parameters need to be recorded.[1,4] Also note that there is no scientific evidence to support that continuous cardiac monitoring has any benefits in patients without underlying heart problems, although many sources recommend continuous monitoring in all patients undergoing PSA.[1,4]

Pulse oximetry is a noninvasive method of continuously monitoring a patient's arterial oxygen saturation and can reliably detect early decreases in saturation, but does not detect decreases in ventilation and thus cannot reliably detect hypercarbia that may precede apnea. There is no clear evidence as to the clinical significance of transient decreases in oxygen saturation; however, continuous pulse oximetry monitoring remains a recommendation during PSA but should not replace clinical monitoring and assessment of a patient's level of consciousness and cardiopulmonary status.[1,3,4] There has been recent literature published regarding the use of capnometry in PSA. Capnometry is a measure of a patient's end-tidal CO_2, thus may detect early decreases in adequacy of ventilation and hypercarbia that are not evident with pulse oximetry monitoring alone. To date there is no clinical evidence to support that the routine use of capnometry has improved outcomes in PSA; however, capnometry is another adjunct that may be used to provide additional information during PSA.[1,4,11,12]

All patients undergoing PSA should be continuously monitored immediately following their procedure. It is during this time period when painful stimuli are removed that patients may become unexpectedly more sedated. Patients may also have prolonged sedation effects secondary to the drugs and dosages used, route of administration (IV, intramuscular [IM], intranasal, rectal, or oral), and the patient's individual pharmacodynamic profile. Level of consciousness, cardiopulmonary status, and vital signs must be monitored and recorded at regular intervals until the patient returns to the presedation baseline. In addition, if any reversal agents such as naloxone or flumazenil were used during PSA, their duration of action must be taken into account.[1-4] "Patients who have not returned to preprocedural baseline status may be discharged under the care of a responsible third party."[1] Although not answered directly in the literature, an important rule of thumb is to ensure that patients who were ambulatory prior to the sedation are able to ambulate with minimal or no support prior to discharge. All patients must be given strict discharge instructions addressing procedural sedation.[1-3]

In conclusion, emergency physicians are uniquely trained in the practice of procedural sedation in the emergency department. Therefore, it is important that emergency physicians are not only actively involved but also provide a leadership role in the policy development for procedural sedation oversight within individual institutions.

REFERENCES

1. American College of Emergency Physicians. Clinical policy: procedural sedation and analgesia in the emergency department. *Ann Emerg Med.* 1998;31:663–677.
2. American Academy of Pediatrics Committee on Drugs. Guidelines for monitoring and management of pediatric patients during and after sedation for diagnostic and therapeutic procedures. *Pediatrics* 1992;89:1110–1115.
3. American Academy of Pediatrics Committee on Drugs. Guidelines for monitoring and management of pediatric patients during and after sedation for diagnostic and therapeutic procedures: addendum. *Pediatrics* 2002;110: 836–838.
4. American Society of Anesthesiologist Task Force on Sedation and Analgesia by a Non-Anesthesiologist. Practice guidelines for sedation and analgesia by a non-anesthesiologists. *Anesthesiology* 2002;96:1004–1017.
5. American College of Emergency Physicians. Clinical policy: evidence-based approach to pharmacologic agents used in pediatric sedation and analgesia in the emergency department. *Ann Emerg Med* 2004;44:342–377.
6. Joint Commission on Accreditation of Healthcare Organizations. *Comprehensive Accreditation Manual for Hospitals, the Official Handbook.* Chicago, IL: JCAHO Publication; 2004.
7. American Society of Anesthesiologist. Continuum of depth of sedation: definition of general anesthesia and levels of sedation/analgesia. Available at *http://www.asahq.org*.
8. American Society of Anesthesiologist Task Force on Preoperative Fasting. Practice guidelines for preoperative fasting and the use of pharmacologic agents to reduce the risk of pulmonary aspiration: application to healthy patients undergoing elective procedures. *Anesthesiology* 1999;90: 896–905.
9. Green SM, Krauss B. Pulmonary aspiration risks during emergency department procedural sedation—an examination of the role of fasting and sedation depth. *Acad Emerg Med.* 2002;9:35–42.
10. Agrawal D, Manzi SF, Gupta R, et al. Preprocedural fasting state and adverse events in children undergoing procedural sedation and analgesia in a pediatric emergency department. *Ann Emerg Med.* 2003;42:636–646.
11. Miner JR, Heegaard W, Plummer D. End-tidal carbon dioxide monitoring during procedural sedation. *Acad Emerg Med.* 2002;9:275–280.
12. McQuillen KK, Steele DW. Capnometry during sedation/ analgesia in the pediatric emergency department. *Pediatr Emerg Care.* 2000;16:401–404.

8

Preprocedural Patient Assessment and Intraprocedural Monitoring

Michael F. Murphy

HIGH YIELD FACTS

- The presedation evaluation ought to evaluate the reserve of the cardiovascular, respiratory, and central nervous systems (CNSs) and answer the following question: How hard will the procedure and the medications to be employed push these systems, and will they tolerate it?
- Select the level of sedation to be sought and titrate slowly to that end point.
- A titratable drug has three features:
  · It is given intravenously (IV).
  · It has a rapid onset and offset.
  · It is so powerful that small doses produce identifiable effects.
- In the face of a patient with compromised vital organ function (e.g., severe chronic obstructive pulmonary disease [COPD] and hypotension), the titration end point may not be a CNS one.
- With the exception of ketamine, caution ought to accompany the use of single non-IV doses of medications to produce moderate and deep sedation.
- In general, use sedative hypnotic drugs to produce sedation and opioids to produce analgesia, not the other way around.

- Evaluate the degree to which the autonomic nervous system is active in each patient, and whether attenuating this activity by medications will permit the patient to sustain viable vital signs.

OVERVIEW

Much like the preoperative evaluation, the evaluation of the patient prior to sedation for a painful procedure is intended to minimize risk and optimize outcome. Thus, the patient under consideration for procedural sedation (PS) must be evaluated for their capacity to withstand the rigors of the procedure, and the effects of the medications to be used for sedation and analgesia. This encounter has the following goals:

- To educate with respect to what is about to occur and obtain consent.
- To obtain pertinent information with respect to:
  - Vital organ system (heart, lungs, and brain) reserve.
  - Existing medications, both licit and illicit, and understand the interplay of these medications in this patient with those to be administered for PS.
  - Medication sensitivities and allergies.
  - Medication elimination pathways.
  - Last meal and aspiration risk.
- To decide what level of sedation (end point) will be sought (light vs. moderate).
- To determine which medications will be employed to achieve the appropriate level of sedation and analgesia (sedative hypnotics, opioids, and dissociative agents).

In order for this to occur, the individual undertaking the PS must appreciate:

- The likely duration of the procedure.
- The amount of pain that will be inflicted by the procedure.
- The degree to which the autonomic nervous system has the capacity to respond.

- The degree to which the cardiovascular system is capable of responding to autonomic nervous system activation (reserve).
- The impact that the administered medications will have on the cardiovascular and respiratory functions of this patient.

In the final analysis, the following risk/benefit analysis ought to occur:

- Will light or moderate sedation suffice in adequately blunting the intensity of the physiologic responses to the degree of stimulation anticipated?
- Will this patient's existing vital organ system reserve (*physiologic reserve*) tolerate the types and doses of medications required to induce the desired level of sedation?
- Will the patient at risk for aspiration (full stomach, reflux) retain protective upper airway reflexes *at all times* during PS?
- Am I capable of detecting (monitoring) and rectifying (skill set) life-threatening complications should they occur?

Even though this is rarely the case, if the answer to any of these questions is *no*, then the case ought to be referred to anesthesia for management.

THE PATIENT

The patient presents with a certain capability with respect to vital organ system performance. Ordinarily, otherwise healthy individuals have more vital organ system reserve than those with coexistent disease. This concept of reserve is crucial to the preprocedural evaluation of the patient. For example, the *disease of ageing* is the loss of vital organ system reserve. This is a major focus of the preprocedural evaluation of the patient.

The question must be asked and answered: will this procedure, the intended PS, or both, place demands on this patient's vital organ systems that are beyond their capacity to respond, i.e., beyond their reserve. An example is the patient with ischemic heart disease and a history of congestive cardiac failure with a dislocated shoulder for reduction. On one hand, one must ensure that sufficient sedation and analgesia is administered to attenuate ischemic stressors. On the other hand, at the same time, ensure that the cardiac depressant actions of the PS medications do not tip the patient into overt heart failure. This assumes that the individual administering the PS has a full understanding of:

1. The patient's functional class with respect to his or her ischemic symptoms. In other words, how much activity does it take to induce angina normally. This gives one some idea of how hard the patient can be *pushed* by the procedure, the PS, or both. This takes on particular significance if with moderate sedation the patient is unable to appreciate or report angina or dyspnea, and emphasizes the crucial role of monitoring. The New York Heart Association (NYHA) Functional Classification (FC) System[1] is often used to describe this degree of reserve for patients with cardiovascular disease, and serves as a surrogate for risk:

   Class I: Patients with cardiac disease but without resulting limitation of physical activity. Ordinary physical activity does not cause undue fatigue, palpitation, dyspnea, or anginal pain.
   Class II: Patients with cardiac disease resulting in slight limitation of physical activity. They are comfortable at rest. Ordinary physical activity results in fatigue, palpitation, dyspnea, or anginal pain.
   Class III: Patients with cardiac disease resulting in marked limitation of physical activity. They are comfortable at rest. Less than ordinary activity causes fatigue, palpitation, dyspnea, or anginal pain.
   Class IV: Patients with cardiac disease resulting in inability to carry on any physical activity without discomfort. Symptoms of heart failure or the anginal syndrome may be present even at rest. If any physical activity is undertaken, discomfort increases.

   These class determinations permit one to characterize the patient with respect to the degree to which cardiovascular disease is present:

   I. No objective evidence of cardiovascular disease.
   II. Objective evidence of minimal cardiovascular disease.
   III. Objective evidence of moderately severe cardiovascular disease.
   IV. Objective evidence of severe cardiovascular disease.

   Patients in the FC III and IV categories must be managed pharmacologically with a high degree of precision, and may require monitoring beyond the capability of the PS location, e.g., arterial lines and multichannel electrocardiography.

2. Though originally intended to reflect the degree of cardiovascular disease, it is a useful construct in describing the functional limitation in patients with any exertionally related disorder such as dyspnea

secondary to underlying pulmonary disease or peripheral vascular disease: The NYHA categories can be distilled to simple language:

NYHA FC I: No symptoms, or symptoms only with maximal exertion.

NYHA FC II: Symptoms with moderate exertion.

NYHA FC III: Symptoms with activities of daily living.

NYHA FC IV: Symptoms at rest.

3. The effects of the various medications to be employed, or that might be employed, on the sympathetic nervous system (SNS), systolic and diastolic cardiac function, ventilation, and so forth.

4. The monitoring modalities and capabilities needed to *discern and warn* when the estimated limits of reserve are being approached.

The pre-PS evaluation is focused on the autonomic nervous system, the cardiovascular system, the respiratory system, and the central nervous system (CNS). It is these systems that will be stressed by the procedure and the PS medications.

The Autonomic Nervous System

Painful procedures induce varying degrees of activation of the autonomic nervous system, most notably the SNS, leading to profound end-organ effects. These normal responses:

- May overtax a patient with underlying cardiovascular disease.

- May lead to undesired CNS effects, particularly in a patient with coexistent brain injury or other intracranial pathology associated with disturbed autoregulation or imperfect control of intracranial pressure (ICP).

The individual undertaking PS ought to have some appreciation as to:

- The degree of SNS activation. Subtle findings such as moderate tachycardia and a narrow pulse pressure may tip one off that the SNS is "turned on." The patient with supramaximal stimulation of the SNS (e.g., incipient shock) will have a pronounced drop in blood pressure (BP) with even tiny doses of opioids and sedative hypnotics, with the possible exception of etomidate. Ketamine may be better tolerated.

- The capacity of the SNS to respond to stimulation. This may be the patient who is already maximally responsive (as described previously) or a patient on

medications that block the end-organ effects (e.g., beta-blockers).

- The threat to end organs in the event an exuberant response is generated.

The Cardiovascular System

The following issues ought to be addressed and documented in the evaluation of the cardiovascular system:

1. *Is there underlying ischemic heart disease; if so:*

   - How is it being managed and how successfully (NYHA FC)?
   - Is it stable, or has it started or worsened over the past 3 months?
   - Are there medications on board that may potentiate the effects of the PS medications (e.g., nitrates, beta blockers, and calcium channel blockers)?

2. *Is there a history of heart failure, and if so how recently?*

   - Systolic or diastolic? If systolic, has the ejection fraction recently been measured?
   - Are there medications on board that may potentiate the effects of the PS medications (e.g., nitrates, beta blockers, and diuretics)?

3. *Does this patient have clinically significant valvular heart disease?*

   - Patients with severe stenotic lesions tend to have a relatively fixed cardiac output and tolerate a fall in systemic vascular resistance poorly (e.g., propofol and midazolam).
   - Patients with regurgitant lesions tolerate tachycardia poorly (e.g., atropine pretreatment with ketamine).

4. *Does this patient have uncontrolled hypertension?*
   - These patients are universally volume depleted and tolerate vasodilators and cardiac depressants poorly.

The Respiratory System

With the exception of patients with Type 2 respiratory failure, elevations in arterial P_{CO_2} are associated with increased minute ventilation. Diseases (e.g., chronic obstructive pulmonary disease [COPD]) and drugs (opioids and sedative hypnotics) blunt this response. The effect of an increasing $PaCO_2$ (produced by inhaling CO_2) on minute ventilation is called a *CO_2 response curve.* Figure 8-1 depicts a normal CO_2 response curve. It should be noted that this curve has a rather steep slope, indicating that rather small increases in $PaCO_2$ result in large increases in minute ventilation. Additionally, the

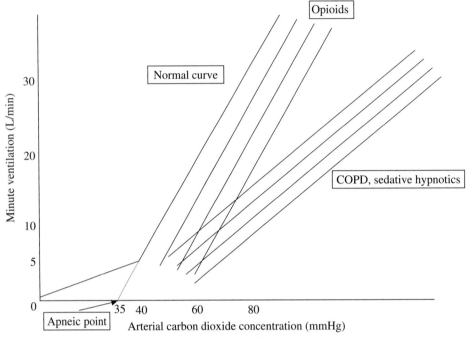

Fig. 8-1. Normal carbon dioxide response curve.

extension of the line to the *x*-axis (extrapolated to the *x*-axis) intersects at the *apneic point*, a point roughly 5 mmHg below the patient's operating $PaCO_2$. The family of curves labeled *opioids* are characteristic of the opioid effect on ventilatory drive. The slope is the same as the normal curve, but shifted progressively more rightward with increasing doses of medication. The family of curves labeled *COPD, sedative hypnotics* are characteristic of patients with a blunted response to inhaled carbon dioxide. This curve is characteristic of patients with COPD. It is also characteristic of sedative hypnotics (e.g., ethanol, midazolam, propofol, etomidate, barbiturates, and chloral hydrate) and anesthetic vapors, in a dose-dependent fashion.

The NYHA FC is a useful model for the evaluation of reserve and for documentation purposes.

It ought to be clear from this discussion that medications used in PS have the potential to induce substantial hypoventilation in patients already on opioids or sedative hypnotics or those with COPD.

The Central Nervous System

It should come as no surprise that patients with compromised cognitive function respond in an exaggerated fashion to CNS depressants. This is manifested by more

sedation with lower doses, longer recovery to alertness, and more postprocedure confusion than their younger and less affected counterparts. The implications with respect to periprocedure mobility, and morbidity, ought to be clear.

The determination of CNS or cognitive reserve is ordinarily gleaned when the history is taken from the patient or from caretakers. A history of prolonged confusion in the past after sedation (e.g., colonoscopy) or general anesthesia is a good indicator of the risk attending the present PS event and the advisability of undertaking it as an outpatient.

Perhaps the most common factor affecting CNS reserve is the presence of coexisting medications, particularly ethanol. The effect of administering sedative hypnotics and opioids to these patients is highly variable and unpredictable, and ought to be approached with the utmost caution and detailed documentation.

Other Areas of Concern

Medication elimination pathways (e.g., hepatic or renal) need to be evaluated, particularly with respect to cumulative dose and anticipated duration of action of the various medications. The last meal and aspiration risk, while important, ought to be of marginal concern in as much as light and moderate sedation are intended to lead to the preservation of airway protected reflexes. It becomes of threshold importance (*go* vs. *no go*) if it is anticipated that the PS will require sedation beyond these end points.

Once one has determined the vital organ system reserve, one is able to decide what level of sedation (end point) will be sought (light vs. moderate), and which medications will be employed to achieve the appropriate level of sedation and analgesia (sedative hypnotics, opioids, and dissociative agents).

ASA PHYSICAL STATUS CLASSIFICATION

The American Society of Anesthesiologists (ASA) Physical Status Classification (Table 1-1) was developed in 1941 with the intent of providing common terminology and to facilitate data collection. The system was modified in 1962 to give us the present format. The ASA Physical Status Classification is intended to grade patients according to *severity of illness* and thus serve as a measure of physiologic reserve. Not surprisingly, it has been demonstrated to be predictive of perioperative mortality.[2] Unfortunately, it has not proven itself to be an accurate measure of anesthetic or operative risk. But then, it was never intended to.

The documentation of the ASA Physical Status, however, is a useful signal that an evaluation of physiologic reserve has taken place. Furthermore, restricting the performance of PS to ASA I and II patients demonstrates some logic as practitioners attempt to limit the risk and maximize the benefits, particularly when potent medications are employed. For example, it has been demonstrated that PS in children who are ASA III and IV is associated with a higher rate of desaturation than those who are ASA I and II.[3]

Table 8-1. ASA Physical Status

Status*	Description
I	Healthy patient
II	Mild systemic disease
III	Severe systemic disease; not incapacitating
IV	Severe systemic disease that is a constant threat to life
V	Moribund; not expected to live 24 hours irrespective of operation

*An *E* added to the status number designates an emergency operation.

MONITORING

To *monitor* means to measure or observe a physiologic parameter either continuously or intermittently. The monitoring device may provide a "snapshot in time" or may detect deterioration, track improvement, or measure the effects of interventions.[4]

Regardless of the sophistication of the equipment, there is no substitute for appropriately trained and experienced personnel in assessing and monitoring the patient undergoing PS. It is specifically recommended that the individual undertaking the procedure and the individual performing the PS, including monitoring, be different individuals.

The following questions are important with respect to monitoring during PS:

1. Which physiologic parameters are important indicators of status or progression?

2. Which technology monitors that parameter?

3. Can the monitoring device be relied on to do so with precision and accuracy in this particular clinical situation? In other words, what are the limitations of the technology?

4. Does the expected standard of care demand a certain level of monitoring?

Line of sight monitoring is ordinarily sufficient for patients undergoing light sedation, provided they are otherwise healthy and remain awake. Monitoring parameters such as clinical observation of color and respiratory action, BP, pulse oximetry, and cardiac monitoring are fundamental monitoring parameters for patients undergoing moderate sedation. The limitations of observation and pulse oximetry in ensuring the adequacy of ventilation during PS have vaulted end-tidal carbon dioxide detection and measurement to a higher profile in PS, albeit an emerging one yet to be widely recommended.

Several organizations have developed recommendations regarding monitoring of patients undergoing moderate sedation.[5–12]

Blood Pressure Monitoring

As in any critical care environment, the importance of the mean BP, the diastolic BP, and the pulse pressure is vital in the patient undergoing PS:

- Cerebral perfusion is dependent on the mean pressure.

- Coronary perfusion is dependent on the diastolic pressure.

- The pulse pressure may reflect systemic vascular resistance and sympathetic tone.

Automatic noninvasive BP measurement has become popular, is widely available, and is recommended during PS. The time interval (and the documentation interval) between measurements is ordinarily 3–5 minutes. In addition to freeing one from repeated manual checks, the advantages of automatic BP readings (depending on the machinery) include a timed repetition of BP measurements, continuous display of the systolic, diastolic, and mean BP, and pulse rate.

The shortcomings of the noninvasive automatic BP technique are those of any cuff measurement technique and usually involve patients with obese arms, uncooperative moving patients, and those with very high or very low BP. Even with these limitations, automatic machines are more accurate, precise, and reliable than auscultation in patients with very low or high BP, primarily because the sensing devices are more sensitive than the human ear.[4]

Pulse Oximetry

The pulse oximeter provides a noninvasive and continuous means of rapidly determining arterial oxygen saturation and its changes, and is the standard of care in patients undergoing moderate sedation. These devices are easy to use and interpret, pose no risk to the patient, and are relatively inexpensive. A reliable interpretation of the information given by these devices requires an appreciation of their limitations in certain situations.

Limitations to the value of pulse oximetry exist with severe vasoconstriction (e.g., shock and hypothermia), excessive movement, synthetic fingernails and nail polish, severe anemia, and the presence of abnormal hemoglobins.[4]

In general, signals are weaker from ears than from fingers, except in hypotension or peripheral vasoconstriction, but ear responses are faster. Nasal bridge probes have been reported to read falsely high.[4]

It must always be remembered that adequate oxygen saturation does not ensure adequate *ventilation*, particularly in patients with decreased levels of consciousness. This explains in part the emergence of end-tidal carbon dioxide as an important monitoring modality in PS.

End-Tidal Carbon Dioxide

CO_2 concentration in exhaled gases is intrinsically linked to tissue metabolism, systemic circulation, and ventilation. Capnography is the graphic record of instantaneous carbon dioxide concentrations (capnogram) in the respired gases during a respiratory cycle. This may be qualitative or quantitative, although typically only the end-tidal ($ETCO_2$) concentration is displayed quantitatively. Capnometry is the measurement and display of CO_2 concentrations on a visual display; again, the usual concentration displayed is the $ETCO_2$.[4]

Capnometers are either sidestream or mainstream in design. Sidestream capnometers work by aspirating a sample of gas through a small catheter into a measuring chamber. The incorporation of a carbon dioxide sampling line into nasal prongs is commercially available and is highly accurate. It is lightweight, reliable, and easily employed during moderate sedation. Disadvantages include plugging by secretions, 2- or 3-second delays in response time, mouth breathing, and air leaks, which can dilute the sample. Mainstream capnometers are useful only in intubated patients, are bulky and heavy, and because they must be heated to prevent condensation, may burn patients.[4]

Colorimetric capnometers, commonly used to confirm endotracheal tube placement are inappropriate for use during moderate sedation. They employ color scales to estimate ranges of $ETCO_2$ but are not accurate enough to give the kind of quantitative measurements necessary during moderate sedation. They use pH-sensitive filter paper impregnated with metacresol purple, which changes color from purple (<4 mmHg CO_2) to tan (4–15 mmHg CO_2) to yellow (>20 mmHg CO_2) depending on the concentration of CO_2, although there is some variability in absolute numbers based on the brand of device.[4] The indicator, housed in a plastic casing, is inserted between an endotracheal tube and the ventilator bag and responds quickly enough to detect changes on a breath-by-breath basis.

Usually, a close correlation exists between $ETCO_2$ and arterial CO_2 partial pressure ($PaCO_2$). In patients who are otherwise normal, the $ETCO_2$ is usually 2–5 mmHg less than the $PaCO_2$ because of the contribution of physiologic dead space to the end-tidal gases. Many conditions that effect ventilation/perfusion ratios can widen the Pa-$ETCO_2$ gradient, including hypotension sometimes seen during moderate sedation. Although the $ETCO_2$ may not always accurately reflect the absolute $PaCO_2$ during moderate sedation, it is still valuable in detecting hypoventilation and sudden airway events, such as apnea.

Cerebral Function Monitors

The titration of medication to a moderate sedation end point is done by clinical observation. This is a highly variable and somewhat inaccurate measure fraught with the risk of overshooting the mark and rendering a patient unable to protect their airway, muster adequate ventilation or maintain BP. Cerebral function monitors have been studied in an attempt to objectify the end point by titrating medication to some composite electroencephalogram (EEG) score as measured and computed by these devices (e.g., bispectral index [BIS]). Most studies have not found these devices to be useful in guiding one to a moderate sedation end point, or in discriminating between mild/moderate sedation and moderate/deep sedation, though they do reliably differentiate sedation from general anesthesia.[13–16]

REFERENCES

1. New York Heart Association. *Nomenclature and Criteria for Diagnosis of Diseases of the Heart and Great Vessels.* 9th ed. Boston, MA: Little, Brown & Co; 1994:253–256.
2. Ross AF, Tinker JH. Anesthesia risk. In: Miller RD, ed. *Anesthesia.* 4th ed. New York: Churchill Livingstone; 1994:791–825.
3. Malviya S, Voepel-Lewis T, Eldevik OP, et al. Sedation and general anaesthesia in children undergoing MRI and CT: adverse events and outcomes. *Br J Anaesth.* 2000;84: 743–748.
4. Murphy MF. Monitoring the emergency patient. In: Marx JA, ed. *Rosen's Emergency Medicine Concepts and Clinical Practice.* 6th ed. NY: Mosby; 2004.
5. Waring JP, Baron TH, Hirota WK, et al. Guidelines for conscious sedation and monitoring during gastrointestinal endoscopy. *Gastrointest Endosc.* 2003;58:317–322.
6. Australasian College for Emergency Medicine, Australian and New Zealand College of Anaesthetists; Faculty of Pain Medicine and Joint Faculty of Intensive Care Medicine. Statement on clinical principles for procedural sedation. *Emerg Med* (Fremantle). 2003;15:205–206.
7. Faigel DO, Baron TH, Goldstein JL, et al. Guidelines for the use of deep sedation and anesthesia for GI endoscopy. *Gastrointest Endosc.* 2002;56:613–617.
8. Hosey MT; UK National Clinical Guidelines in Pediatric Dentistry. UK National Clinical Guidelines in Paediatric Dentistry. Managing anxious children: the use of conscious sedation in paediatric dentistry. *Int J Paediatr Dent.* 2002; 12:359–372.
9. American Society of Anesthesiologists Task Force on Sedation and Analgesia by Non-Anesthesiologists. Practice guidelines for sedation and analgesia by non-anesthesiologists. *Anesthesiology.* 2002;96:1004–1017.
10. Innes G, Murphy M, Nijssen-Jordan C, et al. Procedural sedation and analgesia in the emergency department. Canadian Consensus Guidelines. *J Emerg Med.* 1999;17:145–156.
11. Clinical policy for procedural sedation and analgesia in the emergency department. American College of Emergency Physicians. *Ann Emerg Med.* 1998;31:663–677.
12. American Academy of Pediatrics. Guidelines for monitoring and management of pediatric patients during and after sedation for diagnostic and therapeutic procedures: addendum. *Pediatrics.* 2002;110:836–838.
13. Fatovich DM, Gope M, Paech MJ. A pilot trial of BIS monitoring for procedural sedation in the emergency department. *Emerg Med Australas.* 2004;16:103–107.
14. Gill M, Haycock K, Green SM, et al. Can the bispectral index monitor the sedation adequacy of intubated ED adults? *Am J Emerg Med.* 2004;22:76–82.
15. Singh H. Bispectral index (BIS) monitoring during propofol-induced sedation and anaesthesia. *Eur J Anaesthesiol.* 1999;16:31–36.
16. Gill M, Green SM, Krauss B. A study of the bispectral index monitor during procedural sedation and analgesia in the emergency department. *Ann Emerg Med.* 2003;41:234–241.

9

Postprocedure Evaluation

Alfred D. Sacchetti
Kathleen Hogan

HIGH YIELD FACTS

- Termination of the procedure should precede the cessation of the effect of procedural sedation medications. Traditional teaching has maintained that this time frame may represent the greatest respiratory risk to the patient.
- The same patient monitoring criteria employed during performance of a procedure should be maintained in the immediate postprocedure period.
- Recovery time for drugs such as propofol, etomidate, and remifentanil may be as brief as 5–10 minutes following the completion of a procedure.
- The same postsedation scoring system (e.g., Steward, Aldrete, and postanesthetic discharge scoring system [PADSS]) must be used in all areas of a hospital, i.e., if the postanesthesia care area or endoscopy suite is using one of these scoring systems, then the emergency department (ED) is required to use the same system.
- Cases of children asphyxiating in infant car seats or from snow suits as a result of loss of head control and airway obstruction have been reported following inadequate recovery prior to discharge.
- Persistent effects on motor function are also possible in patients after discharge, particularly with ketamine.

INTRODUCTION

The successful completion of a procedure does not represent the conclusion of a patient's care. Termination of the procedure should precede the cessation of the effect of procedural sedation medications. Patient monitoring will thus continue into the postprocedure period and be governed by the patient's physical assessment parameters, not the status of their procedure.

MONITORING

The same patient monitoring criteria employed during performance of a procedure should be maintained in the immediate postprocedure period.[1-4] Ongoing bedside attendance by a nurse or other appropriately trained clinician is appropriate until a specified degree of recovery has been observed. Painful stimulus during the procedure may offset to some degree the sedation normally seen with opioids or sedatives. Physicians may falsely assume that a patient will remain as alert once that stimulus ends. Instead, once this stimulus is removed, the patient may drift into a deeper state of sedation, increasing the risk of respiratory compromise.[2] This effect is demonstrated repetitively with intoxicated or overdosed emergency department (ED) patients who are subjected to a creative array of noxious stimuli to lighten their state of sedation. Such patients awaken readily with the application of painful stimuli only to return to their depressed status when the stimulus is removed. Further, the longer the time interval between awakening attempts, the greater the stimulus needed to arouse the patient. Similar anecdotal experiences describe deeply sedated patients who nearly awaken with traction on a dislocated shoulder or angulated fracture only to relapse quickly once the painful portion of the procedure is completed.

Ironically, the only study to objectively evaluate this phenomenon failed to demonstrate a significant risk of postprocedure adverse events. In a review of over 1300 procedural sedations in children, 92% of adverse events occurred during the procedure itself, with the median time to occurrence within 2.5 minutes of administration of the sedative medication.[5] In contrast, a review of pediatric sedation-related deaths reported that fatalities occurred following completion of procedures in the out-patient setting while parents were returning home with their child.[6] It is probably prudent therefore to maintain bedside patient monitoring during the immediate postprocedure period.

Once the painful stimulus of a procedure has stopped and the patient is observed to establish an undisturbed level of consciousness, there is little danger for regression back to a deeper degree of sedation. It is safe to design postprocedure observation protocols with gradually lessening bedside nursing attendance corresponding to the observed lightening of a patient's level of sedation.

The specific end point at which it is safe to discontinue intensive bedside patient monitoring has not been clearly identified. Many institutions employ fixed interval monitoring with graded levels of observation determined by time from completion of the procedure. In these models frequent vital signs are performed in the immediate postprocedure period and gradually deceased over time frames of 30–60 minutes. Such protocols make no adjustments for a patient's clinical status and require the same degree of monitoring regardless of the medications employed or level of sedation achieved. Consequently, nursing resources may be unnecessarily tied up monitoring a patient long after the effects of a short-acting sedative have resolved.

With the introduction of nontraditional agents for procedural sedation, the need for extended observation has decreased dramatically. Recovery time for drugs such as propofol, etomidate, or remifentanil may be as brief as 5–10 minutes following completion of a procedure. In these cases, it is more reasonable to use patient-sensitive postprocedure monitoring protocols which adjust the degree and duration of bedside nursing observation with the patient's resolving level of consciousness. Fig. 9-1 presents such a monitoring protocol.

The specific patient parameters followed in the immediate postprocedure period are essentially the same as those during induction of sedation and performance of the procedure. Blood pressure, respiratory rate (RR), heart rate (HR), and pulse oximetry are the most relevant indicators. Most monitoring equipment permits continuous HR and pulse oximetry monitoring, while blood pressure and RR may be recorded at fixed intervals. Some monitoring equipment also permits continuous monitoring of RRs. By convention, charting of all monitored vitals signs is done at the interval selected for the blood pressure observations. Therefore, even though the HR, RR, and pulse oximetry are continuously displayed, they are only recorded on the patient flow sheet at the time the blood pressure is obtained. For patients in whom continuous capnometry is used, monitoring should be documented in the same standardized format.

More important than the measurement of vital signs is the objective assessment of clinical parameters reflective of level of consciousness. A steady improvement toward baseline mental status is the best indicator of the appropriate time to discontinue bedside monitoring. All of a patient's vital signs may be normal with no risk of respiratory compromise, yet a patient may still be confused, and at risk of injury if he or she attempts to climb off a stretcher. For this reason some objective determination of mental capabilities should be incorporated into the

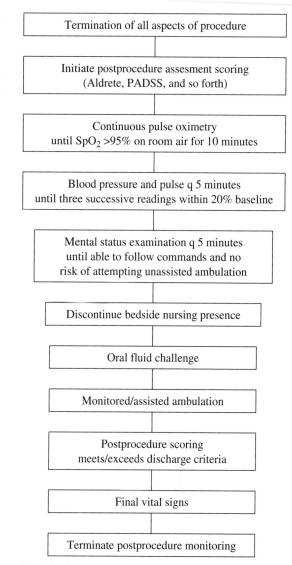

Fig. 9-1. Postprocedure monitoring.

postprocedure observation form even though it may not be included as part of the intraprocedure monitoring.

OBJECTIVE EVALUATION CRITERIA

A number of validated objective scoring systems have been described for patient assessment following same day procedures under general anesthesia.[7–9] Tables 9-1 to 9-3 present three commonly used systems: the Steward, Aldrete, and postanesthetic discharge scoring

Table 9-1. Steward Postanesthetic Recovery Score

Consciousness

Awake	2
Responding to stimuli	1
Not responding	2

Airway

Coughing on command or crying	2
Maintaining good airway	1
Airway requires maintenance	0

Movement

Moving limbs purposefully	2
Nonpurposeful movements	1
Not moving	0

Note: Discharge criteria score 6.

Table 9-2. Aldrete Criteria

Activity

Able to move 4 extremities voluntarily or on command	2
Able to move 2 extremities voluntarily or on command	1
Able to move 0 extremities voluntarily or on command	0

Respiration

Able to cough and deep breathe	2
Dyspnea or limited breathing	1
Apnea	0

Circulation

Systemic blood pressure ±20 mmHg of preanesthetic level	2
Systemic blood pressure ±20–49 mmHg of preanesthetic level	1
Systemic blood pressure ± ≥50 mmHg of preanesthetic level	0

Consciousness

Fully awake	2
Arousal by calling	1
Not responding	0

Oxygen saturation

Able to maintain SpO_2 >92% on room air	2
Need supplemental oxygen to maintain SpO_2 >92%	1
SpO_2 <90% with supplemental oxygen	0

Note: Discharge criteria score 9 or greater.

Table 9-3. Postanesthetic Discharge Scoring System (PADSS)

Vital signs

Within 20% of preoperative value	2
20–40% of preoperative value	1
>40% of preoperative value	0

Activity and mental status

Oriented × 3 and has steady gait	2
Oriented × 3 or has a steady gait	1
Neither	0

Pain, nausea and/or vomiting

Minimal	2
Moderate, having required treatment	1
Neither	0

Surgical bleeding

Minimal	2
Moderate	1
Severe	0

Intake and output

Has had PO fluids and voided	2
Has had PO fluids or voided	1
Neither	0

Note: Score 9 or 10 fit for discharge.

system (PADSS). Although these scoring systems are designed to evaluate patients following general anesthesia, they have been adopted for procedural sedation patients as well. Such an approach is mandated by the Joint Commission on Accreditation of Healthcare Organizations, which requires the same care for similar procedures regardless of the hospital location where they are performed.[10] If the postanesthesia care area or endoscopy suite is using one of these scoring systems, then the ED is required to use the same system.

The point at which a patient is considered stable enough to be left unattended may vary from institution to institution but should include return to baseline mental function, ability to understand and follow verbal commands, and an understanding of the importance of remaining at bed rest. If a reversal agent such as naloxone or flumazenil is used during the procedure, bedside observation should be maintained for the expected duration of action of the reversal drug regardless of the patient's clinical findings. While activity restriction may continue beyond this recovery point, a continuous bedside presence is probably no longer indicated.

DISPOSITION

Eventually, a decision will be made to consider ED discharge or termination of postprocedure monitoring. Again, no standardized criteria have been established for this stage of postrecovery care for ED patients. All postanesthesia scoring systems do have minimum discharge criteria. At a minimum, patients should return to their baseline mental function, baseline ambulatory status taking into consideration any limitations from extremity injuries, and baseline ability to handle food and drink. Table 9-4 lists the minimal criteria considered appropriate for safe discharge. A trial of clear liquids will confirm resolution of any medication-related nausea, while escorted ambulation when possible provides an evaluation of motor function and coordination.

The duration of action of some sedative agents such as chloral hydrate is such that a patient may not return entirely to baseline prior to discharge. For patients receiving these medications, discharge may still be accomplished once they have progressed to a state in which there is no respiratory compromise, ambulation is stable, and they can understand and follow instructions. Most objective scoring systems require this degree of recovery to achieve a minimum discharge score. Cases of children asphyxiating in infant car seats or from snow suits as a result of loss of head control and airway obstruction have been reported following inadequate recovery prior to discharge.[6]

Even after a patient is considered safe for discharge, restrictions on activities may still be appropriate. Some medications may persist with low-level effects even though typical clinical examinations such as Aldrete scores reveal no specific deficits. For these reasons specific postsedation directions should be included in the patient's discharge instructions. Such instructions should

Table 9-4. Minimal Criteria for Consideration for Discharge

Return to baseline mental status
    Capable of understanding events of ED encounter
      and discharge instructions
    or
    If child or underlying cognitive deficits present, the
      patient has responsible adult who understands
      events of ED encounter and discharge instructions
Return to baseline coordination and ambulatory status
    May be compromised by acute extremity problem
Ability to tolerate oral fluids
Ability to contact ED or return should problem arise

Table 9-5. Discharge Instructions

Procedural sedation discharge instructions

Your visit to the ED today required you to be treated with a medicine to care for your pain or allow us to do a procedure on you. That medicine may have included a sedative (sleeping medicine) and/or a narcotic (pain medicine). You may not remember parts of your ED visit, the procedure you had done, or the instructions you were told. This is normal. Most of these effects have worn off but you may continue to have some drowsiness from 6 hours to as long as a day. Because of this, you must be very careful for the next 24 hours and follow the following instructions.

You should have a responsible person watch you for the next 8 hours.

Do not attempt any activity that requires alertness or coordination such as:
    Driving
    Operating heavy or dangerous machinery or tools
    Cooking
    Ironing

You or your child should not attempt any recreational or sports activities such as:
    Swimming
    Bike riding
    Skateboarding
    Swings
    Climbing or monkey bars

Do not drink any alcohol for the next 24 hours.

Your first meal after discharge should be light, e.g., tea and toast and soup.

Do not take medications unless prescribed by the physician especially medicine for pain or sleep.

If the patient is a child, he or she must be watched at all times for the next 16 hours.

Even if they normally play alone, they must be watched.

If the patient is a child, he or she should not be placed into a snowsuit or car seat unless under continuous observation by an adult. The respirations and color must be watched very carefully if the child falls asleep under these circumstances.

Do not make any important decisions over the next 24 hours.

Call or return to the ED with unexpected problems or if not back to usual level activity in 24 hours. If you experience any dizziness, vomiting, passing out, or weakness, call the ED or 911 immediately. Do not stay home with problems!

contain information on both potential cognitive and motor function impairment.[1–6]

Impaired judgment is frequent in those receiving sedative agents or opioid analgesics, and may extend well beyond the therapeutic life of the drug. Although the clinical effects of medications are somewhat known for patient cohorts, the exact duration of these effects on any given patient cannot be precisely predicted. It is considered prudent to caution patients who may have impaired judgment for up to 24 hours following administration of sedative or analgesic agents. For medication such as chloral hydrate, central nervous system (CNS) effects can be detected 72 hours postadministration.

Persistent effects on motor function are also possible in patients after discharge. Predominately manifest as poor coordination, patients should be cautioned to take additional care in navigating potential hazards such as stairs or bathtubs. Children are not immune from these effects. Parents should be advised that children will need closer supervision following discharge. They should refrain from typical high coordination play activities such as bicycle riding or climbing, and should not be left unattended even though they may typically play independently.

Table 9-5 contains sample discharge instructions for the postsedation/analgesic component of a patient's care.

Whenever possible, patients should be discharged into the care of a responsible adult.[1–4] Although frequently quoted, this recommendation originates from the period when the only procedural sedation agents exhibited their effect over hours not minutes. No objective studies have examined the appropriate time to maintain postdischarge observation of patients receiving ultra-short-acting agents such as propofol, etomidate, and remifentanil. Until these data are available, the traditional recommendations on post discharge supervision should be observed.[1–4] Specific discharge instructions for all aspects of the patient's medical care should be reviewed with an individual other than the patient whenever possible.

SUMMARY

Postprocedure care remains an important component of sedation and analgesic management. It remains the final safety evaluation and an opportunity to educate patients or parents on potential problems prior to discharge.

REFERENCES

1. American Academy of Pediatrics. Guidelines for monitoring and management of pediatric patients during and after sedation for diagnostic and therapeutic procedures: addendum. *Pediatrics*. 2002;110:836–838.
2. American Society of Anesthesiologists Task Force on Sedation and Analgesia by Non-Anesthesiologists. Practice guidelines for sedation and analgesia by non-anesthesiologists. *Anesthesiology*. 2002;96:1004–1017.
3. American College of Emergency Physicians. Clinical policy for procedural sedation and analgesia in the emergency department. *Ann Emerg Med*. 1998;31:663–677.
4. Sacchetti AD, Schafermeyer R, Gerardi M, et al. Pediatric analgesia and sedation. *Ann Emerg Med*. 1994;23: 237–250.
5. Newman DH, Azer MM, Pitetti RD, et al. When is a patient safe for discharge after procedural sedation? The timing of adverse effect events in 1367 pediatric procedural sedations. *Ann Emerg Med*. 2003;42:627–635.
6. Cote CJ, Notterman DA, Karl HW, et al. Adverse sedation events in pediatrics: a critical incident analysis of contributing factors. *Pediatrics*. 2000;105:805–814.
7. Chung F, Chan V, Ong D. A post anesthetic discharge scoring system for home readiness after ambulatory surgery. *J Clin Anesth*. 1995;7:500–506.
8. Aldrete JA, Kroulik D. A Postanesthetic recovery score. *Anesth Analg*. 1970;49:924–934.
9. Steward DJ. A simplified scoring system for the post-operative recovery room. *Can Anesth Soc J*. 1975;22:111–113.
10. Joint Commission on Accreditation of Healthcare Organizations. *Comprehensive Accreditation Manual for Hospitals, the Official Handbook*. Chicago, IL: JCAHO Publication; 2003.

10

Evaluation of Pain

Anne-Maree Kelly
Bernie Whitaker

HIGH YIELD FACTS

- Evaluation of pain is complex because pain is an individual experience with physiologic, emotional, cognitive, behavioral, and social dimensions.
- The emergency department (ED) evaluation of pain can be conceptualized as evaluation of pain intensity to guide immediate pain management, establishment of a pain pattern to guide diagnosis, and assessment of other aspects of the impact of pain such as mood and disability that have immediate and ongoing therapeutic implications.
- Health care worker evaluation of pain intensity shows poor agreement with patient self-report of pain intensity. It should only be used when self-report is not possible.
- Language and communication have key roles in pain evaluation and should be optimized.
- Behavioral indicators of pain can be used to assess the presence and severity of pain, but are significantly inferior to self-report.

INTRODUCTION

Evaluation of pain is complex because pain is an individual experience with physiologic, emotional, cognitive, behavioral, and social dimensions (Fig. 10-1). These are integrated into what the patient perceives and reports as pain. For a given potentially painful stimulus, the experience of pain and its severity are not inevitable. Indeed, there will be a range of pain experiences. A good example is labor pain. Some women will report little or no pain during childbirth, while others report "worst imaginable pain."[1] The proportion of women who find labor pain to be severe varies from culture to culture. Other factors identified as contributing negatively to pain experience in childbirth include anxiety, and negative patient expectations while perceived control and confidence in their ability to cope have been found to be associated with a better pain experience.[1,2]

Like other sensorineural inputs such as vision and hearing, pain cannot be explained simply as activation of peripheral pathways that feed up to the brain resulting in pain perception. What actually reaches consciousness as pain is the integration of sensorineural messages and inputs from higher centers. These inputs, including fear, anxiety, understanding of pain, expectations, emotional response, and coping strategies, can modulate what the patient perceives. They may also partially explain the variation in pain reported by patients suffering the same injury or painful condition.[3]

The emergency department (ED) evaluation of pain can be conceptualized as *evaluation* of pain intensity to guide immediate pain management, *establishment* of a pain pattern to guide diagnosis, and *assessment* of other aspects of the impact of pain such as mood and disability that have immediate and ongoing therapeutic implications.

Evaluating Pain Intensity

Pain intensity is a quantification of the severity of pain. Many clinicians believe they can evaluate a patient's pain intensity with minimal interaction with the patient. They report using behavioral and physiologic cues in their evaluation. Both of these are crude and unreliable measures. This partly explains why surrogate pain intensity assessment by nurses, physicians, or parents has been shown to be quite inaccurate when compared to patient self-report.[4-6]

Physiologic changes such as increased heart and respiratory rates and increased blood pressure are measurable autonomic responses that accompany, rather than represent, an individual's response to pain. Moreover, the variation in response between individuals and response to different painful stimuli makes it hard to specify, let alone quantify, a pattern of physiologic responses characteristic of pain.[7] In the ED setting, sympathetically-mediated physiologic changes may be due to anxiety associated with the condition. Complications of the painful condition, for example, blood loss or ventilatory compromise, will also alter these responses, making it impossible to quantify the relative contributions of each to the physiologic parameters observed.

Pain behaviors are actions, both verbal and nonverbal, that communicate pain to others.[8] Unfortunately, there is considerable variability between individuals and situations that also influences these behaviors. Factors such

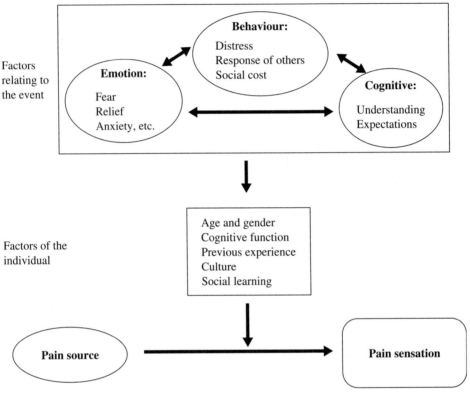

Factors relating to the event

Behaviour:
Distress
Response of others
Social cost

Emotion:
Fear
Relief
Anxiety, etc.

Cognitive:
Understanding
Expectations

Factors of the individual

Age and gender
Cognitive function
Previous experience
Culture
Social learning

Pain source

Pain sensation

Fig. 10-1. A model of the factors that influence pain. (Modified from Turk DC, Melzack R. *Handbook of Pain Assessment.* 2nd ed. New York: Guilford Press; 2001:96.)

as personality traits, cognitive function, and cultural and contextual issues all play a role,[9] contributing to difficulty establishing their reliability and validity.[10] The most important observable pain behavior is facial expression because it is accessible, highly plastic, and rapidly changing.[9] Other observed behaviors associated with pain are protection or limited use of an injured body part, changes in vocalizations, physiologic changes such as pallor, sweating, and muscle tension and withdrawal from usual social functioning. None of these are found consistently. Even expecting social withdrawal may be misleading: many patients with chronic pain make use of distracting measures—such as watching television or talking to others—to decrease their pain perception. Constellations of behavioral observations have been developed into behavioral pain scales primarily used for pain assessment in preverbal and preschool children and the cognitively impaired elderly.

Pain itself is not directly observable. The evaluation of pain by health care workers is further complicated by

personal factors. Clinicians bring their own expectations about how much a given condition "should hurt" to their interaction with the patient, or worse still, fail to make an objective assessment. Clinicians are also coparticipants, rather than simply observers in the pain evaluation process, because of their roles in diagnosis and therapy.[11] These two roles require different, but overlapping, information.

Because of the demonstrated inability of surrogate evaluators (including clinicians) to accurately quantify pain, the most widely accepted method for doing so is by patient self-report. There is a range of methods suitable for use in the ED including verbal rating scales, visual analogue scales, or numerical rating scales. The use and limitations of pain scales are discussed in detail in Chapters 11 and 12.

ESTABLISHING A PAIN PATTERN

The characteristics of pain combined with associated symptoms make up what is known as the pain pattern. Pain patterns are important for guiding investigation and establishing diagnosis. The salient features of a pain pattern include site[s] of pain, radiation, quality/character, severity, duration (including onset and progress), periodicity, aggravating and relieving factors, and associated symptoms. Many conditions are associated with distinct pain patterns. Cardiac ischemia is associated with constant, heavy/pressing, and retrosternal pain radiating to the left arm or jaw and accompanied by sweating, nausea, and vomiting. The pain of bowel obstruction is classically described as severe for a few minutes then abating for several minutes in a recurring pattern associated with abdominal distension, nausea or vomiting, and absolute constipation. The pain of subarachnoid hemorrhage is often described as very sudden, severe ("worst ever") headache reaching a peak pain very quickly that may be associated with loss of consciousness, photophobia, and nausea. There are many others and it is not the aim of this chapter to provide a comprehensive list. It must be remembered, however, that not all patients with a given condition describe the same pain pattern and that not all patients with a given pain pattern have the same illness.

Some of the features of a pain pattern are self-evident (e.g., duration). Pain location and quality are worthy of further discussion, as they are key elements of a pain pattern whose limitations need to be understood.

Location

Perceived location of pain and changes in localization can provide important information about the source of the pain and the underlying pathology. Perceived location will depend on the innervation of the affected structure[s], presence of referred pain, and if pain is associated with complications. Two pertinent examples that illustrate the importance of evaluating the location of pain are appendicitis and myocardial ischemia. In the early stages of appendicitis where the organ is distended but there is no involvement of the parietal peritoneum, pain is poorly localized (usually reported as periumbilical). The involved nerves transmitting pain messages are unmyelinated and cover a large area. When the parietal peritoneum is involved as a result of increased inflammation, pain is more localized (usually to the right iliac fossa) signaling activation of the more discriminating somatic nervous system. The pain of myocardial ischemia is usually reported as retrosternal or epigastric. Pain in the jaw or left arm is also common and is due to the phenomenon of referred pain, where pain is perceived in the cutaneous distribution of a nerve affected by the pathologic process. In this example, the jaw pain is due to referral to the C3 cutaneous distribution while the arm pain is due to referral to the

C4/C5 cutaneous distribution. The same mechanism is responsible for the shoulder tip pain associated with subdiaphragmatic blood or gas.

Pain localization is in part communication dependent, so additional care is required when clinician and patient do not share a common language.

Pain Quality

Pain quality refers to the descriptors used to describe the sensory characteristics of pain such as "dull," "sharp," "like an electric shock," or "pressing." These sensory characteristics are important in differentiating pain patterns associated with pathologic states, but are highly reliant on language. While the English language is rich in pain descriptors, the same is not true of all languages, so a word that translates to sharp in English may actually be more closely aligned with a concept of severity in another language. Cultural factors can also influence the choice of pain descriptors. For these reasons, particular care is necessary in assessing pain quality in patients unable to communicate fluently in a shared language or who are from a different cultural background from the clinician.

While not used in the emergency medicine setting because of their cumbersome nature, there are scales that can be used to formally assess pain quality. They were developed for evaluating patients with chronic pain syndromes and include the sensory scale of the McGill Pain questionnaire and the Neuropathic Pain Scale.[11]

EVALUATING THE IMPACT OF PAIN
The Affective Component

One way of conceptualizing the experience of pain is the pain context model.[11] Four dimensions of pain are considered relevant for evaluation: intensity, quality, location, and affect. The first three of these are readily accepted by clinicians as important and have already been discussed. Although it is recognized that the affective component plays a major role in chronic pain, in particular secondary aspects such as depression, anger, frustration, and anxiety,[11] its role in acute pain is often underappreciated.

Pain affect is the "degree of emotional arousal or change in action readiness caused by the pain experience."[11] Alternatively, it can be thought of as the unpleasantness of pain. It represents the sum of a variety of emotional reactions, the foremost of which is fear. In the ED setting, emotional reactions may be mixed and may also include relief at being safe, expectation of help, and anxiety or depression about long-term outcome.

Statistically, measures of the affective component of pain are distinct from measures of pain intensity, but rarely independent of them.[11] Cognitive factors also play an important part in pain affect, in particular the perceived meaning of this pain in the person's overall context. Provision of information about the cause, treatment, and likely outcome of a painful episode can modify the pain experience by influencing these cognitive factors. Evidence suggests that changing patient's expectations, for example, by explanation or distraction therapy, can alter the experienced unpleasantness of pain without changing its reported intensity.[12]

The affective component of procedure-related pain is likely to be quite different from the affective component when pain is the reason for seeking treatment in the ED. Patient preparation in terms of information, managing expectations, and facilitating coping and control can significantly modify the pain experience associated with procedures. This is well documented with children[13] and is likely to be the case with adults as well.

Pain affect is not often formally measured in emergency medicine practice but can easily be assessed and managed informally. Asking patients about their concerns using questions like "Is there something particular that is worrying you about this pain?" *or* "Is there anything you would like to ask me about your pain?" may elicit fears about dying, having cancer, or not being able to support their family. Even if the news is bad, listening to these fears and responding to them with honest appraisal, information, and support gives the patient better understanding what is happening, facilitates their control of the situation, and assists coping the mechanisms. The approach with children can be more direct because children tend to be more open about what is frightening them. If a health care worker in the ED asks a child "What is the scariest bit about being here/this procedure/what we are doing?," the question itself lets the child know that being frightened is okay but is something that together can be worked through.

Formal measurement of the affective component may be particularly important in chronic pain syndromes. It can be measured using the affective subscale of the McGill Pain Questionnaire, visual analogue, or verbal rating scales with appropriate descriptors or descriptor differential scales.[11]

Evaluating Disability and Impairment

Disability and impairment are related concepts that do not have discrete definitions. As these are often used in assessment for ability to work and compensation, definitions are dependent on the agencies that require them and thus may vary by region or company. In general terms, disability refers to "the inability to perform necessary tasks in an important domain of life."[14] Disability can also be considered to include social functioning outside the workplace and the degree of ability to care for oneself. Impairment, on the other hand, can be defined as "a deviation from normal in a body part or organ and its functionality."[15] Thus evaluation of impairment aims to quantify the medical component of disability. It can be quantified using guides such as *Guides to the Evaluation of the Permanent Impairment* published by the American Medical Association,[15] whose aim is to determine the extent of a patient's impairment and its severity.

Painful conditions pose challenges in assessing disability. A principle underlying the concept of impairment is that it can be objectively quantified. It also assumes that limitations in activities are due to measurable dysfunction of a body part or system. Neither of these is necessarily true for painful conditions. Most impairment guides try to factor pain into impairment ratings, relying on *typical* or *expected* pain levels. As is known, there can be wide variation in pain for a given condition for which the standard impairment rating may not account.

Inevitably, evaluating disability and impairment will incorporate an integration of objective and subjective data. Objective data might include results of investigations such as x-ray, computed tomography (CT), magnetic resonance imaging (MRI), or electromyographic studies. Subjective data might include patient self-report of pain (severity and affective components) and reported restrictions of activity. Semiobjective data such as findings on physical examination might also be included. This integration is not easy as the relative weightings of these components may vary with the type of painful condition, the availability of objective data, and interpersonal issues such as assessment of patient credibility.

This brief discussion of disability and impairment assessment would not be complete without mentioning the ethical issues that can be associated with these assessments. When performing these assessments for a patient with whom one does have a therapeutic relationship, issues such as one's personal attitude toward disability and particular disability types, what one knows about the company/agency for which the assessment is done, and the relative importance one gives to self-report data need to be addressed. For patients with whom one has a therapeutic relationship, the additional issues regarding trust in the doctor-patient relationship and how that evaluation might impact future care arise. Working through these with the patient as appropriate, before a formal evaluation is submitted, is recommended.

SUMMARY

The evaluation of pain is complex and needs to address intensity, pain pattern, and affective and disability components. Whenever possible, patient self-report should be used to assess pain intensity as surrogate evaluations of intensity (including clinicians) have been shown to be inaccurate. Language and communication play key roles in pain assessment and clinicians should aim to do whatever is possible to optimize communication. When effective communication is not possible, behavioral scales may be helpful in assessing the presence and/or severity of pain.

REFERENCES

1. Waldenstrom U, Bergman V, Vasell G. The complexity of labour pain: experience of 278 women. *J Psychosom Obstet Gynaecol.* 1996;17:215–228.
2. Green JM. Expectations and experiences of pain in labour: findings from a large prospective study. *Birth.* 1993; 20:65–72.
3. Mesulam M. From sensation to cognition. *Brain.* 1998; 121:1013–1052.
4. Guru V, Dubinsky I. The patient vs. caregiver perception of acute pain in the emergency department. *J Emerg Med.* 2000;18:7–12.
5. Kelly AM, Powell CV, Williams A. Parent visual analogue scale ratings of children's pain do not reliably reflect pain reported by child. *Pediatr Emerg Care.* 2002;18:159–162.
6. Blomqvist K, Hallberg IR. Pain in older adults living in sheltered accommodation—agreement between older adults and staff. *J Clin Nurs.* 1999;8:159–169.
7. Sternbach R. *Pain: A Psychophysiological Analysis.* New York: Academic Press; 1968.
8. Gagliese L. Assessment of pain in elderly people. In: Turk DC, Melzak R, eds. *Handbook of Pain Assessment.* 2nd ed. New York: Guilford Press; 2001.
9. Craig KD, Prkachin KM, Eckstein-Grunau R. The facial expression of pain. In: Turk DC, Melzak R, eds. *Handbook of Pain Assessment.* 2nd ed. New York: Guilford Press; 2001.
10. Reading AE. Pain measurement and experience. *J Psychosom Res.* 1983;27:415–420.
11. Karoly P, Jensen MP. Self report scales and procedures for assessing pain in adults. In: Turk DC, Melzak R, eds. *Handbook of Pain Assessment.* 2nd ed. New York: Guilford Press; 2001.
12. Price DD, Riley III JL, Wade JB. Psychophysical approaches to measurement of the dimensions and stages of pain. In: Turk DC, Melzak R, eds. *Handbook of Pain Assessment.* 2nd ed. New York: Guilford Press; 2001.
13. Anderson CT, Zeltzer LK, Fanurik D. Procedural pain. In Schechter NL, Berde CB, Yaster M, eds. *Pain in Infants, Children and Adolescents.* Baltimore, MD: Williams & Wilkins; 1993.
14. Robinson JP. Disability evaluation in painful conditions. In Turk DC, Melzak R, eds. *Handbook of Pain Assessment.* 2nd ed. New York: Guilford Press; 2001.
15. American Medical Association. *Guides to the Evaluation of Permanent Impairment.* 5th ed. Chicago, IL: AMA; 2001.

11

Pain Scales

Jacques S. Lee

HIGH YIELD FACTS

- Patient self-report is the most accurate measure of pain severity.
- Pain measurement improves pain management.
- Although pain is a multidimensional experience, existing multidimensional tools may be impractical for use in the emergency department (ED).
- For pain measurement in emergency research, the Visual Analog Scale (VAS) is a valid, reliable scale that exhibits ration-scale properties, allowing the use of parametric statistical analysis.
- The Numeric Rating Scale (NRS) may have advantages for clinical use in the ED.

INTRODUCTION

Challenges in Pain Measurement

Medical science has traditionally relied on objective measurements such as blood pressure or body temperature to quantify patient status. Ideally, pain measurement would also be simple, objective, and standardized. Pain, however, is complex, subjective, and highly individualized. The belief that perturbations in vital signs accurately reflect pain intensity has been disproved. Even relying on something subjective such as behavior to quantify pain severity is problematic, since individual differences in developmental, psychologic, emotional, cultural, and cognitive states modify behavioral expressions of pain. Lacking an objective gold standard for pain measurement, researchers have focused on constructing pain scales, using psychometric techniques developed primarily by psychologists and social scientists. Some physicians, unfamiliar with these methodologies, may be suspicious of the resulting *subjective* scales.[1] Existing pain scales

are based on the assumption that the patient is the most accurate source of information regarding pain intensity. Not all physicians accept this assumption. How else can patients accurately communicate their pain to health care workers?

Why Measure Pain?

Improving pain management is the primary reason to measure pain. No physician would manage hypertension without assessing blood pressure, or diabetes without measuring glucose. Yet pain is often treated based primarily on the physician's subjective impression of the patient's state or response to analgesic therapy. Unfortunately, clinicians consistently underestimate pain severity in comparison to the level reported by patients.[2,3]

Why not ask the patient if the pain has been adequately treated rather than measure pain intensity? This approach may confuse the issues of pain severity and patient acceptance of opioids and other analgesics. Up to 45% of patients believe that a "good" patient would not complain to the health care providers about pain.[4] Many patients and family members are reluctant to accept analgesics due to beliefs that pain is inevitable. They may also be concerned that analgesics may be addictive, unhealthy, or might mask progression of their disease.[4]

In the era of evidence-based medicine, physicians require proof prior to changing practice. Clinical research has documented the positive impact of measuring pain on cancer pain management.[2] Two recent studies have demonstrated that serial use of pain scales improved pain management in the emergency department (ED).[5,6]

WHAT IS PAIN?

Specificity Theory of Pain

To measure pain, it is necessary to first define it. The classic definition of pain as a purely sensory experience was based on the *specificity* theory of pain, first proposed over 200 years ago. According to this model, pain was purely a sensation. Tissue injury stimulates *specific* pain sensors, or *nociceptors*, leading to the transmission of impulses along a dedicated neural pathway to the brain, resulting in the awareness of pain. While the specificity model correctly predicted the existence of sensory nerve pathways before they had been described by anatomists, it also implied that without injury there should be no pain, greater tissue injury should produce greater pain severity, and transection of the specific pain pathway should completely relieve pain.

When clinical observations contradicted this theory, the validity of the observations was questioned. For example, during World War II phantom limb pain among soldiers was attributed to "shell-shock" or malingering; however, it was more difficult to explain the recurrent observation of soldiers in the after-math of a battle who complained of little or no pain despite horrific wounds. These soldiers did not appear to be bearing severe pain stoically; rather, they did not appear to be experiencing pain commensurate with the severity of their injuries. Surgical procedures for chronic pain that interrupted the pain pathway at the level of peripheral nerves, spinal tracts, and the thalamus failed to produce pain relief. Worse, some patients developed new iatrogenic pain syndromes.[7]

Gate-Control Theory of Pain

In 1965, Melzack and Walls developed a new theory to explain mounting evidence that pain perception involved an interactive, rather than the passive "one-way" system described by the specificity theory.[8] Their new gate-control theory proposed a system in which synapses in the spinal cord act like a "gate," controlling how much pain from peripheral nerves is allowed to ascend to the cerebral cortex and consciousness. The degree to which peripheral pain impulses are inhibited or facilitated is influenced by descending impulses from the brain, and are affected by the individual's expectations, emotional state, and previous experience. Although this theory has been updated by new experimental observations,[9] the idea of an interactive or plastic system is now firmly established. Melzack recently commented that "the (gate-control) theory forced the medical and biological sciences to accept the brain as an active system that filters, selects and modulates inputs."[9] Given the highly individual nature of the interaction between noxious stimuli and pain perception, the intensity of a noxious stimulus will be a poor proxy measure for the pain experienced by the patient.[10] Thus, patient self-reports should be used as the best available source of information about pain severity.[11]

Multidimensional Nature of Pain

Fundamental changes in the understanding of the physiologic mechanisms of pain prompted equally fundamental changes in the understanding of the psychologic experience of pain. Rather than being a simple physical sensation that varies in intensity only, Melzack and Casey proposed a new multidimensional model of pain to help explain paradoxical clinical observations. For example,

although patients undergoing frontal lobotomy accurately localized painful stimuli, they rarely complained about pain or requested analgesics. These patients could experience the sensory aspects of pain, but their emotional response to the pain had been blunted, and they did not take action to alleviate pain.

This new model of pain included three dimensions or aspects of the pain experience:

1. The *sensory-discriminative* dimension corresponds to the classic view of pain perception. This dimension is associated with information about the location, intensity, and temporal pattern of pain. Unidimensional scales used in acute pain measure primarily this dimension.

2. The *affective-motivational* dimension is associated with aversion, fear, and other emotional aspects of the pain experience. This dimension has also been called the *unpleasantness* or *suffering* dimension.

3. The *cognitive-evaluative* dimension is associated with an organism's assessment of the significance of painful stimuli and appropriate reaction to pain. This involves interaction of current sensory information, affective dimensions of pain, previous experiences, and higher cognitive functions.

This multidimensional nature of pain is recognized in the International Association of Pain Specialists definition of pain as "an unpleasant sensory and emotional experience associated with actual or potential tissue damage, or described in terms of such damage."

HOW TO MEASURE PAIN

To measure the myriad subjective, multidimensional, and internal experiences of humans, psychologists developed a set of methods called *psychometrics*. Because psychologic experiences can be so subjective, psychometry outlines rigorous methods that allow us to build scales to measure such intangible states as *depression* or *perceived locus of control*. We will briefly review relevant principles of psychometry before describing the strengths and weaknesses of existing pain scales.

PSYCHOMETRICS AND PAIN MEASUREMENT

Properties of scales: A scale can be defined as a progressive system of classification, allowing us to judge relative magnitudes. Ordinal scales are divided into categories of increasing magnitude, but each step is not necessarily equal (e.g., an anger scale ranging from *Calm* to *Irritated* to *'Furious*). In contrast, scales with equal intervals are called *interval scales*. Finally, some interval scales have a meaningful zero point making it is possible to determine the ratio of different measurements on the scale. For example, using the Celsius scale of temperature, air temperature in the summer (30°C) can be said to be double the temperature in the spring (15°C). Parametric statistics should only be applied to ratio and interval scales.

Reliability: Reliability is the ability of a scale to measure something in a reproducible fashion. An automated thermometer that measures widely different temperatures in the same patient minutes apart is likely unreliable, whereas a depression scale that measures similar scores when administered by different users is demonstrating interrater reliability.

Validity: Validity is the ability of a scale to measure what it is intended to measure. For example, a poorly designed automated blood-pressure cuff might be influenced by arm size more than a patient's blood pressure. The machine could be quite reliable, reporting identical blood pressures in patients with similar sized arms. But this measure is invalid—it does not measure what it was designed to. Streiner defines validity as "the degree of confidence we can place in the inferences we draw from scores on a scale."[1] In the absence of a gold standard, it is more difficult to establish the validity of a scale—no single study is likely to do so. Instead, a series of investigations might assess the degree to which the new scale agrees with existing measures (convergent validity), how well the scale predicts expected outcomes (criterion or predictive validity), and how well the scale agrees with the theoretical understanding of what is being measured (construct validity). For example, the validity of a new pain scale might be tested by comparing it to existing scales such as the Visual Analogue Scale (VAS) (convergent validity); however, the motivation for developing a new scale might be dissatisfaction with the existing scale, in which case perfect agreement would be undesirable!

Next, the new scale might be used to measure pain in patients before and after they receive analgesics—a valid scale would be expected to measure the change in pain severity (criterion or predictive validity).

When testing construct validity, you must first specify the theoretical construct you wish to measure. If you accept Melzack's multidimensional construct of pain, you would expect a valid scale to measure both sensory and affective dimensions of pain, and expect the affective dimensions to be more severe in patients with chronic malignant pain compared to patients with superficial lacerations. Once again, the lack of a gold standard complicates issues. Lack of construct validity could mean that the scale is flawed, but it could equally mean that the theoretical construct is wrong! For this reason, it is difficult to state that a scale is valid or not. Instead, validation of a scale should be viewed as an ongoing process, attempting to establish a body of evidence, rather than a dichotomous property.[1]

MULTIDIMENSIONAL PAIN SCALES

McGill Pain Questionnaire (MPQ)

Melzack and Torgerson postulated that the words used to describe pain reflect the underlying multidimensional nature of the experience of pain. In other words, the many pain-associated words in the English language were made necessary to describe the sensory, affective, and evaluative aspects of pain.[12] Unidimensional pain scales, such as the VAS,[13] measure pain intensity or the sensory aspects of pain alone. The MPQ was developed to measure affective and evaluative dimensions as well. The scale was originally derived among a group of healthy university graduates who were asked to group together words from a list of 102 pain descriptors that express similar aspects of the pain experience. The authors selected 78 of 102 words that the subjects most frequently grouped together. This resulted in 16 subgroups which the authors classified into three domains according to their theoretical framework: sensory (10 subgroups), affective (five), and evaluative (one).[14] The authors also included an empirically derived *miscellaneous* domain for four subgroups of words that did not fit into any theoretical group. Study subjects then ranked the words in each of the 20 subgroups in order of severity. For example, the words "sharp, cutting, lacerating" form the *incisive pressure* category, listed from least to most severe. A score of one is assigned for the lowest ranking word, sharp, and three is assigned for choosing *lacerating*. The MPQ is administered by reading the word list to patients, and asking them to choose only those words that describe their pain at present. Pain scores are calculated by summing the rank scores for each category. The sensory pain rating index (PRI) consists of 42 words in 10 subcategories for a range of 0–42. The affective PRI ranges from 0 to 14, the evaluative PRI ranges from 0 to 5, and the miscellaneous PRI ranges from 0 to 17. An overall score can be obtained by summing all four indices to obtain a total ranging from 0 to 78.

Reliability and Validity of McGill Pain Questionnaire

The MPQ has been demonstrated to be reliable in terms of test-retest, alternate versions reliability, and standardized stimulus reliability. Establishing the validity of a measurement tool is more difficult, as the methods used to do so are more controversial. Several authors have tested the validity of the MPQ by showing that similar word groupings are chosen by subjects from different cultural and linguistic groups.[15] The MPQ has been shown to be responsive to analgesic therapies, and seems to be able to discriminate between specific types of pain. In a study of 120 patients, 87% with an identifiable etiology for their back pain used a distinct pattern of words from the MPQ compared with patients with no known cause for their pain. Similarly, in a study of 53 patients with facial pain, specific word-choice patterns on the MPQ allowed correct classification of patients ultimately diagnosed with trigeminal neuralgia (91%) versus atypical pain. This classification performance was validated in a subsequent, independent patient sample.[16]

Application of McGill Pain Questionnaire in Emergency Medicine

Melzack himself was interested in the feasibility of using the MPQ in the ED, and in 1982 studied 138 patients with acute pain.[17] Agitated, intoxicated, or incoherent patients were excluded, as were those with life-threatening injuries. The majority of patients presented with acute injuries (lacerations, 30%; fractures, 20%; sprains, 18%; and bruises, 17%). Significantly, only 82 patients (59%) were able to complete the questionnaire due to time constraints of their treatment in the ED. In its original form, the MPQ was reported to take 15 min to administer and score; however, among elderly cancer patients, the mean time to completion was 24 min.[18] Such a time requirement creates a significant barrier to implementation in the ED setting, and may explain the paucity of ED-based pain studies reporting the MPQ. A literature search using the terms Emergency and McGill revealed that since Melzack's original ED study in 1982, there have been only four studies of emergency patients who used the MPQ.

Short-Form McGill Pain Questionnaire

In view of these shortcomings, a short form of the MPQ (SF-MPQ), which could be completed in 2–5 minutes, was developed for use in acute-care medicine. Only words from the original MPQ that at least 33% of patients had used were included in the SF-MPQ.[19] This yielded 15 words, 11 terms from the sensory domain and 4 from the affective domain. Patients were asked to rate how each of the 15 words applies to their current pain on the following scale: none, mild, moderate, and severe. Both long and short forms of the MPQ were administered to hospitalized patients before and after analgesics. Both forms of the scale were sensitive to analgesic administration and showed high degrees of correlation (coefficient 0.77–0.93).[19] There has been little psychometric analysis of the SF-MPQ to date, with only three studies documenting its use in an acute-care setting.

Other Multidimensional Scales

Multidimensional Affect and Pain Survey (MAPS)

Clarke attempted to revise the MPQ, using a cluster-analysis technique to empirically determine the number of pain dimensions found in the English language, rather than grouping words according to a predetermined theoretical construct.[20] Clark started with a list of 270 English words, including the words used to derive the MPQ, plus more descriptors of emotional states. Healthy volunteers then rated the similarity of different word pairs. Highly correlated words were eliminated as redundant. Next, the remaining pain descriptors were rated for similarity by healthy volunteers from three ethnic groups (African American, Caucasian, and Latino). Pain descriptors that were not used consistently by ethnic or gender groups were also eliminated leaving 101 pain terms. These words were found to cluster into three dimensions: sensory, emotional, and well being. Patients were asked to respond to 101 sentences using a 6-point Likert scale.

The sensation/ pain is	INTENSE	(0 not at all; 5 very much so)
The sensation/ pain is	SPREADING	(0 not at all; 5 very much so)
I feel	DEPRESSED	(0 not at all; 5 very much so)
I feel	ANGRY	(0 not at all; 5 very much so)

While the MAPS has been used in a research setting to assess postoperative pain among cancer patients,[21] the length of this scale limits its potential use in the ED setting.

Brief Pain Inventory (BPI)

The Brief Pain Inventory was designed to be a self-administered survey to measure the prevalence and severity of pain in a large cohort of cancer patients. The authors wanted a brief scale that captured relevant sensory and affective information similar to the MPQ, as well as additional data on pain-associated disability.[22] The BPI includes nine questions: (1) previous history of pain; (2) location of pain, drawn on a body diagram; (3) an 11-point Numeric Rating Scale (NRS) for severity at its worst; (4) least; (5) average; (6) current pain; (7) analgesics used; (8) amount of relief due to analgesics (in percentage); and (9) pain interference with general activity, mood, walking, interpersonal relations, sleep, and enjoyment of life.

Unlike other multidimensional scales, the length of the BPI does not prohibit its potential use in the ED. The reliability and validity of the BPI have been established in cancer and other chronic pain populations.[23] It has not been evaluated in the ED. Postoperative patients and primary care patients with arthritis and low-back pain are the most similar groups studied to date.[23,24] Because of its relative ease of use and multidimensional properties, the BPI is potentially promising for use in ED-based research.

SCALES IN SELECTED PATIENT POPULATIONS

Behavioral Scales

Behavioral pain scales have been developed for use in patients who are unable to communicate their pain severity due to verbal, cognitive, or other barriers, and will be covered in this chapter. The use of pain scales in pediatric populations will be covered in Chapter 12 and geriatric populations in Chapter 44.

Uni versus Multidimensional Scales

Several authors have documented the problems of measuring the pain experience with unidimensional scales. When asked to rate pain severity on a unidimensional scale, one-third of cancer patients expressed primarily the emotional/affective component of pain, one-third expressed primarily the sensory/intensity component, and one-third expressed an average of the two,[25] and yet, unidimensional scales dominate emergency medical research and clinical use. Apart from the poor feasibility of using multidimensional scales in the ED, there is a question regarding the importance of emotional/affective dimensions of pain in the acute-care setting.

In acute pain, several studies have reported significantly decreased affective dimension scores when compared with chronic pain.[17,26] A meta-analysis of 3624 subjects in 51 studies that reported MPQ scores found that the affective dimension scores in chronic pain patients ranged from 30 to 100% of the maximum, while in acute pain, affective scores ranged from 11 to 19%.[27] While factor analyses have tended to support the three-dimensional model in chronic pain, the sensory factor seems to dominate in acute pain.

Putting aside these highly theoretical arguments, we return to two studies that have examined the actual impact of pain scales on pain management in the ED. Despite using unidimensional scales, both studies demonstrated a positive impact on patient care. These findings imply that use of a unidimensional pain scale is superior to not measuring pain. Emergency physicians should not be blind to the potential complexity underlying a patient's report of pain severity on a unidimensional scale.

Unidimensional Pain Scales

Visual Analog Scale (VAS)

The VAS is one of the most commonly used pain measurement tools in emergency-based research, and has been used to measure other psychologic phenomena such as anxiety and depression. Typically, the VAS consists of a 10-cm line bounded at each end by perpendicular stops and descriptors (Fig. 11-1).[28] Patients are asked to place a mark on the line to indicate their pain severity. Pain intensity is determined by measuring the distance from the lower end of the scale to the mark made by the patient. Many variations have been created; however, not all are equivalent. Horizontal lines are preferred, because scores tend to be more normally distributed. Similarly, placing adjectival descriptors or intermediate marks along the line creates artificial clustering of pain severity scores.[29] Descriptors vary as well. In Western culture, the lower bound of pain severity (typically *no pain*) is placed to the left of the vertical stop, and the upper bound (*worst pain ever* or *unbearable pain*) is placed to the right. Slide ruler version of the VAS, or pain *visual analog thermometers* have been developed to increase the ease of use and scoring.[30]

Reliability and Validity of Visual Analogue Scale

The VAS scores have been shown to be reliable measures of pain severity.[31,32] The VAS is responsive to pain therapies among inpatients as well as ED patients.[33] Other evidence of the validity of the VAS is its high correlation with verbal and numeric rating scores,[34] as well as reasonable correlation with the MPQ in acute pain.[35] One distinct advantage of the VAS is that it exhibits the properties of a ratio scale, i.e., a reduction of 4 cm represents twice the

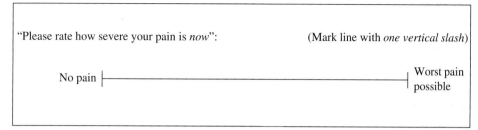

Fig. 11-1. The Visual Analog Scale of pain severity.

decrease in pain severity as a reduction of 2 cm.[36] An important result of the ratio properties of the VAS is that it allows the direct comparison of VAS pain scores at different points in time as well as among different patient populations.

Clinical versus Statistical Significance

Given the ease of use, reliability, validity, and ratio properties of the VAS, it is not surprising that it has enjoyed extensive use. Another unfortunate reason for the popularity of the VAS may be that, when analyzed as a continuous measure, small changes in the VAS may be statistically significant. But are such small differences clinically meaningful? Should patients use a new analgesic because it produces a 5-mm reduction in pain severity more than existing medications? Previous authors have attempted to define the minimum clinically important difference (MCID) by measuring the mean change in VAS that correlates with either patient or physician perception of "a little less pain." Using this method, several studies have reported the MCID to be between 13 and 19 mm.[37–39] This definition for MCID corresponds to the smallest difference that is reliably detectable; however, the minimal detectable difference may not be the ideal standard against which to test new therapies in pain research, given the existence of effective and safe analgesics. Another approach to defining the MCID recently proposed is to measure the mean change in VAS corresponding to a patient's perception of adequate analgesia. The MCID for the VAS using this definition was 30 mm, or a 30% reduction in initial pain scores. This 30-mm reduction in pain severity on the VAS may also be a useful clinical end point for analgesic therapy.[40]

Problems of the Visual Analogue Scale

Despite its apparent simplicity, not all subjects understand the concept underlying the VAS as a graphic representation of pain severity. Approximately 7–11% of adults and up to 25% of the aged are unable to complete it.[31,41] Due to its unidimensional nature, the VAS may not be as sensitive to therapies that alter the affective component of pain. This is particularly important in chronic pain.[42] A 1995 study compared the VAS to the MPQ in postoperative patients given two different doses of analgesics. They found that although the VAS was less sensitive and showed a smaller reduction in pain severity compared with the MPQ, this did not change the conclusion that the higher dose of medication provided the most pain relief.[43]

The Numeric Rating Scale (NRS)

Another rapid and simple pain severity score is the NRS. Patients are asked to rate their current pain severity from a scale of 0 to 10 or 0 to 100. Reliability and validity of the NRS has been established in a manner similar to the VAS.[41,43] Patients prefer the NRS to the VAS, and only 2–4% fail to complete it, compared to 11–19% for the VAS.[41] In a recent study, emergency patients with acute pain were interviewed over the telephone 1 and 7 days after discharge and asked to recall their pain severity on both forms of the NRS. Patient recall of their initial pain score recorded in the ED was excellent, with correlations of 0.96–0.98. Ratio properties of the NRS have not been established. The 0–10 NRS has been found to be less sensitive to therapy than a VAS when used to measure chronic back pain.[44]

Verbal Rating Scales (VRS)

Verbal descriptor scales are among the simplest and most intuitive pain scales. The patient is asked to choose from a list of words that describes increasingly intense pain. One commonly used set is "None…Mild…Moderate… Severe," although many variations exist. VRS have been validated in adult and pediatric patient populations. They are favored by older patients. Verbal scales that use a

Table 11-1. Descriptor Differential Scale

Low Intensity	Low Affect	Medium Intensity	Medium Affect	High Intensity	High Affect
Faint	Slightly unpleasant	Mild	Slightly distressing	Strong	Slightly intolerable
Very weak	Slightly annoying	Barely strong	Very unpleasant	Intense	Very distressing
Very mild	Unpleasant	Moderate	Distressing	Very intense	Intolerable
Weak	Annoying	Slightly intense	Very annoying	Extremely intense	Very intolerable

small number of words (four or five) are the most popular for ease of use, but may not be sensitive to significant changes in pain severity after treatment.[45] Because of variable interpretation of the meaning of descriptor words, there may be more interindividual variability with VRS. The difference between *none* and *mild* is not necessarily the same as between *moderate* and *severe*). Gracely and Doctor carefully tested a series of 12 words to form a VDS with none of these limitations, known as the Descriptor Differential Scales of Pain Intensity (DDS-I) and Affect (DDS-A) (see Table 11-1).

The Descriptor Differential Scales of Pain Intensity (DDS-I) and Affect (DDS-A)

The descriptor differential scales of pain consist of two VRS developed specifically to have ratio-scaling properties.[46] Patients rate the intensity or unpleasantness of their pain relative to 12 pain descriptors on a line with 21 boxes similar to a VAS, with the descriptor word at the center of the line (e.g., "Indicate if your pain is more intense, the same intensity, or less intense than 'mild' pain"). The DDS has been shown to be reliable and sensitive to very small changes in experimental pain intensity. The validity of the DDS has been tested using cross-modal matching techniques, where patients matched the pain intensity suggested by a particular word to grip strength or the length of a line. While the intensity and affect DDS were designed to be used together, most studies have used the DDS-I by itself. The total 24 items have said to take 5–10 minutes to complete. Further study is needed to assess the performance of the scale in acute pain patients, and its acceptability to ED patients and staff.

CHOOSING AN IDEAL PAIN SCALE

The criteria for evaluating pain scales have been proposed by pain researchers. An ideal pain scale for use in emergency medicine should (1) be simple to use in the ED setting; (2) be reliable and valid; (3) be responsive to changes in pain intensity; (4) be free of bias (work the same in mild and severe pain); (5) be useful for both clinical and research settings; (6) assess affective and sensory aspects; (7) have ratio-scale properties; and (8) generalize to different patient populations. Users must prioritize conflicting criteria to determine the most appropriate scale for them. For example, clinicians have traditionally emphasized ease of use over statistical properties, and chronic pain researchers emphasize the importance of multidimensional properties. Table 11-2 shows a detailed comparison of several pain measurement scales.

CONCLUSION

The choice of which measuring tool to use for pain is certainly not as important as the decision to incorporate pain measurement into clinical practice. There are few areas in medicine where we initiate therapy without a specified end point. Yet, analgesics are prescribed routinely in the ED without measuring the initial pain severity, beyond recognizing its presence. Similarly, the effectiveness of analgesic therapy is not routinely verified prior to discharge. Assessment after discharge is almost unheard of.[47] The first property of an ideal measurement tool, ease of use, may need to take priority until pain measurement is more firmly established in emergency medicine. As discussed, there are strong theoretical arguments for the use of multidimensional pain scales in the assessment of pain. The fact that only four emergency-based publications have used multidimensional pain scales, compared with over 150 publications reporting unidimensional pain scales, suggests that existing multidimensional pain scales are impractical for use in the ED.

Further research should replicate the positive impact of pain measurement on patient care, examine methods of promoting pain measurement in the ED, and develop an easy-to-use, valid, reliable, and responsive ED pain measurement scale that is multidimensional.

Table 11-2. Comparison of Pain Measurement Scales

Scale	Ease of Use	Reliability?	Validity	Dimensions	Pros	Cons
MPQ	Poor	Good	Good	Sensory Affective Evaluative	Multidimensional Discriminates cause of pain	Statistical analysis? Not feasible in ED
SF-MPQ	Moderate	Good	Good	Sensory Affective	Multidimensional	Still lengthy
MAPS	Poor	Good	Excellent	Sensory Emotional Well being	Multidimensional Chronic pain	Not feasible in ED
BPI	Moderate	Good	Good	Sensory Emotional Disability	Multidimensional Feasible Assesses pain disability	Generalizes to acute pain?
DDS-I DDS-A	Moderate	Good	Excellent	Sensory Affective	Uni or Multidimensional Ratio scale	Never tested in ED
VAS	Good	Good	Good	Sensory	Ease of use Ratio scale Parametric stats	Unidimensional Requires paper Difficult for elders
NRS	Excellent	Good	Fair	Sensory	Ease of use Clinical use	Unidimensional
VDS	Excellent	Good	Fair	Sensory	Easiest to use	Poor responsiveness

REFERENCES

1. Streiner D. Basic concepts. In: Streiner D, RN N, eds. *Health Measurement Scales. A Practical Guide to Their Development and Use.* 2nd ed. Oxford: Oxford University Press; 1995: 4–14.

2. Cleeland CS, Gonin R, Hatfield AK, et al. Pain and its treatment in outpatients with metastatic cancer. *N Engl J Med.* 1994;330(9):592–596.

3. Lee JS, Stiell IG, Shapiro S, et al. Physicians' attitudes toward opioid analgesic use in acute abdominal pain. *Acad Emerg Med.* 1996;3(5):299.

4. Ward SE, Goldberg N, Miller-McCauley V, et al. Patient-related barriers to management of cancer pain. *Pain.* 1993;52(3):319–324.

5. Silka PA, Roth MM, Moreno G, et al. Pain scores improve analgesic administration patterns for trauma patients in the emergency department. *Acad Emerg Med.* 2004;11(3): 264–270.

6. Thomas SH, Andruszkiewicz LM. Ongoing visual analog score display improves emergency department pain care. *J Emerg Med.* 2004;26(4):389–394.

7. Tasker RR. History of lesioning for pain. *Stereotact Funct Neurosurg.* 2001;77(1–4):163–165.

8. Melzack R, Wall PD. Pain mechanisms: a new theory. *Science.* 1965;150(699):971–979.

9. Melzack R. From the gate to the neuromatrix. *Pain.* 1999;suppl 6:S121–S126.

10. Lee JS. Pain measurement: understanding existing tools and their application in the emergency department. *Emerg Med* (Fremantle). 2001;13(3):279–287.

11. Reading A. Testing pain mechanisms in persons in pain. In: Melzack PWR, ed. *Textbook of Pain.* New York: Churchill-Livingston; 1989:269–280.

12. Melzack R, Torgerson WS. On the language of pain. *Anesthesiology.* 1971;34(1):50–59.

13. Huskisson EC. Measurement of pain. *Lancet.* 1974;2(7889): 1127–1131.

14. Katz J, Melzack R. Measurement of pain. *Surg Clin North Am.* 1999;79(2):231–252.

15. Reading AE, Everitt BS, Sledmere CM. The McGill Pain Questionnaire: a replication of its construction. *Br J Clin Psychol.* 1982;21(pt 4):339–349.

16. Melzack R, Terrence C, Fromm G, et al. Trigeminal neuralgia and atypical facial pain: use of the McGill Pain Questionnaire for discrimination and diagnosis. *Pain.* 1986;27(3):297–302.

17. Melzack R, Wall PD, Ty TC. Acute pain in an emergency clinic: latency of onset and descriptor patterns related to different injuries. *Pain.* 1982;14(1):33–43.

18. McGuire D. Assessment of pain in cancer inpatients using the McGill Pain Questionnaire. *Oncol Nurs Forum.* 1984;11(6):32–37.

19. Melzack R. The short–form McGill Pain Questionnaire. *Pain.* 1987;30(2):191–197.

20. Clark WC, Kuhl JP, Keohan ML, et al. Factor analysis validates the cluster structure of the dendrogram underlying the Multidimensional Affect and Pain Survey (MAPS) and challenges the a priori classification of the descriptors in the McGill Pain Questionnaire (MPQ). *Pain.* 2003;106(3): 357–363.

21. Yang JC, Clark WC, Tsui SL, et al. Preoperative Multidimensional Affect and Pain Survey (MAPS) scores predict postcolectomy analgesia requirement. *Clin J Pain.* 2000; 16(4):314–320.

22. Daut RL, Cleeland CS, Flanery RC. Development of the Wisconsin Brief Pain Questionnaire to assess pain in cancer and other diseases. *Pain.* 1983;17(2):197–210.

23. Keller S, Bann CM, Dodd SL, et al. Validity of the brief pain inventory for use in documenting the outcomes of patients with noncancer pain. *Clin J Pain.* 2004;20(5):309–318.

24. Zalon ML. Comparison of pain measures in surgical patients. *J Nurs Meas.* 1999;7(2):135–152.

25. Knotkova H, Crawford Clark W, Mokrejs P, et al. What do ratings on unidimensional pain and emotion scales really mean? A Multidimensional Affect and Pain Survey (MAPS) analysis of cancer patient responses. *J Pain Symptom Manage.* 2004;28(1):19–27.

26. Reading AE. A comparison of the McGill Pain Questionnaire in chronic and acute pain. *Pain.* 1982;13(2):185–192.

27. Wilkie DJ, Savedra MC, Holzemer WL, et al. Use of the McGill Pain Questionnaire to measure pain: a meta-analysis. *Nurs Res.* 1990;39(1):36–41.

28. Scott J, Huskisson EC. Graphic representation of pain. *Pain.* 1976;2(2):175–84.

29. Husskisson E. Visual analogue scales. In: Melzack RC, ed. *Pain Measurement and Assessment.* New York: Raven; 1983:33–40.

30. Price DD, Bush FM, Long S, et al. A comparison of pain measurement characteristics of mechanical visual analogue and simple numerical rating scales. *Pain.* 1994;56(2): 217–226.

31. McCormack HM, Horne DJ, Sheather S. Clinical applications of visual analogue scales: a critical review. *Psychol Med.* 1988;18(4):1007–1019.

32. Bijur PE, Silver W, Gallagher EJ. Reliability of the Visual Analog Scale for Measurement of Acute Pain. *Acad Emerg Med.* 2001;8(12):1153–1157.

33. Wood V, Christianson J, Innes G, et al. Titrated intravenous meperidine vs. single dose ketorolac in acute renal colic: a randomized clinical trial. *Can J Emerg Med.* 2000; 2:83–89.

34. DeLoach LJ, Higgins MS, Caplan AB, et al. The visual analog scale in the immediate postoperative period: intra-subject variability and correlation with a numeric scale. *Anesth Analg.* 1998;86(1):102–106.

35. Reading AE. A comparison of pain rating scales. *J Psychosom Res.* 1980;24(3–4):119–124.

36. Price DD, McGrath PA, Rafii A, et al. The validation of visual analogue scales as ratio scale measures for chronic and experimental pain. *Pain.* 1983;17(1):45–56.

37. Wells GA, Tugwell P, Kraag GR, et al. Minimum important difference between patients with rheumatoid arthritis: the patient's perspective. *J Rheumatol.* 1993;20(3):557–560.

38. Todd KH, Funk JP. The minimum clinically important difference in physician-assigned visual analog pain scores. *Acad Emerg Med.* 1996;3(2):142–146.

39. Stahmer SA, Shofer FS, Marino A, et al. Do quantitative changes in pain intensity correlate with pain relief and satisfaction? *Acad Emerg Med.* 1998;5(9):851–857.

40. Lee JS, Hobden E, Stiell IG, et al. Clinically important change in the visual analog scale after adequate pain control. *Acad Emerg Med.* 2003;10(10):1128–1130.

41. Kremer E, Atkinson JH, Ignelzi RJ. Measurement of pain: patient preference does not confound pain measurement. *Pain.* 1981;10(2):241–248.

42. Williams ACdC, Davies HT, Chadury Y. Simple pain rating scales hide complex idiosyncratic meanings. *Pain.* 2000; 85(3):457–463.

43. Jenkinson C, Carroll D, Egerton M, et al. Comparison of the sensitivity to change of long and short form pain measures. *Qual Life Res.* 1995;4(4):353–357.

44. Turner JA. Comparison of group progressive-relaxation training and cognitive-behavioral group therapy for chronic low back pain. *J Consult Clin Psychol.* 1982;50(5): 757–765.

45. Jensen MP, Turner JA, Romano JM. What is the maximum number of levels needed in pain intensity measurement? *Pain.* 1994;58(3):387–392.

46. Gracely RH, Kwilosz DM. The descriptor differential scale: applying psychophysical principles to clinical pain assessment. *Pain.* 1988;35(3):279–288.

47. Sivilotti ML, Paris PM, Cantees K, et al. Studying emergency patients outside the emergency department. *Ann Emerg Med.* 1996;27(4):442–447.

12

Pain Assessment and Pain Scales for Pediatric Patients

Sharon E. Mace

HIGH YIELD FACTS

- Pain can be measured in infants and young children as well as in patients with special health care needs, the illiterate, and those speaking another language.
- Patient self-report pain scales can be used in older children and adolescents.
- Pain scales for infants and young children are based on physiologic and behavioral measures.
- QUEST is a pain assessment strategy for pediatric patients.

PAIN ASSESSMENT STRATEGIES IN PEDIATRIC PATIENTS

There are several assessment strategies that have been developed for interviewing patients and their families in order to obtain information regarding their pain. One approach, frequently used for adolescents and adults, is *PQRST*.[1] The P is for what precipitates or provokes and what palliates the pain, Q is for the quality of the pain, R is for the region or location of the pain and radiation of the pain, S is for severity and associated symptoms, and T is for the time course of the pain.[1]

Another strategy for approaching pain in children is QUEST.[2] Q is to question the child and have them describe and locate their pain. Young children and toddlers can generally indicate the location of their pain by pointing to where it hurts. When questioning the child, age/developmental/culturally appropriate terms should be used. The parents or caregivers can relate what words (whether "ouch," "booboo," "owie," "hurt") the child uses and will recognize.

U is to use a pain rating scale that is based on the child's age and developmental level. Do they have abstract reasoning, understand numbers, or the ability to differentiate faces or pictures of people?

E is to evaluate behavior and the physiologic responses to pain especially in infants and nonverbal toddlers or the developmentally delayed.

S is to secure the parents/caregivers' involvement. They know their child and can recognize when the child is in pain. They should also be involved in the medical decision making and care of the child as part of a family-centered care approach.

T means take the cause of the pain into account. Awareness of the etiology of pain and any impending procedures allows for better management of the pain. T is also for taking action using all the appropriate therapeutic options and doing an ongoing assessment of the pain.

MEASUREMENTS OF PAIN IN PEDIATRIC PATIENTS

Of the various measures of pain and pain scales that have been developed, multidimensional (vs. unidimensional) pain scales are generally preferred and patient self-report is considered the most accurate measure of pain severity. The use of such pain scales and self-reporting may not be possible in many patient populations: patients who speak another language, the illiterate, the special needs patient including the developmentally delayed or emotionally disturbed patient, and/or the pediatric patient. Although such patients may not be able to quantify or express their pain by written/graphic or verbal measures, they do experience pain and deserve adequate treatment of their pain. Furthermore, when health care providers or parents estimate pain in a patient or their child, both groups tend to underestimate the severity of the child's pain.[3–6] Inadequate treatment of pain can have negative short and long-term consequences (see Chap. 30).[7–10]

For pediatric patients, measures or scales for pain assessment need to be tailored to the patient's age group and stage of development (Table 12-1). Pain assessment in infants is inferred from behavioral responses (for example, crying and facial expressions) and physiologic parameters (such as vital signs).[10] Simplified pictorial pain scales (such as faces scale) or numerical scales (e.g., hurt thermometer; Fig. 12-1) can be used to obtain a subjective measure of pain in toddlers and young children. Use of such scales must be age specific and developmentally appropriate in that the child must be able to master the task. Use of a numeric scale implies that the child has mastered the abstract concept of numbers. Drawing a picture and/or location of their pain necessitates basic muscle coordination as well as comprehension.

Table 12-1. Pain Scales for Pediatric Patients Based on Age and Development

Newborn/infants
Behavioral or combined behavioral and physiologic
  pain scales
  Premature Infant Pain Profile (PIPP)
  Crying, Requires O_2, Increased Vital Signs,
    Expressions, Sleeplessness (CRIES)
  Pain Assessment Inventory for Neonates (PAIN)
  Neonatal Facial Coding System (NFCS)
  Neonatal Infant Pain Scale (NIPS)
  Nursing Assessment of Pain Intensity (NAPI)
  Infant Pain Behavior Rating Scale (IPBRS)
  Riley Infant Pain Scale (RIPS)
  Facial, Legs, Arms, Cry, Consolability (FLACC)
  Modified Behavioral Pain Scale (MBPS)

Toddlers/preschoolers
Behavioral Pain Scales
  Children's Hospital of Eastern Ontario
    Pain Scale (CHEOPS)
  Face, Legs, Activity, Cry, Consolability (FLACC)
  Child Facial Coding System (CFCS)
Combined Behavioral and Physiologic Pain Scales
  Objective Pain Score (OPS)
Faces/Picture Pain Scales
  Faces
  Oucher
  Bieri
Self-representation
  Drawings

Numeric (analog) Pain Scales
  Poker Chip Tool
  Glasses Tool
  Pain Thermometer (Pain Ladder)
  Numeric Rating Scales

School age
Faces/Picture Pain Scales
  Faces
  Facial Affective Scale (FAS)
  Oucher
  Bieri
Self-Representation
  Drawings
Behavioral and Physiologic Combined Pain Scales
  Objective Pain Score (OPS)
Numeric (Analog) Pain Scales
  Numeric Rating Scales (NRS)
  Verbal Numeric Scales (VNS)
  Word Graphic Numeric Scales (WGNS)
  Color Analog Scales (CAS)
  Visual Analog Scale (VAS)

Adolescents
  Numeric (Analog) Rating Scales (NRS)
  Verbal Numeric Scales (VNS)
  Word Graphic Numeric Scales (WGNS)
  Visual Analog Scale (VAS)

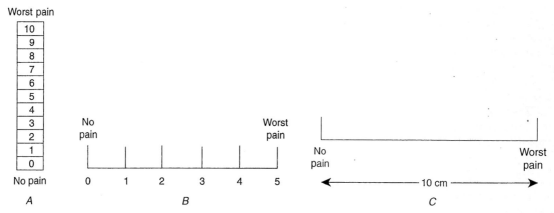

Fig. 12-1. *A.* Pain thermometer. *B.* Numeric rating scale. *C.* Visual analog scale. (Reprinted with permission from Johnston MN, Liebelt EL. Acute pain management and procedural sedation in children. In: Tintinalli JE, Kelen GD, Stapczynski JS, eds. *Emergency Medicine: A Comprehensive Study Guide.* 6th ed. New York: McGraw-Hill; 2004:858–869.)

The gate-control theory of pain by Melzack and Wall has three components of the pain experience: (1) sensory-discriminative, (2) affective-motivational, and (3) evaluative-cognitive.[11,12] Using a unidimensional scale, such as a pain thermometer, the young child may be able to give information about the severity of the pain, but will be unable to express the emotional (*affective-motivational*) dimension. Furthermore, at what age does it become possible to assess the significance of pain and the appropriate reaction to pain (the cognitive-evaluative dimension)?[13]

What is the impact of psychologic, cultural, developmental, and other factors on pain assessment? For example, what effect does peer pressure or self-image have on a teenager's self-report of their pain? Children may minimize their pain because of fear that they may undergo additional painful procedures (for example, parenteral medications), while other children may exaggerate the severity of their pain in order to "guarantee" treatment.[14] Past adverse reactions to medications or pain therapy may lead children to refuse pain medications or underreport their pain severity.

Is there an attention-seeking component? Or conversely, denial in order to please a parent or caregiver? Depressed or withdrawn children may not demonstrate the usual behaviors associated with pain. Whether based on cultural or familial expectations or other reasons, stoic children may not show the expected reactions associated with pain. The child's coping style and temperament, as well as the family's expectation, will all modify the behavioral response to pain. The patient's past experience with pain and similar situations in the past may affect the response to pain.

There are multiple difficulties using self-report scales in pediatric patients. Young children may not be able to verbalize or express their feelings or may not even understand the question. They may be influenced by who is the questioner: the parent/caregiver or the health care provider.[13] The answer may differ, depending on who does the asking.[4] Children may try to please the parent or be so anxious/frightened of the physician that they may not give a valid and reliable answer. The format of the question, whether a checklist or an open ended, may influence the patient response.[15]

TYPES OF PAIN SCALES

In spite of all these variables, evaluation of pain in pediatric patients is possible. Tools for pain assessment in pediatric patients can be grouped into two categories: subjective or self-report and objective which includes behavioral observations and physiologic measures.

Subjective (Self-Report) Pain Scales for Adolescents and Adults

The most frequently used pain assessment tools depend on patient self-report and use only a single dimension (unidimensional) scale.[16] There are many types of self-report scales. Self-report scales can be divided into numeric, word, or picture/faces scales. Numeric scales can be used in patients who have abstract reasoning with a concept of the relative magnitude of numbers. In general these numeric scales can be used in children over 8 years of age and adults.

Verbal descriptor scales use a standard group of words, usually 5–7, that describe the pain severity.[16] The scale should have end points, specifically, no pain (usually denoted 0) to unbearable or worst pain possible.[17] The *five-point global scale* is a verbal descriptor scale. Pain ranges from 0 = none, 1 = a little, 2 = some, 3 = a lot, and 4 = worst possible, with the patient selecting 0, 1, 2, 3, or 4.[18]

The verbal quantitative scale is commonly used in emergency departments. Patients are asked to grade their pain on a 1–10 scale with 0 being no pain and 10 being "the worst pain possible."[16]

The typical numeric rating scale (NRS) consists of a range of numbers with one end point being no pain (represented by zero) and unbearable pain or worst pain possible at the other end.[19] A scale from 0 to 10 is most frequently used, although 0 to 100 has also been used. Patients choose the number that represents the severity of their pain. The 11-point box scale is another single dimension numeric scale.[16] The numbers 0–10 are placed in equal-sized individual boxes. The patient marks the box that represents his or her pain.

Use of these numeric scales implies that the patient has abstract reasoning with the ability to comprehend the concept of numbers and the manual dexterity to mark with a pencil or move a slide rule cursor.

The most common of the numeric scales is the visual analog scale (VAS). The VAS is a horizontal 10 cm line with no pain on the left margin (0 cm mark) and worst pain imaginable or unbearable pain at the right margin (10 cm mark).[16] The patient marks on the line between no pain and worst pain imaginable where the pain is. The distance between the left margin (or no pain mark) to the patient's mark is measured. The VAS can be designed as a 10 cm long slide rule with patients moving the cursor along the slide rule until they reach the point that represents their pain. The other side of the slide rule is marked on a 10 mm scale so patients' pain can be quantified or given a specific number. There is also a 101-point numeric scale going from 0 to 100 where the patient writes down the number between 0 and 100 that represents their pain.

The advantages of these various numeric scales are (1) easy to administer, (2) take very little time, (3) can be done at the patient's bedside, (4) do not need a lot of equipment, (5) require no special training, and (6) are simple to use and record. They can also be used for serial observations or to note changes with therapy. One additional advantage of the VAS is that it yields data that lends itself to parametric analysis. Both the NRS and the visual acuity scale have been validated for reliability and validity as measures of pain intensity. Certain patient populations, specifically cognitively impaired patients and geriatric patients, find it easier to use the numeric scale.[19] Thus, the NRSs are preferred over the visual acuity scales.[19]

Subjective (Self-Report) Pain Scales for School Age Children

Modification of the analog scales can be used in children (about 4 years of age or older) but not in young toddlers or cognitively impaired individuals. One type of analog scale is a graded color scale where the increasing intensity of red color on the horizontal ruler indicates more pain.[13] An analog chromatic continuous scale (ACCS), also called a color analogue scale (CAS), can be used in children over 4 years of age.[13,20,21] This is a horizontal ruler or slide rule with variation in the color red from low to high intensity. An increasing intensity of red color indicates increasing pain. The child can mark on the ruler or adjust the position of the slide rule to indicate the severity of their pain. The CAS can be designed to change in color, width, and length, all to indicate different pain severity.

PAIN ASSESSMENT IN TODDLERS AND YOUNG CHILDREN (AGES 3–7 YEARS)

Toddlers and young children ages 3 to 7 years are developing their speech so they can generally communicate that they are having pain and may even be able to indicate pain severity. They may be able to say ouch, boo-boo, or hurt to indicate pain although they still may not have mastered abstract reasoning and the concept of pain or numbers. Therefore, they are unable to use the standard numerical scales (for example, the VAS) but they can use other means to indicate pain severity from drawings to picture/face scales.

Subjective (Self-Report) Pain Scales for Toddlers and Young Children (Ages 3–7 Years): Numeric Scales

Vertical pain ladders or vertical pain thermometers or blocks are types of analog scales for use in the younger

child or toddler that are adapted from the prototype VAS. The pain ladder or pain thermometer is a numeric single dimension scale that can be used in children over 4 years of age assuming they can count and can grasp the magnitude of numbers.[8] The child places his or her mark on the pain ladder or pain thermometer to indicate the intensity of the pain.[8]

The *poker chip* pain assessment scale uses red plastic poker chips to represent "pieces of hurt."[22,23] The scale goes from one poker chip representing "a little bit of hurt" to four poker chips indicating "a lot of hurt." The child picks the number of poker chips that represents his or her hurt. Another analog pain scale is the *glasses scale*.[22,23] With this scale there are five glasses "filled with pain." The fifth glass is entirely full and the first glass is empty. The child picks the glass that represents the pain.[24] Advantages of these numeric types of pain scales over the faces scales are that multiple photographs or pictures of children representing the various pain intensities are not needed, and it avoids the cultural perceptions associated with some of the faces scales.[10,25]

Subjective Pain Assessment by Self-Representation (Diagrams for Pain Assessment)

Tools for self-report of pain in this age group (≥4 years old) are the use of drawings, pictorial scales using faces or pictures/photos of children, or modified analog scales. Young children who have the manual dexterity to use crayons can be asked to draw a picture of their pain.[26] The location, severity, and type of pain can be inferred from their drawing.

Another method gives the child a printed figure of a body and has the child fill in the body area that contains the hurt[27] with different colors that indicate various pain severity. This pain assessment tool requires the child to have some cognitive development and manual dexterity. It is generally used in children aged ≥6 years.

Subjective Pain Assessment by Picture or Face Pain Scales

The Wong-Baker, Oucher, Bieri, and McGrath scales are all examples of pictorial scales.[28–33] With the *picture* scales, children compare their pain to line drawings of faces or to photos (or pictures) of children.[2–33] The advantages of the pictorial scales are that they can be used in toddlers and younger children. Problems with the faces scale include that selection of the no pain face (whether smiling or neutral) alters the response and cultural effects. Children are influenced by the ethnicity of the child's picture. Race-appropriate versions are available to avoid cultural limitations. One of the scales (e.g., Oucher pain scale) has a Hispanic version.[34] Picture or face scales can also be used in cognitively impaired adults, those who speak another language, or the illiterate.[25]

PAIN ASSESSMENT IN INFANTS AND PREVERBAL CHILDREN

Infants and preverbal children are unable to communicate their pain via linguistic means, so objective (non-self-report) assessment is necessary. Behavioral and physiologic responses are used to assess pain.[7–9,35] Common behavioral responses that are considered to indicate pain are crying, facial expression, and body movements (e.g., withdrawal of the extremities and clenching of the fists in infants). There are some difficulties in using behavioral and physiologic responses for pain assessment. In infants and very young children, behavioral responses such as crying or facial grimacing may be due to fear, anxiety, stress, or illness as well as pain.[36] Behavioral responses to pain can also be affected by many other factors. Some of the variables include the individual's previous painful experience, the environment (including the behavior of others in the environment especially parents or caregivers), cultural influences, and whether the pain is acute or chronic.[35–37] Children with chronic, inadequately relieved pain may react by becoming quiet and withdrawn, which may mislead caregivers or health care providers to conclude that they are not in pain.[35] When their

pain is adequately treated, these children become more alert and interactive.[35] Children with chronic pain may cope or overly compensate by playing normally and engaging in their usual activities.[35] This coping or compensatory behavior may mislead others into thinking children are not in pain.[35]

Many of the pain scales for infants are based on the neonate's typical reaction to pain (Fig. 12-2). The face of a neonate in pain shows the following: eye squeeze, brow bulge, nasolabial furrow, open lips, vertical stretch mouth, pursed lips, taut tongue, and chin quiver.[38,39] Body movements exhibited by infants/children in acute pain include withdrawal or immobility of the painful body part, pulling on the ears (young child), or clenching the fist (neonate).

Physiologic changes that occur with pain include vital sign changes (tachycardia, tachypnea, elevated blood pressure, and decreased oxygen saturation), autonomic signs (pupil dilatation, sweating, flushing, or pallor), nausea, and muscle tension. Physiologic signs of pain like behavioral signs are nonspecific. Physiologic signs can be affected by illness or disease from infections to hypoxia and by medications, all factors not directly related to pain.[36]

Objective (Non-Self-Report) Pain Scales for Infants/Toddlers

Many pain assessment tools for infants and preverbal children are based on a combination of behavioral observations and physiologic parameters.

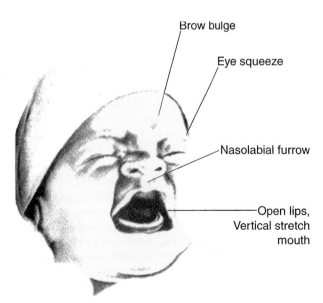

Brow bulge

Eye squeeze

Nasolabial furrow

Open lips, Vertical stretch mouth

Fig. 12-2. Neonate's facial reaction to painful stimulus. (Reprinted with permission from Grunau RVE, Craig KD. Facial activity as a measure of neonatal pain expression. *Adv Pain Res Ther* 1990;15:147.)

Objective (Non-Self-Report) Pain Scales for Infants

The Premature Infant Pain Profile (PIPP) is a pain scale for premature infants based on gestational age that uses behavioral observations and physiologic criteria to assess pain.[40] The physiologic criteria used are heart rate increase per minute and oxygen saturation decrease. The behavioral observation parameters are activity level (from active/awake to quiet/asleep), behavioral state (eyes open or closed), facial movements (yes or no), brow bulge (none, minimum, moderate, or maximum), and eye squeeze (none, minimum, moderate, or maximum). Each indicator, whether gestational age, physiologic variable, or behavioral parameter is scored 0, 1, 2, or 3. All the indicators are summed to derive the total score.

The CRIES (crying, requires O_2, increased vital signs, expressions, and sleepless) also uses behavioral observation plus physiologic measures for pain assessment.[41] There are five parameters, two physiologic and three behavioral. The two physiologic variables are oxygen, required to maintain saturation >95%, and increased vital signs (e.g., heart rate and blood pressure). The three behavioral parameters are crying, expression, and sleeplessness. Each variable receives a score of 0, 1, or 2 and the total score ranges from 0 to 10.

The Neonatal Infant Pain Scale (NIPS) is designed to assess acute pain in neonates and relies on nursing observations of the behavioral changes in neonates with pain.[42] NIPS uses the following behaviors for pain assessment: crying, facial, arms/legs movements, restless/sleep state, and breathing pattern.

Several pain scales are derived from The Children's Hospital of Eastern Ontario Pain Scale (CHEOPS). The NIPS is a modification of the CHEOPS for infants.[42] The NIPS is designed to assess acute pain in neonates and relies on nursing observations of the behavioral changes in neonates with pain.[42] The Nursing Assessment of Pain Intensity (NAPI) is also adapted from the CHEOPS pain rating scale.[43] The behavioral categories of verbal/vocal, body movement, facial, and response to touch are used to assess pain.[43] The Modified Behavioral Pain Scale is a revision of the CHEOPS designed for use with injection pain.[44]

Objective (Non-Self-Report) Pain Scales for Toddlers

CHEOPS is a behavior rating scale designed for evaluating postoperative pain in children ages 1–5 years. It uses six behavioral patterns: crying, facial expression, verbalizing, torso/legs movements, and touching of the wound.[45] The CHEOPS, like most behavioral pain assessment tools, may be more effective measuring acute pain than pain that has been present for several hours. This may be because many behaviors accommodate or habituate after pain has been present for several hours.[46]

The Observational Scale of Behavioral Distress (OSBD) uses verbal, crying, torso movement, arms/legs movement, and other behaviors to assess pain in young children undergoing brief painful procedures such as lumbar puncture or bone marrow biopsy.[47]

The Postoperative Pain Score (POPS), also known as the Postoperative Comfort Score, uses 10 behavioral responses to assess pain.[48]

Other pain assessment tools: FLACC, Objective Pain Scale, Toddler Preschool Postoperative Pain Scale, Infant Pain Behavior Rating Scale, and Infant Body Coding System have been devised to assess acute pain.[49–54] A few pain assessment tools have been developed to evaluate chronic pain including the DEGR and a psychosocial model by Mathews et al.[55,56]

Multidimensional Pain Scales

The McGill Pain Questionnaire (MPQ) evaluates pain experience from a questionnaire utilizing descriptive terms selected by adults. Since the language of children and adolescents likely differs from adults, the MPQ may not be appropriate for pediatric use.[24] Using pain-descriptors from children, a pediatric variant of the MPQ, the Pediatric Pain Questionnaire (PPQ) was developed. Unfortunately, the original descriptors were from pediatric patients with acute pain while the testing and validation was in pediatric patients with chronic pain.[17] Another problem with the multidimensional pain scale is the requirement for an interview with each patient, which makes its use cumbersome and impractical for emergency department use.

SUMMARY

Historically, pain has been undertreated especially in children and infants despite evidence that even the premature infant experiences pain and responds to noxious stimuli with signs of stress and distress. Assessment of pain forms the basis for the recognition and treatment of pain. An approach to the management of pain in pediatric patients may use strategies such as QUEST and pediatric pain scales. Pain scales are either subjective (self-report) or objective, based on behavioral observations and physiologic measures (such as vital signs). Self-report pain assessment tools are available for children as young as three years old. Pain assessment in pediatric patients needs to be age and developmentally appropriate.

Pain assessment in adolescents and older children can use NRSs. Variations of these numeric scales such as the pain ladder, pain thermometer, or a color analog scale can be used in school age children. Patient self-report pain scales for toddlers/preschoolers include: faces/picture scales, and drawings. Objective pain scales in infants may combine behavioral and physiologic parameters. Observers, whether parents or health care providers, generally underestimate the severity of a child or infant's pain. Although there are many barriers to pain assessment and pain management in the pediatric patient, pain assessment tools are available for addressing and treating pain in all ages of patient's even infants. Furthermore, failure to address pain in the young patient can have short- and long-term consequences (see Chap. 43).

REFERENCES

1. Bracken J. Triage. In: *Sheehy's Emergency Nursing Principles and Practice*. St. Louis, MO: Mosby 2003;75–83.
2. Baker CM, Wong DL. Q.U.E.S.T.: a process of pain assessment in children. *Orthop Nurs*. 1987;6(1):11–21.
3. Romsing J. Assessment of nurses judgment for analgesic requirements of postoperative children. *J Clin Pharm Ther*. 1996;21:159.
4. Jylli L, Olsson GL. Procedural pain in a paediatric surgical emergency unit. *Acta Paediatr Scand*. 1995;84:1403–1408.
5. St. Laurent-Gagnon T, Bernard-Bonnin AC, et al. Pain evaluation in preschool children and by their parents. *Acta Paediatr*. 1999;88:422–427.
6. Singer AJ, Thode HC Jr. Parents and practitioners are poor judges of young children's pain severity. *Acad Emerg Med*. 2002;9(6):609–612.
7. Greco CD, Aner MM, LeBel A. Acute pain management in infants and children. In: Warfield CA, Bajwa ZH, eds. *Principles and Practice of Pain Medicine*. New York: McGraw-Hill; 2004:541–552.
8. Bursch B, Zelter LK. Pediatric pain management. In: Behrman RE, Kliegman RM, Jenson HB, eds. *Nelson Textbook of Pediatrics*. Philadelphia, PA: W.B. Saunders; 2004: 358–366.
9. Zempsky WT, Cravero JP. Committee on Pediatric Emergency Medicine and Section on Anesthesiology and Pain Medicine. Relief of pain and anxiety in pediatric patients in emergency medical systems. *Pediatrics*. 2004;114(5):1348–1356.
10. Johnson MN, Liebelt EL. Acute pain management and procedural sedation in children. In: Tintinalli JE, Kelen GD, Stapczynski JS, eds. *Emergency Medicine, A Comprehensive Study Guide*. New York: McGraw-Hill; 2004:858–869.
11. Melzack R. From the gate to the neuromatrix. *Pain*. 1999; (suppl 6):S121–S126.
12. Melzack R, Wall PD. Pain mechanisms: a new theory. *Science*. 1965;150(699):971–979.
13. Desparmet-Sheridan JP. Pediatric pain. In: Raj PP, ed. *Pain Medicine, A Comprehensive review*. St Louis, MO: Mosby; 2003:351–358.
14. Ross DM, Ross SA. The importance of type of question, psychological climate and subject set in interviewing children about pain. *Pain*. 1984;19:71–79.
15. Andrasik F, Burke EJ, Attanasio V, et al. Child, parent and physician reports of a child's headache pain: relationships prior to and following treatment. *Headache*. 1985;25: 421–425.
16. Valley MA. Pain measurement. In: Raj PP, ed. *Pain Medicine A Comprehensive Review*. St. Louis, MO: Mosby; 2003: 173–180.
17. Varni JW, Thompson KL, Hanson V. The Varni/Thompson pediatric pain questionnaire I. Chronic musculoskeletal pain in juvenile rheumatoid arthritis. *Pain*. 1987;28:27–38.
18. Paris P, Yealy DM. Pain management. In: Marx JA, Hockberger RS, Walls RM, eds. *Rosen's Emergency Medicine Concepts and Clinical Practice*. St. Louis, MO: Mosby; 2002: 2555–2576.
19. Todd KH. Pain management in the emergency department. (CME Monograph). Dallas, TX: American College of Emergency Physicians; 2004:1–10.
20. McGrath PA, Seifert CE, Speechley KN, et al. A new analogue scale for assessing children's pain: an initial validation study. *Pain*. 1996;64:435–443.
21. Grossi E, Borghi C, Cerchiari EL, et al. Analogue chromatic continuous scale (ACCS): a new method for pain assessment. *Clin Exp Rheumatol*. 1983;1:337–340.
22. Hester NKD, Foster R, Kristensen K. Measurement of pain in children: generalizability and validity of the pain ladder and the poker chip tool. In: Tyler DC, Krane EJ, eds. *Advances in Pain Research Therapy*. New York: Raven Press; 1990: 79–84.
23. Aradine BT. Children's pain perception before and after analgesia: a study of instrument construct validity and related issues. *J Pediatr Nurs*. 1988;3:11–23.
24. Hain RDW. Pain scales in children: a review. *Palliat. Med.* 1997;11:341–350.
25. Frank AJ, Moll LMH, Hort JF. A comparison of three ways of measuring pain. *Rheumatol Rehabil*. 1982;21: 211–217.
26. Katz ER, Kellerman J, Siegel SE. Behavioral distress in children with cancer undergoing medical procedures: developmental considerations. *J Consult Clin Psychol*. 1980;48: 356–365.
27. Unruh A, McGrath P, Cunningham SJ, et al. Children's drawing of their pain. *Pain*. 1983;17:385–392.
28. Wong DL, Hockenberry-Eaton M, Wilson D, et al. *Whaley and Wong's Nursing Care of Infants and Children*. St. Louis, MO: Mosby; 1999:1153.
29. Beyer A. Convergent and discriminant validity of a self-report measure of pain intensity for children. *Child Health Care*. 1988;16:274–282.

30. Beyer JE, Aradine CR. Patterns of pediatric pain intensity: a methodological investigation of a self-report scale. *Clin J Pain.* 1987;3:130–141.

31. Bieri D, Reeve RA, Champion GD, et al. The faces pain scale for the self- assessment of the severity of pain experienced by children. Development, initial validity and preliminary investigation for ratio scale properties. *Pain.* 1990;41:139–150.

32. Beyer J, Aradine C. Content validity of an instrument to measure young children's perceptions of the intensity of their pain. *J Pediatr Nurs.* 1986;1:386–395.

33. McGrath PA, deVerber LL, Hearn MT. Multidimensional pain assessment in children. In: Fields HL, Dubner R, Cervero F, eds. *Advances in Pain Research and Therapy.* vol 9. New York: Raven Press; 1985:387–393.

34. Villarrael M, Denyes MJ. Hispanic version of Oucher scale. University of Pennsylvania, Philadelphia, PA and Wayne State University, Detroit, MI; 1990.

35. American Academy of Pediatrics Committee on Psychosocial Aspects of Child and Family Health and American Pain Society Task force on Pain in Infants, Children, and Adolescents. The assessment and management of acute pain infants, children, and adolescents. *Pediatrics.* 2001;108(3): 793–797.

36. American Academy of Pediatrics-Committee on Fetus and Newborn, Committee on Drugs, Section on Anesthesiology. Section on Surgery and Canadian Paediatric Society-Fetus and Newborn Committee. *Pediatrics.* 2000;105(2): 454–461.

37. Shaw EG, Routh DK. Effect of mother's presence on children's reaction to aversive procedures. *J Pediatr Psychol.* 1982;7:33–42.

38. Grunau RVE, Craig KD, Facial activity as a measure of neonatal pain expression. *Adv Pain Res Ther.* 1990;15: 147–156.

39. Grunau RVE, Craig KD. Pain expression in neonates: facial action and cry. *Pain.* 1987;28:395–410.

40. Stevens B, et al. Premature infant pain profile: development and initial validation. *Clin J Pain.* 1996;12(1):13–22.

41. Krechel SW, Bildner J. CRIES: a new neonatal postoperative pain measurement score; initial testing of validity and reliability. *Pediatr Anaesth.* 1996;5:53–61.

42. Lawrence J, Alcock D, McGrath PJ, et al. The development of a tool to assess neonatal pain. *Neonatal Netw.* 1993;12:59–66.

43. Stevens B. Development and testing of a pediatric pain management sheet. *Pediatr Nurs.* 1990;16:543–548.

44. Taddio A, Nulman J, Goldbach M, et al. Use of lidocaine-prilocaine cream for vaccination pain in infants. *J Pediatr.* 1994;124:643–648.

45. McGrath PJ, Johnson G, Goodman JT, et al. CHEOPS: a behavioral scale for rating postoperative pain in children. In: Fields HL, Dubner R, Cerveno F, eds. *Advances in Pain Research and Therapy.* vol 9. *Proceedings of the Fourth World Congress on Pain.* New York: Raven Press; 1985: 395–402.

46. McGrath PJ. Behavioral measures of pain. In: Findley GA, McGrath PJ, eds. *Measurement of Pain in Infants and Children. Progress in Pain Research and Management.* vol 10. Seattle, WA: IASP Press; 1998:83–102.

47. Jay SM, Ozolins M, Elliott C, et al. Assessment of children's distress during painful medical procedures. *J Health Psychol.* 1983;2:133–147.

48. Barrier G, Attia J, Mayer MN, et al. Measurement of postoperative pain and narcotic administration in infants using a new clinical scoring system. *Intensive Care Med.* 1989;15: 537–539.

49. Merkel SI, Shayefits JR, Lewis TV, et al. The FLACC: a behavioral scale for scoring postoperative pain in young children. *Pediatr Nurs.* 1997;23:293–297.

50. Norden J, Hannollan R, Getson P, et al. Reliability of an objective pain scale in children [abstract]. *Anesth Analg.* 1991;72:5199.

51. Norden J, Hannallah R, Getson P, et al. Concurrent validation of an objective pain scale in infants and children [abstract]. *Anesthesiology.* 1991;75:A934.

52. Tarbell SE, Cohen T, Marsh JL. The toddler-preschooler postoperative pain scale: an observational scale for measuring postoperative pain in children aged 1–5. Preliminary report. *Pain.* 1992;50:273–280.

53. Craig KD, McMahon RJ, Morison JD, et al. Developmental changes in infant pain expression during immunization injections. *Chron Pain Soc Sci Med.* 1984;19:1331–1337.

54. Craig KD, Whitfield MF, Gruneau RVE, et al. Pain in the preterm neonate: behavioral and phycological indices. *Pain.* 1993;52:287–299.

55. Gauvain-Piquard A, Rodary C, et al. Pain in children aged 2–6 years: a new observational rating scale elaborated in a pediatric oncology unit—a preliminary report. *Pain.* 1987; 31:177–188.

56. Matthews JR, McGrath PJ, Pigeon H. Assessment and measurement of pain in children. In: Schechter N, Berde C, Yaster M, eds. *Pain in Infants, Children and Adolescents.* Baltimore, MD: Williams & Wilkins; 1993:97–111.

13

Barriers to Effective Emergency Department Pain Management

Knox H. Todd

HIGH YIELD FACTS

- Failure to recognize and treat pain may result in anxiety, depression, and sleep disturbances.
- Barriers to superior pain management intrinsic to emergency medicine are inadequate education, a lack of clearly articulated standards, and a lack of health care provider accountability for substandard care.
- We tend to disbelieve pain reports that do not conform to our expectations.
- Emergency physicians may have a fear of regulatory scrutiny and sanctions, as well as a more realistic fear of being duped by patients seeking opioids for nonmedical purposes.
- Inadequate pain management education is a problem at both the medical school and postgraduate levels.
- There is a paucity of treatment guidelines and best practice standards for emergency department (ED) pain care.
- Given that pain cannot be measured in an objective fashion, the clinician is often confronted with the difficulties of differentiating legitimate versus illegitimate complaints of pain.
- The true prevalence of addiction and aberrant drug-seeking behaviors is unknown and unstudied. When the prevalence of such problems is overestimated, oligoanalgesia is the predictable result.

INTRODUCTION

Pain is the single most common reason for seeking medical care and taking medications.[1] As such, it should demand our attention; however, pain is often seemingly invisible to the emergency physician. It is an unspoken presence that, if not acknowledged and managed appropriately, causes dissatisfaction with medical care, hostility toward the physician, unscheduled returns to the emergency department (ED), delayed return to full function, and potentially, an increased risk of litigation. Failure to recognize and treat pain may result in anxiety, depression, sleep disturbances, increased oxygen demands with the potential for end-organ ischemia, and decreased movement with an increased risk of venous thrombosis. Given this state of affairs, it is reasonable to ask what barriers serve to block the adequate treatment of pain in our EDs. This chapter will highlight known or suspected roadblocks to effective ED pain treatment.

The ED serves as a fail-safe mechanism for our fragmented health care system. Pain is but one of the many conditions where we face not only the problem of acute clinical presentations, but also the failures of other sectors of the system that might have prevented patients' presentations to our departments. Patients commonly present to the ED for a variety of chronic medical conditions that could be treated in primary care offices. Our patients face barriers to superior medical care in areas other than pain; however, the treatment of pain seems particularly problematic in this regard and solutions seem for the most part elusive. A number of barriers to adequate pain care are extrinsic to the clinical encounter, including administrative, regulatory, and socioeconomic factors. Emergency medicine has in addition its own set of intrinsic barriers to overcome and it is these that will be considered in this chapter.[2]

Among barriers to superior pain management intrinsic to emergency medicine are inadequate education, a lack of clearly articulated standards, and a lack of health care provider accountability for substandard care.[3] Emergency physicians commonly fail to adequately assess pain. We tend to disbelieve pain reports that do not conform to our expectations. Emergency physicians may have an inappropriate fear of regulatory scrutiny and sanctions, again related to opioid use, and a more realistic fear of being duped by patients seeking opioids for nonmedical purposes. Patients themselves may be reluctant to report pain, or fear our therapeutic recommendations because of their own fears of addiction or adverse effects related to the use of opioids.

INTRINSIC BARRIERS

Education

Training in the techniques of pain management is a much-neglected task in professional schools for physicians, nurses, and allied health professionals. These limitations apply to both the pathophysiology and psychosocial aspects of pain. In particular, the appropriate use of opioids is an area where our medical systems give us little guidance.

Inadequate pain management education is a problem at both the medical school and postgraduate levels. Very few hours of the medical school curriculum are devoted to pain management despite its primacy as a reason for physician visits. Although resident and continuing education levels of pain management instruction have increased of late, it is notable that the model of the clinical practice of emergency medicine does not include a formal pain management curriculum.[4]

It is reasonable to ask whether this lack of emphasis on pain management represents an error of *omission*, or rather that of *commission*, on the part of medical educators. Most medical school applicants express a desire to relieve human suffering. Most laypersons view the relief of pain and suffering as the primary goal of medicine. As noted by Eric Cassell, within medical schools pain relief and palliative care in general are accorded much less importance by both medical students and their teachers.[5] It is *curative*, rather than *palliative* medicine that commands attention and respect within our medical schools and postgraduate training programs.[6]

Within the curative model of medicine, scientific objectivity and rationality may be valued over the seemingly idiosyncratic and subjective pain experience of individual patients.[7] Pain is valued as a symptom and guide to correct diagnoses rather than the appropriate object of medical therapies. This emphasis on accurate diagnoses and clinical objectivity over symptom relief is perhaps best exemplified by the persistence of surgical dogma regarding withholding analgesics in the setting of acute abdominal pain, a practice that persists despite zero evidence regarding its dangers and a growing literature supporting analgesic use.[8] The curative model of medicine would demand overwhelming evidence of the safety of analgesic administration in this setting, given its devaluation of subjective patient experience.

Given the role that teachers of emergency medicine have increasingly assumed in the early medical school curriculum, we have a tremendous opportunity to shape the attitudes of all future physicians regarding pain treatment, not just those who choose to train in emergency medicine. Given our strategic location in the front lines of patient care, and the relative youth of our specialty, we may have particularly pertinent lessons to transmit to medical students regarding pain management practices, with less dogma to obscure a critical examination of current pain management practice.

Assessment of Chronic Pain

Of particular importance to the assessment of pain, we should note that acute and chronic pain may be associated with markedly different pain-related behaviors. While acute pain is usually associated with objective signs of sympathetic nervous system activation and overt signs of physical suffering, patients with chronic pain may not exhibit such typical behaviors and signs of autonomic nervous system over activity. This disparity between observed patient behaviors and physician expectations of such behaviors in the setting of chronic pain may lead to inaccurate determinations of pain intensity and ultimately, undertreatment of pain.

Lack of Practice Standards

There is a paucity of treatment guidelines and best practice standards for ED pain care, in part because of the lack of research in this area by our specialty. Although the American College of Emergency Physicians (ACEP) has adopted a statement of general principles regarding pain management (Table 13-1), our specialty lacks clearly articulated standards to drive pain care.[9] Our care systems do not include adequate mechanisms to ensure accountability for inferior practice.[9]

In 2001, the Joint Commission on Accreditation of Healthcare Organisms issued new standards related to pain management, and it is likely that this effort will increase documentation of ED pain intensity levels; however, it is unclear if these standards will have an effect on pain management practice or patient outcomes.[10]

To facilitate quality improvement, organized emergency medicine must develop more specific definitions of quality pain care. An operational definition of quality pain care beyond the broad principles enumerated in Table 13-1 must be developed and standardized process and outcome measures to evaluate the quality of pain management practice should be adopted. Without such goals and standards, it is unlikely if pain care will improve.

There is evidence from other systems of care that rapid improvements in pain management are achievable. In 1998, Ken Kizer championed the Veterans' Health Administration (VHA) National Pain Management Strategy. The goals of this initiative included the provision of a system-wide standard for pain management as well as processes for

Table 13-1. ACEP Policy Statement: Pain Management in the Emergency Department

The majority of ED patients require treatment for painful medical conditions or injuries. ACEP recognizes the importance of effectively managing ED patients who are experiencing pain and supports the following principles:

ED patients should receive expeditious pain management, avoiding delays such as those related to diagnostic testing or consultation.

Hospitals should develop unique strategies that will optimize ED patient pain management using both narcotic and nonnarcotic medications.

ED policies and procedures should support the safe utilization and prescription writing of pain medications in the ED.

Effective physician and patient educational strategies should be developed regarding pain management, including the use of pain therapy adjuncts and how to minimize pain after disposition from the ED.

Ongoing research in the area of ED patient pain management should be conducted.

---

monitoring and improving pain outcomes.[11] Recent studies demonstrate the effectiveness of such a strategy in producing significant changes in pain management within a complex system such as the VHA.[12] These developments bode well for similar efforts within our specialty.

Fear of Inappropriate Analgesic Use

Federal regulators and state medical boards do not perceive emergency medicine as a specialty prone to inappropriate prescribing and investigations of, or sanctions against, emergency physicians are rare, if not unheard of. Despite this, many emergency physicians express fears of such scrutiny or sanctions related to prescribing or administering opioids. Although this concern is often voiced, it seems likely that this fear represents concern about other, less obvious physician uncertainties related to pain management. Two barriers related to such fears may be the emergency physicians' concern about being overburdened by the inherent difficulties of managing patients with complicated pain syndromes and the clinicians' fears of being "duped" by the drug addict.

Pain cannot be objectively measured with a laboratory test. The validity of patient self-report is often questioned and attempts to "objectify" the pain experience are sought. This search is bound to disappoint the querulous clinician, as blood tests, tissue pathology, diagnostic imaging, physical assessments, or patient behaviors cannot reliably reflect the internal pain experience.

Given that pain cannot be measured in such a fashion, unless a source for the pain is obvious, the clinician is confronted with the difficulties of differentiating legitimate versus illegitimate complaints of pain. The hectic nature of practice often does not allow sufficient time for precisely characterizing such patient complaints. Clinicians may lump legitimate pain complaints with the ploys of those

seeking inappropriate opioids. Both groups of patients are ultimately mistrusted and treated with disdain.

Additionally, in treating pain in patients receiving chronic opioid therapy, confusion over the concepts of physical dependence, tolerance, addiction, and pseudoaddiction may constitute a barrier to appropriate treatment. These phenomena are discrete and standard definitions may be helpful in caring for patients managed with chronic opioids. Table 13-2 contains accepted definitions of these terms.[13]

ED personnel commonly identify patients who are thought to seek opioids for illegitimate purposes. Although drug addiction occurs in all patient populations, EDs are felt to be particularly rife with such patients. Unfortunately, the true prevalence of addiction and aberrant drug-seeking behaviors is unknown and unstudied. There is little research on risk factors for prescription drug abuse to guide the emergency physician. When the prevalence of such problems is overestimated, oligoanalgesia is the predictable result.

A spectrum of aberrant behaviors and their association with addiction are listed in Table 13-3. Many behaviors commonly felt to represent inappropriate drug seeking are felt by experts to be actually less predictive of addiction. Certainly, the presence of an obvious painful condition (e.g., sickle cell and fracture) should preempt concerns about illegitimate drug-seeking behaviors. For patients with recurrent ED visits prompted by less obvious pain complaints, an active case management strategy should be pursued, with involvement of pain or addiction specialists when necessary.

Chronic pain is often accompanied by mood disorders that complicate the management of these challenging patients.[14] Emergency physicians often receive limited training in dealing with such disorders and the specialty's deficiencies in dealing with such problems have been documented.[15]

Table 13-2. Definitions Related to the Use of Opioids for the Treatment of Pain

Addiction is a primary, chronic, and neurobiologic disease, with genetic, psychosocial, and environmental factors influencing its development and manifestations. It is characterized by behaviors that include one or more of the following: impaired control over drug use, compulsive use, continued use despite harm, and craving.

Physical dependence is a state of adaptation that often includes tolerance and is manifested by a drug class-specific withdrawal syndrome that can be produced by abrupt cessation, rapid dose reduction, decreasing blood level of the drug, and/or administration of an antagonist.

Tolerance is a state of adaptation in which exposure to a drug induces changes that result in a diminution of one or more of the drug's effects over time.

Pseudoaddiction is a term that has been used to describe patient behaviors that may occur when pain is undertreated. Patients with unrelieved pain may become focused on obtaining medications, may "clock watch," and may otherwise seem inappropriately "drug seeking." Even such behaviors as illicit drug use and deception can occur in the patient's efforts to obtain relief. Pseudoaddiction can be distinguished from true addiction in that the behaviors resolve when pain is effectively treated.

Attitudes toward Pain Medicine Physicians

Many emergency physicians have jaundiced views of pain management specialists. They are often viewed as either accomplices in patients' aberrant analgesic use behaviors, or as irresponsible practitioners who abandon the most difficult patients, resulting in their inevitable presentations to the ED. Given the current state of health care financing in the United States, pain specialists are better reimbursed for interventional procedures than for other pharmacologic and

Table 13-3. Spectrum of Aberrant Drug-Related Behaviors that Raise Concern about the Potential for Addiction

Less suggestive of addiction
Aggressive complaining about the need for more drug
Drug hoarding during periods of reduced symptoms
Requesting specific drugs
Openly acquiring similar drugs from other medical sources
Occasional unsanctioned dose escalation or other noncompliance
Unapproved use of the drug to treat another symptom
Reporting psychic effects not intended by the clinician
Resistance to a change in therapy associated with "tolerable" adverse effects with
expressions of anxiety related to the return of severe symptoms

More suggestive of addiction
Selling prescription drugs
Prescription forgery
Stealing or "borrowing" drugs from others
Injecting oral formulations
Obtaining prescription drugs from nonmedical sources
Concurrent abuse of alcohol or illicit drugs
Repeated dose escalation or similar noncompliance despite multiple warnings
Repeated visits to other clinicians or emergency rooms without informing prescriber
Drug-related deterioration in function at work, in the family, or socially
Repeated resistance to changes in therapy despite evidence of adverse drug effects

Source: Shalmi CL. Opioids for nonmalignant pain: issues and controversy. In: Warfield CA, Bajwa ZH, eds. *Principles and Practice of Pain Medicine*. 2nd ed. New York, The McGraw-Hill Companies Inc.; 2004:607.)

nonpharmacologic approaches. Patients with insufficient health care insurance or those for whom interventional procedures are not indicated may find themselves abandoned in the many communities that lack balanced, multidisciplinary pain treatment facilities. Patients with pain represent a subset of all patients with unmet medical needs who find themselves in overcrowded EDs.

Nursing Barriers

In addition to physicians, all of the barriers discussed previously are likely applicable to nursing personnel and other allied health professionals practicing in the ED. Given the traditional nursing focus on patient assessment and relief of discomfort, such barriers may be particularly important obstacles to overcome in our efforts to improve patient care. Among pediatric nurses, knowledge deficits and attitudinal barriers regarding the treatment of pain in children have been particularly well documented.[16-19]

Patient Barriers

Patients themselves may be reluctant to report pain presence and intensity and use analgesics that might otherwise improve their well-being and function. To the extent that patients' attitudes regarding pain and its treatment are based on erroneous belief, they may constitute a major barrier to optimal management.

Most of these barriers have been identified among groups of cancer patients with eight specific barriers being well characterized. These include the fear of addiction, fear of becoming tolerant to the effects of analgesics, fear of unmanageable side effects, fear that pain indicates cancer progression, fear of intramuscular injections, as well as a fatalistic belief system maintaining that pain is an inevitable and unavoidable component of cancer, that "good" patients do not complain of pain, and that patients should not distract health care providers by complaining about pain.[20-33] These patient-related barriers to pain management can be measured using the Barriers Questionnaire, a valid and reliable instrument that has been used in numerous studies.[34,35]

Although these barriers have been well characterized among cancer patients, there is no literature addressing their importance among ED patients. It seems likely that such barriers are operative, particularly among ED patients with cancer and other chronic conditions. A better understanding of the role of patient beliefs will be necessary if we are to address what may be an important obstacle to superior pain management in our EDs.

CONCLUSION

Relieving pain and reducing suffering are primary responsibilities of emergency medicine and much can be done to improve the care of patients in pain. We have discussed a number of physician, patient, and system barriers to superior pain treatment. Our specialty should continue to refine our approach to the problem of pain and reduce the current large amount of variability in our practices. We should continue to more precisely define our own standards for excellence in pain practice and promote quality improvement initiatives to achieve these goals. We will find many allies in our attempts to improve ED pain management, but the primary responsibility for surmounting these barriers to superior patient care remains our own.

REFERENCES

1. Cordell WH, et al. The high prevalence of pain in emergency medical care. *Am J Emerg Med.* 2002;20(3):165–169.
2. Rupp T, Delaney KA. Inadequate analgesia in emergency medicine. *Ann Emerg Med.* 2004;43(4):494–503.
3. Todd KH. Emergency medicine and pain: a topography of influence. *Ann Emerg Med.* 2004;43(4):504–506.
4. Hockberger RS, Binder LS, Graber MA, et al. The model of the clinical practice of emergency medicine. *Ann Emerg Med.* 2001;37(6):745–770.
5. Cassell E. The nature of suffering and the goals of medicine. *N Engl J Med.* 1982;206:639–645.
6. Fox E. Predominance of the curative model of medical care—a residual problem. *JAMA* 1997;278:761–763.
7. Rich BA. An ethical analysis of the barriers to effective pain management. *Camb Q Healthc Ethics.* 2000;9:54–70.
8. McHale PM, LoVecchio F. Narcotic analgesia in the acute abdomen—a review of prospective trials. *Eur J Emerg Med* 2001;8(2):131–136.
9. ACEP Board of Directors. Policy statement: pain management in the emergency department. *Ann Emerg Med.* 2004;44:198.
10. Joint Commission for the Accreditation of Healthcare Organizations. Background on the development of the Joint Commission standards on pain management. Available at *http://www.jcaho.org/news+room/health+care+issues/pain.htm.* Accessed July 21, 2004.
11. Veterans Health Administration. *VHA National Pain Management Strategy.* Washington, DC: Veterans Health Administration; 1998.
12. Cleeland CS, Reyes-Gibby CC, Schall M, et al. Rapid improvement in pain management: the Veterans Health Administration and the institute for healthcare improvement collaborative. *Clin J Pain.* 2003;19(5):298–305.
13. American Society of Addiction Medicine. Definitions related to the use of opioids for the treatment of pain.

Consensus document from the American Academy of Pain Medicine, the American Pain Society, and the American Society of Addiction Medicine, February 2001. Available at *http://www.asam.org*. Accessed July 21, 2004.

14. Gureje O, Von Korff M, Simon GE, et al. Persistent pain and well-being: a World Health Organization Study in Primary Care. *JAMA*. 1998;280:147–151.

15. Tse SK, Wong TW, Lau CC, et al. How good are accident and emergency doctors in the evaluation of psychiatric patients? *Eur J Emerg Med* 1999;6:297–300.

16. Broome ME, Slack JF. Influences on nurses/management of pain in children. *MCN*. 1990;15:158–162.

17. Ross RS, Bush JP, Crummette BD. Factors affecting nurses' decisions to administer PRN analgesic medication to children after surgery: an analog investigation. *J Pediatr Psychol*. 1991;16(2):151–167.

18. Hamers JPH, Huijer Abu-Saad H, van den Hout MA, et al. Are children given insufficient pain-relieving medication postoperatively? *J Adv Nurs*. 1998;27:37–44.

19. Read JV. Perceptions of nurses and physicians regarding pain management of pediatric emergency room patients. *Pediatr Nurs*. 1994;20(3):314–318.

20. Cleeland CS. The impact of pain on the patient with cancer. *Cancer*. 1984;54:2635–2641.

21. Jones W, Rimer B, Levy M, et al. Cancer patients' knowledge, beliefs and behavior regarding pain control regimens: implications for education programs. *Patient Educ Couns*. 1984;5:159–164.

22. Hodes R. Cancer patients' needs and concerns when using narcotic analgesics. Hiss CS, Fields WS, eds. Advances in Pain Research and Therapy. Vol 11. New York, NY: Raven Press; 1989:91–99.

23. Melzak R. The tragedy of needless pain. *Sci Am*. 1990;262: 27–33.

24. Ferrel BR, Cohen M, Rhiner M, et al. Pain as a metaphor for illness. *Oncol Nurs Forum* 1991;18(8):1315–1321.

25. Dar R, Beach C, Barden P, et al. Cancer pain in the marital system: a study of patients and spouses. *J Pain Symptom Manage*. 1992;7:87–93.

26. Riddell A, Fitch MI. Patients' knowledge of and attitudes toward the management of cancer pain. *Oncol Nurs Forum*. 1997;24(10):1175–1184.

27. Sherwood G, Adams-McNeil J, Starck PL, et al. Qualitative assessment of hospitalized patients' satisfaction with pain management. *Res Nurs Health*. 2000;23:486–495.

28. Levin DN, Cleeland CS, Dar R. Public attitudes toward cancer pain. *Cancer*. 1985;56:2337–2339.

29. Diekmann JM, Engber D, Wassem R. Cancer pain control: one state's experience. *Oncol Nurs Forum*. 1989;16(2):219–223.

30. Arazathuzik D. Pain experiences for metastatic breast cancer patients. Unraveling the mystery. *Cancer Nurs*. 1991; 14(1):41–48.

31. Twycross R, Lack S. *Symptom Control in Far Advanced Cancer: Pain Relief*. London: Raven Pitman; 1984.

32. Cleeland CS. Barriers to the management of cancer pain. *Oncology*. 1987;April(Suppl):19–26.

33. Zborowski M. *People in Pain*. San Francisco, CA: Josey-Bass, 1969.

34. Ward SE, Goldberg N, Miller-McCauley V, et al. Patient-related barriers to management of cancer pain. *Pain*. 1993;52:319–324.

35. Wells N, Rolanda RN, Johnson L, et al. Development of a short version of the Barriers Questionnaire. *J Pain Symptom Manage*. 1998;15:294–298.

14

Pharmacotherapy in Pain Management

Michael A. Turturro

HIGH YIELD FACTS

- Because of their rapid effectiveness in a variety of painful syndromes, most emergency department (ED) patients with moderate-to-severe pain should be treated with opioids.
- Opioids are often underdosed, consider weight/age/comorbidity when dosing, additional dosages are often needed for titration.
- Use lower doses of opioids in the elderly, those with chronic hepatic or renal dysfunction, and individualize the dose for each specific patient.
- Avoid intramuscular (IM) injections if possible since the onset/peak effects are unpredictable and IM injections are painful and can cause hematomas (subcutaneous [SQ] is less painful).
- All opioids produce analgesia with appropriate dosing and more side effects with escalating doses.
- Avoid meperidine when possible since it can cause seizures/myoclonus/altered mental status, is contraindicated with monoamine oxidase (MAO) inhibitors and selective serotonin reuptake inhibitors (SSRIs).
- Nonopioid analgesics are used for mild-to-moderate pain especially in syndromes with prostaglandin-mediated pain (e.g.,

dysmenorrhea, ureteral colic, and biliary colic)
- Nonopioid analgesics have therapeutic ceiling and side effects including gastrointestinal (GI) bleeding and acute renal failure.
- A major concern with the cyclooxygenase (COX)-2 inhibitors is their association with cardiovascular complications.

OPIOID ANALGESICS

Introduction

The opioid analgesics, sometimes referred to as opiates or narcotic analgesics, have been used for hundreds of years to alleviate a wide range of painful conditions. They are a class of naturally occurring, semisynthetic, and synthetic drugs that have effects related to binding at opioid receptors within the central and peripheral nervous systems. Most of the useful clinical effects of the opioids discussed in this chapter relate to binding at central mu (μ) receptors. The net effect is modulation of the response of the central nervous system (CNS) to a given painful stimulus. These drugs may be pure agonists, partial agonists, mixed agonist-antagonists, and antagonists. A discussion of opioid receptors, agonism, and antagonism is included in Chapter 16.

Basic Principles of Opioid Analgesia

Because of their rapid effectiveness in a variety of painful syndromes, most patients with moderate-to-severe pain in the emergency department (ED) should be treated with opioid analgesics; however, these drugs are frequently underused and underdosed in the ED. This may be related to several factors including a poor understanding of the pharmacologic properties of opioid analgesics, an inappropriate fear of obscuring a diagnosis (particularly in patients with acute abdominal pain), an inordinate fear of side effects, an inappropriate fear of disciplinary action by licensing agencies when using opioids for legitimate medical conditions, and an inappropriate fear of either causing addiction or a heightened suspicion of drug-seeking behavior.[1]

The following principles should be applied when using opioid analgesics in the ED:

1. Use the right dose
Opioids are frequently underdosed in the ED, and one dose for all patients without regard for weight, age, or comorbidity will frequently result in inadequate analgesia in some and excess side effects and potential toxicity in others. In an ED study of high-dose opioid analgesia for painful procedures using meperidine, adult patients received a *mean* dose of 2.5 mg/kg, and although sedation was common, clinically significant respiratory depression did not occur.[2] Reasonable starting doses of commonly used opioid analgesics are listed in Table 14-1. Additional doses are frequently needed to titrate to the desired effect, and some patients may require much higher doses to control their pain. The range of effective doses can be markedly higher in tolerant versus opioid-naïve individuals. The best way to determine if additional doses are needed is the patient's report of pain control. Lower doses should be used in the elderly and those with chronic hepatic or renal dysfunction. Therefore, the dose use must be individualized for each specific patient based on the response to initial doses and balanced between effective analgesia and adverse effects.

2. Use the right route
In patients who require parenteral opioid analgesia, titration to a desired effect is best achieved with intravenous (IV) dosing. This allows for rapid effect and easier determination if the patient requires additional dosing. Intramuscular (IM) dosing should be avoided as the onset of action and time to peak effect are delayed and unpredictable, making individualized titration difficult.[3] Additionally, IM injections are painful and may cause hematomas in patients with coagulopathy. In patients in whom the use of a single dose of opioid analgesic is anticipated, the oral route should be used. In patients who cannot tolerate oral therapy and IV establishment is not possible, the subcutaneous (SQ) route should be used as it is less painful than IM administration. Similar doses can be used.

3. Use the right frequency
After discharge from the ED or if the patient is in the ED for a prolonged period of time, a subsequent dosing schedule should be established. After the patient's pain is initially relieved, additional doses should be administered based on the specific pharmacokinetics of the individual drug. More sustained analgesia occurs with around-the-clock dosing, presumably due to sustained plasma levels of analgesics. Additionally, the dose required to prevent the return of significant pain is less the dose needed to treat uncontrolled pain. Therefore, analgesics should not be prescribed on a *prn* basis.

4. Use the right drug
All opioid analgesics will produce analgesia with appropriate dosing, and more side effects with escalating doses. Therefore, the choice of opioid analgesic should be primarily based on the duration of action desired and side effects specific to the individual drug. For example, fentanyl may be chosen for analgesia for a painful procedure because of its relatively short half-life, whereas morphine may be chosen to reduce the pain of a long bone fracture because of its relatively long half-life. The specific properties of each individual drug are listed below.

Parenteral Opioid Analgesics

Morphine

Morphine is a naturally occurring active ingredient in opium obtained from the poppy plant, and is the analgesic to which all others are compared. It is a direct agonist of μ receptors, resulting in analgesia as well as euphoria, respiratory depression, miosis, and decreased gastrointestinal (GI) motility. It has a rapid onset after IV administration,

Table 14-1. Parenteral Opioid Analgesic Dosing

Drug	Brand Name	Starting Parenteral Dose	Duration
Morphine		0.1 mg/kg	3–5 h
Meperidine	Demerol	1 mg/kg	2–3 h
Hydromorphone	Dilaudid	0.03 mg/kg	2–4 h
Fentanyl	Sublimaze	1.5 µg/kg	1–2 h
Alfentanil	Alfenta	1 µg/kg	30–90 min
Sufentanil	Sufenta	0.1 µg/kg	30–90 min
Remifentanil	Ultiva	0.5 µ/kg	5–10 min

and its duration of action is 3–5 hours. Ninety percent of absorbed morphine is subsequently conjugated in the liver to active and inactive metabolites and excreted through the kidneys. Morphine-induced peripheral vasodilation has been well described. Morphine can cause histamine release resulting in opioid-induced hypotension, skin rash, and flushing. Injectable morphine contains sodium bisulfite (Duramorph is preservative free), which may cause bronchospasm in asthmatics and allergic reactions. Pruritus may occur due to both allergic, and most commonly, non-allergic phenomena (direct histamine release or anaphylactoid reaction). Increased intrabiliary pressure may occur (as it does with virtually all opioids); however, the actual clinical significance of this effect is unclear.[4] The effective dose may vary widely; however, a reasonable IM starting dose in otherwise healthy opioid-naïve patients is 0.1 mg/kg.

Meperidine (Demerol)

Meperidine is a synthetic opioid analgesic with similar effects at μ opioid receptors as morphine. It is commonly used by physicians because they are familiar with the drug, though its duration of action is shorter than morphine. Although commonly believed to cause less spasm at the sphincter of Oddi than morphine, this has only been observed in animal studies, and is likely of no clinical relevance.[4] The major concern with meperidine is its propensity to cause CNS excitability including altered mental status, myoclonus, and seizures. This is due to the metabolism of the parent compound meperidine to normeperidine, which can have a half-life of up to 40 hours in elderly patients, and is renally excreted. Therefore, repeated doses of this drug should be avoided in patients with renal dysfunction, those who require high doses (such as sickle cell patients), and the elderly. Additionally, meperidine is contraindicated in patients who are receiving monoamine oxidase (MAO) inhibitors, in which this drug interaction may result in severe, occasionally fatal, hyperthermia. Although the use of MAO inhibitors in patients with depression is now uncommon, the use of selective serotonin reuptake inhibitors (SSRIs) is common. Patients taking SSRIs may be at risk of developing serotonin syndrome after the use of meperidine due to its potential to increase CNS serotonin levels.[5] Since there are many effective alternatives for use in the ED, meperidine should be avoided when possible.

Hydromorphone (Dilaudid)

Hydromorphone is a semisynthetic μ receptor agonist. As with other μ agonists, dose-dependent analgesia as well as respiratory depression, euphoria, sedation, miosis, and decreased GI motility occurs after its use. It is metabolized in the liver to both active and inactive metabolites, and subsequently excreted by the kidneys. Consequently, it should be used with caution in patients with hepatic or renal dysfunction. In opioid-naïve patients, a starting dose of 0.03 mg/kg IM is reasonable, however, this dose should be lowered in elderly patients.

Fentanyl (Sublimaze)

Fentanyl is a synthetic opioid analgesic with agonist effects at μ opioid receptors. It has several properties that make it attractive for use in the ED. Its relatively short duration of action makes it an ideal agent for use with brief painful procedures or in those in which serial examinations may be required (e.g., patients with acute abdominal pain). It causes no clinically significant histamine release and therefore may be preferred for use in patients with reactive airways disease. Additionally, since histamine-mediated vasodilation and does not significant myocardial depression occur after fentanyl use, it may be a safer choice in patients at risk for hemodynamic instability. Muscular rigidity, involving the muscles of respiration, has been reported at doses much higher than typically used in the ED (>10 μg/kg) particularly if injected rapidly, and can be treated with naloxone or neuromuscular blocking drugs. At high doses, respiratory depression is more profound than CNS depression. An appropriate parenteral starting dose in the ED is 1–1.5 mcg/kg, which can be quickly titrated to the desired effect. Because of its short duration of action, when used in ED patients to treat acute pain, additional doses are often necessary. Fentanyl is well absorbed through the oral mucosa, and consequently an oral transmucosal form is available (Actiq). Transdermal fentanyl in patch form (Duragesic) is frequently used in the management of chronic pain. It is of primary concern to emergency physicians due to the risk of opioid toxicity in children with accidental ingestion and overdose related to abusers who inject extracted fentanyl from patches. Additionally, opioid toxicity may be precipitated by administering opioid analgesics in the ED to patients who are concurrently using transdermal fentanyl.

Alfentanil, Sufentanil, and Remifentanil

Like fentanyl, these are synthetic phenylpiperidine derivatives and act as short-acting μ receptor agonists. As with fentanyl, no clinically significant histamine release occurs after their use, and chest wall rigidity may occur with high doses. All of these agents have a shorter duration of action than fentanyl, and remifentanil has an extremely short duration of action due to rapid hydrolysis by blood and tissue esterases. This may make it useful for procedural sedation in the ED when used in conjunction with short-acting sedatives such as propofol.

Opioid Agonist-Antagonist Analgesics

The opioid agonist-antagonist analgesics are a group of drugs that are believed to stimulate kappa (κ) opioid receptors, causing supraspinal and spinal analgesia like the μ agonists. In contrast, these drugs appear to have antagonist properties at the μ opioid receptors, therefore increasing doses result in a ceiling effect for inducing respiratory depression. They also seem to cause less euphoria and sedation; however, due to the μ antagonism, they can precipitate withdrawal in patients dependent on μ receptor agonists. Due to κ receptor agonism, they may also cause dysphoria and psychotomimetic effects such as disorientation and hallucinations. Abuse is thought to be less common with this group of drugs, however, is occasionally reported. The currently available agonist-antagonists are summarized in Table 14-2.

Pentazocine (Talwin Nx, Talacen)

Pentazocine was the first opioid agonist-antagonist available. At commonly used doses, it is a weak antagonist to pure opioid agonists such as morphine. The most commonly used oral form is manufactured as a combination product with 0.5 mg naloxone added to reduce the potential for IV abuse of the oral form (naloxone has no significant clinical effect at an *oral* dose of 0.5 mg). Pentazocine is metabolized in the liver, and patients with advanced liver disease may consequently be more prone to adverse effects. With long-standing use or abuse cutaneous and muscular fibrosis may occur. It also has been shown to decrease myocardial contractility, and increase pulmonary artery wedge pressure, heart rate, and

systemic vascular resistance, therefore should be avoided in patients with heart failure or advanced coronary disease. Of the agonist-antagonist analgesics, it is thought to have the highest incidence of psychotomimetic reactions, occurring in approximately 2–3% of patients. Because of these issues and the multiple alternatives, pentazocine has limited use in the ED.

Nalbuphine (Nubain)

Nalbuphine acts as a κ receptor agonist and a μ receptor antagonist in the CNS. It is estimated to be equianalgesic to similar doses of morphine sulfate on a mg for mg basis; however, respiratory depression and analgesia hit a ceiling at approximately 30 mg in adult patients. Unlike other parenteral opioids that are classified as pregnancy category C, animal studies have shown no teratogenic effects of nalbuphine, and it is classified as pregnancy category B. Consequently, it is commonly used in obstetric analgesia during labor and delivery. Because of its antagonistic properties, it can precipitate withdrawal in patients dependent on μ opioid agonist analgesics, and should be avoided in such patients. It produces no histamine release and has minimal cardiovascular effects. Psychotomimetic reactions occur less frequently than with pentazocine.

Butorphanol (Stadol)

Butorphanol is available both in parenteral form and as a nasal spray (Stadol-NS). The transnasal form is occasionally used to treat migraine headache; however, side effects are frequent and limit its use.[6] It has similar effects as nalbuphine in the CNS, and cardiovascular effects similar to pentazocine suggesting it ought to be avoided in patients with heart failure or advanced coronary disease. It is cleared more slowly in elderly patients, and in this population half the usual dose is recommended.

Table 14-2. Opioid Agonist-Antagonist Analgesics

Drug	Brand Name	Dosing	Routes
Pentazocine	Talwin Nx (w/Naloxone)	50 mg/0.5 mg q 4–6 h	PO
	Talacen [w/Acetaminophen (APAP)]	25 mg/650 mg q 4–6 h	PO
Nalbuphine	Nubain	10–20 mg q 3–4 h	IV/IM/SQ
Butorphanol	Stadol	1–2 mg q 3–4 h	IV/IM/SQ/transnasal
Buprenorphine	Buprenex	0.3–0.6 mg q 4–6 h	IV/IM/SQ

Buprenorphine (Buprenex)

Although often listed with opioid agonist-antagonist analgesics, buprenorphine is actually a partial μ receptor agonist, with minimal κ receptor effects; however, like opioid agonist-antagonists, a ceiling on respiratory depression is seen with escalating doses. It has a high affinity and slowly dissociates from the μ opioid receptor, therefore high doses of naloxone are required to reverse its effect. The use of buprenorphine in the treatment of opioid addiction is discussed in Chap. 16.

Oral Opioid Analgesics for Acute Pain

The oral opioid analgesics are available alone or in a variety of combination preparations in various doses, and are often combined with various doses of acetylsalicylic acid (ASA), acetaminophen, or ibuprofen. The theoretical advantage of such combinations is that by treating pain both centrally with an opioid and peripherally with a nonopioid, the analgesic properties would be additive, resulting in a lower dose of each agent to achieve the desired effect, and minimizing side effects. In fact, several studies comparing opioid analgesics in combination with a nonopioid have consistently demonstrated improved pain relief when compared to the individual components. Table 14-3 lists the commonly used oral opioid products for acute pain. In appropriate doses, these agents can effectively treat most acute painful conditions; however, as in parenteral opioid analgesia, the effective dose can vary, and finding an optimal dose for an individual patient may involve some trial and error. A specific advantage of the oral opioid

analgesics is that in generic form they are inexpensive, with a supply of 20 tablets typically costing less than $10. It is common for these combination products to have as much as 750 mg of acetaminophen per tablet, therefore in an overdose situation, the potential exists for both opioid and acetaminophen toxicity.

Codeine

Codeine is available alone, but is commonly used in preparation products containing acetaminophen (e.g., Tylenol no. 3) or ASA. Codeine initially gained popularity because it is half as potent orally as parenterally. Its analgesic activity may be related to its demethylation to morphine by cytochrome P-450 enzyme CYP2D6, an enzyme that is not functionally expressed in 7–10% of Caucasian patients. This genetically-mediated phenomenon may explain why some patients do not respond well to the analgesic effects of codeine, but still suffer adverse effects.[7] Additionally, this may partially explain why in many comparative studies of codeine with or without a nonopioid analgesic, codeine provided little or no additional analgesia. Codeine commonly causes nausea, vomiting, and sedation. Its use in the ED should primarily be reserved to patients who have responded well to this drug in the past.

Hydrocodone

Hydrocodone is a semisynthetic codeine derivative that is available in a range of dosages and in combination with various nonnarcotic analgesics, typically acetaminophen

Table 14-3. Oral Opioid Analgesics for Acute Pain

Drug	Brand Names	Drug Enforcement Administration (DEA) Drug Schedule	Doses of Opioid	Doses of Nonopioid
Codeine	Tylenol nos. 2, 3, 4 Empirin w/codeine	III	30–60 mg	APAP: 300 mg Acetylsalicylic acid: 325 mg
Hydrocodone	Vicodin, Lortab, Lorcet, Vicoprofen, Norco, others	III	5–10 mg	APAP: 325–750 mg Acetylsalicylic acid (ASA): 500 mg Ibuprofen: 200 mg
Hydromorphone	Dilaudid	II	1–8 mg	N/A
Pentazocine	Talwin Nx Talacen	IV	25–50 mg	APAP: 650 mg
Propoxyphene	Darvon, Darvocet	IV	50–100 mg	APAP: 325–650 mg Acetylsalicylic acid: 389 mg
Oxycodone	Percocet, Endocet Percodan, Roxicet, OxyIR, others	II	2.5–10 mg	APAP: 325–650 mg Acetylsalicylic acid: 325 mg
Tramadol	Ultram, Ultracet	N/A	37.5–50 mg	APAP: 325 mg

or ibuprofen (Vicodin, Vicoprofen, Lortab, Lorcet, Norco, and others). Comparative studies suggest that at the commonly used doses it is as effective as oxycodone and more effective than codeine or tramadol, with a lower incidence of side effects. Due to its popularity, relatively low side effect profile, and propensity to induce euphoria, it is also a common drug of abuse.

Hydromorphone

Hydromorphone (Dilaudid) is commonly used both parenterally (see previously) and orally. The approximate equianalgesic oral dose is two to four times the parenteral dose. Hydromorphone is not available as a combination product (e.g., with ASA or acetaminophen). Consequently, there is no risk for developing acetaminophen or salicylate toxicity when used in treating opioid-tolerant patients who require regular large doses (e.g., for cancer pain).

Propoxyphene

Although commonly used, most evidence suggests that propoxyphene itself has minimal analgesic effects, but significant CNS side effects. A meta-analysis of 26 randomized controlled trials involving 2231 patients concluded that the addition of propoxyphene to acetaminophen provided minimal additional analgesia to acetaminophen alone.[8] In combination preparations with acetaminophen (Darvocet) and ASA (Darvon), the nonnarcotic component may explain much of the analgesic effect. It is common practice to prescribe propoxyphene to elderly patients in an effort to employ a *mild* analgesic; however, since the elderly population is at risk of adverse outcomes related to CNS depression (such as falls), this practice is best avoided. In overdose, miosis may not occur, obscuring the diagnosis of opioid overdose. Additionally, high doses of naloxone (10 mg or more) are required to reverse the respiratory depression and sedation, and seizures may develop that are difficult to control.

Oxycodone

Oxycodone is available alone or in combination products ranging between 2.5 and 10 mg, with 325–650 mg of acetaminophen or 325 mg of ASA. While an effective and useful analgesic, it is associated with euphoria and a substantial abuse potential. OxyContin, a long-acting oxycodone preparation, has gained notoriety as a frequently abused drug, often due to abusers who crush and inject or inhale the drug. Although an effective analgesic, there are several reasonable alternatives available and its

use in the ED should be limited to patients with well-defined chronic pain syndromes who need to be controlled with this agent.

Tramadol

Tramadol displays a weak affinity for μ opioid receptors and inhibits both serotonin and norepinephrine reuptake in the CNS. The former mechanism explains its potential in treating acute pain, the latter mechanism (similar to the effect of tricyclic antidepressants) explains its potential in treating chronic pain. In acute pain studies, tramadol alone was as effective or marginally more effective than placebo, and less effective than a hydrocodone/acetaminophen[9] combination or ASA with codeine.[10] Its weak μ receptor binding may explain this phenomenon, however, like codeine it is also metabolized to an active metabolite by cytochrome P-450 enzyme CYP2D6. Therefore, some patients may not respond due to an inability to convert tramadol to the active metabolite. Tramadol is now available in a combination product with acetaminophen (Ultracet). It is unclear if the acetaminophen component accounts for the majority of the analgesic effects of this product. Side effects with tramadol are frequent, and dizziness, nausea, constipation, headache, and somnolence are commonly reported. Seizures may occur at commonly used doses, and the risk seems to be increased in patients taking SSRIs, tricyclic antidepressants or similar compounds (e.g., cyclobenzaprine), MAO inhibitors, and patients with a known seizure disorder. In tramadol overdose, administration of naloxone may precipitate seizures. Since many alternatives exist, tramadol use in the ED should be limited to patients who have successfully been treated with this drug in the past and have no known contraindications to its use.

Meperidine

Oral meperidine is available in 50 or 100 mg tablets for use in both acute and chronic pain. Due to first-pass hepatic metabolism, the typical effective oral dose is twice the effective parenteral dose. The cautions with meperidine are similar with parenteral use, particularly with repeated doses. The oral form drug is rarely needed and should rarely be prescribed from the ED.

Oral Opioid Preparations for Chronic Pain

Certain opioid preparations are specifically used to manage chronic pain. In addition to OxyContin, several long-acting morphine preparations are available in doses from 15 to 200 mg (Avinza, Kadian, MS Contin, MSIR, Oramorph SR), which can be dosed based on the patient's individual requirement from once to three times daily. Levorphanol (Levo-Dromoran), a long-acting synthetic opioid, is available parenterally and orally, and may be used in acute pain, but is commonly used to treat chronic pain. It may cause fewer GI side effects than morphine or meperidine. It is supplied as 2 mg tablets, and can be used every 6–8 hours. Dextromethorphan, commonly used as an antitussive, is a derivative of levorphanol and has been studied in high doses for the treatment of chronic pain syndromes, particularly neuropathic pain. Its mechanism of action is thought to be due to its blocking effect on central *N*-methyl-D-aspartate (NMDA) receptors; however, the side effects encountered at the doses required to produce analgesia limit its use. Methadone (Dolophine) is occasionally used effectively to treat chronic pain; however, due to its long half-life, sedation is common when multiple daily doses are used. Typical doses for the management of chronic pain are 2.5–10 mg every 4–6 hours.

NONOPIOID ANALGESICS

Introduction

The nonopioid analgesics are a group of drugs which primarily inhibit prostaglandin synthesis, both centrally and peripherally. These medications are often considered first-line drugs in the management of mild-to-moderate pain, and are effective in a wide variety of painful conditions. Their use is often preferred in clinical syndromes associated with known prostaglandin-mediated pain such as dysmenorrhea, ureteral colic, and biliary colic. Unlike the majority of the members of the opioid class, the analgesic effects of nonopioids have a therapeutic ceiling in which escalating doses do not enhance pain relief. Specific advantages of the nonopioid analgesics are lack of tolerance, lack of dependence, low abuse potential, and lack of significant respiratory depression or sedation; however, they can be associated with serious and occasionally fatal side effects, most notably GI bleeding and acute renal failure related to nonsteroidal anti-inflammatory drug (NSAID) use. This class of drugs includes acetaminophen, salicylates, cyclooxygenase (COX)-2-specific inhibitors, and other NSAIDs agents. Each class of agent will be discussed separately. Individual agents with their typical analgesic doses are summarized in Table 14-4.

An understanding of the mechanism of action of the nonopioids is essential before discussing the individual categories. Most appear to mediate their effects by inhibiting the enzyme COX, which has a key role in

prostaglandin and leukotriene synthesis. Two isoforms of COX have been described (COX-1 and COX-2). COX-1 is responsible for prostaglandin synthesis in gastric mucosa and platelets. COX-2 is responsible for prostaglandin synthesis accompanying inflammation or injury in the CNS. Salicylates and nonselective NSAIDs inhibit both isoforms of COX, thereby decreasing inflammation, but also inhibiting platelet activity and gastroprotective prostaglandin synthesis. Specific COX-2 inhibitors are thought to primarily inhibit the isoform responsible for prostaglandin synthesis associated with inflammation, without significantly affecting COX-1, maintaining gastroprotective prostaglandin synthesis.

Acetaminophen

Acetaminophen has well-established antipyretic and analgesic actions. Although commonly referred to as a peripheral analgesic, acetaminophen is also thought to have a mechanism of action in the CNS. The precise mechanism is unknown, though it is a weak inhibitor of COX-1 and COX-2. A recently described variant of COX-1, often referred to as COX-3, is thought to be inhibited by acetaminophen in the CNS, and is currently being investigated as a possible key in determining acetaminophen's mechanism of action.[11] The lack of significant peripheral prostaglandin inhibition likely explains minimal anti-inflammatory effects of acetaminophen and low risk of GI side effects.

Because of its effectiveness, low side effect profile and relative safety if used at appropriate doses, acetaminophen should be considered first-line therapy in the management of mild-to-moderate pain. It is also considered first-line therapy in the management of osteoarthritis, and there is scant evidence that any of the NSAIDs provide significantly better pain relief than acetaminophen alone in patients with osteoarthritis.[12]

Toxicity due to acetaminophen misuse is well-known to emergency physicians, and a discussion is beyond the scope of this chapter. In long-term alcoholics, misuse or chronic therapeutic use may result in hepatotoxicity, even at recommended doses, so alcoholics who present to the ED with liver failure should be questioned about acetaminophen use.

Salicylates

Salicylates are nonsteroidal anti-inflammatory agents which are derivatives of salicylic acid. Several of the salicylates are used therapeutically, including ASA or aspirin, methyl salicylate (Oil of Wintergreen), salsalate (Disalcid), sulfasalazine, diflunisal (Dolobid), and others. No particular salicylate has been shown to be any more

Table 14-4. Nonopioid Analgesics

Chemical Class	Drug	Brand Names	Analgesic Dose*
Acetaminophen		Tylenol, others	500–1000 mg q 4 h
Salicylates	Aspirin	Various	325–650 mg q 4 h
	Diflunisal	Dolobid	500 mg q 12 h
	Salsalate	Disalcid, Salflex	1000 mg q 8 h
Acetic acids	Diclofenac[†]	Voltaren, Cataflam	50 mg q 8 h
	Etodolac[†]	Lodine	200–400 mg q 6–8 h
	Indomethacin	Indocin	50 mg q 8 h
	Ketorolac	Toradol	10 mg q 6 h
	Nabumetone[†]	Relafan	1 g q 12 h
	Sulindac	Clinoril	150 mg q12h
	Tolmetin	Tolectin	200–400 mg q 8 h
Propionic acids	Fenoprofen	Nalfon	200 mg q 4–6 h
	Flurbiprofen	Ansaid	50–100 mg q 8–12 h
	Ibuprofen Advil, others	Motrin, Rufen	400 mg q 4–6 h
	Ketoprofen	Orudis, Oruvail	25–50 mg q 6–8 h
	Naproxen	Naprosyn, Anaprox Alleve	250–500 mg q 12 h
	Oxaprozin	Daypro	1200 mg q 24 h
Oxicams	Meloxicam[†]	Mobic	7.5 mg q 24 h
	Piroxicam	Feldene	20 mg q 24 h
Fenamates	Meclofenamate	Meclomen	50–100 mg q 4–6 h
	Mefenamic acid	Ponstel	250 mg q 6 h
Pyrazole	Celecoxib[‡]	Celebrex	200 mg q 12 h
Isoxazole	Valdecoxib[‡]	Bextra	20 mg q 12 h

*Typical loading dose for analgesia is twice the usual analgesic dose.

[†]COX-2 selective.

[‡]COX-2 specific.

effective as an analgesic than any other. All pose similar antipyretic and anti-inflammatory activity. Like most other NSAIDs, they are nonselective COX inhibitors, and consequently inhibit platelet aggregation and gastric prostaglandin synthesis. They also carry the same risks as other NSAIDs, most notably GI bleeding, renal failure, and anaphylactoid reactions. Diflunisal is less likely to cause salicylism in overdose, and patients taking diflunisal may have falsely elevated serum salicylate levels.

NSAIDs

Nonselective COX inhibitors are collectively known as NSAIDs. All are thought to have a similar mechanism of action and a therapeutic ceiling of analgesia. None have been shown to be a superior analgesic to any other; however, certain patients may respond better to one class than another.[13] It is therefore reasonable to try a different

chemical class of NSAID if the patient has responded well. The dose required to treat inflammatory conditions is typically higher than analgesic doses, and in treating acute pain a loading dose (usually twice the typical analgesic dose) should be administered. The major differences in NSAIDs relate to the pharmacokinetics of the individual drugs, their activity in inhibiting COX, and their cost. Of note is that certain NSAIDS are more COX-2 selective than others, specifically diclofenac, etodolac, meloxicam, and nabumetone, and with chronic use these agents may be less prone to cause gastric ulceration.[14]

The use of NSAIDs is widespread, with approximately 70 million prescriptions and 30 billion over-the-counter tablets sold annually in the United States[15] and there is a common perception among patients that these are relatively safe drugs.[16] While the lack of respiratory depression, significant sedation, dependence, and tolerance are advantages of the NSAIDs, side effects can be frequent, severe, and occasionally life threatening. Although NSAIDs are usually well tolerated, approximately 10–20% of patients develop dyspepsia. NSAID-induced GI bleeding is common, accounting for over 100,000 hospitalizations and 16,500 deaths annually in the United States.[17] All NSAIDs carry the risk of GI bleeding; however, the risk appears to be lowest with ibuprofen[18] and highest with ketorolac.[19] Anaphylactoid reactions and renal failure may occur after NSAID use, and heart failure may be exacerbated. Since NSAIDs are not without the risk of serious adverse consequences, in patients at risk for developing such adverse effects (elderly, history of peptic ulcer disease, concomitant corticosteroid use, anticoagulant use, history of renal failure, or allergy to NSAIDs), opioid analgesics are safer, and therefore preferred.

Although typically administered orally, indomethacin may be administered rectally and both ketorolac and diclofenac are available as topical ophthalmic solutions. Ketorolac is the only NSAID available for parenteral administration in the United States. Its use is widespread in emergency medicine for a variety of painful conditions; however, there is no evidence of improved analgesia with this drug versus other NSAIDs, and comparative studies between parenteral ketorolac and oral NSAIDs have shown no analgesic advantage of this drug.[20] Since is it an NSAID, it has a ceiling effect of analgesia, unlike opioids. It is expensive, carries a higher risk of GI bleeding than other NSAIDs, and can be associated with renal dysfunction and platelet inhibition even with a single dose. Its use should be limited to conditions in which NSAID therapy is desirable (e.g., dysmenorrhea, ureteral colic, and biliary colic) and the patient is unable to tolerate oral therapy.

COX-2 Inhibitors

The currently available specific COX-2 inhibitors, celecoxib (Celebrex) and valdecoxib (Bextra), were developed in an effort to produce drugs that had the desirable effects of decreasing inflammation by inhibiting COX-2, while maintaining the synthesis of gastroprotective prostaglandins by not significantly inhibiting COX-1 in vivo. Their benefit seems to be in limiting the development of gastric ulceration with chronic use.[21] This advantage is not seen in patients concomitantly taking aspirin. There appears to be no decrease in the risk of developing renal failure or anaphylactoid reactions with COX-2 inhibitors versus NSAIDs. Additionally, there is no proven reduction in the incidence of dyspepsia when using these drugs. Bextra was withdrawn from the market by Pfizer Pharmaceutical on April 7, 2005.

While primarily used to treat the pain of osteoarthritis, they are also marketed for the treatment of acute pain. Most studies comparing these drugs to older NSAIDs for a variety of painful conditions have suggested that they are weaker analgesics. In a randomized controlled trial in ED patients in acute pain, celecoxib was associated with less pain reduction than ibuprofen, however, the study was not powered to detect a significant difference.[22]

The major concern with the COX-2 inhibitors is their association with cardiovascular complications. This may be related to their lack of inhibition of thromboxane A_2, thus reducing any cardioprotection, in addition to a prothrombotic effect.[23] The increased risk of thromboembolic events resulted in the withdrawal of the COX-2 inhibitor rofecoxib (Vioxx) in September 2004. This risk appears to be less with celecoxib and valdecoxib, possibly due to less selective inhibition of COX-2; however, there appears to be an increased risk of stroke and myocardial infarction in patients undergoing coronary artery bypass grafting who receive valdecoxib. It is likely that the cardiovascular risk is a class effect of the COX-2 inhibitors.

Parecoxib is a parenteral COX-2 inhibitor similar to valdecoxib that may become available for the treatment of acute pain. Etoricoxib is a COX-2 inhibitor available in Europe that may become available in the United States for acute pain management. These drugs could be potentially used to treat acute pain, since the cardiovascular complications only seem to occur with chronic use; however, due to safety concerns with all COX-2 inhibitors, they may never become available in the United States.

OTHER ANALGESICS AND ADJUNCTIVE AGENTS

Skeletal Muscle Relaxants

The class of drugs commonly used in the ED to treat pain and discomfort related to muscular spasm and pain is the centrally acting skeletal muscle relaxants, summarized in Table 14-5. Although chemically diverse, they all share the common property of having their major site of action in the CNS rather than in the peripheral muscle fibers; however, the precise mechanism by which skeletal muscle relaxants act is not known, and there is no objective evidence that they actually do relax skeletal muscle. Their sedating side effects may substantially contribute to pain relief. Many were developed in the 1960s and 1970s at a time when rest, instead of early mobilization, was commonly recommended for acute myofascial strain, consequently their sedative effects were thought to be beneficial. In comparative studies versus placebo, they do

Table 14-5. Skeletal Muscle Relaxants

Drug	Brand Name	Dose	Comment
Carisoprodol	Soma	350 mg PO q 6–8 h	Occasionally reported as a drug of abuse
	Soma compound (w/ASA)	1–2 PO q 6–8 h	
	Soma with Codeine (w/ASA/codeine)	1–2 PO q 6–8 h	
Chlorzoxazone	Parafon Forte	250–500 mg q 6–8 h	
Cyclobenzaprine	Flexeril	5–10 mg PO q 8 h	Structurally similar to TCAs, caution in overdose
Metaxolone	Skelaxin	800 mg PO q 6–8 h	
Methocarbamol	Robaxin	1000 mg PO/IV q 6 h	Parenteral form available
Orphenadrine	Norflex	100 mg PO q 12 h	Parenteral form available
		60 mg IV/IM q 12 h	
	Norgesic (w/ASA/caffeine)	1–2 PO q 6–8 h	
	Norgesic Forte (w/ASA/caffeine, at twice the dose or Norgesic)	0.5–1 PO q 6–8 h	

TCA: Tricyclic antidepressants.

appear to have some analgesic activity, however, no specific agent has ever been demonstrated to be superior to another. Additionally, many of these trials were flawed by the inclusion of patients with both acute and chronic muscle spasms, unblinding, and subjective determination of outcome. A meta-analysis of the muscle relaxant cyclobenzaprine (Flexeril) in the treatment of back pain concluded that it is significantly better at relieving back pain than placebo; however, the effect is modest, the greatest effect is seen in the first few days of treatment, and adverse effects (usually drowsiness) are experienced by more than 50% of the patients.[24]

The common practice of adding cyclobenzaprine to ibuprofen was studied in an ED population and was associated with increased sedation, but not increased pain relief.[25] The 1994 clinical practice guideline on acute lower back problems in adults issued by the Agency for Health Care Policy and Research (now the Agency for Healthcare Research and Quality) concluded that despite their sedative effects, skeletal muscle relaxants have not been shown to be more effective than NSAIDs, and no additional benefit is gained by using muscle relaxants in combination with NSAIDs alone.[26]

Butalbital

Butalbital is a barbiturate found in combination products with caffeine, ASA, acetaminophen, and/or codeine (Esgic, Fiorinal, Fioricet, and Fiormar) and commonly used to treat the pain associated with muscle contraction and migraine; however, the butalbital component of these products appears to add little analgesia, produces sedation, may cause drug-induced headaches, may be habit forming, and withdrawal may result if abruptly discontinued.[27] Acute barbiturate poisoning in addition to salicylism or acetaminophen toxicity may be seen in overdose. Its use in the ED should be limited to patients who have achieved prior success with this drug and are not at risk of dependence.

Capsaicin

Capsaicin (Zostrix) is a topical compound available without a prescription for the treatment of a variety of chronic painful conditions. It is made from chili peppers and when applied topically, produces a local burning sensation, primarily from local substance P release by afferent nerve fibers. It is hypothesized that with repeated application the area becomes desensitized, presumably due to depletion of substance P. Additionally, the counterirritation may activate inhibitory fibers in the CNS.

Capsaicin is often used to treat neuropathic pain (particularly from postherpetic neuralgia and diabetic neuropathy), osteoarthritis, and rheumatoid arthritis. In these conditions, it seems to have a modest analgesic effect, although this benefit may be transient. A meta-analysis confirmed these findings from smaller studies, demonstrated that greater than 50% of patients develop adverse effects, and that 13% discontinue therapy due to these adverse effects.[28]

Salmon Calcitonin

Vertebral compression fractures in the elderly are often problematic, as the pain associated with these fractures may result in long-term use of opioids with consequent CNS and GI side effects such as sedation and constipation. Salmon calcitonin, often used to attenuate osteoporosis and increase bone density, has gained attention as a treatment for the pain associated with vertebral compression fractures. It is known to inhibit bone resorption by reducing the activity of osteoclasts; however, the exact mechanism of its analgesic activity is unknown, and may be a combination of central and peripheral factors, such as the release of beta-endorphins.[29] In studies in which salmon calcitonin was used following vertebral compression fractures, treated patients had less pain, less analgesic requirements, and greater mobility.[30] In patients seen in the ED with these fractures, it is reasonable to begin therapy on discharge with salmon calcitonin (Miacalcin), 200 IU (one spray) daily, and alternating nostrils. Side effects are minimal, and the most common is rhinitis.

REFERENCES

1. Rupp T, Delaney KA. Inadequate analgesia in emergency medicine. *Ann Emerg Med.* 2004;43:494–503.
2. Barsan W. Safety of high-dose narcotic analgesia for emergency department procedures. *Ann Emerg Med.* 1993;22:1444–1449.
3. Erstad BL, Meeks ML, Chow HH, et al. Site-specific pharmacokinetics and pharmacodynamics of intramuscular meperidine in elderly postoperative patients. *Ann Pharmacother.* 1997;31:23–28.
4. Thompson DR. Narcotic analgesic effects on the sphincter of Oddi: a review of the data and therapeutic implications in treating pancreatitis. *Am J Gastroenterol.* 2001;96:1266–1272.
5. Weiner AL. Meperidine as a potential cause of serotonin syndrome in the emergency department. *Acad Emerg Med.* 1999;6:156–158.
6. Hoffert MJ, Couch JR, Diamond S, et al. Transnasal butorphanol in the treatment of acute migraine. *Headache.* 1995;35:65–69.
7. Eckhardt K, Li S, Ammon S, et al. Same incidence of adverse drug events after codeine administration irrespective of the genetically determined differences in morphine formation. *Pain.* 1998;76:27–33.
8. Po ALW, Zhang WY. Systematic overview of co-proxamol to assess analgesic effects of addition of dextropropoxyphene to paracetamol. *BMJ.* 1997;315:1565–1571.
9. Turturro MA, Paris PM, Larkin GL. Tramadol versus hydrocodone-acetaminophen in acute musculoskeletal pain: a randomized, double–blind clinical trial. *Ann Emerg Med.* 1998;32:139–143.
10. Moore PA, Crout RJ, Jackson DL, et al. Tramadol hydrochloride: analgesic efficacy compared with codeine, aspirin with codeine, and placebo after dental extraction. *J Clin Pharmacol.* 1998;38:554–560.
11. Davies RM, Good RL, Roupe KA, et al. Cyclooxygenase-3: axiom, dogma, anomaly, enigma or splice error—not as easy as 1, 2, 3. *J Pharm Pharm Sci.* 2004;7:217–226.
12. Zhang W, Jones A, Doherty M. Does paracetamol (acetaminophen) reduce the pain of osteoarthritis? A meta-analysis of randomized clinical trials. *Ann Rheum Dis.* 2004;63:901–907.
13. Brooks PM, Day RO. Nonsteroidal anti-inflammatory drugs—similarities and differences. *N Engl J Med.* 1991; 324:1716–1725.
14. Hooper L, Brown T, Elliott R, et al. The effectiveness of five strategies for the prevention of gastrointestinal toxicity induced by non-steroidal anti-inflammatory drugs: systematic review. *BMJ.* 2004;329:948–951.
15. Lichtenstein DR, Syngal S, Wolfe MM. Nonsteroidal anti-inflammatory drugs and the gastrointestinal tract: the double-edged sword. *Arthritis Rheum.* 1995;38:5–18.
16. Fraenkel L, Wittink DR, Concato J, et al. Informed choice and the widespread use of antiinflammatory drugs. *Arthritis Rheum.* 2004;51:210–214.
17. Wolfe MM, Lichtenstein DR, Singh G. Gastrointestinal toxicity of nonsteroidal anti-inflammatory drugs. *N Engl J Med.* 1999;340:1888–1899.
18. Lewis SC, Langman MJ, Laporte JR, et al. Dose-response relationships between individual nonaspirin nonsteroidal anti-inflammatory drugs (NANSAIDs) and serious upper gastrointestinal bleeding: a meta-analysis based on individual patient data. *Br J Clin Pharmacol.* 2002;54: 320–326.
19. Laporte JR, Ibanez L, Vidal X, et al. Upper gastrointestinal bleeding associated with the use of NSAIDs: newer versus older agents. *Drug Saf.* 2004;27:411–420.
20. Turturro MA, Paris PM, Seaberg DC. Intramuscular ketorolac versus oral ibuprofen in acute musculoskeletal pain. *Ann Emerg Med.* 1995;26:117–120.
21. Silverstein FE, Faich G, Goldstein JL. Gastrointestinal toxicity with celecoxib vs. nonsteroidal anti-inflammatory drugs for osteoarthritis and rheumatoid arthritis. *JAMA* 2000;284:1247–1255.
22. Salo DF, Lavery MA, Varma V, et al. A Randomized, Clinical Trial Comparing Oral Celecoxib 200 mg, Celecoxib 400 mg, and Ibuprofen 600 mg for Acute Pain. *Acad Emerg Med* 2003;10:22–30.
23. Fitzgerald GA. Coxibs and cardiovascular disease. *N Engl J Med.* 2004;351:1709–1711.
24. Browning R, Jackson JL, O'Malley PG. Cyclobenzaprine and back pain—a meta-analysis. *Arch Intern Med.* 2001; 161:1613–1620.
25. Turturro MA, Frater CF, D'Amico FJ. Cyclobenzaprine with ibuprofen versus ibuprofen alone in acute myofascial strain: a double-blind clinical trial. *Ann Emerg Med.* 2003;41:818–826.

26. Bigos S, Bowyer O, Braen G, et al. Clinical Practice Guideline 14: Acute Lower Back Problems in Adults. Rockville, MD: Agency for Health Care Policy and Research, Public Health Service, US Dept of Health and Human Services; 1994. AHCPR Publication No. 95-0642.

27. Silberstein SD, McCrory DC. Butalbital in the treatment of headache: history, pharmacology, and efficacy. *Headache.* 2001;41:953–967.

28. Mason L, Moore RA, Derry S, et al. Systematic review of topical capsaicin for the treatment of chronic pain. *BMJ.* 2004;328:991.

29. Gennari C. Analgesic effect of calcitonin in osteoporosis. *Bone.* 2002;30(suppl 5):67S–70S.

30. Blau LA, Hoehns JD. Analgesic efficacy of calcitonin for vertebral fracture pain. *Ann Pharmacother.* 2003;37(4): 564–570.

Part 1: PROCEDURAL SEDATION

15

Adjunct Medications: Atropine and Glycopyrrolate

Sharon E. Mace

HIGH YIELD FACTS

- Muscarinic receptor antagonists competitively antagonize the action of acetylcholine (Ach)/ other parasympathomimetic drugs and/or the vagal nerve at these receptors.
- Decreased salivary gland secretions:
  · Improve efficacy of topical anesthesia in those areas subject to salivary secretions.
  · May decrease the incidence of laryngospasm (laryngospasm may be precipitated by salivary secretions).
- Affect many organs including cardiovascular, respiratory, gastrointestinal (GI), genitourinary, and central nervous system (CNS) systems.
- Effects include ↑ heart rate, bronchodilation, ↓ GI/genitourinary peristalsis, and dry mouth.
- Glycopyrrolate preferred over atropine: greater antisialagogue effect and fewer side effects (less tachycardia, fewer dysrhythmias, and no CNS side effects).

The antimuscarinic agents, atropine and glycopyrrolate, are commonly used drugs. In anesthesia they are used as a premedication when topical upper airway anesthesia and awake intubation is contemplated and during surgery to counter vagal tone and bradycardia. In emergency medicine they are used primarily to reverse vagally mediated bradycardia, reduce salivary secretions suspected as contributing to ketamine-induced laryngospasm during procedural sedation, and as ACLS drugs.[1–4]

Atropine, derived from the plant *Atropa belladonna* (*deadly nightshade*), is a naturally occurring alkaloid, while glycopyrrolate is a semisynthetic derivative of atropine. Both agents antagonize the actions of acetylcholine (Ach) at the cholinergic muscarinic receptor, and are colloquially known as members of the *anticholinergic* class of compounds. Members of this broader class are used widely in emergency medicine as mydriatics, antispasmodics, and bronchodilators for asthma therapy and other indications.[4,5]

RECEPTOR PHYSIOLOGY

Ach is the endogenous neurotransmitter synthesized and then released from cholinergic neurons in both the peripheral and central nervous systems (CNSs)[6,7] (Table 15-1). The actions of Ach are referred to as *cholinergic*. There are four types of synapses where Ach serves as the neurotransmitter:

1. Autonomic effector sites innervated by postganglionic parasympathetic fibers.
2. Parasympathetic and sympathetic ganglia (including adrenal medulla).
3. Skeletal muscle motor end plates, innervated by somatic motor nerves.
4. Selected peripheral and central nervous system synapses, both presynaptic and postsynaptic.[4]

For the most part, particularly outside the CNS, Ach's actions are mediated by two types of receptors: nicotinic and muscarinic cholinergic receptors.[8,9]

Though muscarinic receptors *are* found in high concentrations in specific areas of the brain such as the thalamus, hippocampus, and cortex, most of the cholinergic neurotransmission in the CNS is neither muscarinic nor nicotinic.[4] Cholinergic receptors are also found in the spinal cord as well as in the CNS and in the periphery. Ach serves as an excitatory neurotransmitter in the CNS. The neural pathways in the CNS mediated by Ach regulate awareness or the

Table 15-1. Acetylcholine Receptors and Antagonists

Acetylcholine (Cholinergic Neurotransmitter)*

Muscarinic (parasympathomimetic) (muscarinic cholinergic) receptors	Nicotinic (nicotinic cholinergic) receptor
Location	Location
Central nervous system	Skeletal muscle neuromuscular junction
Peripheral nervous system	Ganglia (parasympathetic and sympathetic innervation)
Autonomic effector cells with postganglionic parasympathetic innervation	
Ganglia	
Blood vessel endothelial cells	
Adrenal medulla	

Acetylcholine Antagonists (Cholinergic Blockers)

Muscarinic receptor antagonist	Nicotinic receptor antagonist
Blocks actions of acetylcholine at muscarinic receptor sites (i.e., are parasympatholytic)	Blocks actions of acetylcholine at nicotinic receptors (skeletal muscle neuromuscular junction)
Atropine = natural occurring alkaloid	Two types of neuromuscular blockers: do or do not depolarize motor end plate
Glycopyrrolate = semisynthetic alkaloid	Succinylcholine = depolarizing neuromuscular blocker
Act at autonomic effector sites	Vecuronium/pancuronium = nondepolarizing (competitive, stabilizing) neuromuscular blocker

*Actions are terminated by hydrolysis by cholinesterases.

level of consciousness and the degree of consciousness. The process starts in the midbrain (e.g., midbrain reticular formation), goes to the thalamus, then throughout the cerebral cortex via two major cholinergic neural pathways in the brain. The two cholinergic projections are the basal forebrain pathway and the pedunculopontine pathway. The thalamus acts as the coordinating or synchronizing center. The three neurotransmitters, Ach, γ-aminobutyric acid (GABA), and glutamate, control the cholinergic neurons in these two neural pathways. Consciousness or awareness depends on the interactions of (1) Ach in the thalamus and cerebral cortex and (2) the three neurotransmitters which control the cholinergic neurons in the two pathways. This is important because most anesthetic agents inhibit the Ach and/or glutamate receptors in the CNS, thereby causing loss of consciousness or loss of awareness (Fig. 15-1).

Muscarinic receptors in the peripheral nervous system are mainly located on autonomic effector cells innervated by postganglionic parasympathetic nerves. They are also found in ganglia and various other cells including blood vessel endothelium.[4]

Cholinergic agonists such as the cholinomimetic agent bethanechol (Urecholine) mimic the effects of Ach at both muscarinic and nicotinic receptor sites. Cholinergic blockers or antagonists (anticholinergic agents generally) block the effect of Ach at muscarinic (antimuscarinic agents) and nicotinic (antinicotinic agents) receptor sites.[7] Some drugs are fairly nonselective and will have actions on both nicotinic and muscarinic receptor sites; however, there are a few pharmacologic agents that act almost exclusively at muscarinic sites or at nicotinic sites. Atropine and glycopyrrolate are muscarinic receptor antagonists.

The actions of Ach (or similar drugs) on autonomic effector sites are denoted as muscarinic (or muscarinic cholinergic or parasympathomimetic). The actions of Ach (or related drugs) on the neuromuscular junction of skeletal muscle and autonomic ganglia are denoted nicotinic or nicotinic cholinergic.[10] The neuromuscular blocking agents are classified according to whether or not they cause depolarization of the motor end plate. Succinylcholine is the prototype of the depolarizing agents, while pancuronium and vecuronium are agents in the nondepolarizing or competitive (stabilizing) class of neuromuscular blockers[11,12] (see Chap. 28). Ach combines with the nicotinic receptor on the muscle to initiate the end-plate potential (EPP) or in the nerve to begin the excitatory postsynaptic potential (EPSP).

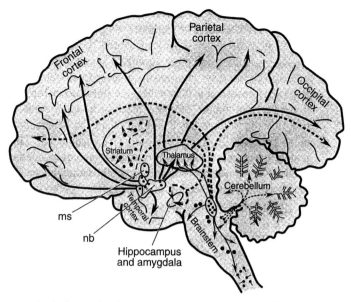

Fig. 15-1. Cholinergic systems in the human brain. Two major pathways project widely to different brain areas: basal forebrain cholinergic neurons (solid lines) (including the nucleus basalis [nb] and medial septal nucleus [ms]) and pedunculopontine-lateral dorsal tegmental neurons (dashed lines). Other cholinergic neurons include striatal interneurons, cranial nerve nuclei, vestibular nuclei, and spinal cord preganglionic and motoneurons. (Reprinted with permission from Beattie C. History and principles of anesthesiology. In: Hardman JG, Limbird LE, eds. *Goodman & Gilman's The Pharmacological Basis of Therapeutics.* 10th ed. New York: McGraw-Hill; 2001:321–335.)

In summary, muscarinic receptors are found mainly in peripheral visceral organs. Nicotinic receptors are located on the neuromuscular junction of the skeletal muscle and both sympathetic and parasympathetic ganglia.[13] Atropine and glycopyrrolate are muscarinic receptor antagonists (part of the anticholinergic category of drugs). They block Ach's actions at the muscarinic receptor sites, which are mostly in peripheral organs.

Ach is inactivated by hydrolysis by the cholinesterase enzymes: acetylcholinesterase and butylcholinesterase.[6,7,13]

CLINICAL EFFECTS OF MUSCARINIC RECEPTOR AGONISTS (ACETYLCHOLINE AND DERIVATIVES)

Ach, the chemical mediator or neurotransmitter of the parasympathetic nervous system, has wide-ranging effects[6] (Table 15-2). Ach's main cardiovascular effects are a negative chronotropic effect (↓ heart rate), a negative inotropic effect (↓ contractility), a negative dromotropic effect (↓ rate of conduction in the sinoatrial node [SAN] and atrioventricular node [AVN]), and vasodilatation.[4,7]

If a small dose of Ach is given intravenously, there is a transient decrease in blood pressure (from vasodilatation) followed by a reflex tachycardia.[4]

Bronchoconstriction and increased tracheobronchial secretions occur with vagal stimulation of the respiratory tract.[4,7] Vagal (parasympathetic) stimulation of the GI tract increases peristalsis by increasing the strength of contractions and the tone of the stomach and the intestines as well as increasing their secretory activity.[4,7] Similarly, vagal stimulation increases peristalsis in the genitourinary tract, increases voiding pressure, and contraction of the bladder's musculature.[4,7]

Increased secretions of the tracheobronchial, digestive, salivary, lacrimal, and exocrine sweat glands (all glands innervated by the vagal nerves) occur with vagal or parasympathetic stimulation. Ach or parasympathetic stimulation also causes miosis[4,7] (Table 15-2).

Ach is rarely used clinically because it has varied effects and somewhat transient or limited effects because of rapid hydrolysis of Ach by the cholinesterases[4]; however, derivatives of Ach that have more selective actions are used clinically (Table 15-3).

Table 15-2. End-Organ Actions of Acetylcholine and Antimuscarinic Agents*

Organ	Acetylcholine	Antimuscarinic Agents
Cardiovascular	↓ HR ↓ contractility ↓ conduction of SAN, AVN, vasodilatation	↑ HR (blocks vagal effects) No change in BP or cardiac output if given alone (but counteracts Ach's ↓ BP) ↑ conduction of SAN, AVN
Respiratory	Bronchoconstriction ↑ tracheobronchial secretions Stimulates aortic/carotid bodies chemoreceptors	Bronchodilatation ↓ tracheobronchial secretions Dry mouth, dry mucous membranes ↓ laryngospasm precipitated by secretions
GI (stomach, intestines)	↑ peristalsis (↑ tone, ↑ strength of contractions) ↑ secretions	↓ peristalsis (↓ tone, ↓ strength of contractions ↓ secretions) (uses: antispasmodic, ↓ acid secretions)
Genitourinary	↑ ureter peristalsis ↑ voiding pressure ↑ bladder (detrusor muscle) contractions	↓ peristalsis ↓ voiding pressure ↓ bladder contractions
Ophthalmologic	Miosis	Mydriasis, cycloplegia
Sweat glands (sympathetic cholinergic innervation)	↑ sweating	↓ sweating (hot dry skin)
CNS	Cortical arousal response	Restlessness Irritability
Toxic doses	Severe bradycardia Asystole	Respiratory failure Circulatory collapse (if toxic dose)
Treatment of overdose	Atropine (epinephrine for bronchospasm)	Physostigmine (for central effects) Neostigmine (for peripheral effect)
Glands: lacrimal, salivary, digestive, exocrine sweat glands, tracheobronchial	↑ secretion (↑ sweating)	↓ secretion (↓ sweating)

*Acetylcholine (cholinergic neurotransmitter) or parasympathomimetics; antimuscarinic: parasympatholytics atropine and glycopyrrolate.

CLINICAL EFFECTS OF MUSCARINIC RECEPTOR ANTAGONISTS (ANTIMUSCARINIC AGENTS ATROPINE AND GLYCOPYRROLATE)

Atropine and its analogs, including glycopyrrolate, block the muscarinic actions of Ach (or parasympathetic stimulation) by competitively occupying muscarinic receptor sites on the autonomic effector cells and ganglion cells.[13] Other drugs block Ach's nicotinic effects: competitive blocking agents (e.g., curare and pancuronium) block

Ach at the skeletal muscle's neuromuscular junction and trimethaphan blocks Ach at autonomic ganglia[10] (Table 15-2).

Various subtypes of muscarinic receptors have been identified.[4] This holds promise for the future development of drugs that act on a specific subtype of muscarinic receptor(s) which would narrow the effects of a given drug thereby limiting the drug's side effects.[4]

The muscarinic receptor antagonists, atropine and glycopyrrolate, are used in anesthesia as preoperative antimuscarinics to decrease secretions in the respiratory

Table 15-3. Commonly Used Drugs: Muscarinic Receptor Agonists and Antagonists

Muscarinic (Acetylcholine) Receptor Agonists	Muscarinic (Acetylcholine) Receptor Antagonists
Mimic actions of acetylcholine or parasympathetics or vagal nerve stimulation at muscarinic receptors	Blocks actions of acetylcholine, parasympathomimetics, or vagal nerve stimulation at muscarinic receptors
Acetylcholine	Naturally occurring alkaloids (from belladonna plants, nightshade plant):
Natural alkaloids:	Atropine
Pilocarpine	Scopolamine
Arecoline	Semisynthetic analog:
Muscarine	Glycopyrrolate
Cholinomimetic choline esters:	Synthetic analogs:
Methacholine	Homatropine
Carbachol	Ipratropium
Bethanechol	Tiotropium
Urecholine	Pirenzepine
Side effects:	Tolterodine
Hypotension	Tropicamide
Wheezing	Clinical uses:
Sweating	Atropine–
Flushing	Abolishes reflex vagal HR slowing/asystole
Abdominal cramps	Causes bronchodilation
Visual disturbance	$\downarrow$ tracheobronchial secretions ($\downarrow$ occurrence of laryngospasm)
Problem with accommodation	
Headache	Antispasmodic agent
Salivation	Ipratropium/Tiotropium–
Contraindications:	Aerosols for treatment of bronchospasm with asthma/COPD
Asthma (precipitates bronchospasm)	
Hyperthyroidism (precipitates atrial fibrillation)	Glycopyrrolate
Coronary insufficiency	$\downarrow$ tracheobronchial secretions
Hypotension ($\downarrow$ coronary blood flow)	Blocks vagal effects on heart/respiratory tract
Aulcer disease ($\uparrow$ acid secretions)	$\downarrow$ GI motility
Clinical uses:	Belladonna alkaloids/synthetic derivatives
Bethanechol	Treat diarrhea, diseases with $\uparrow$ GI motility, Parkinson's disease
$\uparrow$ GI peristalsis, used in gastroparesis, gastric atony, others	
	Ophthalmic preparations (atropine, homatropine)
Urecholine–	
$\uparrow$ emptying of bladder in neurogenic bladder	Causes mydriasis (pupillary dilation for eye examination)
Methacholine–	
Causes bronchoconstriction, used to cause wheezing to test for asthma	Antihistamines
	Antimuscarinic effect—$\downarrow$ nasal secretions, drying effect of cold remedies
Pilocarpine–	
Causes constriction of pupils, used in ophthalmology, treatment of xerostomia	Scopolamine–
	Prevents motion sickness
	Benztropine–
	Treat dystonia from antipsychotic drugs
	Atropine as an antidote–
	Treat anticholinesterase organophosphate poisoning/certain mushroom poisonings, antagonizes parasympathomimetic effects of neostigmine/other anticholinesterase agents

(Continued)

Table 15-3. Commonly Used Drugs: Muscarinic Receptor Agonists and Antagonists (*Continued*)

Muscarinic (Acetylcholine) Receptor Agonists	Muscarinic (Acetylcholine) Receptor Antagonists
	Side effects
	Visual disturbance (from pupil dilatation)
	Dry mouth
	Drowsiness
	↓ sweating
	Central anticholinergic syndrome (with atropine but not glycopyrrolate)
	Contraindications
	Ileus, megacolon, GI obstruction
	Myasthenia gravis
	Heat stroke
	↓ sweating lead to ↑ temperature
	Glaucoma
	Obstructive uropathy

COPD: chronic obstructive pulmonary disease

tract and salivary glands, to decrease gastric secretions, and to block the cardiac vagal reflexes (especially the bradycardia and hypotension) that occur during intubation and the induction of anesthesia. They are also coadministered with ketamine to decrease tracheobronchial secretions, which has been associated with the occurrence of laryngospasm.[14] Their use as an antisialagogue improves conditions for intubation.[1,2,15]

Atropine is a standard ACLS drug used to increase the heart rate.[16–18] It is indicated for the treatment of symptomatic bradycardia, high nodal AV block, and cardiac arrest associated with asystole or pulseless electrical activity.[16–18] The increase in heart rate is due to a vagolytic effect. In patients with a denervated heart (e.g., heart transplant patients) atropine loses its positive chronotropic effect.

The antimuscarinics, atropine and glycopyrrolate, are used prior to some airway procedures as they enhance topical anesthesia by providing better mucosal contact with local anesthetic agents and decreasing the dilution of local anesthetics by saliva.[2]

Atropine and glycopyrrolate also cause dilatation of the pupils, decreased motility of the GI and urinary tract, and inhibit gastric acid secretion.[7,13] These anticholinergic effects are dose-related[4] (Table 15-2). As such, they have been used as antispasmodics to treat pylorospasm and other GI spasmodic conditions.[4] In the past, atropine was used to treat biliary and ureteral colic and to inhibit gastric

acid secretions, but newer drugs have replaced it for these indications.[4] (Table 15-3).

CONTRAINDICATIONS AND SIDE EFFECTS OF MUSCARINIC RECEPTOR ANTAGONISTS: ATROPINE AND GLYCOPYRROLATE

Contraindications to atropine and glycopyrrolate include a known hypersensitivity to the drug, glaucoma, obstructive GI disease (such as ileus or toxic megacolon), obstructive uropathy (as with bladder neck obstruction from prostatic hypertrophy), and myasthenia gravis.[19,20]

Tachycardia (by causing increased myocardial oxygen demand) may aggravate the condition of patients with disorders such as ischemic heart disease or congestive heart failure, particularly if they are also exhibiting any tachydysrhythmia or significant tachycardia.[19,20] Therefore, the muscarinic receptor antagonists should be used with caution in such patients. There is concern that decreased bronchial secretions occurring with the muscarinic receptor antagonists may lead to inspissated mucous plugs in some patients such as those with COPD. Other patients in whom atropine should be used with caution include those with hyperthyroidism, autonomic neuropathy, prostatic hypertrophy, and renal disease.[19,20] As with many medications, the antimuscarinics should be used with caution in children with special health care needs and the elderly.[19,20]

OVERDOSE/TOXICITY WITH MUSCARINIC RECEPTOR ANTAGONISTS: ATROPINE/ GLYCOPYRROLATE

Overdosage, whether intentional or accidental, can lead to blurred vision, dilated pupils, photophobia, dry mouth, nausea, vomiting, abdominal distention, fever (due to decreased sweating), and urgency/difficulty with urination.[8,21] Cardiovascular symptoms may include tachycardia, weak pulse, hypertension, and circulatory failure.[4]

In addition to the peripheral side effects/toxicity noted above, central CNS side effects and toxicity with atropine can include signs/symptoms of CNS stimulation: restlessness, dizziness, headache, drowsiness, delirium, stupor, tremor, seizures, ataxia, hallucinations, psychosis, and coma. With large doses, nicotinic receptor blockade can possibly occur causing a curare-like effect with neuromuscular weakness and paralysis. Central anticholinergic syndrome can occur with atropine since it crosses the blood barrier.[21] It is an acute psychosis or delirium due to inhibition of central cholinergic transmission.[8]

Since glycopyrrolate is a quaternary ammonium compound and has limited passage across lipid membranes including the blood-brain barrier, the occurrence of CNS side effects/toxicity is lower compared to atropine and other anticholinergics, which are tertiary amines that readily pass across the blood-brain barrier.

TREATMENT OF ATROPINE OR GLYCOPYRROLATE OVERDOSE

The usual supportive and symptomatic therapy, as with any overdose, is indicated. For atropine overdose, physostigmine 1–3 mg intravenously (IV) has been used to treat the central CNS symptoms, but its use is controversial.[3,8] The occurrence of bradycardia, asystole, and seizures has been reported. To reverse the peripheral anticholinergic effects of atropine or glycopyrrolate, neostigmine can be used, but its use is also controversial. Neostigmine does not cross the blood-brain barrier. The dose in adults is 0.25 mg IV repeated every 5–10 minutes to a maximum of 2.5 mg or until the excessive anticholinergic activity is reversed.[3,8]

DRUG DOSE: ATROPINE

The dose of atropine varies depending on its indication. Atropine or glycopyrrolate and ketamine are compatible and can be mixed. It is recommended by some to give atropine or glycopyrrolate with ketamine intramuscular (IM) in the same syringe to avoid two IM injections instead of one.[22]

Although because of different pharmacodynamics including onset, this is illogical because ketamine's effect may occur before the antimuscarinic agent.

Atropine is indicated for various dysrhythmias. It is the drug of choice for symptomatic sinus bradycardia (class I) and is a class IIa drug for second-degree heart block (Mobitz type I or Wenckebach). It is a second line drug (after epinephrine or vasopressin) for asystole or pulseless electrical activity (class indeterminate) and it is a class II drug for infranodal second-degree heart block Mobitz type II.[16–18] For asystole or pulseless electrical activity, the dose in adults is 1 mg IV every 3–5 minutes to a maximum of 0.03–0.04 mg/kg (or in a 70-kg adult, about 2.1–2.8 mg maximum). The bradycardia dose in adults is 0.5–1 mg IV every 3–5 minutes up to a maximum of 0.04 mg/kg.[3,16] For tracheal administration 2–3 mg is diluted in 10 cc normal saline.

The pediatric dose is usually 0.01–0.02 mg/kg up with a minimum dose of 0.1 mg and a maximum dose of 1 mg. A minimum dose of atropine is recommended in order to avoid paradoxical bradycardia.[13,17] As with adults, higher doses are used when atropine is used as an antidote for cholinergic crisis with an initial dose of 1 mg IV/IM followed by 0.5–1 mg every 5–10 minutes until muscarinic symptoms resolve or signs of atropine toxicity occur.

Atropine is also used as an antidote for significant organophosphate poisoning. Since atropine is a competitive antagonist of Ach or a cholinergic blocker of Ach at its CNS and peripheral muscarinic receptors, it is used to reverse the effects of excessive parasympathetic stimulation caused by the organophosphates.

Organophosphate compounds can be used as nerve agents. Atropine is recommended drug therapy for various nerve agent exposures, whether by an inhalational or dermal route of exposure.

DRUG DOSE: GLYCOPYRROLATE

When given with ketamine for its antisialagogue effect the dose is the same as atropine, 0.01 mg/kg.[20,23] The doses to reverse vagal-induced bradycardia and prevent the bradycardia associated with the reversal of neuromuscular blockade are approximately one-half of that used for atropine.[20] It has also been given in adults for peptic ulcer disease in a 0.1 mg dose.

In pediatric patients, the dose is 0.01 mg/kg in children (age 1 month to 12 years) and occasionally younger children (1 month to 2 years) may require a higher dose, 0.02 mg/kg.

PREGNANCY CATEGORY

Both atropine and glycopyrrolate are pregnancy category B drugs.[19,20]

WHICH PREMEDICATION: ATROPINE OR GLYCOPYRROLATE?

Glycopyrrolate does not cross the blood-brain barrier, so the CNS side effects that can occur with atropine (or scopolamine) are avoided.[8] Glycopyrrolate also produces a more gradual increase in heart rate and a lower peak heart rate than an equipotent dose of atropine. There is also a decreased incidence of dysrhythmias.

Atropine when given with ketamine has been reported to increase the frequency of unpleasant dreams compared to ketamine alone, suggested to be because of its CNS effects,[24] though others have disputed this finding.[25] There is conflicting evidence regarding which antimuscarinic, atropine, or glycopyrrolate has a lesser incidence of nausea and vomiting.[26]

Central anticholinergic syndrome is a rare but serious complication that can occur with the use of the naturally occurring muscarinic receptor antagonists, atropine, and scopolamine, which are alkaloids from the belladonna plants.[1,27] The hallmarks of the central anticholinergic syndrome are restlessness, confusion, delirium, and obtundation.[1] Although it is more frequent when scopolamine is used, the syndrome can also occur when large doses (>2 mg) of atropine are administered.[1] Patients with increased susceptibility to central anticholinergic syndrome are those who are experiencing pain and are geriatric.[1] The use of physostigmine in the management of this syndrome has been recommended by some clinicians. Since glycopyrrolate does not cross the blood-brain barrier, this syndrome is not a concern when glycopyrrolate is used.

Because of its use as an ACLS drug, emergency physicians probably are more familiar with atropine than glycopyrrolate. Some experts prefer glycopyrrolate because it has greater antisialagogue effects and fewer side effects: less tachycardia, fewer dysrhythmias, and lack of CNS side effects such as the central anticholinergic syndrome.[28]

SUMMARY

The muscarinic receptor antagonists, atropine and glycopyrrolate, have widespread effects throughout the body including tachycardia, bronchodilation, dry mouth, and decreased GI/genitourinary peristalsis. Glycopyrrolate is preferred over atropine by some because it has a greater antisialagogue effect and fewer cardiac/CNS side effects.

REFERENCES

1. Porter BR, Gomez MN. Premedication. In: Longnecker DE, Tinker JH, Morgan GE Jr, eds. *Principles and Practice of Anesthesiology.* St. Louis, MO: Mosby; 1998:52–72.
2. Gal TJ. Airway management. In: Miller RD, ed. *Miller's Anesthesia.* Philadelphia, PA: Elsevier Churchill Livingstone; 2005:1617–1652.
3. Clements EA, Kuhn BR. Pharmacology of antidysrhythmic and vasoactive medications. In: Tintinalli JE, Kelen GD, Stapczynski JS, eds. *Emergency Medicine. A Comprehensive Study Guide.* New York: McGraw-Hill; 2004:203–218.
4. Brown JH, Taylor P. Muscarinic receptor agonists and antagonists. In: Hardman JG, Limbird LE, Gilman AG, eds. *Goodman and Gilman's The Pharmacological Basis of Therapeutics.* New York: McGraw-Hill; 2001:155–174.
5. Delaney KA. Anticholinergics. In: Marx JA, Hockberger RS, Walls RM, et al, eds. *Rosen's Emergency Medicine Concepts and Clinical Practice.* St. Louis, MO: Mosby; 2002:2080–2087.
6. Parenteau AR, Maktabi MA. Basic physiology and pharmacology of the autonomic nervous system. In: Longnecker DE, Tinker JH, Morgan GE Jr, eds. *Principles and Practice of Anesthesiology.* St. Louis, MO: Mosby; 1998:721–754.
7. The autonomic nervous system and its central control. In: Berne RM, Levy MN, Koeppen BM, et al, eds. *Physiology.* St. Louis, MO: Mosby; 2004:206–220.
8. Kirk MA. Anticholinergics and antihistamines. In: Haddad LM, Shannon MW, Winchester JF, eds. *Clinical Management of Poisoning and Drug Overdose.* Philadelphia, PA: W.B. Saunders; 1998:641–649.
9. Wax PM. Anticholinergic toxicity. In: Tintinalli JE, Kelen GD, Stapczynski JS, eds. *Emergency Medicine A Comprehensive Study Guide.* New York: McGraw-Hill; 2004:1143–1145.
10. Taylor P. Agents acting at the neuromuscular junction and autonomic ganglia. In: Hardman JG, Limbird LE, Gilman AG, eds. *Goodman and Gilman's The Pharmacologic Basis of Therapeutics.* New York: McGraw-Hill; 2001:193–214.
11. Pino RM, Basta SJ. Pharmacology of neuromuscular blocking drugs. In: Longnecker DE, Tinker JH, Morgan GE Jr, eds. *Principles and Practice of Anesthesiology.* St. Louis, MO: Mosby; 1998:765–790.
12. Haspel KL, Ali HH. Physiology of neuromuscular transmission and mechanism of action of neuromuscular blocking agents. In: Longnecker DE, Tinker JH, Morgan GE Jr, eds. *Principles and Practice of Anesthesiology.* St. Louis, MO: Mosby; 1998:755–764.
13. Moss J, Glick D. The autonomic nervous system. In: Miller RD, ed. *Miller's Anesthesia.* Philadelphia, PA: Elsevier Churchill Livingstone; 2005:617–677.
14. Cunningham SJ, Crain EF. Conscious sedation. In: Henretig FM, King C, eds. *Textbook of Pediatric Emergency Procedures.* Baltimore, MD: Williams & Wilkins; 1997:445–454.
15. Brookman CA, The HP, Morrison LM. Anticholinergics improve fiberoptic–intubating conditions during general anesthesia. *Can J Anaesth.* 1997;44:165–167.

16. Pharmacology 2: agents for control of rate and rhythm. In: Cummins RO, Field JM, Hazinski MF, eds. *ACLS: Principles and Practice*. Dallas, TX: American Heart Association; 2003:239–259.

17. Rhythm disturbances. In: Hazinski MF, Zaritsky AL, Nadkarni VM, et al. *PALS Provider Manual*. Dallas, TX: American Heart Association; 2002:185–228.

18. ACLS drugs, cardioversion, defibrillation, and pacing. In: Cummins RD, Field JM, Hazinski MF, eds. *ACLS Provider Manual*. Dallas, TX: American Heart Association; 2002: 285–299.

19. Atropine. Stat: REF Online Electronic Medical Library [database online]. *Mosby's Drug Consult*. 14th ed. 2004. Section II—Drug Information.

20. Glycopyrrolate. Stat: REF Online. Electronic Medical Library [database on line]. *Mosby's Drug Consult*. 14th ed. 2004. Section II—Drug Information.

21. Sutin KM, Kaufman B. Neuromuscular blocking agents. In: Goldfrank LR, Flomenbaum NE, Lewin NA, et al, eds. *Goldfrank's Toxicologic Emergencies*. New York: McGraw-Hill; 2002:806–823.

22. Chudnofsky CR, Lozon MM. Sedation and analgesia for procedures. In: Marx JA, Hockberger RS, Walls RM, et al, eds. *Rosen's Emergency Medicine Concepts and Clinical Practice*. St. Louis, MO: Mosby; 2002:2577–2590.

23. Johnson MN, Liebelt EL. Acute pain management and procedural sedation in children. In: Tintinalli JE, Kelen GD, Stapczynski JS, eds. *Emergency Medicine. A Comprehensive Study Guide*. New York: McGraw-Hill; 2000:858–869.

24. Bovill JG, Dundee JW, Coppel DL, et al. Current status of ketamine anaesthesia. *Lancet*. 1971;1:1285–1288.

25. Mogensen F, Muller D, Valentin D. Glycopyrrolate during ketamine/diazepam. Anaesthesia. *Acta Anaesthesiol Scand*. 1986;30:332–336.

26. Nelskyla K, li-Hankala A, Soikkeli A, et al. Neostigmine with glycopyrrolate does not increase the incidence or severity of postoperative nausea and vomiting in outpatients undergoing gynecological laparoscopy. *Br J Anaesth*. 1998; 81:757–760.

27. Brown DV, Heller F, Barkin R. Anticholinergic syndrome after anesthesia: a case report and review. *Am J Ther*. 2004;11:144–153.

28. Pruitt JW, Goldwasser MS, Sabol SR, et al. Intramuscular ketamine, midazolam, and glycopyrrolate for pediatric sedation in the emergency department. *J Oral Maxillofac Surg*. 1995;53:13–17.

16

Reversal Agents

Michael F. Murphy

HIGH YIELD FACTS

- Opiates are drugs derived from opium (natural: morphine, codeine or semisynthetic: heroin, hydrocodeine, hydromorphone).
- Opioids are compounds related to opium (natural, semisynthetic, synthetic, or endogenous: enkephalins, endophorins, dynorphins).
- Opioids are substances that interact with opioid receptors (agonists, antagonists, agonist/antagonists). There are three opioid receptors: mu (μ), kappa (κ), delta (δ).
- Mu agonism causes supraspinal/spinal analgesia, euphoria δ a, respiratory depression, physical dependence, ↓ gut motility. Kappa agonism causes spinal/supraspinal analgesia, dysphoria. Delta agonism causes spinal analgesia.
- Antagonists can be pure antagonists (for all three receptors) (e.g., naloxone and naltrexone); agonist/antagonists: antagonistic at μ receptors, agonist at κ receptors (e.g., nalbuphine and nalorphine); partial agonist at μ receptor, full agonist at κ receptors (e.g., butorphanol and pentazocine).
- Naloxone is used to reverse μ receptor overstimulation (respiratory depression, sedation) from opioids.
- The benzodiazepine receptor antagonist, flumazenil, antagonizes the actions of benzodiazepines at the γ-aminobutyric acid (GABA)$_A$ receptor.
- Flumazenil is indicated for uncomplicated iatrogenic benzodiazepine overdose in adults if no chronic benzodiazepine use, no seizure history, and no tricyclic overdose.

OPIOID RECEPTOR ANTAGONISTS

Overview and Definitions

Neither the term *opiate* nor *opioid* is particularly specific. Opiates are drugs that are derived from opium, including natural substances such as morphine and codeine, and the semisynthetic agents derived from them, such as heroin, hydrocodone, hydromorphone, and thebaine (precursor to oxycodone and naloxone).[1]

Opioid is a general term that is applied to all compounds related to opium whether endogenous (e.g., enkephalins, endorphins, and dynorphins), natural, semisynthetic, or synthetic in origin. The synthetic agents include such drugs as the piperadine derivatives (meperidine, fentanyl, sufentanyl, and so forth), pentazocine, nalbuphine, butorphanol, and others. Perhaps more specifically, the term opioid is applied to all substances that interact with opioid receptors (agonists, antagonists, and agonist/antagonists).

Opioid Receptors and Antagonism

To understand opioid *receptor* antagonists, one must understand opioid receptors. Three opioid receptor types are classically described: mu (μ), kappa (κ) and delta (δ). Though this tends to oversimplify the situation, it is useful for discussion. Mu receptor agonism produces supraspinal and spinal analgesia, euphoria, respiratory depression, physical dependence, and decreased gut motility. Kappa agonism also produces spinal and supraspinal analgesia, but dysphoria as opposed to euphoria. Delta agonism produces spinal analgesia.[2]

Morphine, hydromorphone, meperidine, fentanyl, and most other clinically useful opioid analgesics are μ receptor agonists. They also produce euphoria and a sense of well-being. Kappa receptor agonists produce analgesia mediated primarily at spinal sites, result in less respiratory depression, and produce dysphoric and psychotomimetic effects. Butorphanol, pentazocine, and nalbuphine are predominantly κ receptor agonists. While δ receptor agonists are potent analgesics, most of the currently available agents are peptides (such as the endogenous endorphins and enkephalins) and do not cross the blood-brain barrier, so to be effective they require intraspinal injection.

This chapter deals with opioid receptor antagonists rather than opioid receptor agonists, which are discussed in detail in Chapter 14. Opioid receptors do not ordinarily have a baseline level of agonism or antagonism. Thus the administration of a receptor antagonist has little effect. However, when endogenous opioid systems are activated, such as in shock or other forms of stress, or exogenous receptor agonists have been administered, there may be perceptible consequences.

Antagonists may:

- Be *pure* antagonists, i.e., for all receptor subtypes (e.g., naloxone and naltrexone).

- Be antagonistic at μ receptors and agonistic at κ receptors (e.g., nalbuphine and nalorphine). These medications are called agonist/antagonists, and as might be expected, tend to produce a degree of dysphoria, moreso when endogenously or exogenously-induced μ receptors agonism exists.

- Be partial agonists at μ receptors and fully agonistic at κ receptors (e.g., butorphanol and pentazocine). These agents act like agonist/antagonists when the patient already has a pure μ receptor on board or the endogenous opioid system is activated due to the competition they establish for the μ receptor.

By and large, opioid antagonists are produced by altering the structure of an opioid agonist in a minor way. Examples are minor chemical substitutions to change morphine to nalorphine, and oxymorphone to naloxone and naltrexone.

Pharmacologic Properties

Naloxone: Although this medication is absorbed readily from the gastrointestinal (GI) tract, it is almost completely metabolized by the liver before reaching the systemic circulation. For this reason it is ordinarily given intravenously. Though the half-life is about 1 hour, the clinically effective duration of action may be much less. Virtually all of the opioids of abuse and used clinically have longer elimination half-lives than naloxone, explaining why an infusion of naloxone is ordinarily required in overdose situation. The hourly dose of naloxone by infusion is two-thirds of the dose required to reverse the respiratory depression, titrated as required.[2]

Naltrexone: It retains more of its efficacy when given orally reaching peak plasma concentrations within 1–2 hours. The half-life is approximately 3 hours and the duration of action approaches 24 hours.

Alvimopan: It is a novel, peripherally restricted, opioid antagonist that after oral administration has activity specific to the GI tract. It has low systemic absorption and a high affinity for gut μ opioid receptors. There is little information available regarding the pharmacokinetics of this medication.

Methylnaltrexone: It is a quaternary opioid antagonist with a limited ability to cross the blood-brain barrier. Pharmacokinetic analysis reveals an elimination half-life

of 117.5 minutes ($\pm$53.2), and a clearance of 38.8 L/h ($\pm$17.4) with a methylnaltrexone dose of 0.64 mg/kg.

Clinical Uses

The clinical use of an antagonist or agonist/antagonist is dependent on several factors including the following:

- The degree to which endogenous opioid systems have been activated.

- The opioid receptor-specific profile of any exogenous opioid that has been administered.

- The opioid receptor-specific profile of the agonist/antagonist to be administered.

- The degree to which physical dependence on an opioid has occurred.

Like any other receptor system, agonists and antagonists compete for the receptor. Among agonists, some are more potent than others, thus if a weak μ receptor agonist (e.g., pentazocine) is administered to a patient already taking a potent μ receptor agonist, the result will be attenuated analgesia, euphoria, and a feeling of well-being; interpreted by the patient as unpleasant and the patient will be displeased at the result. However, if this same medication (in this case, pentazocine) is administered to a μ receptor naive patient in pain, μ receptor stimulation will produce analgesia and the patient will be grateful.

This competition for receptors explains why naloxone can be titrated in small amounts (0.1 mg/dose) to reverse some undesirable effects of μ receptor over stimulation (e.g., respiratory depression and sedation) while preserving the analgesic effects, or avoid precipitating an overt opioid withdrawal syndrome in a physically opioid-dependent patient suffering a respiratory arrest from an opioid overdose.

Opioid receptor antagonists and agonist/antagonists have been studied in a variety of conditions where the mobilization of endogenous opioids is thought to occur with potentially deleterious results including the following:

Shock: There is some evidence that endogenous opioid peptides play a role in the pathophysiology of shock and that naloxone may play a role in treatment. While naloxone has been shown to improve blood pressure it is not clear that outcome is improved.[3]

Opioid-induced ileus, post-operative ileus, and perhaps irritable bowel syndrome: The peripheral μ receptor antagonists, alvimopan and methylnaltrexone, have shown promise in the management of these very difficult conditions. These agents have been shown in healthy subjects to antagonize loperamide-induced changes in GI transit and prevent morphine-induced delays in oral-cecal transit time without antagonizing centrally mediated opioid effects, such as analgesia or pupillary constriction. In the treatment of opioid-naive patients who underwent surgery and received opioids for acute pain, these agents improved the management of postoperative ileus by shortening the time to achieve normal bowel function and, ultimately, hospital stay.[4–10]

Alcoholism: It is generally felt that ethanol increases opioid neurotransmission and that this activation may reinforce the positive drive to imbibe excessively. Opioid antagonists have been studied to determine if they antagonize this positive reinforcement and reduce the drive to drink. Results have been conflicting.[11–14]

Opioid dependence: The agonist/antagonist buprenorphine and the antagonist naltrexone have both been studied in the treatment of opioid dependence. Buprenorphine, a partial agonist at the μ receptor and an antagonist at the κ receptor, produces typical morphine-like effects at low doses. At higher doses, it produces opiate effects that are less than those of full opiate agonists. Subutex and suboxone are the Food and Drug Administration (FDA)-approved formulations of buprenorphine for treatment of opiate dependence. Suboxone contains a mixture of buprenorphine and naloxone. The naloxone is poorly absorbed sublingually and is designed to discourage intravenous use. Subutex, buprenorphine only, is intended to be used primarily as an initial test dose.[15–20]

BENZODIAZEPINE RECEPTOR ANTAGONIST: FLUMAZENIL

Specific subunits of the γ-aminobutyric acid $(GABA)_A$ receptor are responsible for the specific pharmacologic properties of the benzodiazepines. Flumazenil antagonizes the action of benzodiazepines at this receptor.[21–28]

Pharmacologic Properties

Flumazenil is only available for intravenous administration owing to an extensive first pass hepatic metabolism if taken orally. Like naloxone, it has a half-life of approximately 1 hour, and the duration of clinical effect is only 30–60 minutes.[28]

Clinical Uses

The primary indication for flumazenil is iatrogenic overdose of a benzodiazepine (usually in the setting of procedural sedation) in a patient who is not benzodiazepine habituated. It is generally felt that individuals who overdose on benzodiazepines are those that are on them chronically and perhaps have developed physical dependence raising the specter of inducing status seizures and death should flumazenil be administered in this setting.[29] This is of particular concern if tricyclic antidepressants have also been taken. Having said this, in a monitored setting, adults who have overdosed that meet low-risk criteria for flumazenil administration *may* be treated. These low-risk criteria include the following[30]:

- Clinical picture compatible with an uncomplicated benzodiazepine overdose.
- Absence of findings suggestive of tricyclic antidepressant overdose (e.g., anticholinergic signs and electrocardiogram [ECG] findings).
- History negative for a seizure disorder.
- History negative for long-term benzodiazepine use.

The dose of flumazenil is 0.5–5 mg (0.005–0.2 mg/kg in children) infused over 3–5 minutes in a titrated fashion (0.1 mg/dose). Because of its short half-life compared to virtually all benzodiazepines a continuous infusion of 0.1–0.3 mg/kg/h[31] is recommended.

Several trials have assessed flumazenil in patients suffering from hepatic encephalopathy with conflicting results. Flumazenil has not been shown to significantly impact recovery or survival from hepatic encephalopathy, though in cirrhosis patients with a favorable prognosis it has been demonstrated to produce short-term improvement in hepatic encephalopathy. Because of the fluctuating nature of hepatic encephalopathy, future trials will need to determine if treatment with flumazenil leads to a sustained improvement and improved recovery and survival.[32]

Positron emission tomography (PET) has an established role in the noninvasive localization of epileptic foci during presurgical evaluation. 11C Flumazenil, used as a tracer, has been used to enhance image neurotransmission related to γ-aminobutyric acid and pinpoint epileptogenic foci.[33]

REFERENCES

1. Gutstein HB, Akil H. Opioid analgesics. In: Hardman JG, Limbird LE, Gilman AG, eds. *Goodman and Gilman's The Pharmacologic Basis of Therapeutics.* 10th ed. New York: McGraw-Hill; 2001:569–619.
2. Kleinschmidt KC, Wainscott M, Ford M. Opioids. In:Ford M, Delaney KA, Ling LJ, et al, eds. *Clinical Toxicology.* Philadelphia, PA: W.B. Saunders; 2001:627–639.
3. Boeuf B, Poirier V, Gauvin F, et al. Naloxone for shock. *Cochrane Database Syst Rev.* 2003(4):CD004443.
4. Cremonini F, Talley NJ. Diagnostic and therapeutic strategies in the irritable bowel syndrome. *Minerva Med.* 2004;95:427–441.

5. Greenwood-Van Meerveld B, Gardner CJ, et al. Preclinical studies of opioids and opioid antagonists on gastrointestinal function. *Neurogastroenterol Motil.* 2004;16(Suppl 2): 46–53.

6. Yuan CS. Clinical status of methylnaltrexone, a new agent to prevent and manage opioid-induced side effects. *J Support Oncol.* 2004;2:111–117.

7. Tamayo AC, Diaz-Zuluaga PA. Management of opioid-induced bowel dysfunction in cancer patients. *Support Care Cancer* [Epub]. 2004;19.

8. Holte K, Kehlet H. Postoperative ileus: progress towards effective management. *Drugs.* 2002;62:2603–2615.

9. Azodo IA, Ehrenpreis ED. Alvimopan (Adolor/ GlaxoSmithKline). *Curr Opin Investig Drugs.* 2002;3:1496– 1501.

10. Kurz A, Sessler DI. Opioid-induced bowel dysfunction: pathophysiology and potential new therapies. *Drugs.* 2003; 63:649–671.

11. Anton RF, Pettinati H, Zweben A, et al. A multi-site dose ranging study of nalmefene in the treatment of alcohol dependence. *J Clin Psychopharmacol.* 2004;24:421–428.

12. Rohsenow DJ. What place does naltrexone have in the treatment of alcoholism? *CNS Drugs.* 2004;18:547–560.

13. Mann K. Pharmacotherapy of alcohol dependence: a review of the clinical data. *CNS Drugs.* 2004;18:485–504.

14. Oswald LM, Wand GS. Opioids and alcoholism. *Physiol Behav.* 2004;81:339–358.

15. Sporer KA. Buprenorphine: a primer for emergency physicians. *Ann Emerg Med.* 2004;43:580–584.

16. Comer VG, Annitto WJ. Buprenorphine: a safe method for detoxifying pregnant heroin addicts and their unborn. *Am J Addict.* 2004;13:317–318.

17. Doran CM, Shanahan M, Bell J, et al. A cost-effectiveness analysis of buprenorphine-assisted heroin withdrawal. *Drug Alcohol Rev.* 2004;23:171–175.

18. Martin J. Evolving use of buprenorphine in the treatment of addiction. *J Psychoactive Drugs.* 2004;(Suppl 2):129–137.

19. Wesson DR. Buprenorphine in the treatment of opiate dependence: its pharmacology and social context of use in the *U.S. J Psychoactive Drugs.* 2004;(Suppl 2):119–128.

20. Rea F, Bell JR, Young MR, et al. A randomised, controlled trial of low dose naltrexone for the treatment of opioid dependence. *Drug Alcohol Depend.* 2004;75:79–88.

21. Seger DL. Flumazenil—treatment or toxin. *J Toxicol Clin Toxicol.* 2004;42:209–216.

22. Als-Nielsen B, Kjaergard LL, Gluud C. Benzodiazepine receptor antagonists for acute and chronic hepatic encephalopathy. *Cochrane Database Syst Rev.* 2001(4):CD002798.

23. Proudfoot AT. Antidotes: benefits and risks. *Toxicol Lett.* 1995;82–83:779–783.

24. Hoffman RS, Goldfrank LR. The poisoned patient with altered consciousness. Controversies in the use of a 'coma cocktail.' *JAMA.* 1995;274:562–569.

25. McDuffee AT, Tobias JD. Seizure after flumazenil administration in a pediatric patient. *Pediatr Emerg Care.* 1995;11: 186–187.

26. McCloy RF. Reversal of conscious sedation by flumazenil: current status and future prospects. *Acta Anaesthesiol Scand Suppl.* 1995;108:35–42.

27. Whitwam JG, Amrein R. Pharmacology of flumazenil. *Acta Anaesthesiol Scand Suppl.* 1995;108:3–14.

28. Charney DS, Mihic SJ, Harris RA. Hypnotics and sedatives. In: Hardman JG, Limbird LE, Gilman AG, eds. *Goodman and Gilman's The Pharmacologic Basis of Therapeutics.* 10th ed.. New York: McGraw-Hill; 2001:399–427.

29. Seger DL. Flumazenil—treatment or toxin. *J Toxicol Clin Toxicol.* 2004;42:209–216.

30. Gueye PN, Hoffman JR, Taboulet P, et al. Empiric use of flumazenil in comatose patients: limited applicability of criteria to define low risk. *Ann Emerg Med.* 1996;27: 730–735.

31. Farrell SE. Benzodiazepines. In: Ford M, Delaney KA, Ling LJ, et al, eds. *Clinical Toxicology.* Philadelphia, PA: W.B. Saunders; 2001:575–581.

32. Als-Nielsen B, Gluud LL, Gluud C. Benzodiazepine receptor antagonists for hepatic encephalopathy. *Cochrane Database Syst Rev.* 2004(2):CD002798.

33. Juhasz C, Chugani HT. Imaging the epileptic brain with positron emission tomography. *Neuroimaging Clin N Am.* 2003;13:705–716.

Part 2: AGENTS FOR PROCEDURAL SEDATION (SEDATIVE DRUGS)

17

Propofol

Sharon E. Mace

HIGH YIELD FACTS

- Propofol has negative cardiovascular effects that are dose and rate of administration dependent: vasodilatation, bradyarrhythmias, and negative inotrope. So, use cautiously in volume-depleted or hypotensive patients.

- Respiratory depression/apnea can occur especially if given in high dose, as a rapid bolus, or with other drugs such as opioids that can also be respiratory depressants.

- Neurologic events such as posturing, myoclonus, seizure-like activity, and seizures may be seen.

- Generally, geriatric patients (patients with reduced vital organ system reserve; see Chap. 8) require lower doses and pediatric patients require higher doses.

- Dosage does not have to be adjusted in patients with renal disease or liver disease.

- Avoid using propofol in patients with an egg, soybean, or EDTA allergy.

- Pain on injection is common.

- Bacterial contamination in the syringe following ampule violation can occur if allowed to stand for prolonged periods.

INDICATIONS

Propofol is used for procedural sedation, rapid sequence intubation (RSI), sedation after intubation, sedation in the intensive care unit (ICU) including benzodiazepine-resistant agitation, and for the induction/maintenance of general anesthesia.[1–7] It may be combined with ketamine or midazolam for procedural sedation.

PHARMACOLOGY

Propofol is an ultra-short-acting sedative hypnotic drug with no analgesic effect and a variable dose-dependent amnestic effect.[1–3] Propofol interacts with the γ-aminobutyric acid (GABA) receptor system and prolongs the duration of contact between GABA and its receptor site. This causes an extended influx of chloride into the neuron, resulting in hyperpolarization of the neuronal cell membrane.[8,9] Propofol is an alkyl phenol (2,6-diisopropylphenol)[10] that is rapidly metabolized by the liver to inactive forms via conjugation to glucuronides and sulfides, which are excreted by the kidneys. Extrahepatic metabolism probably does occur to a minor extent.[1,11–13] Table 17-1 contains dosage information and Table 17-2 contains administration information.

CLINICAL EFFECTS

Propofol has a very rapid onset and offset of action.[14–16] Sedation occurs within 1 minute of administration and recovery occurs within 5–15 minutes.[17–20] Propofol has a smooth recovery (e.g., rapid awakening with mental clearness).[3,20] Patients recover very quickly and can be discharged soon after completion of the surgery or procedure allowing for a fast turn around and rapid discharge.[21] Propofol also has antiemetic, and possibly euphoric properties.[15]

Cardiopulmonary depression can occur with propofol. Propofol has a relatively high incidence of respiratory depression including hypoventilation, upper airway obstruction, and apnea. With induction doses of propofol, apnea 30–60 seconds in duration occurs in 24% in adults and 10% of children, and apnea > 60 seconds, in 12% of adults and 5% of children.[22] Another study reported the incidence of apnea on induction to exceed 40%.[17]

The incidence of hypoxia varies depending on the definition of hypoxia or respiratory depression, the dose administered, and the type of patient/setting. In an emergency department (ED) setting when propofol was used for procedural sedation, oxygen desaturation (<93%) occurred in 11.6% of patients with no treatment required except supplemental oxygen.[23] Similar results with a 5–10% incidence of hypoxia were noted in two radiology studies using propofol for sedation of pediatric patients undergoing magnetic resonance imaging (MRI) scans.[24,25] In numerous studies of pediatric patients[26–37] and adults in the ED[38–41] undergoing procedural sedation with

Table 17-1. Propofol: Dosage Information

Dose (mg/kg)	Usual dose	Maximum dose	Onset (min)	Duration (min)
0.5–1.5 IV initially* followed by additional 0.5 IV * or continuous infusion 50–200 ug/kg/min	Difficult to estimate; probably close to 1.5–2 mg/kg	None	<1	8 (5–15) minutes

*Titrate to effect, avoid rapid IV push, use higher dose for rapid sequence intubation (RSI).

propofol, there were no instances where intubation was necessary and the incidence of bag mask ventilation (BMV) was low (≤2.5% in the pediatric patients[42] and 3.9% in the largest ED adult series).[38] One adult ED study found a higher incidence of respiratory depression, but this was a small series which included geriatric patients (mean patient age 62.5 years) who often had comorbid factors (valvular and/or ischemic heart disease).[40] In one critical care study where high doses of propofol were used, there was a 20% incidence of hypoxia with 19% of the patients needing assisted ventilation.[37] This may be an exception to the previously mentioned studies due to the higher doses of propofol administered, and the higher patient acuity and American Society of Anesthesiologists (ASA) status with increased comorbidity.[37]

The clinical evaluation of a medication such as propofol for respiratory depressant features is typically characterized by constructing a carbon dioxide response curve (Chap. 8); however, clinical studies involving these medications that are undertaken in practice situations need to consider several questions:

How is respiratory depression characterized?

- Hypoxia
- Hypercarbia
- Apnea
- Laryngospasm

What is the definition of a side effect or an adverse event and how is it measured?

- Respiratory frequency and subjective assessment of depth of respiration.
- By oxygen saturation and, if so, at what level: a pulse oximeter saturation <95 or 93 or 90%.
- By capnometry or capnography: a rise in $ETCO_2 \geq$ 10 mm or loss of waveform.

Table 17-2. Propofol: Administration Information

Practical Tips	Administration	Advantages	Side Effects/ Disadvantages
Used as antiemetic Used to treat refractory status epilepticus Lower doses in elderly Higher doses in pediatric patients Try the ketamine propofol combination	Check for allergies to eggs, soybean oil, EDTA ↓ pain on injection by giving with lidocaine in a larger vein, with premedication	Rapid onset/offset Smooth recovery, clearness Can use in patients with renal or liver disease (no dose change) Lesser incidence of myoclonus than etomidate Can be used in malignant hyperthermia patients	Causes cardiorespiratory depression Use with caution in hypotensive patients, shock, impaired cardiac function (consider NS bolus) Be ready to treat for hypoxia, apnea, bradycardia, hypotension Use with caution if increased intracranial pressure, pulmonary hypertension

Is it clinically significant?

- Respiratory system intervention required: (a) supplemental oxygen only, (b) sustained versus transient BMV, and (c) intubation.
- A brief hypotensive episode needing only a bolus of normal saline intravenously (IV).

What is the patient's age, overall condition, and comorbidity?

In general, patients at the extremes of age and those with a higher ASA class ought to be expected to display adverse events more frequently.[43–46]

What is the procedure being performed and could this affect the incidence of side effects or complications?

For example, bronchoscopy and other shared airway procedures typically lead to a higher frequency of adverse respiratory events including hypoxemia and laryngospasm.

The Miner study of propofol versus methohexital for procedural sedation in adult patients in an ED suggests that transient subclinical respiratory depression (as indicated by capnography) probably does occur in up to 49% of patients, although the incidence of hypoxia is much lower (10.7% = 11/103 patients receiving propofol or methohexital).[38] This finding ought not to be surprising. The use of supplemental oxygen may mask subtle early respiratory depression and argues for the use of end-tidal CO_2 monitoring or capnography[38]; however, the incidence of intervention was low (BMV in 7.7% = 4/52 patients receiving methohexital vs. 3.8% = 2/51 patients receiving propofol).[38] In none of the ED studies (adult[38–41] or pediatric[23,26,29,31,32]) using propofol for procedural sedation was intubation necessary.

Studies of procedural sedation using propofol in settings other than the ED such as the gastroenterology suite,[47,48] bronchoscopy unit,[43] dental office,[49] and the cardiac unit (pediatric transesophageal echocardiography and cardioversion)[50,51] have noted similar findings regarding the incidence of propofol-induced cardiorespiratory depression and the minimal incidence of required intervention.

Propofol's cardiovascular effects include the following:

- A decrease in the systemic vascular resistance.
- Negative inotropic effect.[1,13,16]
- A decrease in cardiac output.
- A resetting of the baroreflex resulting in a blunted compensatory heart rate response.[1,13,16]

- Enhancement of central vagal tone resulting in bradycardia or even asystole when administered with other drugs that affect cardiac chronotropic function (e.g., fentanyl and succinylcholine).[1,13,16]

These effects may lead to significant hypotension, particularly in hypovolemic patients. Some clinicians will empirically give a normal saline bolus prior to administering propofol because of concern over propofol's hypotensive side effects. When given in induction doses, dose and rate of administration related decreases in systolic blood pressure of up to 25–40% have been noted[1]; however, in ED studies of pediatric[23,26,29,31,32] and adult patients[38,41] undergoing procedural sedation with propofol (as well as in other non-ED settings[47–51]) the overwhelming majority of patients had clinically insignificant and transient decreases in blood pressure requiring no intervention. In the four adult ED studies,[38–41] only one patient had a significant drop in blood pressure (systolic BP = 80 for less than 1 minute) which required no treatment.[40]

It can be concluded that the respiratory and cardiac depressive effects of propofol are accentuated:

- When higher doses are administered.[12,15,19,27,49]
- It is given by a rapid IV bolus.[12,19,45]
- When other respiratory depressant drugs are coadministered.[3,16]
- In specific populations (e.g., the elderly[1,15] and patients in higher ASA classes 3 and 4).[43,46]

The undesirable cardiopulmonary effects of propofol when used for procedural sedation can be mitigated by combining it with ketamine and titrating both together. This confers an element of analgesia and augments the amnestic effect of propofol to the procedure (see further).

Undesirable neurologic side effects can occur with propofol: myoclonus, opisthotonic posturing, and seizure-like activity (without electroencephalogram [EEG] evidence of epileptiform activity).[52,53] Propofol has been advocated for the treatment of refractory status epilepticus,[54,55] although there are reports of seizures associated with propofol therapy.[52]

Propofol, when used in euvolemic patients with increased intracranial pressure (ICP), has produced a decrease in ICP[52] suggesting that it can be used in head injured patients provided the cerebral perfusion pressure is maintained.[52]

Propofol has mild antiemetic properties, so the occurrence of nausea and emesis with its use is rare.[13,14] It has been used by subanesthetic infusion as an antiemetic in oncology patients and for postoperative nausea and vomiting.[56,57]

ADVERSE EFFECTS

Several of the side effects of propofol are related to its formulation as a lipid emulsion containing egg lecithin, soybean oil, glycerol, and disodium edetate (EDTA). Anaphylactoid and anaphylactic reactions to propofol have been reported, with a higher incidence of this complication occurring in patients with multiple drug and food allergies, and allergies to any of its constituents (eggs, soybean, or EDTA).[1,9,45] Because it is a lipid emulsion, hypertriglyceridemia may occur[16] and rare occurrences of pancreatitis have been reported.[2,53,58]

Bradycardia and hypotension can occur even at doses used for procedural sedation. It may be related to the concurrent administration of sedative hypnotics or opioids.[14] Fortunately, both of these rarely occur.[14]

Hypoventilation is the most important and frequent of the adverse effects seen with propofol in the context of procedural sedation. Patients with a blunted response to inhaled carbon dioxide (e.g., COPD and those on respiratory depressant medications) are at particular risk. Because of the high incidence of respiratory depression with resultant hypercapnia associated with propofol, it should be avoided in patients with pulmonary hypertension or increased ICP,[14] both of which may be exacerbated by hypercarbia.

Propofol is an excellent growth media for bacteria. The medication must be administered immediately after being drawn up and not left to stand in the syringe.[14] After reports of life-threatening infections including sepsis occurred from bacterial contamination of propofol, EDTA was added to the formulation.[13]

Propofol, like all of the sedative hypnotic class of agents, at low doses that maintain consciousness may cause dysphoric reactions.[15,59]

The propofol infusion syndrome while not an acute care issue, occurs with prolonged administration of high doses of propofol, and is associated with metabolic acidosis, cardiac failure, and death.[53,60] It is characterized by:

- Muscle necrosis leading to marked elevations of creatine kinase (CK) and myoglobinuria.
- Lipemic serum.
- Metabolic acidosis.
- Hepatomegaly (from fatty infiltration of the liver).
- Myocardial failure with marked bradycardia resistant to treatment progressing to asystole and death.

The propofol infusion syndrome has generally been described in pediatric patients less than 4 years of age,[60] but has also been reported in adults. Risk factors for the propofol infusion syndrome are propofol administration for >48 hours and doses >4 mg/kg/h.[9,53]

ADMINISTRATION OF THE DRUG

After the IV administration of propofol, the plasma concentration equilibrates quickly with the brain concentration (within one arm to brain circulation time),[17] causing a rapid onset of sedation (about 40 seconds) with a duration of approximately 8 minutes.[11,12] Pediatric patients (especially <3 years of age)[1] require larger doses than adults probably because of a greater volume of distribution while geriatric patients require a lower dose due to their attenuated physiologic reserve.[13,17] Similarly, smaller doses are required when used with other CNS depressant drugs such as opioids or benzodiazepines.[11,18]

Propofol is a pregnancy category B drug.[61] Propofol is not Food and Drug Administration (FDA) approved for patients <3 years of age although it has been used in infants and children <3 years of age.[4,5,22,28,31] Propofol administration is associated with pain at the injection site and can cause phlebitis.[14] The pain on injection can be limited by using a larger vein with a rapidly running IV fluid and by mixing the propofol with lidocaine (0.5 mg/kg or 0.05 mL/kg of a 1% lidocaine solution up to 10 mg) or administering 1 mg/kg of lidocaine IV immediately before the administration of the propofol.[14,62] A lower lipid emulsion of propofol (ampofol) has been developed which has equivalent anesthetic properties to Diprivan, but an increased incidence of pain on injection.[63,64]

DOSE

For procedural sedation, propofol can be given by two techniques: an initial bolus followed by repeat boluses or IV drip. Initial boluses doses equal to 10% of the induction dose (1.5 mg/kg) are given, followed by additional equivalent boluses until the desired end point is achieved. Some authors have described continuous infusion methods, which is generally not the preferred technique for ED procedural sedation.

Propofol for procedural sedation may be combined with ketamine (in the same or separate syringes) to minimize the cardiorespiratory hazards seen when propofol alone is used.[65–73] The typical preparation is a 5 mg/mL solution of each titrated 1–2 mL at a time to the desired end point. Combinations of propofol and midazolam, and propofol and fentanyl, have also been employed.[74–78]

SUMMARY

Propofol has several uses including procedural sedation, RSI, sedation in the ICU including benzodiazepine-resistant agitation, and for general anesthesia. It has a very rapid onset and offset of action and a smooth recovery; however, dose-dependent cardiopulmonary depression can occur with propofol, which can lead to hypoventilation, bradycardia, and hypotension, especially in hypovolemic patients. These adverse effects are accentuated when given by rapid IV bolus, at higher doses, when coadministered with other respiratory depressant drugs, and in at-risk populations (geriatric patients, those with higher ASA classes 3 and 4). Other side effects include myoclonus, posturing, seizure-like activity, pain on injection, and the propofol infusion syndrome. Propofol in subanesthetic doses has been used as an antiemetic. It can be used in euvolemic head injured patients so long as the cerebral perfusion pressure is maintained. It is formulated as a lipid emulsion containing egg lecithin, soybean oil, glycerol, and disodium edetate (EDTA), so avoid its use in patients with true allergies to any of its constituents. It has not been FDA approved for patients <3 years of age although it has been used in infants and children <3 years old.

REFERENCES

1. Reeves JG, Glass PA, Lubarsky DA. Nonbarbiturate intravenous anesthetics. In: Miller RD, Cuehiara RF, Miller ED, et al, eds. *Anesthesia*. Philadelphia, PA: Churchill Livingstone; 2000:228–272.
2. McKeage K, Perry CM. Propofol—a review of its use in intensive care sedation of adults. *CNS Drugs*. 2003;17(4):235–272.
3. Nicolaou DD. Procedural sedation and analgesia. In: Tintinalli JE, Kelen GD, Stapczynski JS, eds. *Emergency Medicine. A Comprehensive Study Guide*. New York: McGraw-Hill; 2004:275–280.
4. Sivilotti MLA, Filbin MR, Murray HE, et al. Does the sedative agent facilitate rapid sequence intubation? *Acad Emerg Med*. 2003;10:612–620.
5. Cornfield D, Tegtmeyer K, Nelson MD, et al. Continuous propofol infusion in 142 critically ill children. *Pediatrics*. 2002;110(6):1177–1181.
6. Simon L, Trifa M, Mokhtari M, et al. Premedication for tracheal intubation: a prospective survey in 75 neonatal and pediatric intensive care units. *Crit Care Med*. 2004;32 (2):565–568.
7. Wetzel RC. Anesthesia and perioperative care. In: Behrman RE, Kliegman RM, Jenson HB, eds. *Nelson's Textbook of Pediatrics*. Philadelphia, PA: W.B. Saunders; 2004:342–357.
8. Lewis KP, Stanley GD. Pharmacology. In: Gilbertson LI, ed. *Conscious Sedation. International Anesthesiology Clinics*. Philadelphia, PA: Lippincott Williams & Wilkins; 1999:73–86.
9. Tobias JD. Pharmacology of sedative agents. In: Malviya S, Naughton NN, Tremper KK, eds. *Sedation and Analgesia for Diagnostic and Therapeutic Procedures*. Humana Totowa, NJ: 2003: 125–132.
10. Propofol. Package insert. Deerfield, IL: Baxter Healthcare Corporation; . 2002; and Diprivan. Package insert. Wilmington, DE: Astra-Zeneca Pharmaceuticals LP; 2001.
11. Chu JW, White PF. Nonopioid intravenous anesthesia. In: Barash PG, Cullen BF, Stoelting RK, eds. *Clinical Anesthesia*. Philadelphia, PA: Lippincott Williams & Wilkins; 2001: 327–343.
12. Blackburn P, Vissers R. Pharmacology of emergency department pain management and conscious sedation. *Emerg Clin North Am*. 2000;18:803–827.
13. Evers AS, Crowder CM. General anesthetics. In: Hardman JG, Limbird LE, Gilman AG, eds. *Goodman & Gilman's The Pharmacological Basis of Therapeutics*. New York: McGraw-Hill; 2001:337–365.
14. Litman R. Sedatives/hypnotics. In: Kraus B, Brustowicz RM, eds. *Pediatric Procedural Sedation and Analgesia*. Philadelphia, PA: Lippincott Williams & Wilkins; 1999:39–46.
15. Green SM, Krauss B. Procedural sedation and analgesia. In: Roberts JR, Hedges JR, Canmugam AS, et al, eds. *Clinical procedures in Emergency Medicine*. Philadelphia, PA: W.B. Saunders; 2004:596–620.
16. Barr J. Propofol: a new drug for sedation in the intensive care unit. *Int Anesthesiol Clin*. 1995;23:131–154.
17. Sacchetti A, Schafermeyer R, Gerardi M, et al. Pediatric analgesia and sedation. *Ann Emerg Med*. 1994;23:237–250.
18. Hopson LR, Kronen SC. Pharmacologic agents to intubation. In: Roberts JR, Hedges JR, Chanmugam AS, et al, eds. *Clinical Procedures in Emergency Medicine*. Philadelphia, PA: W.B. Saunders; 2004:100–114.
19. Green SM. Propofol for emergency department procedural sedation—not yet ready for prime time. *Acad Emerg Med*. 1999;6:975–978.
20. Rothermel LK. Newer pharmacologic agents for procedural sedation of children in the emergency department—etomidate and propofol. *Curr Opin Pediatr*. 2003;15:200–203.
21. Chudnofsky CR, Lozon MM. Sedation and analgesia for procedures. In: Marx JA, Hockberger RS, Walls RM et al, eds. *Rosen's Emergency Medicine: Concepts and Clinical Practice*. St Louis, MO: Mosby; 2002:2577–2590.
22. Propofol. *Lexi-Drugs Online*. Lexi-Comp; 2005. Last accessed on June 29, 2005, at www.lexi.comp.
23. Havel CJ Jr, Strait RT, Hennes H. A clinical trial of propofol vs midazolam for procedural sedation in a pediatric emergency department. *Acad Emerg Med*. 1999;6:989–997.
24. Kain ZN, Gaal DJ, Kain TS, et al. A first-pass cost analysis of propofol versus barbiturates for children undergoing magnetic resonance imaging. *Anesth Analg*. 1994;79:1102–1106.
25. Bloomfield EL, Masaryk TJ, Caplin A, et al. Intravenous sedation for MR imaging of the brain and spine in children: pentobarbital versus propofol. *Radiology*. 1993;183:93–97.

26. Godambe SA, Elliot V, Matheny D, et al. Comparison of propofol/fentanyl versus ketamine/midazolam for brief orthopedic procedural sedation in a pediatric emergency department. *Pediatrics*. 2003;112:116–123.

27. Keidan I, Berkenstadt H, Sidi A, et al. Propofol/remifentanyl versus propofol along for bone marrow aspiration in paediatric hemato-oncological patients. *Paediatr Anaesth*. 2001;23: 290–293.

28. Levati A, Columbo N, Arosio EM, et al. Propofol anaesthesia in spontaneously breathing paediatric patients during magnetic resonance imaging. *Acta Anesthesiol Scand*. 1996; 40:561–565.

29. Skokan ED, Pribble C, Bassett KE, et al. Use of propofol sedation in a pediatric emergency department: a prospective study. *Clin Pediatr*. 2001;40:663–671.

30. Hertzog JH, Dalton HJ, Anderson BV, et al. Prospective evaluation of propofol anesthesia in the pediatric intensive care unit for elective oncology procedures in ambulatory and hospitalized children. *Pediatrics*. 2000;106;742–747.

31. Guenther E, Pribble CG, Junkins EP Jr, et al. Propofol sedation by emergency physicians for elective pediatric out-patient procedures. *Ann Emerg Med*. 2003;42:783–791.

32. Bassett KE, Anderson JF, Pribble CG, et al. Propofol for procedural sedation in children in the emergency department. *Ann Emerg Med*. 2003;42:773–782.

33. Jayabose S, Levendoglu-Tugal O, Giamelli J, et al. Intravenous anesthesia with propofol for painful procedures in children with cancer. *J Pediatr Hematol Oncol*. 2001;23:290–293.

34. Merola C, Albarracin C, Lebowitz P, et al. An audit of adverse events in children sedated with chloral hydrate or propofol during imaging studies. *Paediatr Anaesth*. 2001;11:297–301.

35. Scheiber G, Ribeiro FC, Karienski H, et al. Deep sedation with propofol in preschool children undergoing radiation therapy. *Paediatr Anaesth*. 1996;6:209–213.

36. McDowell RH, Scher CS, Barst SM. Total intravenous anesthesia for children undergoing brief diagnostic or therapeutic procedures. *J Clin Anesth*. 1005;7:273–280.

37. Vardi A, Salem Y, Padeh S, et al. Is propofol safe for procedural sedation in children? A prospective evaluation of propofol versus ketamine in pediatric critical care. *Crit Care Med*. 2002;30:1231–1236.

38. Miner JR, Biros M, Krieg S, et al. Randomized clinical trial of propofol versus methohexitol for procedural sedation during fracture and dislocation reduction in the emergency department. *Acad Emerg Med*. 2003;10:931–937.

39. Swanson ER, Seaberg DC, Matias S. The use of propofol for sedation in the emergency department. *Acad Emerg Med*. 1996;3:324–328.

40. Coll–Vincent B, Sala X, Fernandez C, et al. Sedation for cardioversion in the emergency department: analysis of effectiveness in four protocols. *Ann Emerg Med*. 2003;42: 767–772.

41. Totten VY, Zambito RF. Propofol bolus facilitates reduction of luxed temporomandibular joints. *J Emerg Med*. 1998;16: 467–470.

42. Mace SE, Barata IA, Cravero JP, et al. Clinical policy: evidence-based approach to pharmacologic agents used in pediatric sedation and analgesia in the emergency department. *Ann Emerg Med*. 2004;44(4):342–377.

43. Perrin G, Colt HG, Martin C, et al. Safety of interventional rigid bronchoscopy using intravenous anesthesia and spontaneous assisted ventilation–a prospective study. *Chest*. 1992;102:1526–1530.

44. Proudfoot J. Analgesia, anesthesia, and conscious sedation. *Emerg Med Clin North Am*. 1995;13:357–379.

45. Rodriquez E, Jordan R. Contemporary trends in pediatric sedation and analgesia. *Emerg Med Clin North Am*. 2002;20: 199–222.

46. Malviya S, Voepel-Lewis T, Eldevik OP, et al. Sedation and general anaesthesia in children undergoing MRI and CT: adverse events and outcomes. *Br J Anaesth*. 2000;84:743–748.

47. Kulling D, Rothenbuhler R, Inauden U. Safety of non-anesthetic sedation with propology for outpatient colonoscopy and esophagogastroduodenoscopy. *Endoscopy*. 2003;35: 679–682.

48. Vargo JJ, Zuccaro G, Dumot JA, et al. Gastroenterologist-administered propofol versus meperidine and midazolam for ERCP and EIS: a prospective randomized trial with cost effectiveness analysis. *Gastroenterology*. 2002;123;8–16.

49. Johns FR, Sandler NA, Buckley MJ, et al. Comparison of propofol and methohexital continuous infusion techniques for conscious sedation. *J Oral Maxillofac Surg*. 1998;56: 1124–1127.

50. Heard CMB, Gunnarson B, Heard AMB, et al. Anaesthetic technique for transesophageal echocardiography in children. *Paediatr Anaesth*. 2001;11:181–184.

51. Herregods LL, Bossuyt GP, De Baerdemaeker LE, et al. Ambulatory electrical external cardioversion with propofol or etomidate. *J Clin Anesth*. 2002;15:91–96.

52. Urwin SC, Menon DK. Comparative tolerability of sedative agents in head-injured adults. *Drug Saf*. 2004;27:107–103.

53. Short TG, Young Y. Toxicity of intravenous anaesthetics. *Best Pract Res Clin Anaesthesiol*. 2003;17:77–89.

54. Claassen J, Hirsch LJ, Emerson RG, et al. Treatment of refractory status epilepticus with pentobarbitol, propofol or midazolam: a systematic review. *Epilepsia*. 2002;43:146–153.

55. Stecker MM, Kramer TH, Raps EC, et al. Treatment of refractory status epilepticus with propofol: clinical and pharmacokinetic findings. *Epilepsia*. 1998;39:18–26.

56. Apfel CC, Korttila K, Abdalla M, et al. A factorial trial of six interventions for the prevention of postoperative nausea and vomiting. *N Engl J Med*. 2004;350:2441–2451.

57. Scher CS, Amar D, McDowell RH, et al. Use of propofol for the prevention of chemotherapy induced nausea and emesis in oncology patients. *Can J Anaesth*. 1992;39:170–172.

58. Jawaid Q, Presti ME, Neuschwander-tetri BA, et al. Acute pancreatitis after single-dose exposure to propofol. *Dig Dis Sci*. 2002;47:614–618.

59. Ducharme J. Procedural sedation in the ED: how, when, and which agents to choose. *Emerg Med Pract*. 2000;2:1–20.

60. Kang TM. Propofol infusion syndrome in critically ill patients. *Ann Pharmacother*. 2002;36:1453–1456.

61. Briggs GG, Freeman RK, Yaffe SJ, eds. *Propofol Drugs in Pregnancy and Lactation.* Williams & Wilkins; 2002:112–113.

62. Madenoglu H, Yildiz K, Dogru K, et al. Efficacy of different doses of lidocaine in the prevention of pain due to propofol injection: a randomized open-label trial in 120 patients. *Curr Ther Res.* 2003;64:310–316.

63. Song D, Hamza MA, White PF, et al. The pharmadynamic effects of a lower-lipid emulsion of propofol: a comparison with the standard propofol emulsion. *Anesth Analg.* 2004;98:687–691.

64. Song D, Hamza MA, White PF, et al. Comparison of a lower-lipid propofol emulsion with the standard emulsion for sedation during monitored anesthesia care. *Anesthesiology.* 2004;100:1072–1075.

65. Frey K, Sukhani R, Pawlowski J, et al. Propofol versus propofol-ketamine sedation for retrobulbar nerve block: comparison of sedation quality, intraocular pressure changes, and recovery profiles. *Anesth Analg.* 1999;89:317–321.

66. Frizelle HP, Duranteau J, Samii K. A comparison of propofol with a propofol-ketamine combination for sedation during spinal anesthesia. *Anesth Analg.* 1997;84:1318–1322.

67. Mortero RF, Clark LD, Tolan MM, et al. The effects of small-dose ketamine on propofol sedation: respiration, postoperative mood, perception, cognition, and pain. *Anesth Analg.* 2001;92:1465–1469.

68. Friedberg BL. Propofol-ketamine technique. *Aesthetic Plast Surg.* 1993;17:297–300.

69. Friedberg BL. Propofol-ketamine technique: dissociative anesthesia for office surgery (a 5-year review of 1264 cases). *Aesthetic Plast Surg.* 1999;23:70–75.

70. Palermo S, Cammardella MP, Vallebona C, et al. Clinical evaluation of propofol-ketamine anesthesia in general surgery [Italian]. *Minerva Anestesiol.* 1991;57:91–96.

71. Scarrone S, Vivaldi N, D'Amico G, et al. A propofol-ketamine combination in short-term anesthesia [Italian]. *Minerva Anestesiol.* 1990;56:809–811.

72. Gianuario L, Luongo C, Vicario C, et al. The ketamine-propofol combination in the voluntary termination of pregnancy [Italian]. *Minerva Anestesiol.* 1991;57:554–555.

73. Badrinath S, Avramov MN, Shadrick M, et al. The use of a ketamine-propofol combination during monitored anesthesia care. *Anesth Analg.* 2000;90:858–862.

74. Chudnofsky CR, Weber JE, Stoyanoff PJ, et al. A combination of midazolam and ketamine for procedural sedation and analgesia in adult emergency department patients. *Acad Emerg Med.* 2000;7:228–235.

75. Seigler RS, Avant MG, Gwyn DR, et al. A comparison of propofol and ketamine/midazolam for intravenous sedation of children. *Pediatr Crit Care Med.* 2001;2:20–23.

76. Riavis M, Laux-End R, Carvajal-Busslinger MI, et al. Sedation with intravenous benzodiazepine and ketamine for renal biopsies. *Pediatr Nephrol.* 1998;12:147–148.

77. Cammardella MP, Palermo S, Vallebona C, et al. Propofol-ketamine versus propofol-fentanyl in air/O_2 in general surgery [Italian]. *Minerva Anestesiol.* 1990;56:817–819.

78. Yoho R. Regarding propofol-ketamine and propofol-fentanyl sedation technique. *Dermatol Surg.* 1999;25:974.

18

Etomidate

Sharon E. Mace

HIGH YIELD FACTS

- Etomidate provides considerable "downside protection" in patients who are incipiently or actually hemodynamically unstable (e.g., patients with hypotension, hypovolemia, shock, and cardiomyopathy). It does not prevent postintubation hypertension and tachycardia.

- Etomidate causes myoclonus. The use of an induction agent in induction doses to facilitate intubation should *always* include a neuromuscular blocking agent. This is particularly true when using etomidate where orofacial myoclonus may occur.

- Premedication with opioids or benzodiazepines decreases the incidence of myoclonic movements.

- Avoid prolonged infusions of etomidate, which have been associated with suppression of the adrenocortical stress response, and also avoid etomidate in patients with adrenal insufficiency.

- Etomidate's central nervous system (CNS) effects decrease intracranial pressure and although etomidate is often used to facilitate intubation in head-injured patients, the risk of tachycardia and hypertension must be balanced with the risk of further increasing intracranial pressure.

- In some studies, etomidate is a proconvulsant so use with caution in patients with known focal seizures.

- Pain on injection can occur with etomidate, so give with lidocaine, run the intravenous (IV) wide open and use a larger vein to reduce the pain on injection.

- The manufacturer does not recommend its use in children <10 years of age, although its use in children/infants has been documented in many studies.

INDICATIONS

Etomidate is used for procedural sedation, rapid sequence intubation, and the induction and maintenance of general anesthesia.

PHARMACOLOGY

Etomidate is an ultra-short-acting sedative hypnotic drug[1] with an amnestic[2,3] effect but no analgesic effect. It is a nonbarbiturate carboxylated imidazole compound[2] that exerts its effects via depression of the ascending reticular activating system. Its hypnotic properties are mediated by inhibition of neurotransmission by γ-aminobutyric acid (GABA) via increased chloride conductance across cell membranes, causing hyperpolarization of the neuronal cell membrane.[4] It is protein bound and rapidly metabolized in the liver but the duration of the drug's action is terminated by redistribution from the brain to inactive tissues.[1,4] Table 18-1 contains dosage information and Table 18-2 contains administration information.

CLINICAL EFFECTS

It lacks the hypotensive inducing properties of other commonly used sedative hypnotic induction agents, such as propofol and thiopental,[5–7] making it ideal for patients who are incipiently or actually hemodynamically unstable (e.g., cardiomyopathy, hypotension, hypovolemia, shock, and trauma).[6] The usual induction doses of etomidate produce no real change in heart rate, blood pressure, cardiac output, or coronary perfusion pressure, and it decreases myocardial oxygen consumption.[1] Its use as an induction agent to facilitate endotracheal intubation in patients with coronary artery disease needs to be balanced with the risk of postintubation tachycardia and hypertension, which it does not attenuate.

The effect of etomidate on the central nervous system (CNS) is to decrease intracranial pressure,[1] since the systemic blood pressure is maintained, the cerebral perfusion pressure and cerebral oxygen consumption are also decreased. During tracheal manipulation, a significant decrease in intracranial pressure with minimal effects on cerebral perfusion pressure was noted.[8] The same precaution regarding postintubation hypertension is reiterated here, especially in patients with imperfect autoregulation (e.g., acute severe head injury) and intracranial pressure (ICP) control. Because of these CNS effects, use of etomidate as a protective drug mitigating against cerebral ischemia has been suggested. Unfortunately, there have

Table 18-1. Etomidate: Dosage Information

Dose (mg/kg)	Usual Dose (mg/kg)	Maximum Dose (mg/kg)	Onset (min)	Duration (min)
0.1–0.3 IV	0.2 PSA 0.3 RSI	0.6	<1	3–10

PSA, procedural sedation and analgesia; RSI, rapid sequence intubation.

been no controlled human clinical trials and animal studies have not consistently demonstrated a benefit.[1]

ADVERSE EFFECTS

Myoclonus is the most common side effect of etomidate occurring in about one out of three patients, although higher incidences from 50 to 80% when used as a single agent have been reported.[9–13] Like most potent induction agents, the theory explaining etomidate-induced myoclonus is based on its suppression of cortical function resulting in disinhibition-mediated myoclonus.[2] Pretreatment with opioids (such as fentanyl, morphine, or sufentanil)[11–13] or benzodiazepines (e.g., midazolam)[14,15] has been demonstrated to inhibit myoclonus producing subcortical stimuli thereby decreasing (but not necessarily eliminating) such myoclonus.[16] The use of a paralytic during RSI will mask the myoclonus.[17]

Myoclonus may be important for the emergency physician when etomidate is employed without a paralytic to facilitate endotracheal intubation and orofacial myoclonus results.[6,7,18] Several studies have noted a higher incidence of more difficult intubation (e.g., multiple attempts and failed intubations) when etomidate is used as the sole agent for facilitating intubation. In a recent case report, dantrolene in a 1 mg/kg dose was used to terminate severe myoclonic movements secondary to etomidate.[19] Though these studies recommend *rescue*

drugs or *pretreatment* drugs (such as paralytics, benzodiazepines, or opioids), when etomidate is used for intubation[7,18] it needs to be reiterated that the use of a neuromuscular blocking agent (e.g., succinylcholine and rocuronium) is a routine and necessary component of RSI.

In a study of intubation in an aeromedical setting, intubation success rates for etomidate alone were 86.9% (53/61) versus 98.2% (216/220) for etomidate plus succinylcholine ($P < 0.001$) with rescue succinylcholine needed in 11.7% of the etomidate intubations.[18] Furthermore "etomidate only patients were more likely to require multiple (intubation) attempts."[18] An emergency department (ED) study using only etomidate prior to intubation noted a 70% incidence of myoclonus (60%, mild; moderate or severe in another 10% of all patients) and an intubation failure rate of 25% due to orofacial myoclonus or medication-induced trismus.[6] These authors advocated the concomitant administration of either opioids or benzodiazepines when using etomidate to facilitate intubation,[6] though a neuromuscular blocking agent should always be used.

The incidence and intensity of etomidate-induced myoclonic movements are probably dose-related and unassociated with seizure-like activity on electroencephalogram (EEG)[10] though one report described electroencephalographic spikes in 22% of patients with etomidate-induced myoclonus, suggesting otherwise.[20]

Table 18-2. Etomidate: Administration Information

Practical Tips	Administration	Advantages	Side Effects/Disadvantages
↓ myoclonic movements by premedicating with opioids or benzodiazepines, for RSI use paralytic to avoid orofacial myoclonus	↓ pain on injection by giving with lidocaine, in a larger vein, with premedications No analgesic effect, add opioid if painful procedure	Limited CV/respiratory depression (use if patient has shock) ↓ intracranial pressure	Myoclonic movements Pain on injection Phlebitis Nausea, vomiting Adrenal suppression (with prolonged use) Propylene glycol toxicity (with prolonged use)

According to some reports, etomidate has been associated with seizures.[21] Therefore, one may consider using another sedative or using etomidate with caution in patients with a known seizure disorder.[1,22]

Etomidate has minimal respiratory depressant effects,[1,22] although oxygen desaturation from hypoventilation or short duration apnea (from 5 to 90 seconds with spontaneous recovery), as well as laryngospasm has been reported.[2,3,18,22] The incidence of such adverse respiratory events is low,[20] probably <1%. Concomitant use of other respiratory depressants, especially opioids, increases the risk of oxygen desaturation.[2,15,23]

Etomidate does have a negative effect on adrenal steroid production via inhibition of the enzyme 11-β-hydrolase, which converts cholesterol to cortisol and aldosterone.[1] Prolonged etomidate infusions in an intensive care unit setting have been associated with adrenal suppression and increased mortality, probably from adrenal insufficiency.[24] Even after a single induction dose,[25-28] the normal stress-induced rise in cortisol is depressed for about 8 hours, perhaps lasting up to 24 hours in debilitated and/or elderly patients. A prospective, randomized, controlled trial of patients intubated in the ED using a 0.3 mg/kg induction dose of etomidate documented an abnormal response to exogenous cosyntropin (cosyntropin stimulation test [CST]). Patients receiving etomidate had significantly depressed cortisol levels in response to CST (30% vs. 100% for controls, $P < 0.004$), resolving by 12 hours as documented by a normal CST.[25] No significant clinical sequelae after a single induction dose of etomidate have been reported.[25-28]

Gastrointestinal side effects of etomidate include a relatively high incidence of nausea and vomiting (~30–40% incidence) on emergence from anesthesia, and occasionally hiccups (1–10%).[2,3,15,18,29]

The incidence of side effects is probably greater when higher dosages of etomidate are used, and in geriatric patients. An overdose of etomidate can cause respiratory arrest, hypotension, and/or coma with supportive treatment given until the drug is cleared.[1]

Because of limited data, the manufacturer does not recommend the use of etomidate in children less than 10 years of age. However, this should not be considered as a contraindication since numerous studies have demonstrated its safe and effective use in neonates, infants, and children[3,28,30-32] It is a pregnancy category C drug.

ADMINISTRATION OF THE DRUG

Localized pain at the injection site occurs 30–80% of the time with etomidate.[1] Giving etomidate through a larger vein with a rapid intravenous (IV) infusion rate and/or giving it after an injection of 3–5 mL of lidocaine 1% immediately before the etomidate may decrease the pain of injection, local irritation, and phlebitis.[1,29] The propylene glycol diluent is thought to be responsible for the local irritation.[33] Osmolal gap metabolic acidosis from propylene glycol toxicity associated with a prolonged etomidate infusion has rarely been reported.[34] Superficial thrombophlebitis (up to 20%) can occur 2–3 days after etomidate injection.

DOSE

The dose of etomidate for rapid sequence intubation is 0.2–0.6 mg/kg[1] IV given over 30–60 seconds with a usual dosage of 0.3 mg/kg.[6,7] For procedural sedation and analgesia (PSA) 0.2 mg/kg[4,23] titrated to the moderate sedation end point is generally used. Occasionally, for RSI or PSA, additional doses are needed and are titrated up to a maximum of 0.6 mg/kg.[3,4,18,25]

SUMMARY

Etomidate is used for procedural sedation, rapid sequence intubation, and general anesthesia. It is an excellent choice for patients who are incipiently or actually hemodynamically unstable and frequently produces myoclonus, and is associated with postuse nausea and vomiting and pain at the injection site. Etomidate does have a negative effect on adrenal steroid production, although this has not been shown to have any clinical significance following a single induction dose. The manufacturer does not recommend the use of etomidate in children <10 years old, although multiple pediatric studies have documented the safety and efficacy of etomidate in neonates, infants, and children.

REFERENCES

1. Evers AS, Crowden CM. General anesthetics. In: Hardman JG, Limbird LE, eds. *Goodman and Gilman's The Pharmacological Basis of Therapeutics*. New York: McGraw-Hill; 2001:337–365.
2. Ruth WJ, Burton JW, Bock AJ. Intravenous etomidate for procedural sedation in emergency department patients. *Acad Emerg Med*. 2001;8:13–18.
3. Vinson DR, Bradbury DR. Etomidate for procedural sedation in emergency medicine. *Ann Emerg Med*. 2002; 39:592–598.
4. Davis PJ, Cook DR. Clinical pharmacokinetics of the newer intravenous anaesthetic agents. *Clin Pharmacokinet*. 1986; 11:18–35.
5. Gooding JM, Weng JT, Smith RA, et al. Cardiovascular and pulmonary responses following etomidate induction in patients with demonstrated cardiac disease. *Anesth Analg*. 1979;58:40–41.

6. Plewa MC, King R, Johnson D, et al. Etomidate use during emergency intubation of trauma patients. *Am J Emerg Med.* 1997;15:98–100.

7. Swanson ER, Fosnocht DE, Neff RJ. The use of etomidate for rapid sequence intubation in the air medical setting. *Prehosp Emerg Care.* 2001;5:142–146.

8. Modica PA, Tempelhoff R. Intracranial pressure during induction of anaesthesia and tracheal intubation with etomidate-induced EEG burst suppression. *Can J Anaesth.* 1992;39:236–241.

9. Giese JL, Stanley TH. Etomidate: a new intravenous anesthestic induction agent. *Pharmacotherapy.* 1983;3:251–258.

10. Doenicke AW, Roizen MF, Kugler J, et al. Reducing myoclonus after etomidate. *Anesthesiol.* 1999;90:112–119.

11. Stockham RJ, Stanley TH, Pace NL, et al. Fentanyl pretreatment modifies an anaesthetic induction with etomidate. *Anaesth Intensive Care.* 1988;16:171–176.

12. Helmers JH, Adam AA, Giezen J. Pain and myoclonus during induction with etomidate. A double-blind, controlled evaluation of the influence of droperidol and fentanyl. *Acta Anaesthesiol Belg.* 1981;32:141–147.

13. Hueter L, Schwarzkoff K, Simon M, et al. Pretreatment with sufentanil reduces myoclonus after etomidate. *Acta Anaesthesiol Scand.* 2003;47:482–484.

14. Schwarzkoff KRG, Hueter L, Simon M, et al. Midazolam pretreatment reduces etomidate-induced myoclonic movements. *Anaesth Intensive Care.* 2003;31:18–20.

15. Burton JH, Bock AJ, Strout TD, et al. Etomidate and midazolam for reduction of anterior shoulder dislocation: a randomized controlled trial. *Ann Emerg Med.* 2002;40:496–504.

16. Van Keulen SG, Burton JH. Myoclonus associates with etomidate for ED procedural sedation and analgesia. *Am J Emerg Med.* 2003;21:556–558.

17. Smith DC, Bergen JM, Smithline H, et al. A trial of etomidate for rapid sequence induction in the emergency department. *J Emerg Med.* 2000;18:13–16.

18. Kociszewski C, Thomas SH, Harrison T, et al. Etomidate vs succinylcholine for intubation in air medical setting. *Am J Emerg Med.* 2000;18:757–763.

19. Greenberg M, Hilty C. Myoclonus after prolonged infusion of etomidate treated with dantrolene. *J Clin Anesth.* 2003;15:489–490.

20. Reddy RV, Moorthy SS, Dierdorf SF, et al. Excitatory effects and electroencephalographic correlation of etomidate, thiopental, methohexital, and propofol. *Anesth Analg.* 1993;77:1008–1011.

21. Hanson HC, Drenck NF. Generalized seizures after etomidate anaesthesia. *Anaesthesia.* 1988;43:805–806.

22. Mace SE, Barata IA, Cravero JP, et al. Clinical Policy: evidence-based approach to pharmacologic agents used in pediatric sedation and analgesia in the emergency department. *Ann Emerg Med.* 2004;44:342–377.

23. Keim SM, Erstad BL, Sakles JC, et al. Etomidate for procedural sedation in the emergency department. *Pharmacotherapy.* 2002;22:586–592.

24. Ledingham IM, Watt I. Influence of sedation on mortality in critically ill multiple trauma patients. *Lancet.* 1983;1:1270.

25. Schenarts CL, Burton JH, Riker RR. Adrenocortical dysfunction following etomidate induction in emergency department patients. *Acad Emerg Med.* 2001;8:1–7.

26. Allolio B, Stuttmann R, Leonhard U, et al. Adrenocortical suppression by a single induction dose of etomidate. *Klin Wochensch.* 1984;62:1014–1017.

27. Allolio B, Dorr H, Stuttman R, et al. Effect of a single bolus of etomidate upon eight major corticosteroid hormones and plasma ACTH. *Clin Endocrinol* (oxf). 1985;22:281–286.

28. Absalom A, Pledger D, Kong A. Adrenocortical function in critically ill patients 24 hours after a single dose of etomidate. *Anaesthesia.* 1999;54:861–867.

29. McDowell RH, Scher CS, Barst SM. Total intravenous anesthesia for children undergoing brief diagnostic or therapeutic procedures. *J Clin Anesth.* 1995;7:273–280.

30. Guldner G, Schultz J, Sexton P, et al. Etomidate for rapid-sequence intubation in young children: hemodynamic effects and adverse events. *Acad Emerg Med.* 2003;10:134–139.

31. Dickinson R, Singer AJ, Carrion W. Etomidate for pediatric sedation prior to fracture reduction. *Acad Emerg Med.* 2001;8:74–77.

32. Sokolove PE, Price DD, Okada P. The safety of etomidate for emergency rapid sequence intubation of pediatric patients. *Pediatr Emerg Care.* 2000;16:18–21.

33. Doenicke AW, Roizen MF, Hoeinecki R, et al. Solvent for etomidate may cause pain and adverse effects. *Br J Anaesth.* 1999;83:464–465.

34. Bedickeck E, Kirschbaum B. A case of propylene glycol toxic reaction associated with etomidate infusion. *Arch Intern Med.* 1991;151:2297–2298.

19

Barbiturates

Sharon E. Mace

HIGH YIELD FACTS

- Decrease intracranial and intraocular pressure → ideal for use in head injury patients.
- Can cause profound cardiac/respiratory depression.
- Can cause histamine release so should be used with caution in hypotension and asthma.
- Stimulation of respiratory reflexes can occur causing coughing, gagging, hiccups, and laryngospasm.
- Avoid intra-arterial injection (may cause gangrene) and avoid extravasation (may cause tissue necrosis).
- Give with analgesics during painful procedures.
- Absolute contraindication: porphyria.

INDICATIONS

Barbiturates are one of the oldest classes of anesthetics with a broad safety profile[1-3]; however, they have largely been replaced in emergency practice by newer agents. Barbiturates may still be used for:

- Procedural sedation in patients of all ages.
- Rapid sequence intubation particularly in the head-injured patient.
- Sedation in the intensive care unit (ICU) in both adults and children including during extracorporeal membrane oxygenation (ECMO).
- For the induction of general anesthesia.[4-10]
- *Barbiturate coma* (generally *pentobarbital coma*) has been used to treat patients with head injuries and various central nervous system (CNS) diseases who have increased intracranial pressure.[11]

Barbiturates are often used for cerebroprotection when ischemic/hypoxic or traumatic brain injury is expected.[1,7,12-14] Thiopental is the most commonly used of the barbiturates for RSI and induction, though it has largely been replaced by propofol, etomidate, and midazolam in emergency practice over the past decade.[14-16] Barbiturates are considered by some to be the "drug of choice" for diagnostic imaging in older children (>3 years of age).[2] Pentobarbital may be the most frequently used sedative for radiology procedures, specifically computed tomography (CT) and magnetic resonance imaging (MRI) scans,[14,17] though some in emergency medicine prefer the shorter acting methohexital and thiopental.[18-20] However, generally the intravenous (IV) titration of methohexital and thiopental by emergency physicians to facilitate diagnostic studies has been replaced by midazolam, propofol, etomidate, and ketamine.

PHARMACOLOGY

Barbiturates belong to the sedative-hypnotic class of agents. They are derived from barbituric acid, a potent anticonvulsant. Hypnotic and amnestic activities are produced by adding a side chain (preferably branched) to the barbituric acid structure.[21] Generally, structural modifications that increase lipid solubility will shorten the onset and duration of action, hasten metabolic degradation, and usually increase hypnotic potency.[21] Barbiturates, like other sedative-hypnotics have no analgesic properties, and may in fact, be antianalgesic.

γ-Amino butyric acid (GABA) is the main inhibitory neurotransmitter in the human CNS.[22] Barbiturates' mechanism of action on the GABA receptor is to increase the influx of chloride ions into neuronal cells causing hyperpolarization and inhibition of postsynaptic neurons.[21] This results in a decreased rate of GABA dissociation from its receptor, thereby prolonging GABA's inhibitory effect.[22,23] This causes depression of the reticular activating system, which is responsible for wakefulness, and the induction of hypnosis or sleep.[24,25] At high drug levels, barbiturates directly activate chloride channels even in the absence of GABA.[22]

The sedative-hypnotic effects of barbiturates are likely mediated by enhancement of the GABA system, while the anesthetic effects are probably due to the direct activation of chloride channels.[23] In addition to activating the inhibitory GABA receptors, barbiturates also inhibit the excitatory amino-3 hydroxy-5-methyl-4-isoxazole propionic acid (AMPA) subtypes of the glutamate receptor.[26] Barbiturates reversibly suppress the activity of all excitable tissue with weak effects on peripheral tissue and more marked effects on the CNS including central respiratory depression.[3]

Barbiturates are classified according to their duration of action: ultrashort, short, intermediate, and long acting.[27,28] Ultra-short-acting anesthetic agents include methohexital, thiopental, and thiamylal.[10,27,28] Pentobarbital is a short-acting agent.[27,29] Butabarbital is an intermediate acting agent.[27] Phenobarbital is a long-acting barbiturate used as an anticonvulsant.[29] The ultra-short- and short-acting barbiturates are preferred for emergency department (ED) usage because of a rapid onset and short duration.[18]

Following administration, barbiturates rapidly accumulate in highly vascular organs such as the brain.[21,30] The relatively rapid redistribution of the ultra-short- and short-acting barbiturates to less vascular depots such as skeletal muscle and fat is responsible for these drugs duration of action and explains their relatively long elimination half-life and large volume of distribution.[21,31] Barbiturates undergo degradation in the liver to inactive metabolites, which are then excreted in the urine, with the exception of the less lipid-soluble pentobarbital which also undergoes renal excretion.[26,31] Table 19-1 contains dosage information and Table 19-2 contains administration information.

CLINICAL EFFECTS

Central Nervous System Effects

Barbiturates cause a dose-dependent decrease in cerebral metabolic rate, cerebral blood flow, intracranial pressure, and intraocular pressure.[9,32] Because of these effects they have been employed:

- As neuroprotective agents in cases of cerebral ischemia/hypoxia (especially thiopental).
- During neurosurgical or ophthalmologic procedures.[4,21,22,30,31]
- In patients with acute severe head injury.[4,14,33]

They are potent anticonvulsants and have been used to treat status epilecticus.[12,34,35]

Cardiorespiratory Effects

The cardiorespiratory effects of barbiturates depend on several factors: the dose of the drug, the rate at which it is administered, the patient's underlying clinical condition, the activity of the sympathetic nervous system which affects vascular tone, volume status, and whether other drugs are coadministered.[1,23,31] In otherwise healthy

Table 19-1. Barbiturates: Dosage Information

Dose (mg/kg)	Usual Dose (mg/kg)	Maximum Dose	Onset (min)	Duration (min)
Methohexital	Methohexital	Methohexital	Methohexital	Methohexital
1–3 IV	1–1.5 IV	3 mg/kg IV	IV 1	IV 10
10 IM	Pentobarbital	Pentobarbital	PR 2–5 (sleepy)	PR 45–60
25 PR	2 IV	6 mg/kg or	10–15 (for	Pentobarbital
Pentobarbital	Adjust in	200 mg	procedural	IV 15–60
1–6 IV	increments	IV or PO	sedation)	IM 60–120
2–6 PO/PR	of 1–2	150 mg IM	Pentobarbital	PO/PR 60–240
4–6 IM	Larger doses may	or PR	IV 5	Thiopental
Thiopental	be needed in	Thiopental	IM 10	IV 15
3–5 IV	older children	1 g or 1000 mg PR	PO/PR 15–60	PR 60–120
25 PR			Thiopental	
			IV 1	
			PR 10–15	

IM, intramuscular; IV, intravenous; PO, oral; PR, per rectum.

Table 19-2. Barbiturates: Administration Information

Practical Tips	Administration	Advantages	Side Effects Disadvantages
Good choice for patients with head injury if stable	Incompatible with other drugs	Decreases intracranial/ intraocular pressure	Contraindication: porphyria
Use thiopental for RSI if stable and methohexital for procedural sedation	Low incidence of pain on injection	Ideal for head injury patients if stable	Can cause cardiac/ respiratory depression
↓ dose of barbiturate and the opioid or benzo- diazepine dose when given together (synergistic effect)	Subcutaneous infiltration can cause phlebitis	Commonly used for radiology procedures	In subtherapeutic doses can get paradoxical reaction
All of the barbiturates may be used to treat status epilepticus	Discontinue immediately if extravasates → tissue necrosis can occur	Can give IV, IM, PO, PR	Can stimulate laryngeal reflexes
	Avoid intra-arterial injection → arterial vasospasm	May be used in patients with malignant hyperthermia	Avoid if severe hepatic function
			Avoid methohexital in patients with temporal lobe epilepsy

IM, intramuscular.

individuals without hypovolemia, cardiopulmonary disease, or concomitant depressant medications; sedative doses (10–20% of the induction dose) of barbiturates titrated gradually do not significantly produce hypotension, apnea, or loss of airway protective reflexes.[25,31] Substantial hypotension and respiratory depression may occur with:

- High doses, particularly if given rapidly.
- Hypovolemia.
- The coadministration of other cardiorespiratory depressants (such as opioids or benzodiazepines).
- Cardiopulmonary disease.[24]

The cardiovascular depressant effects of barbiturates are due to both a direct negative inotropic effect on the heart and peripheral vasodilatation.[22,29] In patients with normal sympathetic tone and reflexes, the drop in cardiac output, peripheral vascular resistance, and systemic arterial pressure that occurs when barbiturates are given may be somewhat mitigated by a mild compensatory tachycardia.[22,29] In patients with decreased preload (hypovolemia), who have an inability to respond with compensatory tachycardia (for example, patients on beta-blockers or calcium channel blockers), or in whom tachycardia may be harmful (ischemic heart disease,

severe heart failure, and so forth), barbiturates should be used with extreme caution.[21,24]

ADVERSE EFFECTS

Barbiturate-induced cardiac and respiratory depression is dose and rate of administration dependent. The coadministration of depressant medications (including opioids and benzodiazepines) may produce additive or potentiating effects.[21,22,26] Barbiturates depress the CNS respiratory centers and can produce respiratory depression and apnea, particularly in patients with underlying respiratory disease (e.g., chronic obstructive pulmonary disease [COPD])[24,26,36–42] Though apnea may resolve rapidly with the ultra-short-acting agents and the respiratory pattern may return to normal, responses to hypercarbia/hypoxia remain depressed for a longer time.[21]

Barbiturates tend to result in greater laryngeal reflex sensitivity than with other drugs such as propofol.[22] This increased airway reactivity can precipitate hiccups, gagging, coughing, or even laryngospasm.[25,40,41] The bronchospasm and laryngospasm seen with barbiturates (and other sedative-hypnotics) is ordinarily associated with airway manipulation in underanesthetized patients.[22,43]

A study of the use of methohexital alone, without a paralytic agent, for airway management in the ED found that increased airway reflexes and inadequate jaw relaxation impaired its performance in some patients.[41] This is a common finding in studies that have looked the use of induction agents alone to facilitate intubation and should not be taken to imply that methohexital should be avoided in RSI, it simply demonstrates that paralytic agents are an essential component RSI.[6,7,44,45]

Thiopental can cause histamine release so it should be used with caution in asthmatics.[32,45,46] Pruritus from histamine release can occur with the use of methohexital.[24]

Like all sedative-hypnotics, the administration of sub-anesthetic doses of barbiturates may produce paradoxical responses or hyperactivity (*nembutal rage*) with restlessness, delirium, and excitement, particularly in the presence of pain.[47–49] Therefore, analgesics should be coadministered when barbiturates are given for painful procedures.[16–24,50] This paradoxical reaction occurs more frequently in debilitated or elderly patients.[3] There are anecdotal reports of oral caffeine used as a treatment for such paradoxical reactions.[51]

The inducible porphyrias (variegate, acute intermittent, and hereditary coproporphyria) constitute an absolute contraindication to barbiturates since barbiturates (among others, such as diazepam, lidocaine, pentazocine, phenytoin, and sulfonamides) increase porphyrin synthesis.[3,21] Use of barbiturates in patients with porphyria results in demyelination of cranial and peripheral nerves causing weakness and paralysis.[24]

Although barbiturates have been used to treat status epilepticus,[34,35] methohexital has been associated with seizures.[4,41,52] Methohexital has a ring *N*-methyl group that is thought to account for its tendency to precipitate seizures in patients with epilepsy.[41]

SPECIFIC BARBITURATES

Thiopental (Pentothal)

Introduced into clinical practice in 1934, thiopental is the "most commonly used barbiturate for IV induction."[15] Because of its propensity to cause hypotension in hypovolemic patients it was said to ". . . have killed more Americans in Pearl Harbor than the Japanese."

Thiopental is an ultra-short-acting barbiturate. This ultrashort duration of action makes it well suited for procedural sedation. Though it is typically administered intravenously, the rectal route has been used,[53] though not as extensively as either methohexital or pentobarbital for outpatient procedural sedation. This is probably because it has a longer duration of action than methohexital when given by this route (duration = 60 minutes

for methohexital PR vs. 60–120 minutes for thiopental, and 60–240 minutes for pentobarbital PR).[7]

Thiopental is typically supplied as a powder, which when mixed with sterile water produces a 2.5% solution (25 mg/mL). The solution is highly alkaline (pH >10) and must be used within 24 hours of mixing. This very alkaline pH explains the danger that occurs with subcutaneous extravasation or inadvertent intra-arterial injection. It also explains why precipitates often form in the IV line when thiopental is administered with other medications in the same line and even with Ringer's lactate.

Methohexital (Brevital)

Methohexital is an ultra-short-acting barbiturate It has a rapid onset of action (<1 minute)[54] and a brief duration of action (<10 minutes) when given IV.[37,38,41] Methohexital via the IV,[37,41,42] PR,[55,56] and IM[57] routes has been used effectively and safely for procedural sedation in the ED and other outpatient settings especially for painless diagnostic studies (e.g., CT or MRI scans).

Methohexital is also supplied as a powder, which when reconstituted with sterile water produces a 1–2% solution (10–20 mg/mL). These solutions are stable for up to 6 weeks once constituted.

Pentobarbital (Nembutal)

Pentobarbital is a short-acting barbiturate with an onset of sedation in 5 minutes and duration of 15–45 minutes when given IV.[58–63] It can also be given IM, PO, or PR.[2,10,47,49] Of the barbiturates, pentobarbital is the most widely used for pediatric procedural sedation (particularly radiology procedures).[4,17,50,64–66] Pentobarbital has also been used for sedation in the ICUs.[8–10,67]

Pentobarbital is supplied as 50 mg/mL solution. Propylene glycol is used as a preservative and the pH is adjusted to 9.5.

ADMINISTRATION

Neither thiopental nor methohexital is associated with as much pain on IV injection as other commonly used IV sedative–hypnotics such as propofol or etomidate. Local tissue reaction to extravasation of thiopental produces marked pain, erythema, edema, and even tissue necrosis. Accidental intra-arterial injection of the barbiturates causes arterial spasm and severe pain in the distribution of the artery.[21] Clinical signs of arterial vasospasm include absent or diminished pulses, blanching or cyanosis of the extremity that may lead to irreversible tissue damage, and necrosis.

Treatment involves immediate injection of normal saline into the artery to dilute the injected barbiturate, and perhaps the injection of a vasodilator such as phentolamine, phenoxybenzamine, or papaverine to relieve arterial spasm and restore arterial blood flow.[24] Lidocaine and heparin may also be injected as required.[24] If the upper limb is involved, a stellate ganglion block creating a sympathectomy of the upper extremity has also been done in some cases.[24]

The category for use in pregnancy is pentobarbital-D, phenobarbital-D, thiopental-C, and methohexital-B.[68,69]

DOSE

Both thiopental and methohexital are used for moderate sedation. The safest manner of using these medications for this indication is by IV titration to the moderate sedation end point. Ordinarily, one begins with 10–20% of the induction dose of the medication and administers additional doses based on the rapidity and degree of CNS change noted. Since the sedatives cannot be titrated with oral or rectal administration, patients should be monitored closely for oversedation.

The induction dose of methohexital is 1 mg/kg IV (usual starting dose 1–1.5 mg/kg with additional 1 mg/kg given as needed up to 3 mg/kg total) given over 1 minute, 25 mg/kg PR, or 10 mg/kg IM. The induction dose of thiopental is 3–5 mg/kg IV and 25 mg/kg PR. The dose of pentobarbital for procedural sedation is 1–6 mg/kg IV, 2–6 mg/kg PO/PR/IM with a maximum dose of 150 mg.

For barbiturate coma, an IV loading dose of 10–15 mg/kg pentobarbital is given slowly over 1–2 hours followed by IV maintenance starting at 1–3 mg/kg/h. When given for sedation during ECMO, pentobarbital is given in a loading dose of 1–2 mg/kg followed by a continuous infusion at 1–2 mg/kg/h with repeat boluses and increasing the infusion as necessary.[6]

Opioids and benzodiazepines have synergistic effects with the barbiturates so the doses of both the barbiturate and the opoid or benzodiazepine should be decreased when given together.

SUMMARY

Barbiturates cause a decrease in cerebral metabolic rate, cerebral blood flow, intracranial pressure, and intraocular pressure. That is why they have been used as anticonvulsants, to treat status epilepticus, and to treat patients with increased intracranial pressure from head injuries or CNS disease (barbiturate coma or pentobarbital coma). Barbiturates are also used for procedural sedation, RSI,

sedation in the ICU, and induction of general anesthesia especially in patients with severe head injuries. Barbiturates can cause cardiac and respiratory depression, apnea, increased airway reactivity (resulting in hiccups, coughing, and laryngospasm), and paradoxical reactions. Methohexital and thiopental are preferred over pentobarbital in the ED because they are short acting. Methohexital can precipitate seizures so it should not be used in patients with epilepsy. Porphyria is an absolute contraindication to the use of the barbiturates.

REFERENCES

1. Rodriquez E, Jordan R. Contemporary trends in pediatric sedation and analgesia. *Emerg Med Clin North Am.* 2002;20: 199–222.
2. Silvilotti MLA, Filbin MR, Murray HE, et al. Does the sedative agent facilitate emergency rapid sequence intubation? *Acad Emerg Med.* 2003;10:612–620.
3. Gerardi MJ, Sacchetti AD, Cantor RM, et al. Rapid-sequence intubation of the pediatric patient. *Ann Emerg Med.* 1996; 28:55–74.
4. Luten RC, Stenklyft PH. Rapid-sequence induction in children. In: Harwood-Nuss A, Wolfson AB, Linden CH, et al. *The Clinical Practice of Emergency Medicine.* Philadelphia, PA: Lippincott Williams & Wilkins; 2001:1133–1137.
5. Liu LL, Gropper MA. Postoperative analgesia and sedation in the adult intensive care unit. *Drugs.* 2003;63:755–767.
6. Tobias JD. Sedation and analgesia in pediatric intensive care units. *Pediatr Drugs.* 1999;1:109–125.
7. Green SM, Krauss B. Procedural sedation and analgesia. In: Roberts JR, Hedges JR, Chanmugam AS, eds. *Clinical Procedures in Emergency Medicine.* Philadelphia, PA: W.B. Saunders; 2004:596–620.
8. Allen CH, Ward JD. An evidence-based approach to management of increased intracranial pressure. *Crit Care Clin.* 1998;14:485–495.
9. Urwin SC, Menon DK. Comparative tolerability of sedative agents in head-injured adults. *Drug Saf.* 2004;27:107–133.
10. Wadbrook PS. Advances in airway pharmacology. *Emerg Med Clin North Am.* 2000;18:767–788.
11. Tobias JD. Pharmacology of sedative agents. In: Malviya S, Naughton NN, Tremper KK, eds. *Sedation and Analgesia for Diagnostic and therapeutic Procedures.* Totowa, NJ: Humana Press; 2003:125–152.
12. Rubin M, Sadoonikoff N. Pediatric airway management. In: Tintinalli JE, Kelen GD, Stapczynski JS, eds. *Emergency Medicine—A Comprehensive Study Guide.* New York: McGraw-Hill; 2004:88–94.
13. Wetzel RC. Anesthesia and perioperative care. In: Behrman RE, Kliegman RM, Jensen HB, eds. *Nelson's Textbook of Pediatrics.* Philadelphia, PA: W.B. Saunders; 2004:342–357.
14. Decker JM, Lowe DA. Rapid sequence induction. In: Henretig FM, King C, eds. Textbook of Pediatric Emergency Procedures. Baltimore: Williams & Wilkins, 1997:141–159.

15. Krauss B, Green SM. Sedation and analgesia for procedures in children. *N Engl J Med.* 2000;342:939–945.

16. Cook BA, Bass JW, Nomizus, et al. Sedation of children for technical procedures: current standard of practice. *Clin Pediatr.* 1992;31:137–142.

17. Kester S, Benator RM, Weinberg SM, et al. Sedation in pediatric CT: national survey of current practice. *Radiology.* 1990;175:745–752.

18. Sacchetti A, Schafermeyer R, Gerardi M, et al. Pediatric analgesia and sedation. *Ann Emerg Med.* 1994;23:237–250.

19. Glauser J, Cullen B. Procedural sedation: definitions and review of systemic agents. *Emerg Med Rep.* 2002;23: 247–261.

20. Chiu JW, White PF. Nonopiod intravenous anesthesia. In: Barash PG, Cullen BF, Stoelting RK, eds. *Clinical Anesthesia.* Philadelphia, PA: Lippincott Williams & Wilkins 2001:327–343.

21. Kennedy SK. Pharmacology of intravenous anesthetic agents. In: Longnecker DE, Tinker JH, Morgan GE Jr, eds. *Principles and Practice of Anesthesiology.* St. Louis, MO: Mosby; 1998:1211–1232.

22. Malviya S. Barbiturates. In: Krauss B, Brustowicz RM, eds. *Pediatric Procedural Sedation and Analgesia.* Philadelphia, PA: Lippincott Williams & Wilkins 1999:33–38.

23. Blackburn P, Vissers R. Pharmacology of emergency department pain management and conscious sedation. *Emerg Med Clin North Am.* 2000;18:803–827.

24. Charney DS, Mihic SJ, Harris RA. Hypnotics and sedatives. In: Hardman JG, Limbird LE, Goodman AG, eds. *Goodman & Gilman's The Pharmacological Basis of Therapeutics.* New York: McGraw-Hill; 2001:399–427.

25. Urwin SC, Menon DK. Comparative, tolerability of sedative agents in head-injured adults. *Drug Saf.* 2004;27:107–133.

26. Evers AS, Crowder CM. General anesthetics. In: Hardman JG, Limbird LE, Gilman AG, eds. *Goodman & Gilman's The Pharmacological Basis of Therapeutics.* New York: McGraw-Hill; 2001:337–366.

27. Cunningham SJ, Crain EF. Conscious sedation. In: Henretig FM, King C, eds. *Textbook of Pediatric Emergency Procedures.* Baltimore, MD: Lippincott Williams & Wilkins; 1997: 445–454.

28. Alexander SM, Tobias ID. The use of sedation and muscle relaxation in the ventilated infant. *Clin Perinatol.* 1998;25: 63–78.

29. Kennedy RM, Luhmann JD. The "ouchless emergency department". *Pediatr Clin North Am.* 1999;46:1215–1247.

30. Fragen RJ, Avram MJ. Barbiturates. In: Miller RD, Cuehiora RF, Milar ED Jr, et al, eds. *Anesthesia.* Philadelphia, PA: Churchill Livingston; 2000:209–227.

31. Lewis KP, Stanley GD. Pharmacology. *Int Anesthesiol Clin.* 1999;37:73–86.

32. Proudfoot J. Analgesia, anesthesia, and conscious sedation. *Emerg Med Clin North Am.* 1995;13:357–379.

33. Danzl DF, Vissers RJ. Tracheal intubation and mechanical ventilation. In: Tintinalli JE, Kelen GD, Stapczynski JS, eds. *Emergency Medicine A Comprehensive Study Guide.* New York: McGraw-Hill; 2004:108–119.

34. Clausen J, Hirsch LJ, Emerson RG, et al. Treatment of refractory status epilepticus with pentobarbital, propofol, or midazolam: a systematic review. *Epilepsia.* 2002;43:146–153.

35. Osborn IP. Intravenous conscious sedation for pediatric patients. *Int Anesthesiol Clin.* 1999;37:99–111.

36. Morse RB, Arteaga G. Rapid sequence intubation. In: Strange GR, Ahrens WR, Lelyveld S, et al, eds. *Pediatric Emergency Medicine.* New York: McGraw-Hill; 2002:28–36.

37. Lerman B, Yoshida D, Levitt MA. A prospective evaluation of the safety and efficacy of methohexital in the emergency department. *Am J Emerg Med.* 1996;14:351–354.

38. Miner JR, Biros M, Krieg S, et al. Randomized clinical trial of propofol versus methohexital for procedural sedation during fracture and dislocation reduction in the emergency department. *Acad Emerg Med.* 2003;10:931–937.

39. Gale DW, Grissom TE, Mirenda JV. Titration of intravenous anesthetics for cardioversion: a comparison of propofol, methohexital, and midazolam. *Crit Care Med.* 1993;21: 1509–1513.

40. Chudnofsky CR, Lozon MM. Sedation and analgesia for procedures. In: Marx J, Hockberger RS, Walls RM, et al, eds. *Rosen's Emergency Medicine Concepts and Clinical Practice.* St Louis, MO: Mosby; 2002:2577–2590.

41. Sanderson PM. A survey of oral pentobarbital sedation for children undergoing abdominal CT scans after oral contrast medium. *Pediatr Anesth.* 1997;7:309–315.

42. Zink BJ, et al. The efficacy and safety of methohexital in the emergency department. *Ann Emerg Med.* 1991;20:1293–1298.

43. Schwanda AE, Freyer DR, Sanfilippo DJ, et al. Brief unconscious sedation for painful pediatric oncology procedures. *Am J Pediatr Hematol Oncol.* 1993;15:370–376.

44. White PF, Schlobohm RM, Pitts LH, et al. A randomized study of drugs for preventing increases in intracranial pressure during endotracheal suctioning. *Anesthesiology.* 1982;62:135–139.

45. Walls RM. Airway. In: Marx JA, Hockberger RS, Walls RM, et al, eds. *Rosen's Emergency Medicine Concepts and Clinical Practice.* St. Louis, MO: Mosby; 2002:2–21.

46. Sacchetti A, Gerardi MJ. Emergency department procedural sedation and analgesia. In: Strange GR, Ahrens WR, Lelyveld S, et al, eds. *Pediatric Emergency Medicine.* New York: McGraw-Hill; 2002:185–196.

47. Karian VE, Burrows PE, Zurakowski D, et al. Sedation for pediatric radiological procedures: analysis of potential causes of sedation failure and paradoxical reactions. *Pediatr Radiol.* 1999;29:869–873.

48. Slovis TL, Parks C, Reneau D, et al. Pediatric sedation: short-term effects. *Pediatr Radiol.* 1993;23:345–348.

49. Karian VE, Burrows PE, Zurakowski, D, et al. The development of a pediatric radiology sedation program. *Pediatr Radiol.* 2002;32:348–353.

50. Hopson LR, Dronen SC. Pharmacologic adjuncts to intubation. In: Roberts JR, Hedges JR, Chanmugam AS, et al, eds. *Clinical Procedures in Emergency Medicine.* Philadelphia, PA: W.B. Saunders; 2004:100–114.

51. Bunt C, Towlin R. Treatment of pentobarbital sodium (nembutal) hyperactivity: a new approach. *Pediatr Radiol.* 2000;30:204.

52. Male CG. Methohexitone-induced convulsions in epileptics. *Anaesth Intensive Care.* 1977;5:226–230.

53. Sedik H. Use of intravenous methohexital as a sedative in pediatric emergency departments. *Arch Pediatr Adolesc Med.* 2001;155:665–668.

54. Pomeransy ES, Chudnofsky CR, Deegans TJ, et al. Rectal methohexital for computed tomography imaging of stable pediatric emergency department patients. *Pediatrics.* 2000; 105:1110–1114.

55. Manuli MA, Davies L. Rectal methohexital for sedation of children during imaging procedures. *AJR Am J Roentgenol.* 1993;160:577–580.

56. Varner PD, Ebert JP, McKay RD, et al. Methohexital sedation of children undergoing CT scan. *Anesth Analg.* 1985;64:643–645.

57. Moro-Sutherland DM, Algren JT, Louis PT, et al. Comparison of intravenous midazolam with pentobarbital for sedation for head computed tomography imaging. *Acad Emerg Med.* 2000;7:1370–1375.

58. Greenburg SB, Adams RC, Aspinall CL. Initial experience with intravenous pentobarbital sedation for children undergoing MRI at a tertiary care pediatric hospital: the learning curve. *Pediatr Radiol.* 2000;30:689–691.

59. Kain ZN, Gaal DJ, Kain TS, et al. A first pass cost analysis of Propofol versus barbiturates for children undergoing magnetic resonance imaging. *Anesth Anal.* 1994;79:1102–1106.

60. Egelhoff JC, Ball WS Jr, Koch BL, et al. Safety and efficacy of sedation in children using a structured sedation program. *AJE.* 1997;168:1259–1262.

61. Strain JD, Campbell JB, Harvey LA, et al. IV Nembutal: safe sedation for children undergoing CT. *AJR Am J Roentgenol.* 1988;151:975–979.

62. Mason KP, Zurakowski D, Karian VE, et al. Sedatives used in pediatric imaging: comparison of IV pentobarbital with IV pentobarbital with midazolam added. *AJR Am J Roentgenol.* 2001;177:427–430.

63. Bloomfield EL, Masaryk TJ, Caplin A, et al. Intravenous sedation for MR imaging of the brain and spine in children: pentobarbital versus propofol. *Radiology.* 1993;186:93–97.

64. Sanderson PM. A survey of pentobarbital sedation for children undergoing abdominal CT scans after oral contrast medium. *Paediatr Anaesth.* 1997;7:309–315.

65. Rooks VJ, Chung T, Connor L, et al. Comparison of oral pentobarbital sodium (nembutal) and oral chloral hydrate for sedation of infants during radiologic imaging: preliminary results. *AJR Am J Roentgenol.* 2003;180:1125–1128.

66. Tobias JD. Pentobarbital for sedation during mechanical ventilation in the Pediatric ICU patient. *J Intens Care Med.* 2000;15:115–120.

67. Okutan V, Lenk MK, Sarici SU, et al. Efficacy and safety of rectal thiopental sedation in outpatient echocardiographic examination of children. *Acta Paediatr.* 2000;89:1340–1343.

68. Briggs GG, Freeman RK, Yaffe SJ, eds. *Pentobarbital, Phenobarbital Drugs in Pregnancy and Lactation.* Philadelphia, PA: Lippincott Williams & Wilkins 2002;1087, 1097–1105.

69. Thiopental, methohexitol. In: *Mosby's Drug Consult.* 15th ed. St. Louis, MO: Mosby; 2005; pp II-1900 and II-2783.

20

Ketamine

Sharon E. Mace

HIGH YIELD FACTS

- Causes minimal respiratory depression (patients maintain spontaneous respiration/ airway reflexes).
- Has analgesic as well as sedative/amnestic effects so it can be used for painful or painless procedures.
- Can use with an antisialagogue (preferably glycopyrrolate) to ↓ secretions (perhaps ↓ incidence of laryngospasm) if time and circumstances permit.
- May increase intracranial pressure (ICP) in patients with elevated ICP or imperfect ICP control so may want to avoid if ventilation is not controlled.
- Sympathomimetic effects make it a good choice in patients with hypotension, bradycardia, or shock; and a poor choice with thyrotoxicosis, uncontrolled hypertension, and ischemic heart disease.
- Coadministering midazolam does not ↓ emergence reactions.
- Causes bronchodilation so excellent choice in patients with asthma/other bronchospastic diseases and may prevent intubation in some.
- Include "fall" precautions in discharge instructions since it can cause disequilibrium.

INDICATIONS

Ketamine is used for procedural sedation in pediatric and adult patients.[1,2] Because it is a *dissociative* anesthetic agent, sedation produced with this agent is generally termed *dissociative sedation*, particularly if the patient becomes dissociated.

The dissociative state is *qualitatively* much different from the sedation produced by conventional sedative hypnotic agents. Once dissociated, patients do not respond purposefully to painful stimuli, much like patients under general anesthesia, though unlike patients under general anesthesia they maintain muscle tone (catalepsy), ventilation, and protective airway reflexes. In high doses, ketamine abolishes ventilatory drive, loses its cataleptic property, no longer supports the maintenance of protective airway reflexes, and produces hypotension, like other general anesthetic agents. Sedation without dissociation is possible with lower doses of ketamine that is *qualitatively* similar to the sedation produced by sedative hypnotics. Thus, ketamine conforms poorly to conventional definitions of moderate and deep sedation if given in sufficient doses to produce dissociation. In lower (sedative) doses it conforms rather better.

Ketamine is also employed in rapid sequence induction (particularly valuable with severe bronchospastic disease,[3–5] and in the hypovolemic or hypotensive patient, or critically ill patient),[6–9] sedation in the intensive care unit (in adult, pediatric, and even neonatal patients),[10–12] and for the induction/maintenance of general anesthesia.[13]

Ketamine is unique among commonly used sedatives in that it has analgesic properties,[14] so it has been used for refractory acute and chronic pain management.[15] It also has bronchodilating properties which account for its recommendation for the treatment of acute, severe asthma or status asthmaticus.[16,17] Unlike the sedative hypnotics and opioids, ketamine maintains protective airway reflexes.[13,18] Because of ketamine's remarkable airway and cardiovascular stability, it has been extremely valuable in the developing world where it is used for minor and major surgery, particularly in regions where anesthesia providers are unavailable.[19] Ketamine is the anesthetic of choice on the battlefield or during disasters when general anesthesia is not possible for various reasons, including time and lack of anesthesia equipment.[20]

PHARMACOLOGY

Ketamine is a dissociative anesthetic that has sedative effects with amnestic and analgesic properties.[21] Sedation, analgesia, and amnesia are all produced before dissociation in a dose-related fashion. Ketamine is unlike other anesthetics that produce a sleep-like state characterized by the depression of brain wave activity secondary to depression of the reticular activating system due to inhibition of neurotransmission by γ-aminobutyric acid (GABA).[22]

Ketamine produces a trance-like cataleptic state in which the brain's higher centers are disassociated from, and prevented from perceiving painful, visual, or auditory stimuli. Catalepsy simply means the maintenance of muscle tone. When dissociated with ketamine, patients often

Table 20-1. Ketamine: Dosage Information

Dose (mg/kg)	Usual Dose (mg/kg)	Maximum Dose	Onset (min)	Duration (min)
1-2 IV initial (repeat 0.5–1.0 bolus for longer procedures) 4 IM 7 PO 10–15 PR	1.5 IV 4 IM 7 PO 15 PR (higher dose 2 IV for RSI)	Need higher doses PO, PR with less predictable effect, and ↑ incidence of side effects (best to avoid PO, PR, and intranasal)	1 IV 5 IM 20 PO, PR	15 IV 30 IM 30–60 PO, PR

IV, intravenous; IM, intramuscular; PR, per rectum; RSI, rapid sequence intubation.

keep their eyes open and maintain many reflexes, especially the protective airway reflexes: swallowing, glottic closure, and cough. It does not depress electroencephalogram (EEG) activity. Patients dissociated with ketamine are often described as "The lights are on but nobody is home."[20]

There is a functional and electrophysiologic dissociation between the cortex and the limbic system.[23] In addition to depression of the reticular activating system via inhibition of GABA neurotransmission, ketamine acts on the halmoneocortical projection system. The drug stimulates areas of the limbic system, especially the hippocampus while selectively depressing areas of the cerebral cortex including the thalamus and cortical association areas. Ketamine exerts its action via interaction with the *N*-methyl-D-aspartate (NMDA) receptor and the μ-receptor.[10,13,24]

Ketamine is an arylcyclohexylamine (2-*O*-chlorophenyl-2-methylaminocyclohexamine) whose structure resembles both phencyclidine hydrochloride (PCP) and cyclohexamine.[23,25] It is an analogue of PCP, and has properties similar to PCP including nystagmus and the occasional emergence reaction with the undesirable side effects of dysphoria, delirium, and psychosis. Hence, its popularity as an illicit drug of abuse.[26] After a parenteral dose, ketamine is rapidly absorbed by the highly perfused nervous system leading to rapid onset with redistribution into the peripheral tissues.[27] Ketamine is metabolized by the hepatic microsomal enzyme system to norketamine with the degradation products then excreted by the kidneys.[27] Table 20-1 contains dosage information and Table 20-2 contains administration information.

Table 20-2. Ketamine: Administration Information

Practical Tips	Administration	Advantages	Side Effects/Disadvantages
Has analgesic effects (may not need additional pain medication) Use in patients with bronchospasm (e.g., asthma) Discharge instructions should include fall precautions because of ataxia Use in disasters, battlefield, developing world if no anesthesia provider available	May use glycopyrrolate to ↓ secretions Do not administer midazolam since it does not ↓ incidence of emergence reactions Titrate IV to end point. No pain on injection with ketamine	Respiratory/cardiovascular stability (maintains airway reflexes) Excellent safety profile Bronchodilator (use with asthmatics) Sympathomimetic effects (use if hypotension, shock, bradycardia) Provides sedation, amnesia, and analgesia Can be used as sole agent for painless or painful procedures Can be given IM as well as IV (no need for IV start if given IM)	Emergence reaction Vomiting Rarely, laryngospasm, avoid if respiratory disease (e.g., pneumonia) present or age <3 months Sympathomimetic effects: avoid if ↑ ICP and unventilated, ↑ intraocular pressure, severe head injury other than induction for intubation, severe cardiovascular disease, severe thyroid disease Avoid in patients with psychosis (↑ emergence reaction)

IM, intramuscular; IV, intravenous; URI, upper respiratory infections.

CLINICAL EFFECTS

Ketamine has an excellent safety profile.[18,28] Ketamine's major advantage is that at sedative and dissociative doses it maintains cardiovascular/respiratory stability, causes minimal respiratory depression, and does not result in loss of protective airway reflexes with the patient maintaining spontaneous ventilation.[3,21,28,29]

Ketamine's mild sympathomimetic effects lead to bronchodilation, mild tachycardia, and a slight increase in the systolic blood pressure. Because of its bronchodilating effects, ketamine has been used in induction doses to facilitate intubation and by continuous low-dose infusion to avoid intubation in patients with acute severe asthma.[16,17,30–35] The tachycardia and increased blood pressure occurring with ketamine may be advantageous in patients with hypotension and/or bradycardia but can be a disadvantage in patients with significant hypertension or tachycardia.[5–8,36] The sympathomimetic effects are probably due to ketamine's ability to block the reuptake of catecholamines,[20,36] and may be mediated through the CNS.[6,37]

Ketamine does cause increases in cardiac output and myocardial oxygen consumption as well as increasing the heart rate and blood pressure.[6] This may be an undesirable side effect in patients with coronary artery disease, although the true risk is unknown since there has been limited use of ketamine in patients with coronary artery disease.[18] Ketamine does not cause dysrhythmias.

Ketamine causes an increase in cerebral metabolism, cerebral blood flow, and intracranial pressure (ICP) due to cerebral vasodilation and the rise in systemic blood pressure, particularly if ventilation is not controlled.[13,38–40] Ketamine has been said to be contraindicated (e.g., for rapid sequence intubation [RSI]) in the face of elevated ICP or imperfect ICP control (e.g., acute severe head injury), though this advice is probably overstated provided ventilation and arterial blood pressure is controlled. It can also cause an increase in intraocular pressure. Thus, ketamine may be contraindicated in patients with increased intraocular pressure or open globe eye injuries.[28,41]

As with other sedatives such as propofol, ketamine has antiepileptic activity,[20,36,42] although there have been instances of seizures temporally associated with the use of ketamine in patients with seizure disorders.[20]

Occasionally patients will vocalize or have random meaningless movements including turning the neck leading to partial airway obstruction and snoring respirations after receiving ketamine.[36] Head/neck repositioning ought to resolve this problem and rarely interferes with the performance of procedures.[36]

ADVERSE EFFECTS

The most common side effect of ketamine is probably the emergence reaction.[41] This is thought to be caused by the drug's depression of CNS visual/auditory relay nuclei causing altered perception and interpretation of visual and auditory stimuli.[13] The occurrence of emergence reactions is associated with age (adults > children), gender (females > males), anxiety level and psychologic state prior to the procedure, and underlying medical conditions.[41,43,44] The incidence varies but may be as high as 10–30% in adults[13] with a much lower occurrence in children.[43] Severe agitation occurs in 1.6% and mild agitation in 17.6% of the pediatric patients.[43] Emergence reactions are less common in older children (12.1% in those >5 years vs. 22.5% in children <5 years of age).[43]

Small doses of midazolam have been used to treat severe emergence reactions[41]; however, prophylactic coadministration of benzodiazepines is not recommended since they have no proven benefit,[18,28,45–48] delay ketamine metabolism thereby prolonging recovery,[23,49,50] may actually increase the incidence of recovery agitation in specific patient populations,[47] and increase the risk of respiratory depression.[20] These recommendations differ from earlier reports that suggest prophylactic coadministration of benzodiazepines (either diazepam, lorazepam, or preferably midazolam) are effective in suppressing the emergence reaction.[17,51–55] One study found that the incidence of emergence reactions actually increased in patients over 10 years of age when midazolam was given with ketamine (recovery agitation = 5.7% for ketamine vs. 35.7% for ketamine plus midazolam)[47]; however, the addition of midazolam did decrease the incidence of vomiting.[48] A second study also found no difference in recovery agitation between ketamine alone versus ketamine and midazolam, although the addition of midazolam was again noted to decrease the incidence of vomiting.[48] Such differing conclusions may at least be partly explained by different patient populations: pediatric patients versus adults. Midazolam has been suggested as the preferred drug since it has a short duration of action and powerful amnestic effects.[17]

There has also been a debate on whether a quiet secluded environment which limits stimuli during the postrecovery period decreases the incidence of emergence reactions.[20,23,28] Some suggest that preprocedure discussions with the patient (adult or child) will decrease the occurrence of recovery agitation.[20,23]

Vomiting occurs in 6.7% of patients, often persists into the recovery phase, and is also age-related, being more common in younger children (12.5% incidence in children <5 years vs. 3.5% in those >5 years)[43,56–59]; however, there have been no documented reports of *clinically significant* aspiration with ketamine when used in patients without contraindications.[18]

Clinically significant respiratory depression is rare but has occurred when ketamine has been accidentally given:

- In massive doses (>22 mg/kg intramuscular [IM])
- By rapid intravenous (IV) bolus
- To specific types of patients (e.g., those with CNS injury/disease or ill neonates)
- In combination with the respiratory depressant drugs[20,28]

It is generally more difficult for infants and neonates to maintain an airway with any sedative agent than it is for older children and adults.[20] There are several reasons for this, which are not unique to ketamine, including anatomical differences and increased laryngeal reactivity. The suggestion has been to avoid using ketamine in patients <3 months old and to use it with caution in infants aged 3–12 months.[20]

Laryngospasm is a rare occurrence with ketamine use. In fact, laryngospasm is associated with all of the sedative hypnotics to some extent. The incidence is about 1% (0.017, 0.4, 0.9, and 1.4%, respectively in various studies including studies with data from over 11,000 patients).[42,43,60,61] It manifests as a transient stridor. It is likely due to ketamine-induced sensitization of laryngeal reflexes and in some cases is thought to be related to excessive upper respiratory secretions.[20] Hence, the recommendation by some for the administration of an antisialagogue drug such as glycopyrrolate or atropine with ketamine.[36] Risk factors for laryngospasm include respiratory infection (fivefold increase) and age (three times greater risk in infants aged 1–3 months than the average).[28] In one report of nearly 1200 cases of laryngospasm, the incidence of complications were: (1) hypoxia: 3.2%; aspiration: 1.1%; and (3) cardiac arrest: 0.5%.[62]

Laryngospasm occurring with ketamine or other sedatives is generally transient and best treated by repositioning the head, administering supplemental oxygen, applying positive pressure to the upper airway or bag-valve-mask-assisted ventilation, and rarely intubation.[63]

The laryngeal musculature is exquisitely sensitive to neuromuscular blocking agents, so much so that 10% of a paralyzing dose of succinylcholine is recommended if required to break deadly laryngospasm.

Laryngospasm has been reported during procedures in which posterior pharyngeal stimulation occurs.[63] This has

lead to the recommendation that such procedures are a relative contraindication to the use of ketamine.[42,60] However, recent studies suggest otherwise, that ketamine can be used safely during procedures that stimulate the posterior pharynx such as dental procedures, airway management, esophagoscopy, and bronchoscopy.[64–66] The earlier study of pediatric patients undergoing gastroenterology procedures with an 8.2% incidence of transient laryngospasm had a very high number of American Society of Anesthesiologists (ASA) status III or greater patients.[63] Almost half the patients in this earlier study were ASA status III or greater.[63] This may be one explanation for the disparity between this study[63] and the recent studies.[64–66]

If used, glycopyrrolate is preferred because it produces less tachycardia, has a somewhat greater antisialogic effect, does not cross the blood-brain barrier (quaternary substituted ammonium compound) so it does not have CNS effects, and is not associated with the recovery agitation sometimes seen with atropine.[30,67] The glycopyrrolate and atropine dose is 0.01 mg/kg with a maximum dose of 0.25 mg. The onset and peak effect profiles of concomitantly IM-administered ketamine and an antimuscarinic agent are an imperfect match calling into question the rationale of the practice though some still advise that both drugs can be combined in the same syringe and given IM so only one injection is necessary.

A recent report challenges the dictum of avoiding ketamine in infants <3 months old and/or procedures that stimulate the posterior pharynx. In this study, ketamine sedation was used safely and effectively in infants (<12 months old) for bronchoscopy.[66] These authors suggest that the respiratory complications such as hypoxia, apnea, and laryngospasm may be more a function of a *higher risk* population (such as greater ASA class) and the type of procedure.[66] In this study, the majority of complications were related to the procedure itself, and occurred after the bronchoscope passed below the vocal cords.[66]

Ataxia commonly occurs during the recovery phase with ketamine use.[45] To prevent falling, patients recovering from ketamine sedation should be watched closely by family or friends and should not be allowed to walk unassisted for several hours until the disequilibrium resolves.

Because ketamine has mild sympathomimetic effects, it may be advisable to avoid ketamine in patients on thyroid medicines, with hyperthyroidism, or porphyria, though the contraindication for ketamine use in patients on thyroid medications or with thyroid disease is founded on anecdotal evidence.[20]

Other relative contraindications to ketamine use are based on:

1. Its sympathomimetic effects (avoid in patients with increased intracranial or intraocular pressure, severe head injury, and significant cardiovascular disease).
2. Increased risk for laryngospasm (increased occurrence in patients with pulmonary disease such as pneumonia and/or infants <3 months old).
3. Underlying psychiatric disease (predisposition for emergence reactions).

ADMINISTRATION

Ketamine may be given IV, IM, PO, PR, and intranasally. Higher doses of ketamine are required to achieve a similar effect when it is given via the oral, rectal, or intranasal routes. Moreover, the onset, peak, duration, and intensity of effect are less predictable than when the drug is titrated intravenously. This increase in dose is associated with an increased incidence of side effects. IV or IM administration is preferable to the PO, PR, and intranasal routes.[20] Ketamine does not cause pain with IV administration. Like the sedative hypnotics, ketamine when employed for procedural sedation ought to be titrated to the desired end point. Ketamine is a category B drug during pregnancy.[68] (Note: The manufacturer and micromedex do not list a pregnancy category for ketamine and lexi-compon line lists ketamine as a category D drug. However, other sources including textbooks[68] list ketamine as a category B drug).

Of the medications used as a single PO, PR, or IM dose (e.g., chloral hydrate and pentobarbital) to produce moderate sedation, ketamine is widely considered the safest as it tends to best preserve respiration and airway protective reflexes. In other words, the margin of safety is greatest.

Though there is some disagreement on this matter, it is generally felt that the establishment of IV access as a safety precaution is unnecessary when using IM, PO, or PR ketamine unless patient condition warrants it (e.g., ischemic heart disease).

As described in Chapter 17 (Propofol), ketamine for procedural sedation may be combined with propofol (in the same or separate syringes) to minimize the cardiorespiratory hazards seen when propofol alone is used. The typical preparation is a 5 mg/mL solution of each titrated 1–2 mL at a time to the desired end point. This is a very useful preparation and technique.

DOSE

As with any medication used intravenously for procedural sedation, ketamine is best titrated in small doses to achieve the desired end point (sedated or dissociated). Large bolus doses are unsafe and not recommended. Start with 10% of the induction dose (1.5 mg/kg) given over 30–60 seconds and repeat as needed. Depending on the response to the initial dose and its time course to effect, one may adjust the dose or interval to achieve the desired end point.

The IM dose of ketamine is 4 mg/kg ideal body weight and 2 mg/kg <2 years of age. With the IM route, sedation followed by dissociation will onset in 5–10 minutes and persist for 15–30 minutes. The PO dose is 7 mg/kg ideal body weight. The PO route is somewhat slower in onset and ought to be given a full 20 minutes prior to the procedure to allow the full effect of the dose. Repeated doses should to be no more than 50% of the initial dose and repeated no more than once to preserve safety.

SUMMARY

Ketamine is a dissociative anesthetic agent that is used for procedural sedation, rapid sequence induction/intubation, the treatment of acute severe asthma, and acute/chronic pain management. It is unique among the commonly used sedatives in that it has analgesic properties. Ketamine maintains cardiorespiratory stability, has minimal respiratory depression, and is a bronchodilator. These properties make it a good choice in patients with bronchospasm, hypovolemia, hypotension, and for those who are hemodynamically unstable or in respiratory distress. Ketamine doses have mild sympathomimetic effects resulting in a mild tachycardia, a slight increase in the systolic blood pressure, cardiac output, and myocardial oxygen consumption. It also causes an increase in ICP and intraocular pressure so may be contraindicated in patients with severe head or eye injuries. The most common side effect is the emergence reaction, which is not prevented by the prophylactic coadministration of benzodiazepines. Laryngospasm is associated with all of the sedative hypnotics including ketamine but is a rare occurrence with an incidence of <1% with ketamine use. Coadministration of an antisialogogue (glycopyrrolate or atropine) with ketamine has been recommended by some to decrease secretions and the incidence of laryngospasm.

REFERENCES

1. Cunningham SJ, Crain EF. Conscious sedation. In: Henretig FM, King C, eds. *Textbook of Pediatric Emergency Procedures.* Baltimore, MD: Williams & Wilkins; 1997:445–454.
2. Chudnofsky CR, Weber JE, Stoyanoff PJ, et al. A combination of midazolam and ketamine for procedural sedation and analgesia in adult ED patients. *Acad Emerg Med.* 2000; 7:228–235.

3. Walls RM. Airway. In Marx JA, Hockberg RS, Walls RM, et al, eds. *Rosen's Emergency Medicine—Concepts and Clinical Practice.* St. Louis, MO: Mosby; 2002:2–21.

4. Silvilotti MLA, Filbin MR, Murray HE, et al. Does the sedative agent facilitate rapid sequence intubation? *Acad Emerg Med.* 2003;10:612–620.

5. Danzl DF, Vissers RJ. Tracheal intubation and mechanical ventilation. In: Tintinalli JE, Kelen GD, Stapczynski JS, eds. *Emergency Medicine a Comprehensive Study Guide.* New York: McGraw-Hill; 2004:108–119.

6. Wadbrook PS. Advances in airway pharmacology. *Emerg Med Clin North Am.* 2000;18(4):767–788.

7. Luten RC, Stenklyfgt PH. Rapid-sequence induction in children. In: Harwood-Nuss A, Wolfson AB, Linden CH, et al. *The Clinical Practice of Emergency Medicine.* Philadelphia, PA: Lippincott Williams & Wilkins; 2001:1133–1137.

8. Decker JM, Lowe DA. Rapid sequence induction. In: Henretig FM, King C, eds. *Textbook of Pediatric Emergency Procedures.* Baltimore, MD: Williams & Wilkins; 1997:141–159.

9. Johnston MN, Lisbelt EL. Acute pain management and procedural sedation in children. In: Tintinalli JE, Kelen GB, Stapczynski JS, eds. *Emergency Medicine A Comprehensive Study Guide.* New York: McGraw-Hill; 2004:858–869.

10. Liu LL, Gropper MA. Postoperative analgesia and sedation in the adult intensive care unit. *Drugs.* 2003;63:755–767.

11. Tobias JD. Sedation and analgesia in pediatric intensive care units. *Pediatr Drugs.* 1999;1:109–126.

12. Alexander SM, Todres ID. The use of sedation and muscle relaxation in the ventilated infant. *Clin Perinatol.* 1998; 25:63–78.

13. Reeves JG, Glass PA, Lubarsky DA, et al. Intravenous nonopioid anesthetics. In: Miller RD, ed. *Miller's Anesthesia.* Philadelphia, PA: Elsevier Churchill Livingstone; 2005: 317–378.

14. Murphy MF. Anaesthesia and analgesia in the emergency department. *Can J Anaesth.* 1997;44:R52–R59.

15. Short TG, Young Y. Toxicity of intravenous anesthetics. *Best Pract Res Clin Anesthesiol.* 2003;17:77–89.

16. Morse RB, Arteaga G. Rapid sequence induction. In: Strange GR, Ahrens WR, Lelyveld S, et al, eds. *Pediatric Emergency Medicine.* New York: McGraw-Hill; 2002:28–36.

17. Hopson LR, Dronen SC. Pharmacologic agents to intubation. In: Roberts JR, Hedges JR, Chanmugam AS, et al, eds. *Clinical Procedures in Emergency Medicine.* Philadelphia, PA: W.B. Saunders; 2004:100–114.

18. Green SM, Krauss B. Procedural sedation and analgesia. In: Roberts JR, Hedges JR, Chanmugam AS, et al, eds. *Clinical Procedures in Emergency Medicine.* Philadelphia, PA: W.B. Saunders 2004:596–620.

19. Ketcham DW. Where there is no anesthesiologist: the many uses of ketamine. *Trop Doct.* 1990;20:163–166.

20. Green SR. Dissociative agents. In: Kraus B, Bructowicz RM, eds. *Pediatric Procedural Sedation and Analgesia.* Philadelphia, PA: Lippincott Williams & Wilkins; 1999: 47–54.

21. Krauss B. Management of acute pain and anxiety in children undergoing procedures in the emergency department. *Pediatr Emerg Care.* 2001;17:115–122.

22. Kennedy SK. Pharmacology of intravenous anesthetic agents. In: Longnecker DE, Tinker JH, Morgan GE Jr, eds. *Principles and Practice of Anesthesiology.* St. Louis, MO: Mosby; 1998:1211–1252.

23. White PF, Way WL, Trevor AJ. Ketamine—it's pharmacology and therapeutic uses. *Anesthesiology.* 1982;56:119–136.

24. Irifune M, Sato T, Kamata Y, et al. Evidence for GABA (A) receptor agonistic properties of ketamine: convulsive and anesthetic behavioral models in mice. Anesth Analg. 2000; 91:230–236.

25. Evers AS, Crowder CM. General anesthetics. In: Hardman JG, Limbird LE, Gilman AG, eds. *Goodman & Gilman's The Pharmacological Basis of Therapeutics.* New York: McGraw-Hill; 2001:337–365.

26. Hansen KN, Prybys KM. Hallucinogens. In: Tintinalli JE, Kelen GD, Stapczynski JS, eds. *Emergency Medicine. A Comprehensive Study Guide.* New York: McGraw-Hill; 2004: 1079–1085.

27. Nicolaou DD. Procedural sedation and analgesia. In: Tintinalli JE, Kelen GD, Stapczynski JS, eds. *Emergency Medicine. A Comprehensive Study Guide.* New York: McGraw-Hill; 2004:275–280.

28. Sachetti A, Gerardi MJ. Emergency department procedural sedation and analgesia. In: Strange GR, Ahrens WR, Lelyveld S, et al. *Pediatric Emergency Medicine.* New York: McGraw-Hill; 2002:185–196.

29. Kim G, Green SM, Denmark TK, et al. Ventilatory response during dissociative sedation in children—a pilot study. *Acad Emerg Med.* 2003;10:140–145.

30. Petrillo TM, Fortenberry JD, Linzer JF, et al. Emergency department use of ketamine in pediatric status asthmaticus. *J Asthma.* 2001;38:657–664.

31. Bohn D, Kalloghlian A, Jenkins J, et al. Intravenous salbutamol in the treatment of status asthmaticus in children. *Crit Care Med.* 1984;12:892–896.

32. Sarma VJ. Use of ketamine in acute severe asthma. *Acta Anaesthesiol Scand.* 1992;36:106–107.

33. Strube PJ, Hallam PL. Ketamine by continuous infusion in status asthmaticus. *Anaesthesia.* 1986;41:1017–1019.

34. Hemming A, MacKenzie I, Finfer S. Response to ketamine in status asthmaticus resistant to maximal medical treatment. *Thorax.* 1994;49:90–91.

35. Rock MJ, Reyes de la Rocha S, L'Hommedieu CS, et al. Use of ketamine in asthmatic children to treat respiratory failure refractory to conventional therapy. *Crit Care Med.* 1986;14:514–516.

36. Chudnofsky CR, Lozon MM. Sedation and analgesia for procedures. In: Marx JA, Hockberger RS, Walls RM, et al, eds. *Rosen's Emergency Medicine Concepts and Clinical Practice.* St. Louis, MO: Mosby; 2002:2577–2590.

37. Rubin M, Sadovnikoff N. Pediatric airway management. In: Tintinalli JE, Kelen GD, Stapczynski JS, eds. *Emergency Medicine. A Comprehensive Study Guide.* New York: McGraw-Hill; 2004:88–94.

38. Werner C. Effects of analgesia and sedation on cerebrovascular circulation, cerebral blood volume, cerebral metabolism

and intracranial pressure. *Anaesthetist*. 1995;44 (suppl 3): S566–S572.

39. Gremmelt A, Braun U. Analgesia and sedation in patients with head-brain trauma. *Anaesthetist*. 1995;44(suppl 3): S559–S565.

40. Kolenda H, Gremmelt A, Rading S, et al. Ketamine for analgosedative therapy in intensive care treatment of head-injured patients. *Acta Neurochir* (Wien). 1996;138(10):1193–1199.

41. Muse DA. Conscious and deep sedation. In: Harwood–Nuss A, Wolfson AB, Linden CH, et al, eds. *The Clinical Practice of Emergency Medicine*. Philadelphia, PA: Lippincott Williams & Wilkins; 2001:1758–1762.

42. Green SM, Johnson NE. Ketamine sedation for pediatric procedures. Part 2. Review and implications. *Ann Emerg Med*. 1990;19:1033–1046.

43. Green SM, Kupperman N, Rothrock SG, et al. Predictors of adverse events with ketamine sedation in children. *Ann Emerg Med*. 2000;35:35–42.

44. Hostetler MA, David CO. Prospective age-based comparison of behavioral reactions occurring after ketamine sedation in the ED. *Am J Emerg Med*. 2002;20:463–468.

45. Dachs RJ, Innes GM. Intravenous ketamine sedation of pediatric patients in the emergency department. *Ann Emerg Med*. 1997;29:146–150.

46. Mace SE, Barata LA, Cravero JP, et al. Clinical policy: evidence-based approach to pharmacologic agents used in pediatric sedation and analgesia in the emergency department. *Ann Emerg Med*. 2004;14(4):342–377.

47. Wathen JE, Roback MG, Mackenzie T, et al. Does midazolam alter the clinical effects of intravenous ketamine sedation in children? A double-blind, randomized, controlled, emergency department trial. *Am Emerg Med*. 2000;36:579–588.

48. Sherwin TS, Green SM, Khan A, et al. Does adjunctive midazolam reduce recovery agitation after ketamine sedation for pediatric procedures? A randomized, double blind, placebo- controlled trial. *Ann Emerg Med*. 2000;36:579–588.

49. Lo JN, Cumming JF. Interaction between sedative premedicants and ketamine in man and in isolated perfused rat livers. *Anesthesiology*. 1975;43:307–312.

50. Reich DL, Silvay G. Ketamine: an update on the first twenty-five years of clinical experience. *Can J Anaesth*. 1989;36:186–197.

51. White PF. Pharmacologic interactions of midazolam and ketamine in surgical patients. *Clin Pharmacol Ther*. 1982; 31:280–281.

52. Dundee JW, Liburn JK. Ketamine-lorazepam: attenuation of the psychic sequelae of ketamine by lorazepam. *Anaesthesia*. 1978;32:312–314.

53. Liburn JK, Dundee JW, Nair SG, et al. Ketamine sequelae—evaluation of the ability of various premedicants to attenuate its psychic actions. *Anaesthesia*. 1978;33:307–311.

54. Dundee JW, McGowan AW, Lilburn JK, et al. Comparison of the actions of diazepam and lorazepam. *Br J Anaesth*. 1979;51:439–446.

55. Kothary SP, Pandit SK. Orally administered diazepam and lorazepam—sedative and amnestic effects. *Anesthesiology*. 1980;53:S18.

56. Kennedy RM, Porter FL, Miller JP, et al. Comparison of fentanyl/midazolam with ketamine/midazolam for pediatric orthopedic emergencies. *Pediatrics*. 1998;102:956–963.

57. Parker RI, Mahan RA, Guigliano D, et al. Efficiency and safety of intravenous midazolam and ketamine as sedation for therapeutic and diagnostic procedures in children. *Pediatrics*. 1997;99:427–431.

58. McDowell RH, Scher CS, Barst SM. Total intravenous anesthesia for children undergoing brief diagnostic or therapeutic procedures. *J Clin Anesth*. 1995;7:273–280.

59. Godambe SA, Elliot V, Matheny D, et al. Comparison of Propofol/fentanyl versus ketamine/midazolam for brief orthopedic procedural sedation in a pediatric emergency department. *Pediatrics*. 2003;112:116–123.

60. Green SM, Nakamura R, Johnson NE. Ketamine sedation for pediatric procedures: part 1. A prospective series. *Ann Emerg Med*. 1990;19:1024–1032.

61. Green SM, Rothrock SG, Lynch EL, et al. Intramuscular ketamine for pediatric sedation in the emergency department: safety profile in 1,022 cases. *Ann Emerg Med*. 1998;31: 688–697.

62. Olsson GL, Hallen B. Laryngospasm during anesthesia—a computer aided incidence study in 136, 929 patients. *Acta Anaesthesiol Scand*. 1984;28:567–575.

63. Green SM, Klooster M, Harris T, et al. Ketamine sedation for pediatric gastroenterology procedures. *J Pediatr Gastroenterol Nutr*. 2001;32:26–33.

64. Pruitt JV, Goldwasser MS, Sabol SR, et al. Intramuscular ketamine, midazolm, and glycopyrrolate for pediatric sedation in the emergency department. *J Oral Maxillofac Surg*. 1995;53:13–17.

65. Hostetler MA, Barnard JA. Removal of esophageal foreign bodies in the pediatric ED: is ketamine an option? *Am J Emerg Med*. 2002;20:96–98.

66. Berkenbosch JW, Graff GR, Stark JM. Safety and efficacy of ketamine sedation for infant flexible fiberoptic bronchoscopy. *Chest*. 2004;125:1132–1137.

67. Decker JM, Lowe DA. Rapid sequence induction. In: Henretig FM, King C, eds. *Textbook of Pediatric Emergency Procedures*. Baltimore, MD: Williams & Wilkins; 1997:1 41–159.

68. Ketamine. Briggs GG, Freeman RK, Yaffe SJ, eds. *Drugs in Pregnancy and Lactation*. Philadelphia, PA: Lippincott Williams & Wilkins; 2005:875–878.

21

Benzodiazepines

Sharon E. Mace

HIGH YIELD FACTS

- Midazolam, the benzodiazepine of choice for emergency department (ED) procedural sedation, can be given intravenous (IV), intramuscular (IM), PO, PR, intranasal (IN), and sublingual (SL).
- Effects can be reversed by antagonist flumazenil.
- Minimal cardiovascular effects (unless patient is hypovolemic).
- Can use in patients with coronary artery disease, has a positive nitroglycerin-like effect in heart failure patients which decreases the elevated ventricular filling pressure.
- Are used to treat seizures, status epilepticus.
- Can cause respiratory depression, apnea, paradoxical agitation, emesis, hiccups, and coughing.
- Wide variation in dosing; ↓ dose if elderly, significant liver disease, renal failure, severe heart disease, and coadministering opioids.
- Metabolism of midazolam and diazepam is affected by hepatic disease/P-450 system, be aware of drug interactions.

INDICATIONS

Benzodiazepines are used for procedural sedation either alone for nonpainful procedures or with an analgesic, commonly an opioid such as fentanyl, for painful procedures.[1,2] Benzodiazepines have also been used for rapid sequence intubation, treatment of seizures, status epilepticus, behavioral emergencies (especially when intravenous [IV] access is unavailable), hypnotics, sedation in intensive care units (ICUs), and for induction of anesthesia.[3–10] Benzodiazepines are the most commonly used sedatives in the ICU[9–13] and have been considered by many clinicians as the *sedative of choice for most emergency department (ED) activities.*[14]

Benzodiazepines, like barbiturates, are classified according to their duration of action, which is a function of their pharmacokinetics: ultrashort acting, short acting, intermediate, and long acting.[15] Midazolam is short acting, lorazepam intermediate, and diazepam a long-acting benzodiazepine. Although there are many benzodiazepines available, three benzodiazepines are commonly used for sedation: midazolam, lorazepam, and diazepam.[16,17] Of the three, midazolam is the most commonly used benzodiazepine for procedural sedation and is preferred for several reasons.[18,19] Midazolam has a rapid onset, short duration, does not cause pain when given intravenously, and can be given by multiple routes.[18–20] In comparison with diazepam, midazolam had a faster onset, fewer adverse effects, better amnestic properties, and a potency three to four times that of diazepam.[20]

The effects of benzodiazepines are reversed by the antagonist flumazenil (see Chap. 16).[15]

PHARMACOLOGY

Benzodiazepines have anxiolytic, amnestic, sedative, hypnotic, muscle relaxant, and anticonvulsant properties but no analgesic effect.[21–24] They exert their effect on the γ-amino butyric acid (GABA) receptor complex by binding to a receptor site different from the barbiturate or GABA binding sites.[15] When they bind to the specific benzodiazepine receptor site on the GABA receptor complex, it opens a chloride channel causing hyperpolarization of the cell membrane.[15,24–26] The net result is inhibition of the neuron.[15,24–26] Benzodiazepines exert their effect by increasing the frequency of opening of these chloride channels, while barbiturates exert their effect by prolonging the opening of these chloride channels.[24,27]

Benzodiazepines consist of a benzene ring fused to a seven-membered diazepine ring. The clinically significant benzodiazepines have a 5-aryl substituent (ring C) and a 1,4-diazepine ring so they are 5-aryl-1,4-benzodiazepines.[15] Changes in the structure of the ring systems gives various compounds.[15]

Midazolam is an imidazobenzodiazepine.[15,28] This unique ring structure accounts for its lipophilicity and water solubility. At a physiologic pH midazolam's ring structure is closed, which imparts lipophilicity.[28,29] At a pH <4, its ring is open which makes it water soluble.[28,29] Water solubility is a desirable characteristic because it eliminates the need for solvents. The presence of solvents, such as propylene glycol, causes a higher frequency of pain on injection and phlebitis as occurs with the non-water-soluble benzodiazepines: lorazepam and diazepam.[8,28]

Eliminating solvents may also decrease the incidence of dysrhythmias.[28]

The lipophilicity of benzodiazepines accounts for their rapid onset of action.[24] Redistribution of drugs from the central nervous system (CNS) to peripheral tissues accounts for the termination of their action.[25]

Benzodiazepines are metabolized by the liver with the metabolites then excreted by the kidneys.[16,19] Some of the metabolites are active and can have clinical effects.[24] Benzodiazepines are lipid soluble and are widely distributed throughout the body.[1,24] The protein binding and the volume of distribution are similar for three benzodiazepines: midazolam, lorazepam, and diazepam.[24,25]

Multiple variables affect benzodiazepine pharmacokinetics including age, gender, ethnicity, obesity, liver disease, and renal disease.[24] The elderly have an increased volume of distribution and decreased clearance of benzodiazepines. The volume of distribution is also greater in women than in men and during pregnancy. Obese individuals have an increased volume of distribution and an increased plasma half-life due to the increased depot of drug in the adipose tissue. This delayed return of the drug from adipose tissue into the plasma leads to an increased elimination half-life.[30]

Benzodiazepines have a high enterohepatic first-pass effect with loss of half of the oral or rectal drug dose. This can cause erratic absorption, variable blood levels, and inconsistent effects of oral and rectally administered benzodiazepines. This is a disadvantage of the oral and rectal routes of administration and one reason why the parenteral route is preferred. Table 21-1 contains dosage information and Table 21-2 contains administration information.

CLINICAL EFFECTS

Benzodiazepines when given in the usual sedative doses have minimal cardiovascular effects.[24] A slight decrease in systemic blood pressure due to a decrease in systemic vascular resistance may occur with midazolam.[15,24] The decrease is dose-related. There is a greater drop in blood pressure if opioids are given concomitantly with benzodiazepines due to a synergistic effect.[24,31,32] In patients with an elevated left ventricular filling pressure (as with congestive heart failure), the combination of benzodiazepines with opioids has the beneficial effect (like nitroglycerin) of lowering the filling pressure thereby, improving cardiac performance.[24] Conversely, in hypovolemic or hypotensive patients, there may be a greater undesirable cardiodepressant effect with a more marked drop in blood pressure; however, benzodiazepines do not have a negative effect on coronary blood flow or cardiac output in most patients with cardiovascular disease.

Benzodiazepines, like barbiturates and propofol, decrease cerebral blood flow and cerebral metabolic rate[33] and raise the seizure threshold and are used as anticonvulsants[33]; however, a neuroprotective effect against cerebral hypoxia/ischemia has not been demonstrated in humans.[33]

The stresses accompanying endotracheal intubation and surgery may not be entirely attenuated by midazolam so adjuvant agents, generally the opioids, are also given.[34]

Clinical Effects in Specific Patient Populations

The metabolism of benzodiazepines has clinical importance. For example, the elderly and patients with impaired liver and/or kidney function are easily oversedated.[24,35–38] A geriatric patient has an increased sensitivity to benzodiazepines for several reasons.[24,38] The age-related diminished hepatic blood flow and hepatic enzyme activity along with an increased volume of distribution and altered protein binding results in a decreased clearance of specific benzodiazepines (e.g., diazepam and midazolam but not lorazepam) and a decreased first-pass metabolism.[24,25,38,39] Therefore, the dose of midazolam should be decreased by about half in the elderly.[8,29,38,40]

Differences in protein binding can affect benzodiazepine metabolism.[25] Both hepatic and/or renal disease and certain drugs (for example, heparin) displace the benzodiazepine from its protein-binding sites which increases the free (unbound) fraction of the benzodiazepine, though this is rarely of clinical significance in the setting of procedural sedation.[25]

Another factor that can have a clinical effect is the presence of active metabolites.[24,25] For example, midazolam is metabolized to hydroxymidazolam, which has biologic activity.[24] Generally, these metabolites undergo conjugation and then are excreted in the urine. In patients with renal failure, these metabolites may accumulate and cause prolonged sedation though again, this is rarely of clinical significance in the setting of procedural sedation.[29] Diazepam also has active metabolites, while lorazepam's key metabolites are inactive.[24]

In clinical practice, the dose of midazolam should be decreased in patients who are chronically ill such as those with liver and/or kidney disease or higher American Society of Anesthesiologists (ASA) classes (e.g., classes 3 and 4).[30,40]

Table 21-1. Benzodiazepines: Dosage Information

Dose (mg/kg)*,†	Usual Dose*,†	Maximum Dose*,†	Onset (min)	Duration (min)
Midazolam				
0.05–0.1 adult/child (6 months to 5 years) IV/IM	If giving with opioids: 0.02 mg/kg IV midazolam plus 1 mcg/kg fentanyl IV	6 mg (age ≤5 years) 10 mg (child >6 years and adults)	3 IV	60 IV
Child (>6 years) 0.025–0.05 (may give 0.02–0.03 IV, repeat as needed) 0.1–0.3 IV (for RSI)	If midazolam alone 0.05 mg/kg IV, unless at-risk patient‡ then 0.02 mg/kg IV	Child (6 months to 5 year)	5–30 IM	60–90 IM/PO/ PR/IN
0.5–1.0 PO/PR 0.3–0.5 IN/SL 0.05–1 mcg/kg/min infusion	1–2 mg IV/IM (adult)	Maximum 0.6 mg/kg Child (6–12 years) Maximum 0.4 mg/kg	10–30 PO/PR	
↓ dose in at-risk patients and if giving with opiates/other respiratory depressant drugs			3–5 IN	
Lorazepam				
0.02–0.05 IV/IM 0.025 mg/kg/h infusion	1–2 mg IV/IM/ PO (adult) 0.05–1 mg elderly	4 mg IV/IM 2 mg/h infusion	15 IV	120
Diazepam				
0.05–0.2 IV/IM 0.5 PO/PR	2–4 mg IV/IM (adult) 2, 5, 10 mg PO (adult)	5–10 mg	3–5 IV	90 IV

IN, intranasal; SL, sublingual; RSI, rapid sequence intubation.

*Doses will vary with individual patients.

†Some patients will need doses greater than the typical maximum doses. When higher doses are needed, it is advisable to titrate them with appropriate monitoring.

‡At-risk patients include the elderly, patients with chronic renal failure, severe hepatic disease, and significant heart failure.

Because benzodiazepines are metabolized in the liver and then excreted by the kidneys,[15,41] the presence of severe hepatic disease and/or chronic renal disease may affect the pharmacokinetics (and thus, the duration of effect) of benzodiapezines.[28,29,35,36] This is dependent on the specific drug and the type of hepatic metabolism the drug undergoes, whether oxidation then glucuronide conjugation or direct conjugation.[24] Oxidation reactions are affected by hepatic dysfunction and the cytochrome P-450 system, while glucuronidation is not affected by the cytochrome P-450 system.[24]

Benzodiazepine metabolism occurs either by hepatic oxidation via the cytochrome P-450 system for midazolam and diazepam, or by glucuronidation for lorazepam.[24] Since the glucuronidation pathways are not via the P-450 system, lorazepam is not affected by liver disease or by other medications[24]; however, both midazolam and diazepam are metabolized by the P-450 system and

Table 21-2. Benzodiazepines: Administration Information

Practical Tips	Administration	Advantages	Side Effects/Disadvantages
Give with analgesic for painful procedures	↓ Dose of both drugs if giving with opioid	Minimal CV effects (unless hypovolemic)	No analgesic effect → need analgesic (opioid) for painful procedure
Effects can be reversed by flumazenil	↓ Dose in elderly, liver or renal disease, severe heart failure	↓ LV filling pressure, ↑ CO in CHF patients (NTG effect)	Can cause respiratory depression, apnea
Used to treat seizures, status epilepticus		Can use in patients with CAD	Paradoxical agitation can occur
Midazolam is the benzo-diazepine of choice for PSA	Drugs affecting hepatic P-450 system affect midazolam/diazepam metabolism	Raises seizure threshold	Vomiting, coughing, hiccups can occur
Wide variation in dosing	Avoid using if patient on protease inhibitor drugs	Decreases CBF, ICP Can be given by many routes. IV, IM, PO, PR, IN, SL	Does not block stress of intubation/surgery → need adjacent drugs (opioid)

PSA, procedural sedation and analgesia; CV, cardiovascular; LV, left ventricle; CO, cardiac output; NTG, nitroglycerin; CBF, cerebral blood flow; ICP, intracranial pressure; IN, intranasal; SL, sublingual.

therefore, may be affected by hepatic dysfunction and other medications.[10,40,41]

Inhibitors of the cytochrome P-450 system may slow the metabolism of midazolam and diazepam, thereby, decreasing the drug's clearance and increasing the serum concentration.[25,28] Inhibitors of the P-450 system include antibiotics (e.g., macrolides: erythromycin and clarithromycin), anticonvulsants, oral contraceptives, antifungals (e.g., ketoconazole and itraconazole), calcium channel blockers, antiulcer drugs (e.g., H_2 blockers: cimetidine and ranitidine; proton pump inhibitors: omeprazole), protease inhibitors, and even components of our diet (grapefruit juice).[42–46] Protease inhibitors commonly used in the therapy of human immunodeficiency disease can impact benzodiazepines' effects. For example, the protease inhibitor, ritonavir, can modify P-450 activity leading to higher plasma levels of midazolam. Conversely, drugs that enhance the P-450 oxidase system, such as rifampin, will accelerate the metabolism of midazolam and diazepam.[47] It may be best to avoid the use of benzodiazepines in patients on such drugs.

ADVERSE EFFECTS

Benzodiazepines cause a dose-related central respiratory depression up to and including apnea, as do most if not all IV anesthetics as a function of dose, route, and rate of administration.[24,48,49] The respiratory depression caused by benzodiazepines is more significant in patients with chronic obstructive pulmonary disease (COPD).[24] The apnea that can occur with benzodiazepines[32,48–51] has an increased frequency: in the elderly, in patients with debilitating disease, with higher doses of benzodiazepines, and when given with opioids and other respiratory depressant drugs.[24]

Paradoxical agitation, similar to that occurring with the barbiturates, can be a side effect of benzodi-azepines.[52–54] Vomiting, coughing, hiccups, and headache are other side effects.[29,53]

CLINICAL EFFECTS: BENZODIAZEPINES AND ANALGESICS

The preferred benzodiazepine for ED sedation for painless procedures is midazolam. An opioid is commonly coadministered for painful procedures, most often fentanyl. This coadministration of benzodiazepines with opioids results in a synergistic effect for both the desired effects (sedation, amnesia, anxiolysis, hypnosis, and muscle relaxation) and the unwanted side effects (respiratory depression and hypotension).[51,55] This is true in both adults and children.[32,48,51]

A randomized, blinded, placebo-controlled study in adults undergoing dental procedures found a 3% occurrence of apnea with midazolam alone versus 63% with midazolam plus fentanyl.[51] In one study of 12 healthy adult volunteers, the individual drugs (fentanyl = F or midazolam = M) were compared with the combination of fentanyl plus midazolam (FM).[32] The relative incidences of hypoxia (oxygen saturation <90%) were M = 0%, F = 50%, FM = 92%, and apnea M = 0%, F = 0%, FM = 50%.[32]

Two pediatric studies also found a greater risk of respiratory depression with the combination of fentanyl and midazolam.[48,56] One study measured the end-tidal carbon dioxide ($ETCO_2$) during sedation with midazolam (M) alone, midazolam and ketamine (MK), and midazolam and an opioid (MO). An increased $ETCO_2$ >10 mmHg occurred in 9% M, 35% MK, and 50% MO.[48] Another report of pediatric patients noted hypoxia (oxygen saturation <90%) in 6% of the patients receiving ketamine/midazolam sedation versus 25% of those receiving fentanyl/midazolam.[56]

However, other studies have documented no significant complications from the coadministration of fentanyl and midazolam.[53,55] One large prospective study of 1180 patients found only a 2.3% incidence of adverse events for fentanyl/midazolam ($N = 391$): 0.8% ($N = 10$) oxygen desaturation, 0.6% ($N = 7$) paradoxical reaction, 0.17% ($N = 2$) patients given supplemental oxygen, and 0.25% ($N = 3$) emesis.[53] The 1.8% adverse events for ketamine/midazolam ($N = 220$) were: oxygen desaturation ($N = 2$), laryngospasm ($N = 1$), and emesis ($N = 1$).[53]

Differences in the conclusions of the various studies is probably, at least partly, a function of the definitions for respiratory depression and side effects. For example, respiratory depression defined as an increase of ≥10 mm $ETCO_2$ yields a higher incidence than hypoxemia (oxygen saturation <90%), which in turn, occurs more frequently than need for supplemental oxygen or bag-valve-mask ventilation. The need for intervention with fentanyl-midazolam, specifically bag-valve-mask ventilation or intubation, is a rare occurrence.[57] There is a 10–20% incidence of a mild respiratory event needing oxygen or stimulation, a rare need for respiratory assistance, and a near zero incidence of life-threatening events.[57] However, there are reports of respiratory arrest in patients, particularly those at the extremes of age, who were coadministered high doses of both a benzodiazepine and an opioid.[58–60] The majority of the respiratory arrests occurred in patients who were not monitored closely.[58–60] This emphasizes the need for close monitoring with the appropriate personnel and equipment for all procedural sedations.

ADMINISTRATION

For all instances of procedural sedation when opioids are to be coadministered with sedative hypnotics, it is wise to establish the adequacy of analgesia (e.g., pain scores of 1–2)

produced by the opioid before embarking on the titration of the sedative hypnotic agent. This is especially true for potent agents such as midazolam.

Midazolam can be given by multiple routes: parenteral (IV/IM), oral, transmucosal (nasal or rectal), and sublingual (SL).[61–73] The IV route is most commonly used, and only the parenteral (IV/IM) routes are approved by the Food and Drug Administration (FDA). One problem with alternate (nonparenteral) routes of access is that titration of the sedation is difficult. So a consistent reliable depth of sedation is not always possible.[1,23] It should also be remembered that complications including respiratory depression can occur with any route of administration. As with other sedatives, when administering midazolam IV do not give as a rapid bolus, as rapid IV bolus administration has been associated with respiratory depression and respiratory arrest. Administer the medication as a "slow IV push" over 30–60 seconds. Additionally, remember to wait for 2 minutes following the completion of the infusion to permit peak neurologic effect to ensue. This is important in selecting the size and timing of subsequent doses.

In the elderly (age >60 years) and patients with chronic illness, the benzodiazepine dose should be reduced by 30–50%.[3,18,29] Patients with end-stage renal disease, significant congestive heart failure, and liver failure eliminate midazolam slowly and may have prolonged sedation.[26] The apnea and the respiratory depressant effect of benzodiazepines are synergistic with the opioids and other respiratory depressant drugs so the dose of both the benzodiazepine and the opioid or other drug may need to be reduced.[24–26] Avoid using benzodiazepines in patients with acute alcohol intoxication since both benzodiazepines and alcohol are sedative hypnotic agents and act as respiratory depressants. Similarly in patients with chronic obstructive pulmonary disease, the respiratory depressant effect of benzodiazepines is enhanced.[25]

Benzodiazepines (e.g., midazolam, lorazepam, and diazepam) are a class D drug during pregnancy.[74] They are possibly teratogenic in the first trimester of pregnancy.[16]

The parenteral form of midazolam can be used orally but has a bitter taste that often limits patient compliance, so it is generally diluted in kool-aid or a noncitrus juice.[23] A better tasting commercial oral preparation of midazolam is now available.[16] With the oral route, sedation usually occurs in 20–25 minutes.

Midazolam may be administered IM in uncooperative patients with special health care needs. Rectal administration may not always be accepted by the patient. Infrequently, defecation may occur with the medication being expelled, and variable absorption occurs. The rectal dose is diluted in 5 cc normal saline before administering.

Transmucosal routes have also been used. The intranasal route has been used successfully, especially in infants. A needless tuberculin syringe is used to inject half the volume of medication in each nostril. Burning and irritation can occur with intranasal administration. In patients with an upper respiratory infection and/or copious nasal secretions, absorption of the intranasal medication may be suboptimal. The SL route has also been used to administer midazolam by placing the dose of midazolam into the SL space (see Chap. 47).

IV preparations of diazepam have been formulated with propylene glycol, which can cause pain on injection, thrombophlebitis, and even toxicity at very high doses. An emulsified formulation of diazepam appears to have a decreased occurrence of such adverse effects.[75]

DOSAGE

For moderate sedation, the dose of midazolam is 0.05–0.1 mg/kg IV given slowly over 30–60 seconds, which may be repeated if needed to a maximum of 6 mg (age ≤5 years) and 10 mg (adults and children >6 years).[76–79] In selected populations (e.g., elderly, renal failure, hepatic disease, severe heart failure, and the chronically ill), the dose should be decreased by as much as half.[8,18,29,40] Alternatively, some physicians use titrated doses of 0.02–0.03 mg/kg of midazolam and repeat the dose as needed[18,80]; however, when this lower dose of 0.02 mg/kg was used, about one-third (36%) of the patients needed an additional dose of midazolam.[80] For rapid sequence intubation (RSI), the recommended dose is 0.1–0.3 mg/kg.[81,82]

The wide variation in dose of midazolam depends, at least partly, on patient characteristics such as age and comorbidity and on whether other medications are coadministered. A "healthy" child undergoing procedural sedation for a painless procedure receiving only midazolam is quite different from a geriatric patient with COPD on diuretics who is also receiving opioids for sedation. The induction dose is also larger than that used for procedural sedation. There is also much individual variation.

Some physicians also vary the dose based on the child's age.[83] For age 6 months to 5 years, a higher initial dose of 0.05–0.1 mg/kg IV up to a maximum of 0.6 mg/kg is used.[83] For age 6–12 years, the initial dose is 0.025–0.05 mg/kg IV up to a maximum of 0.4 mg/kg.[83]

When using in combination with an opioid, the dose is generally decreased. For example, a dose of 0.02 mg/kg IV midazolam is combined with fentanyl 1 mg/kg IV. The IM dose is usually the same as the IV dose. Administration by other routes requires a higher dose. The oral or rectal dose is about 10 times that of the parenteral (IV/IM) dose at 0.5–1.0 mg/kg. Intranasal administration has an onset almost as quickly as IV administration. A dose of 0.3–0.5 mg/kg is used for intranasal or SL administration.

SUMMARY

Benzodiazepines have many clinical uses: as a sedative, for the treatment of seizures and status epilepticus, for the management of behavioral emergencies, as a hypnotic, for procedural sedation, and for the induction of anesthesia. The most commonly used benzodiazepines for sedation are midazolam, lorazepam, and diazepam. Midazolam is preferred for procedural sedation because it has a rapid onset, short duration, fewer side effects, better amnestic properties, and greater potency. There is a wide variation in dosage based on such factors as age, comorbidity, and on whether other drugs are coadministered. Benzodiazepines cause a dose-related central respiratory depression including apnea. The benzodiazepine dose should be decreased in geriatric patients, chronically ill patients, and when other respiratory depressant drugs are also given. The coadministration of benzodiazepines with opioids results in synergistic effects for both the desired effects and the side effects (respiratory depression and hypotension).

REFERENCES

1. Green SM, Krauss B. Procedural sedation and analgesia. In: Roberts JR, Hedges JR, Chanmugam AS, et al, eds. *Clinical Procedures in Emergency Medicine*. Philadelphia, PA: W.B. Saunders; 2004:596–619.
2. Sacchetti A, Gerardi MJ. Emergency department procedural sedation and analgesia. In: Strange GR, Ahrens WR, Lelyveld S, et al. *Pediatric Emergency Medicine A Comprehensive Study Guide*. New York: McGraw-Hill; 2002: 185–196.
3. Walls RM. Airway. In: Marx JA, Hockberger RS, Walls RM, et al, eds. *Rosen's Emergency Medicine Concepts and Clinical Practice*. St. Louis, MO: Mosby; 2002:2–20.
4. Gerardi MJ, Sacchetti AD, Cantor RM, et al. Rapid sequence intubation of the pediatric patient. *Ann Emerg Med*. 1996; 28:55–74.
5. Silvilotti MLA, Filbin MR, Murray HE, et al. Does the sedative agent facilitate emergency rapid sequence intubation? *Acad Emerg Med*. 2003;10:612–620.
6. Luten RC, Stenklyft PH. Rapid-sequence induction in children. In: Harwood-Nuss A, Wolfson AB, Linden CH, et al, eds. *The Clinical Practice of Emergency Medicine*. Philadelphia, PA: Lippincott Williams & Wilkins; 2001: 1133–1137.
7. Liu LL, Gropper MA. Postoperative analgesia and sedation in the adult intensive care unit. *Drugs*. 2003;63:755–767.

8. Blackburn P, Vissers R. Pharmacology of emergency department pain management and conscious sedation. *Emerg Med Clin North Am.* 2000;18:803–826.

9. Gelbach BK, Kress JP. Sedation in the intensive care unit. *Curr Opin Crit Care.* 2002;8:290–298.

10. Hansen Flaschen JH, Bradzinsky S, et al. Use of sedating drugs and neuromuscular blocking agents in patients requiring mechanical ventilation for respiratory failure: a national survey. *JAMA.* 1991;266:2870–2875.

11. Urwin SC, Menon DK. Comparative tolerability of sedative agents in head-injured adults. *Drug Saf.* 2004;27:107–133.

12. Tobias JD. Sedation and analgesia in pediatric intensive care units. *Pediatr Drugs.* 1999;1:109–125.

13. Burns AM, Shelly MP, Park GR. The use of sedative agents in critically ill patients. *Drugs.* 1992;43:507–515.

14. Sacchetti A, Schafermeyer R, Gerardi M, et al. Pediatric analgesia and sedation. *Ann Emerg Med.* 1994;23:237–250.

15. Charney DS, Mihic SJ, Harris RA. Hypnotics and sedatives. In: Hardman JG, Limbird LE, Gilman AG, eds. *Goodman & Gilman's The Pharmacological Basis of Therapeutics.* New York: McGraw-Hill; 2001:399–??

16. Tobias JD. Pharmacology of sedative agents. In: Malviya S, Naughton NN, Tremper KK, eds. *Sedation and Analgesia for Diagnostic and Therapeutic Procedures.* Totowa, NJ: Humana Press; 2003:125–149.

17. Alexander SM, Todres ID. The use of sedation and muscle relaxation in the ventilated infant. *Clin Perinatol.* 1998;25: 63–78.

18. Glauser J, Cullinson B. Procedural sedation: definition and review of systemic agents. *Emerg Med Rep.* 2002;23:247–261.

19. Lewis KP, Stanley GD. Pharmacology. In: Gilbertson LI, ed. *Conscious sedation. International Anesthesiology Clinics.* Philadelphia, PA: Lippincott Wilkins & Williams; 1999:73–86.

20. Wright SW, Chudnofsky CR, Dronen SC, et al. Comparison of midazolam and diazepam for conscious sedation in the emergency department. *Ann Emerg Med.* 1993;22:201–205.

21. Osborn IP. Intravenous conscious sedation for pediatric patients. *Int Anesthesiol Clin.* 1999;37:99–111.

22. Kennedy RM, Luhmann JD. The "ouchless emergency department". *Pediatr Clin North Am.* 1999;46:1215–1245.

23. Rodriquez E, Jordan R. Contemporary trends in pediatric sedation and analgesia. *Emerg Clin North Am.* 2002;20: 199–222.

24. Reves JG, Glass PSA, Lubarsky DA. Nonbarbiturate intravenous anesthetics. In: Miller RD, Cuchiara RF, Milar ED, et al, eds. *Anesthesia.* Philadelphia, PA: Churchill Livingstone; 2000:228–272.

25. Kennedy SK. Pharmacology of intravenous anesthetic agents. In: Longnecker DE, Tinker JH, Morgan GE Jr, eds. *The Principles and Practice of Anesthesiology.* St. Louis, MO: Mosby; 1998:1211–1232.

26. Chiu JW, White PF. Nonopioid intravenous anesthesia. In: Barash PG, Cullen BF, Stoelting RK, eds. *Clinical Anesthesia.* Philadelphia, PA: Lippincott, Williams & Wilkins; 2001: 327–343.

27. Study RE, Barber JL. Cellular mechanisms of benzodiazepine action. *JAMA.* 1982;247:2147–2151.

28. Dundee JW, Halliday NJ, Harper KW, et al. Midazolam: a review of its pharmacological properties and therapeutic use. *Drugs.* 1984;28:519–543.

29. Chudnofsky CR, Lozon MM. Sedation and analgesia for procedures. In: Marx JA, Hockberger RS, Walls RM, et al, eds. *Rosen's Emergency Medicine.* St. Louis, MO: Mosby; 2002;2577–2590.

30. Nordt SP, Clark RF. Midazolam: a review of the therapeutic uses and toxicity. *J Emerg Med.* 1997;15:357–365.

31. Reeves JG, Fragen RJ, Vinik R, et al. Midazolam: pharmacology and uses. *Anesthesiology.* 1985;62:310–324.

32. Bailey PL, Pace NL, Ashburn MA, et al. Frequent hypoxemia and apnea after sedation with midazolam and fentanyl. Anesthesiology 1990;73:826–830.

33. Urwin SC, Menon DK. Comparative tolerability of sedative agents in head-injured adults. *Drug Saf.* 2004;27: 107–133.

34. Samuelson PN, Reves JG, Kouchoukos NT, et al. Hemodynamic responses to anesthetic induction with midazolam or diazepam in patients with ischemic heart disease. *Anesth Analg.* 1981;60: 802–809.

35. Shelley MP, Mendel L, Park JR. Failure of critically ill patients to metabolize midazolam. *Anesthesia.* 1987;42: 619–626.

36. Bauer TM, Ritz R, Haberthur C, et al. Prolonged sedation due to accumulation of conjugated metabolites of midazolam. *Lancet.* 1995;346:145–147.

37. Vree TB, Shimoda M, Driessen JJ. Decreased plasma albumin concentration results in increased volume of distribution and decreased elimination of midazolam in intensive care patients. *Clin Pharmacol Ther.* 1989;46:537–544.

38. Harper RW, Collins PS, Dundee JW, et al. Age and nature of operation influence the pharmacokinetics of midazolam. *Br J Anaesth.* 1985;57:866–871.

39. Nicolaou DD. Procedural sedation and analgesia. In: Tintinalli JE, Kelen GD, Stapczynski JS, eds. *Emergency Medicine A Comprehensive Study Guide.* New York: McGraw-Hill; 2004:275–280.

40. Muse DA. Conscious and deep sedation. In: Harwood-Nuss A, Wolfson AB, Linden CH, et al, eds. *The Clinical Practice of Emergency Medicine.* Philadelphia, Lippincott, Williams & Wilkins; 2001:1758–1762.

41. Greenblatt DJ, Abernethy DR. Midazolam pharmacology and pharmacokinetics. *Anaesth Rev.* 1985;12:17–20.

42. Hiller A, Olkkola KT, Isohanni P, et al. Unconsciousness associated with midazolam and erythromycin. *Br J Anaesth.* 1990;65(6):826–828.

43. Klotz U, Arvela P, Rosenkranz B. Effect of single doses of cimetidine and ranitidine on the steady state plasma levels of midazolam. *Clin Pharmacol Ther.* 1985;38:652–655.

44. Fee JPH, Collier PS, Howard PJ, et al. Cimetidine and ranitidine increase midazolam bioavailability. *Clin Pharmacol Ther.* 1987;41:80–84.

45. Gugler R, Jensen JC. Omeprazole inhibits oxidative drug metabolism studies with diazepam and phenytoin in vivo and 7—ethoxycoumadin in vitro. *Gastroenterology.* 1985; 89:1235–1241.

46. Abernethy DR, Greenblatt DJ, Divoli M, et al. Impairment of diazepam metabolism by low-dose estrogen-containing oral-contraceptive steroids. *N Engl J Med.* 1982;306: 791–792.

47. Ohnhaus EE, Brockmeyer N, Dylewicz P, et al. The effect of antipyrine and rifampin on the metabolism of diazepam. *Clin Pharmacol Ther.* 1987;42:148– 156.

48. McQuillen KK, Steele DW. Capnography during sedation/ analgesia in the pediatric emergency department. *Pediatr Emerg Care.* 2000;16:401–404.

49. Hart LS, Berns SD, Houck CS, et al. The value of end-tidal CO_2 monitoring when comparing three methods of conscious sedation for children undergoing painful procedures in the emergency department. *Pediatric Emerg Care.* 1997;13: 189–193.

50. Graff KJ, Kennedy RM, Jaffe DM. Conscious sedation for pediatric orthopedic emergencies. *Pediatric Emerg Care.* 1996;12:31–35.

51. Milgrom P, Beirne OR, Fiset L, et al. The safety and efficacy of outpatient midazolam intravenous sedation for oral surgery with and without fentanyl. *Anaesth Prog.* 1993;40: 57–62.

52. Shane SA, Fuchs SM, Khine H. Efficacy of rectal midazolam for the sedation of preschool children undergoing laceration repair. *Ann Emerg Med.* 1994;24:1065–1073.

53. Pena BM, Krauss B. Adverse events of procedural sedation and analgesia in a pediatric emergency department. *Ann Emerg Med.* 1999;34:483–491.

54. Kovoor P, Porter R, Uther RB, et al. Efficacy and safety of a new protocol for continuous infusion of midazolam and fentanyl and its effects on patient distress during electro-physiological studies. *PACE.* 1997;20:2765–2774.

55. Wright SW, Chudnofsky CR, Dronen SC, et al. Midazolam use in the emergency department. *Am J Emerg Med.* 1990;8: 97–100.

56. Kennedy RM, Porter FL, Miller JP, et al. Comparison of fentanyl/midazolam with ketamine/midazolam for pediatric orthopedic emergencies. *Pediatrics.* 1998;102:956–963.

57. Mace SE, Barata IA, Cravero JP, et al. Clinical policy: evidence-based approach to pharmacologic agents used in pediatric sedation and analgesia in the emergency department. *Ann Emerg Med.* 2004;44(4):342–377.

58. Yaster M, Nichols DG, Deshpande JK, et al. Midazolam—fentanyl intravenous sedation in children: case report of respiratory arrest. *Pediatrics.* 1990;86:463–467.

59. Claussen DC, Pestonik SL, Evans RS, et al. Intensive surveillance of midazolam use in hospitalized patients and the occurrence of cardiopulmonary arrest. *Pharmacotherapy.* 1992;12:213–216.

60. Anonymous. Midazolam—is antagonism justified? *Lancet.* 1988;2:388–389.

61. Sievers TD, Yee JD, Foley ME, et al. Midazolam for conscious sedation during pediatric oncology procedures: safety and recovery parameters. *Pediatrics.* 1991;88:1172–1179.

62. Sandler ES, Weyman C, Conner K, et al. Midazolam versus fentanyl as premedication for painful procedures in children with cancer. *Pediatrics.* 1992;89:631–634.

63. Godambe SA, Elliot V, Matheny D, et al. Comparison of propofol/fentanyl versus ketamine/midazolam for brief orthopedic procedural sedation in a pediatric emergency department. *Pediatrics.* 2003;112:116–123.

64. Fragen RJ, Funk DI, Avram MJ, et al. Midazolam versus hydroxyzine as intramuscular premedicant. *Can Anaesth Soc J.* 1983;30:136–141.

65. Younge PA, Kendall JM. Sedation for children requiring wound repair: a randomized controlled double blind comparison of oral midazolam and oral ketamine. *Emerg Med J.* 2001;18:30–33.

66. McMillan CO, Spahr-Schopfer IA, Sikich N, et al. Premedication of children with oral midazolam. *Can J Anaesth.* 1992;39: 545–550.

67. Feld LH, Negus JB, White PF. Oral midazolam preanesthetic medication in pediatric outpatients. *Anesthesiology.* 1990; 73:831–834.

68. McGlone RG, Ranasinghe S, Durham S. An Alternative to "brutacaine": a comparison of low dose intramuscular ketamine with intranasal midazolam in children before suturing. *J Accid Emerg Med.* 1998;15:231–236.

69. Acworth JP, Purdie D, Clark RC. Intravenous ketamine plus midazolam is superior to intranasal midazolam for emergency pediatric procedural sedation. *Emerg Med J.* 2001;18:39–45.

70. Theroux MC, West DW, Corddry DH, et al. Efficacy of intranasal midazolam in facilitating suturing of lacerations in preschool children in the emergency department. *Pediatrics.* 1993;91:624–627.

71. Beebe DS, Belani KG, Chang P, et al. Effectiveness of preoperative sedation with rectal midazolam, ketamine, or their combination in young children. *Anesth Analg.* 1992;39: 545–550.

72. Lejus C, Renaudin M, Testa S, et al. Midazolam for premedication in children: intranasal vs intrarectal administration. *Anesth Analg.* 1993;76:S217

73. Karl HW, Rosenberger JL, Laravch MG, et al. Transmucosal administration of midazolam for premedication of pediatric patients: comparison of the nasal and sublingual routes. *Anesthesiology.* 1993;78:885–891.

74. Briggs GG, Freeman RK, Yaffe SJ, eds. Diazepam, lorazepam, midazolam. Drugs in pregnancy and lactation. Philadelphia, PA: Lippincott Williams & Wilkins; 2002:390, 810, 931.

75. Forrest P, Galletly D. A double-blind comparative study of three formulations of diazepam in volunteers. *Anaesth Intensive Care.* 1988;16:158–163.

76. Cunningham SJ, Crain EF. Conscious sedation. In: Henretig FM, King C, eds. *Textbook of Pediatric Emergency Procedures.* Baltimore, MD: Williams & Wilkins; 1997:445–454.

77. Havel CJ, Strait RT, Hennes H, et al. A clinical trial of propofol vs midazolam for procedural sedation in a pediatric emergency department. *Acad Emerg Med.* 1999;6: 989–997.

78. Parker RI, Mahan RA, Giugliano D, et al. Efficacy and safety of intravenous midazolam and ketamine sedation for

therapeutic and diagnostic procedures in children. *Pediatrics.* 1997;99:427–431.

79. Gunn VL, Nechyba C. Drug doses. In: Gunn VL, Nechyba C, eds. *The Harriet Lane Hand Book*. Philadelphia, PA: Mosby; 2002:761.

80. Coll-Vinent B, Sala X, Fernandez C, et al. Sedation for cardioversion in the emergency department: analysis of effectiveness in four protocols. *Ann Emerg Med.* 2003;42: 767–772.

81. Sagarin MJ, Barton ED, Sakles JC, et al. Underdosing of midazolam in emergency endotracheal intubation. *Acad Emerg Med.* 2003;10:329–338.

82. Decker JM, Lowe DA. Rapid sequence induction. In: Henretig FM, King C, eds. *Textbook of Pediatric Emergency Procedures*. Baltimore, MD: Williams & Wilkins; 1997: 141–159.

83. Krauss B, Green SM. Sedation and analgesia for procedures in children. *N Engl J Med.* 2000;342:938–945.

22

Chloral Hydrate

Sharon E. Mace

HIGH YIELD FACTS

- Most effective in young children and infants (age <3 years).
- Can cause respiratory depression, apnea, cardiovascular toxicity (dysrhythmias, hypotension), especially if in high doses.
- Use with caution if significant renal or hepatic disease, severe cardiac disease, and gastritis/esophagitis/ulcers.
- Can have gastrointestinal (GI) side effects (vomiting, diarrhea, and gastric/esophageal irritation) and neurologic side effects (prolonged sedation, paradoxical reactions, and sedation hangover).
- Decreased oxygen saturation may occur in patients with acute pulmonary disorders (e.g., bronchiolitis).
- Special needs children have an increased risk of exaggerated reactions (prolonged sedation, paradoxical reaction).
- Use with caution and avoid prolonged use in neonates, especially in premature infants, because of delayed elimination, possible hypotension, ↑ bilirubin.
- Drug interactions can occur: coadministration of epinephrine or pressors with chloral hydrate may cause dysrhythmias.

INDICATIONS

Chloral hydrate is used for procedural sedation in pediatric patients for painless procedures.[1-3] It is one of the oldest sedative-hypnotic agents having been synthesized in 1832, and introduced as a hypnotic drug in 1869.[4] It has *a well-established safety profile.*[5-8] It has no analgesic properties.[9-12] It is most effective in children <3 years[13-16] and can be given orally or rectally.[17-21] With the advent of many newer sedatives, its current usage is generally limited to infants and children ≤3 years of age for painless procedures in whom an intravenous line is not possible or desirable and an oral route of administration is preferred.[5,12,22]

Chloral hydrate has generally been used as a sedative for painless outpatient diagnostic procedures such as radiology studies (e.g., computed tomography [CT] or magnetic resonance imaging [MRI] scans), electroencephalograms, and echocardiograms in young children and infants in order to eliminate the need for an intravenous line.[13,23-28] It has also been used for outpatient dentistry with the addition of local anesthesia and/or systemic analgesia.[29-31] Chloral hydrate has been the most frequently used sedative for outpatient pediatric radiology procedures in both children's hospitals and general community hospitals.[32,33] It has been used in infants and even in neonates for hypnosis/sedation.[34] In neonatal intensive care units, it has been used to treat agitation.[4,35]

Chloral hydrate has been used as a hypnotic in adults but has been replaced by newer hypnotics.[36] Chloral hydrate is a mild antiemetic that can be used in low doses (e.g., 10–20 mg) when standard antiemetic therapy has been unsuccessful.[8] It has also been employed to treat pruritus.[8] A recent report has suggested the use of chloral hydrate as a second-line drug in the treatment of myoclonus.[37]

PHARMACOLOGY

Chloral hydrate is a sedative-hypnotic agent without analgesic properties that induces sleep (i.e., a hypnotic).[9,11] It is a small halogenated hydrocarbon[10] compound created by adding a molecule of water to the carbonyl group of 2,2,2-trichloroacetaldehyde.[38] It is also formed as a byproduct of the chlorination of water[39] and is a metabolite of various industrial solvents, specifically, trichloroethylene and tetrachloroethylene.[40,41] This initially raised concerns that chloral hydrate might be a carcinogen.[12,22] However, the American Academy of Pediatrics has determined that there is insufficient data in this regard to withdraw its approval for use as a single dose for sedation.[7]

After an oral or rectal dose, chloral hydrate, $CCl_3CH(OH)_2$ is quickly reduced in the liver by the enzyme alcohol dehydrogenase to its active compound, trichlorethanol (CCl_3CH_2OH).[38] Chloral hydrate's effects are probably due to this active metabolite, trichloroethanol (TCE),[8,38] TCE has barbiturate- like effects on γ-aminobutyric acid (GABA) receptor channels so this may account for its sedative-hypnotic properties.[42] Chloral hydrate and TCE are slightly lipid soluble. Both substances cross the blood-brain barrier leading to their sedative-hypnotic activity.

TCE undergoes hepatic degradation via conjugation with glucuronic acid to trichlorethanol-glucuronide (urochloralic acid) which is water soluble and also excreted in the urine.[8,38] TCE also undergoes degradation in the liver via the enzyme aldehyde dehydrogenase to trichloroacetic acid (TCA) which is also water soluble and eliminated in the urine[8] (Figs. 22-1 and 22-2). A recent report has also identified dichloroacetate as a metabolic byproduct of chloral acetate in children.[43]

The chloral hydrate metabolites, TCE and TCA are 40% and 85% protein bound, respectively.

Significant hepatic or renal disease will impair the metabolism and elimination of chloral hydrate and are relative contraindications to the use of the drug. Table 22-1 contains dosage information and Table 22-2 contains administration information.

CLINICAL EFFECTS

Chloral hydrate is a central nervous system (CNS) depressant causing drowsiness and sedation followed by a sound sleep. Postsedative "hangover" occurs less frequently than with many barbiturates and some of the benzodiazepines.[38] At therapeutic dosages, chloral hydrate generally does not cause respiratory depression and maintains protective airway reflexes since it causes a fairly "light" level of sleep.[1,8,12]

Similarly, at usual doses, chloral hydrate does not significantly affect the blood pressure or heart rate[12] and has been used safely even in patients with all types of acyanotic and cyanotic congenital heart diseases.[11] However, chloral hydrate can have depressant cardiac actions. It decreases myocardial contractility and also decreases the threshold for dysrhythmias by shortening the refractory period and

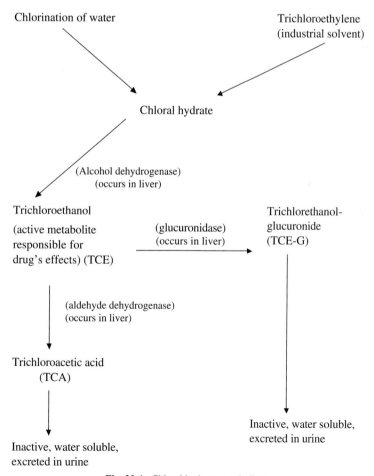

Fig. 22-1. Chloral hydrate metabolism.

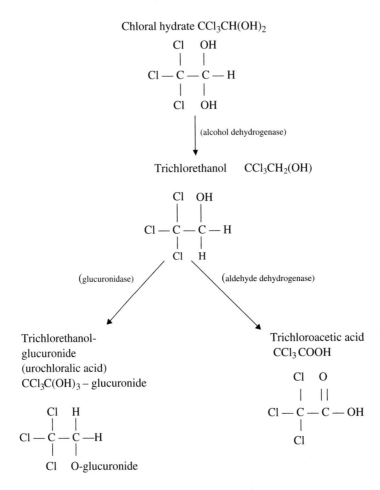

Chloral hydrate CCl$_3$CH(OH)$_2$

(alcohol dehydrogenase)

Trichlorethanol   CCl$_3$CH$_2$(OH)

(glucuronidase)   (aldehyde dehydrogenase)

Trichlorethanol-
glucuronide
(urochloralic acid)
CCl$_3$C(OH)$_3$ – glucuronide

Trichloroacetic acid
CCl$_3$COOH

Derivatives of trichlorethanol and trichloroacetic acid

Ethanol CH$_3$CH$_2$OH

Acetic acid CH$_3$COOH

Fig. 22-2. Chemical structure of chloral hydrate and its metabolites.

increasing the heart's sensitivity to catecholamines.[44] Chloral hydrate is relatively contraindicated in patients on pressor drugs and the administration of medications such as epinephrine or pressors should be avoided in patients who have received it.[8] Its cardiac effects are presumed to be the etiology for the many of the deaths associated with its use, both in therapeutic and overdose situations.[4]

With high doses and/or when combined with other respiratory depressant drugs (such as alcohol, opioids, or barbiturates), and in high-risk patients, respiratory depression and upper airway obstruction can occur.[15,29,45–47] Vulnerable patients include infants and children with upper airway obstruction (e.g., sleep apnea, tonsillar hypertrophy, adenoidal hypertrophy, laryngomalacia, and large tongue),

Table 22-1. Chloral Hydrate: Dosage Information

Dose (mg/kg)	Usual Dose (mg/kg)	Maximum Dose	Onset (min)	Duration (min)
25–100 PO/PR	Low dose 25–50 may repeat in 30 min High dose 80–100	100 mg/kg or 2 g (whichever is lowest)	15–30 PO/PR	Usually may be prolonged

those with congenital anomalies (e.g., Down syndrome), certain acquired disorders (e.g., muscular dystrophy and other neuromuscular disorders), and the very young.[8,15,29] It is theorized that the relaxation of the muscles that support the tongue and upper airway leads to airway obstruction and respiratory compromise even if respiratory depression does not occur.[48] Patients with bronchiolitis, who are administered chloral hydrate, experience a decrease in their oxygen saturation that is felt to be related to respiratory depression.[8]

Children with special health care needs tend to have unusual reactions to chloral hydrate characterized by either an exaggerated response (with a very prolonged sedation) or a dysphoric/paradoxical reaction (with agitation).[8] Such prolonged sedation and paradoxical reactions can occur in any patient[46] but occur more frequently in special needs children.[13,49]

Chloral hydrate has been used in infants and even in neonates.[8,34,35] However, there are several concerns:

1. The drug has a prolonged half-life in newborns.
2. Chloral hydrate's active metabolites compete for the liver enzyme involved in its glucuronidation. This could theoretically aggravate hyperbilirubinemia, and has been observed with prolonged chloral hydrate use in neonates.[8,37]

Several studies have documented a decreased effectiveness of chloral hydrate in older children (>3 years of age)[46,47,49,50] leading to the recommendation that the use

Table 22-2. Chloral Hydrate: Administration Information

Practical Tips	Administration	Advantages	Disadvantages
Use in infants/young children (best if ≤3 years of age) Special needs children are prone to unusual reactions Nausea, vomiting can occur Can cause neurologic side effects: sedation hangover, prolonged sedation, and paradoxical reactions.	Avoid giving with epinephrine/ vasopressors Can give in low dose, wait 30 minutes, if no effect, repeat dose Avoid prolonged administration in neonates (↑ bilirubin, hypotension, and so forth) Drug interactions occur (alcohol, warfarin, others)	Can give PO (may avoid IV start in infant/ young child) Extensive use in pediatrics One of oldest sedatives Use approved for infants/ newborns	Can cause dysrhythmias Can cause respiratory depression and upper airway obstruction (especially high doses with other drugs, neonates) Can cause ↓ oxygen saturation in bronchiolitis patients Metabolism and elimination affected by severe liver or kidney disease Can cause GI mucosal irritation (gastritis, esophagitis)

of chloral hydrate be limited to infants and children ≤3 years of age.[5,12,22]

ADVERSE EFFECTS

The most serious side effects of chloral hydrate are related to respiratory depression/loss of airway reflexes, CNS depression/toxicity, and cardiovascular toxicity.[51-60] In several large series of patients receiving chloral hydrate in therapeutic doses, the incidence of hypoxia (oxygen saturation ≤90% or >5% decrease from baseline in patients with cyanotic congenital heart disease) ranges from 0.4 to 7.1%.[13-15,46,47,61,62] In most cases, repositioning of the head and neck, administering supplemental oxygen, and suctioning the airway was all that was required and the hypoxia resolved without sequelae. This incidence of hypoxia is comparable to that for other sedative-hypnotics. In other studies, for example, the reported incidence of hypoxia (oxygen saturation <90%) was 8.3% for etomidate,[63] 13% for midazolam ± opioid,[64] 7% for methohexital,[65] and 6% for pentobarbital.[66]

Deaths have been reported with intentional overdoses as well as the clinical use of chloral hydrate.[51,52,54,60,67,68] Most deaths are associated with an overdose of the drug, the drug in combination with other drugs, or in patients who were unmonitored.[51,54,60,67,68] In a review of deaths from chloral hydrate, there was only one case where a child received a standard dose and in this case the child was unmonitored. Lack of appropriate monitoring of patients who receive sedation has been cited as a key factor accounting for adverse events and even deaths occurring from sedative drugs. The takeaway message is obvious.[67-70] Monitoring allows trained personnel to respond to any adverse events with appropriate interventions, thereby minimizing or eliminating morbidity and mortality.[67-72]

Chloral hydrate is one of the oldest sedative drugs and had been used for sedation long before monitoring of patients receiving sedation and analgesia had been recommended and accepted. This may, at least partly, explain some of the deaths from chloral hydrate. If these patients had been monitored, then the respiratory depression, airway obstruction, or dysrhythmias might have been detected and interventions undertaken to avert death. The practice of allowing parents to administer a sedative at home (with the parents sometimes overdosing the drug), and then traveling to the hospital or office for their outpatient test is a dangerous outdated practice that was responsible for some adverse effects and deaths from chloral hydrate use.

CNS depression, cardiac dysrhythmias, and hypotension have all been reported with chloral hydrate, usually in overdose situations.[51-60] The dysrhythmias will generally respond to beta-blockers and are worse with vasopressors and epinephrine.[8,53-55] Hemodialysis/hemoperfusion has been used to successfully treat chloral hydrate toxicity/overdoses.[54,58]

Chloral hydrate can cause irritation of the mucous membranes.[73] This is responsible for such side effects as bitter taste and gastritis with accompanying nausea and vomiting, particularly if taken on an empty stomach. More severe manifestations of GI mucosal membrane irritation, including hemorrhagic gastritis, esophagitis, and enteritis have occurred after overdoses of chloral hydrate.[38] Thus, a relative contraindication for oral chloral hydrate may be the presence of known gastritis, esophagitis, or ulcers.

In addition to the occasional prolonged sedation, paradoxical reactions and sedation hangover can occur with chloral hydrate. Other uncommon neurologic side effects include nightmares, headaches, ataxia, dizziness, and seizures.[8,38,59] A chloral hydrate overdose can lead to coma, usually with miotic pupils.[53,54,59] Rashes, leukoplakia, and eosinophilia have also been reported with chronic chloral hydrate use.[8]

EFFICACY OF CHLORAL HYDRATE COMPARED TO SEDATIVE AGENTS

Several studies have compared chloral hydrate to other sedatives.[23,24,34,62,74] In one study of 2857 patients, chloral hydrate, pentobarbital, midazolam, diazepam, and other sedatives were compared.[74] The conclusion was that "the overall safety and efficacy were quite good with all the regimens. Oral chloral hydrate, intravenous midazolam, and oral diazepam had the fewest side effects."[74] Hyperactivity, and the highest incidences of prolonged sleep and prolonged drowsiness after awakening occurred with pentobarbital.[74]

A small-randomized prospective double-blind study comparing chloral hydrate with midazolam sedation for neuroimaging found that "efficacy was significantly improved for the chloral hydrate group" (100% = 11/11 patients for chloral hydrate vs. 50% = 11/22 for midazolam).[23] A small crossover study of seven hospitalized term neonates found "chloral hydrate to be more efficacious than midazolam" (100% sedation for chloral hydrate vs. 42.9% for midazolam) for neuroimaging sedation in the same infants with equivalent side effects. This study of hospitalized stable but not healthy neonates found a high incidence of adverse effects (57%) including hypoxia (oxygen saturation <90%), hypotension, agitation, hiccups, and tachycardia.[34]

Some studies have found a sedation failure rate as high as 40% although these studies included older patients, a group known to have a high sedation failure rate with chloral hydrate.[47,75] However, another review article cites the sedation success rate for chloral hydrate at 89–100%,[4] which agrees with most reported studies. Reasons for this discrepancy include the dose used, the age of the patients, whether the patient is a special needs child, and the end point or measure of sedation.

With the advent of newer sedative agents, chloral hydrate has fallen out of favor for use in the emergency department (ED). It is a poor first choice in the ED for many reasons: a delayed onset and offset (long duration of effect), potential cardiac/respiratory adverse effects, occurrence of prolonged sedation in some patients and paradoxical reaction in others, and variable success rate.

ADMINISTRATION OF THE DRUG

Chloral hydrate can only be given PO or PR and the dose is the same by either route. The absorption of chloral hydrate when given rectally is erratic, so this route of administration is not recommended.[6,22] It is a category C drug in pregnancy.[76]

Chloral hydrate does have various drug interactions. Because of its cardiac effects and the possibility of dysrhythmias, it is best to avoid giving chloral hydrate in patients receiving vasopressors, epinephrine, and stimulant medications.[48,77]

Coadministration of flumazenil or naloxone with chloral hydrate may also precipitate dysrhythmias.[78] When given with other respiratory depressants, there is a synergistic depression of the CNS. Prolonged sedation can also occur with the concomitant administration of chloral hydrate and fluoxetine. Though variable and unpredictable, the administration of chloral hydrate to patients on coumadin may produce an elevated prothrombin time. The interaction of chloral hydrate with furosemide causes a degree of vasomotor instability in some patients, likely by the displacement of furosemide from protein-binding sites by chloral hydrate.[4]

The metabolism of chloral hydrate is affected by ethanol and vice versa because both compete for the enzyme alcohol dehydrogenase. Furthermore, chloral hydrate's active metabolite, TCE, inhibits the oxidation of ethanol, while ethanol inhibits the conjugation of TCE.[4] Ethanol metabolism produces nicotinamide adenine dinucleotide (NADH), a cofactor in the metabolism of chloral hydrate to TCE.[4] Taken together these factors enhance the sedative effects of the ethanol/chloral hydrate combination, commonly known as a "Mickey Finn."

DOSAGE

The dosage of chloral hydrate required to induce moderate sedation is extremely variable ranging between 25 and 100 mg/kg PO or PR. The drug's onset is 15–30 minutes by either route. If there is no effect in 30 minutes, a second dose is often given up to the maximum. The maximum dose also varies. Some clinicians use a maximum of 100 mg/kg while others will give up to 1, 2, or even 3 g.

SUMMARY

Chloral hydrate is one of the oldest sedative-hypnotic agents. It can be given PO or PR. It has an especially high sedation failure rate in older children (≥3 years of age) and in special needs children. Serious adverse effects associated with chloral hydrate include respiratory depression, loss of airway reflexes, CNS depression, and cardiovascular toxicity (dysrhythmias, hypotension). Currently, its only indication is for painless procedures in infants/children ≤3 years of age in whom an IV line is not possible and oral administration of the sedative is preferred. With the advent of many newer better sedatives, the use of chloral hydrate has justifiably experienced a precipitous decline.

REFERENCES

1. Osborn IP. Intravenous conscious sedation for pediatric patients. *Int Anesthesiol Clin.* 1999;37:99–111.
2. Binder LS, Leake LA. Chloral hydrate for emergent pediatric procedural sedation: a new look at an old drug. *Am J Emerg Med.* 1991;9:530–534.
3. Sacchetti A, Gerardi MJ. Emergency department procedural sedation and analgesia. In: Strange GR, Ahrens WR, Lelyveld S, et al. *Pediatric Emergency Medicine.* New York: McGraw-Hill; 2002:185–196.
4. Pershad J, Palmisano P, Nichols M. Chloral hydrate: the good and the bad. *Pediatr Emerg Care.* 1999;15:432–435.
5. Krauss B, Green SM. Sedation and analgesia for procedures in children. *N Engl J Med.* 2000;342:938–945.
6. Krauss B. Management of pain and anxiety in children undergoing procedures in the emergency department. *Pediatr Emerg Care.* 2001;17:115–122.
7. American Academy of Pediatrics Committee on Drugs and Committee on Environmental Health. Use of chloral hydrate for sedation in children. *Pediatrics.* 1993;92:471–473.
8. Litman R. Sedatives and hypnotics. In: Krauss B, Brustowicz RM, eds. *Pediatric Procedural Sedation and Analgesia.* Philadelphia, PA: Lippincott Williams & Wilkins; 1999:39–46.
9. Johnson MN, Liebelt EL. Acute pain management and procedural sedation in children. In: Tintinalli JE, Kelen GD, Stapczynski JS, eds. *Emergency Medicine: A Comprehensive Study Guide.* New York: McGraw-Hill; 2004:858–869.

10. Kennedy RM, Luhmann JD. The "Ouchless Emergency Department". *Pediatr Clin North Am.* 1999;46:1215–1247.
11. Sacchetti A, Schafermeyer R, Gerardi M, et al. Pediatric analgesia and sedation. *Ann Emerg Med.* 1994;23:237–250.
12. Rodriquez E, Jordan R. Contemporary trends in pediatric sedation and analgesia. *Emerg Med Clin North Am.* 2002;20:199–222.
13. Napoli KL, Ingall CG, Martin GR. Safety and efficacy of chloral hydrate sedation in children undergoing echocardiography. *J Pediatr.* 1996;129:287–291.
14. Malviya S, Voepel-Lewis T, Eldevik OP, et al. Sedation and general anesthesia in children undergoing MRI and CT: adverse events and outcomes. *Br J Anesth.* 2000;84:743–748.
15. Malviya S, Voepel-Lewis T, Tait AR. Adverse events and risk factors associated with the sedation of children by non-anesthesiologists. *Anesth Analg.* 1997;85:1207–1213.
16. Ronchera-Oms CL, Casillas C, Marti-Bonmati L, et al. Randomized double-blind clinical trial of intermediate- versus high dose chloral hydrate for neuroimaging of children. *Neuroradiology.* 1995;37:687–691.
17. Egelhoff JC, Ball WS, Koch BL, et al. Safety and efficacy of sedation in children using a structured sedation program. *Am J Roentgenol.* 1997;168:1259–1262.
18. Karien VE, Burrows PE, Zurakowski D, et al. Sedation for pediatric radiological procedures: analysis of potential causes of sedation failure and paradoxical reactions. *Pediatr Radiol.* 1999;29:869–873.
19. Ziegler MA, Fricke BL, Donnelly LF. Is administration of enteric contrast material safe before abdominal CT in children who require sedation? Experience with chloral hydrate and pentobarbital. *Am J Roentgenol.* 2003;180:13–15.
20. Volle E, Park W, Kaufmann HJ. MRI examination and monitoring of pediatric patients under sedation. *Pediatr Radiol.* 1996;26:280–281.
21. Thoresen M, Henrickson O, Wannag E, et al. Does a sedation dose of chloral hydrate modify the EEG of children with epilepsy? *Electroencephalogr Clin Neurophysiology.* 1997;102:152–157.
22. Green SM, Krauss B. Procedural sedation and analgesia. In: Roberts JR, Hedges JR, Chanmugan AS, et al, eds. *Clinical Procedures in Emergency Medicine.* Philadelphia, PA: W.B. Saunders; 2004:596–619.
23. D'Augustino JD, Terndrup TE. Chloral hydrate versus midazolam for sedation of children for neuroimaging: a randomized clinical trial. *Pediatr Emerg Care.* 2000;16:1–4.
24. Chung T, Hoffner FA, Connor L, et al. The use of oral pentobarbital sodium (nembutal) versus oral chloral hydrate in infants undergoing CT and MR imaging—a pilot study. *Pediatr Radiol.* 2000;30:332–335.
25. Keengwe IN, Hegde S, Dearlove O, et al. Structured sedation programme for magnetic resonance imaging examination in children. *Anesthesia.* 1999;54:1069–1072.
26. Kao SC, Adamson SD, Tatman LH, et al. A survey of post-discharge side effects of conscious sedation using chloral hydrate in pediatric CT and MR imaging. *Pediatr Radiol.* 1999;29:287–290.
27. Olson DM, Sheehan MG, Thompson W, et al. Sedation of children for encephalograms. *Pediatrics.* 2001;108:163–165.
28. Campbell RL, Ross GA, Campbell JR, et al. Comparison of oral chloral hydrate with intramuscular ketamine, meperidine, and promethazine for pediatric sedation-preliminary report. *Anesth Prog.* 1998;45:46–50.
29. Wilson S, Easton J, Orchardson R, et al. A retrospective study of chloral hydrate, meperidine, hydroxyzine, and midazolam regimens used to sedate children for dental care. *Pediatr Dent.* 2000;22:107–112.
30. Dallman JA, Ignelzi MA Jr, Briskie DM. Comparing the safety, efficacy and recovery of intranasal midazolam vs oral chloral hydrate and promethazine. *Pediatr Dent.* 2001;23:424–430.
31. Reeves ST, Wiedenfeld KR, Wrobleski J, et al. A randomized double-blind trial of chloral hydrate/hydroxyzine versus midazolam/acetaminophen in the sedation of pediatric dental outpatients. *J Dent Child.* 1996;63:95–100.
32. Malis DJ, Burton DM. Safe pediatric outpatient sedation: the chloral hydrate debate revisited. *Otolaryngol Head Neck Surg.* 1997;116:53–57.
33. Krauss B, Zurakowski D. Sedation patterns in pediatric and general community hospital emergency departments. *Pediatr Emerg Care.* 1998;14:99–103.
34. McCarver-May DG, Kang J, Aouthmany M, et al. Comparison of chloral hydrate and midazolam for sedation of neonates for neuroimaging studies. *J Pediatr.* 1996;128:573–576.
35. Alexander SM, Todres ID. The use of sedation and muscle relaxation in the ventilated infant. *Clin Perinatol.* 1998;25:63–78.
36. Hypnotic drugs. *Med Lett.* 2000;42(1084):71.
37. Pranzatelli MR, Tate ED. Chloral hydrate for progressive myoclonus epilepsy: a new look at an old drug. *Pediatr Neurol.* 2001;25:385–389.
38. Charney DS, Mihic SJ, Harris RA. Hypnotics and sedatives. In: Hardman JG, Limbird LE, Goodman Gilman A, eds. *Goodman & Gilman's The Pharmacological Basis of Therapeutics.* New York: McGraw-Hill; 2001:399–428.
39. Miller JW, Uden PC. *Environ Sci Technol.* 1983;17:150–157.
40. Brunner M, Albertini S, Wurgler FE. *Mutagenesis.* 1991;6:65–70.
41. Sanders VM, Kauffmann BM, White KL Jr, et al. *Environ Health Perspect.* 1982;44:137–146.
42. Lovinger DM, Zimmerman SA, Levitin M, et al. Trichloroethanol potentiates synaptic transmission mediated by gamma-aminobutyric acid A receptors in hippocampal neurons. *J Pharmacol ExpTher.* 1993;264:1097–1103.
43. Henderson GH, Yan Z, James MO, et al. Kinetics and metabolism of chloral hydrate in children: identification of dichloroacetate as a metabolite. *Biochem Biophys Res Commun.* 1997;235:695–698.
44. Graham SR, Day RO, Lee R, et al. Overdose with chloral hydrate: a pharmacological and therapeutic review. *Med J Aust.* 1988;149:686–688.
45. Litman RS, Kottra JA, Verga KA, et al. The additive sedative and respiratory depressant effects of nitrous oxide. *Anesth Analg.* 1998;86:724–728.

46. Greenberg SB, Faerber EN, Aspinall CL, et al. High dose chloral hydrate sedation for children undergoing MR imaging: safety and efficacy in relation to age. *Am J Roentgenol.* 1993;161:639–641.

47. Vade A, Sukhani R, Dolenga M, et al. Chloral hydrate sedation in children undergoing CT and MR imaging: safety as judged by American Academy of Pediatrics (AAP) guidelines. *Am J Roentgenol.* 1995;165:905–909.

48. Hershenson M, Brouillette RT, Olsen E, et al. The effect of chloral hydrate on genioglossus and diaphragmatic activity. *Pediatr Res.* 1984;18:516–519.

49. Rumm PD, Takao RT, Fox DJ, et al. Efficacy of safety of children with chloral hydrate. *South Med J.* 1990;83: 1040–1043.

50. Weir MR, Segapel JH, Tremper JL. Sedation for pediatric procedures. *Mil Med.* 1986;151:181–184.

51. Engelhart DA, Lovins ES, Hazenstab CB, et al. Unusual death attributed to the combined effects of chloral hydrate, lidocaine, and nitrous oxide. *J Anal. Toxicol.* 1998;22:246–247.

52. Caksen H, Odabas D, Unerune A, et al. Respiratory arrest due to chloral hydrate in an infant. *J Emerg Med.* 2003;24: 342–343.

53. Zahed A, Grant MH, Wong DT. Successful treatment of chloral hydrate toxicity with propranolol. *Am J Emerg Med.* 1999;17:490–491.

54. Ludwigs U, Divino Filho JC, et al. Suicidal chloral hydrate poisoning. *Clin Toxicol.* 1996;34:97–99.

55. Sing K, Erickson T, Amitai Y, et al. Chloral hydrate toxicity from oral and intravenous administration. *Clin Toxicol.* 1996;34:101–106.

56. Kirimi E, Huseyin C, Cesur Y, et al. Chloral hydrate intoxication in a newborn infant. *J Emerg Med.* 2002;22: 104–105.

57. Rokicki W. Cardiac arrhythmias in a child after the usual dose of chloral hydrate. *Pediatr Cardiol.* 1996;17:419–420.

58. Anyebuno MA, Rosenfeld CR. Chloral hydrate toxicity in a term infant. *Dev Pharmacol Ther.* 1991;17:116–120.

59. Munoz M, Gomez A, Soult JA, et al. Seizures caused by chloral hydrate sedative doses. *J Pediatr.* 1997;131: 787–788.

60. Gaulier JM, Merle G, Lacassie E, et al. Fatal intoxications with chloral hydrate. *J Forensic Sci.* 2001;46: 1507–1509.

61. Greenberg SN, Faerber FN, Aspinall CT. High dose chloral hydrate sedation for children undergoing CT. *J Comput Assist Tomogr.* 1991;15:467–469.

62. Pereira JK, Burrows PE, Richards HM, et al. Comparison of sedation regimens for pediatric outpatient CT. *Pediatr Radiol.* 1993;23:341–343.

63. Ruth W, Burton J, Bock A. Etomidate for procedural sedation in emergency department patients. *Acad Emerg Med.* 2001;8: 13–18.

64. Sievers TD, Yee JD, Foley ME, et al. Midazolam for conscious sedation during pediatric oncology procedures: safety and recovery parameters. *Pediatrics.* 1991;88:1172–1179.

65. Pomeranz ES, Chudnofsky CR, Deegan TJ, et al. Rectal methohexital sedation for computed tomography imaging of stable emergency department patients. *Pediatrics.* 2000;105: 1110–1114.

66. Greenberg SB, Adams RC, Aspinall CL. Initial experience with intravenous pentobarbital sedation for children undergoing MRI at a territory care pediatric hospital: the learning curve. *Pediatr Radiol.* 2000;30:689–691.

67. Cote CJ, Notterman DA, Karl HW, et al. Adverse sedation events in pediatrics: a critical incident analysis of contributing factors. *Pediatrics.* 2000;105:805–814.

68. Cote CJ, Karl HW, Notterman DA, et al. Adverse sedation events in pediatrics: analysis of medications used for sedation. *Pediatrics.* 2000;106:633–644.

69. Cote CJ. Letter to the editor. *Pediatrics.* p.825.

70. Malviya S, Tait AR, Voeppel-Lewis T, et al. Oranges and apples: sedation and analgesia. *Pediatrics.* p.824.

71. American College of Emergency Physicians. Clinical policy for procedural sedation and analgesia in the emergency department. *Ann Emerg Med.* 1998;31:663–677.

72. Mace SE, Barata IA, Cravero JP, et al. Clinical policy: evidence-based approach to pharmacologic agents used in pediatric sedation and analgesia in the emergency department. *Ann Emerg Med.* 2004;44:342–377.

73. Caksen H, Odabas D. Pierioral skin lesions due to chloral hydrate. *Pediatr Dermatol.* 2001;18:454–455.

74. Slovis TL, Parks C, Reneau D, et al. Pediatric sedation: short term effects. *Pediatr Radiol.* 1993;23:345–348.

75. Seiler G, DeVol E, Kha Fagg Y, et al. Evaluation of the safety and efficacy of repeated sedations for the radiotherapy of young children with cancer: a prospective study of 1033 consecutive sedations. *Int J Radiat Oncol Biol Phy.* 2001;49: P771–P783.

76. Chloral hydrate. Briggs GG, Freeman RK, Yaffe SJ, eds. *Drugs in Pregnancy and Lactation.* Philadelphia, PA: Lippincott Williams & Wilkins; 2002

77. Seger D, Schwartz G. Chloral hydrate: a dangerous sedative for overdose patients? *Pediatr Emerg Care.* 1994;10: 349–350.

78. Donovan KL, Fisher DJ. Reversal of chloral hydrate overdose with flumazenil. *BMJ.* 1989;298:1253.

23

Nitrous Oxide and Volatile Agent Analgesia

Michael F. Murphy

HIGH YIELD FACTS

- Nitrous oxide (N_2O) continues to be a valuable analgesic agent in procedural sedation in a variety of clinical settings, both in hospital and prehospital.
- With N_2O the principle of self-administration is a crucial safety feature.
- Be aware of the contraindications and precautions when using N_2O:
  - Trapped air (e.g., bowel obstruction and severe emphysema).
  - Diffusion hypoxia.
- Volatile anesthetic agents currently have no role in providing procedural analgesia.

The history of painless surgery is inextricably entwined in the evolution of vapors and gases to induce insensibility to pain. Though the precise origins of inhaled anesthesia seem to be lost in the vapors of time and controversy, it is clear that diethyl ether emerged in the mid-1800s as an effective and safe, albeit explosively flammable and nauseating agent. It was used to induce and maintain deep levels of anesthesia while maintaining stable vital signs. The fact that this agent survived in clinical practice into the 1960s is a testament to its clinical efficacy.

Other gases such as N_2O and cyclopropane, and vapors such as chloroform and methoxyflurane entered clinical practice over the years. Only the methyl-ethyl ethers (enflurane, isoflurane, sevoflurane, and desflurane) and N_2O persist in clinical practice to this day. Even long-used agents such as the alkane halothane have faded into history.

VOLATILE ANESTHETIC AGENTS

In a similar fashion to opioids and sedative hypnotics, inhaled volatile anesthetic agents have enjoyed popularity over the years as analgesic agents in subanesthetic concentrations. General anesthesia is an amalgam of hypnosis (sleep), analgesia, and muscle relaxation. Volatile anesthetic agents produce all three to varying degrees. Though hypnosis predominates, the analgesic properties of these medications is considerable and has been exploited over the years to facilitate painful procedures such as minor surgery and to relieve the pain of labor, albeit in subanesthetic concentrations.

Perhaps the best example is the *Penthrane Whistle*. This device, containing methoxyflurane, was used as a self-administered device during labor to provide a measure of analgesia, and in the process, pioneered the concept of *patient-controlled analgesia*. The principle was simple: when the pain of labor became unbearable, the parturient sucked on the whistle inducing analgesia. When consciousness became compromised, the hand fell from the mouth limiting the dose administered. This is no different from the modern concept of patient-controlled analgesia: patient obtundation precludes overdose.

In subanesthetic concentrations, all of the modern volatile anesthetic agents provide some measure of analgesia. At present there are no volatile anesthetic agents routinely employed to produce procedural analgesia.

NITROUS OXIDE

As an analgesic for adults and children, N_2O, either alone or in conjunction with other agents, has been extensively studied in anesthesia and emergency medicine in a variety of hospital and outpatient settings.

History

Joseph Priestly, a Unitarian minister from Yorkshire, England, first reported the use of *nitrous air* in 1772, 50 years before ether was used.[1] Between 1800 and 1845, it was used primarily for its entertaining and pleasurable effects. It was not until the mid-1880s that the analgesic properties of the gas were recognized. Even so, N_2O did not become a supplement to inhaled anesthesia until the early 1900s.

Chemical and Physical Properties

N_2O is a colorless and odorless gas at room temperature that is 1.5 times as heavy as air. It does seem to have a vaguely sweet taste when inhaled. Though it is nonflammable, it supports combustion.[2]

Pharmacokinetics

N_2O is quite insoluble in blood, particularly in comparison to nitrogen, the major component of air. This feature of N_2O has several important implications:

- Rapid equilibration between delivered concentration and alveolar concentration of the gas. This confers a rapid onset and offset of its analgesic effect.[2]
- When discontinued N_2O diffuses rapidly from the blood, diluting the concentration of oxygen in alveoli. This may lead to *diffusion hypoxia* unless the oxygen concentration is supplemented (as is the case with commercial 50/50 N_2O/O_2 preparations).[2]
- The rapid diffusion of N_2O from blood to air-filled cavities in the body (e.g., bowel, pneumothorax, intracranial air, middle ear, and air embolism) before an equivalent volume of nitrogen can diffuse back into the blood may cause expansion of this gas volume with deleterious results (e.g., tension pneumothorax).

N_2O is entirely (99.9%) eliminated by the lungs. Virtually none of the gas is metabolized. However, N_2O can be degraded by intestinal bacteria through a reaction with vitamin B_{12}. With chronic use this may result in vitamin B_{12} deficiency.[2]

Clinical Use

As mentioned previously, N_2O has been used extensively in clinical practice as a moderate analgesic and mild sedative.[3–9] It may be used alone or in conjunction with other intravenous agents and reduces the amount of those agents employed proportionate to the concentration of N_2O delivered. It is typically self-administered to prevent hypoventilation and loss of airway protective reflexes. The importance of this self-administration safety feature cannot be emphasized too strongly, particularly to well-meaning parents, spouses, and others.

The equipment to deliver this agent is usually commercially prepared to deliver a 50%/50% oxygen/N_2O mix, though equipment to vary the concentrations of oxygen and N_2O are also available (the upper limit of N_2O ought not exceed 70%).

N_2O/O_2 can be used for almost any procedural sedation, provided there are no contraindications. However, the most commonly encountered scenarios where N_2O/O_2 analgesia may be employed include the following:

- Fracture and dislocation reductions
- Management of painful perirectal conditions
- Large bowel disimpaction
- Foley catheter insertion
- Dental pain
- Insertion of central venous catheters in children
- Emergency D&C
- Renal colic (but not bowel colic due to the solubility characteristics of N_2O)
- Prehospital pain management

Side Effects and Monitoring

N_2O is a mild cardiac depressant, though this is usually of no consequence in the setting of procedural sedation. It also causes mild elevations in venous resistance that may be clinically significant in patients with preexisting pulmonary hypertension. There is little effect on ventilatory drive, though if side-stream CO_2 detection devices are available they ought to be employed when N_2O is being self-administered. This is particularly true when other systemic analgesics or sedatives are concurrently administered. Continuous pulse oximetry monitoring is advised, particularly in the event that diffusion hypoxia supervenes at the intervals during the procedure when self-administration ceases or at the end of the procedure when N_2O/O_2 is discontinued.

N_2O is not a trigger for malignant hyperthermia.

CONCLUSION

N_2O is a mild sedative and moderate analgesic when administered as a 50/50 mix with oxygen. It has a long history of safety in clinical practice and is an effective agent, both alone and when supplemented with adjunctive intravenous medications.

REFERENCES

1. Frost EAM. A history of nitrous oxide. In: Eger EI, ed. *Nitrous Oxide*. New York: Elsevier Science; 1985:1–22.
2. Evers AS, Crowder CM. General anesthetics. In: Hardman JG, Limbird LE, Gilman AG, eds. *Goodman and Gilman's The Pharmacologic Basis of Therapeutics*. 10th ed. New York: McGraw-Hill; 2001:337–365.

3. Abdelkefi A, Abdennebi YB, Mellouli F, et al. Effectiveness of fixed 50% nitrous oxide oxygen mixture and EMLA cream for insertion of central venous catheters in children. *Pediatr Blood Cancer*. 2004;43:777–779.

4. Kennedy RM, Luhmann JD, Luhmann SJ. Emergency department management of pain and anxiety related to orthopedic fracture care: a guide to analgesic techniques and procedural sedation in children. *Paediatr Drugs*. 2004;6: 11–31.

5. O'Sullivan I, Benger J. Nitrous oxide in emergency medicine. *Emerg Med J*. 2003;20:214–217.

6. Borland ML, Jacobs I, Rogers IR. Options in prehospital analgesia. *Emerg Med* (Fremantle). 2002;14:77–84.

7. Kennedy RM, Luhmann JD. Pharmacological management of pain and anxiety during emergency procedures in children. *Paediatr Drugs*. 2001;3:337–354.

8. Blackburn P, Vissers R. Pharmacology of emergency department pain management and conscious sedation. *Emerg Med Clin North Am*. 2000;18:803–827.

9. Gall O, Annequin D, Benoit G, et al. Adverse events of premixed nitrous oxide and oxygen for procedural sedation in children. *Lancet*. 2001;358:1514–1515.

24

Neuraxial Analgesia and Anesthesia

Michael F. Murphy

HIGH YIELD FACTS

- Blocks performed on the neuraxis include epidural, spinal, and caudal (an epidural block performed through the sacral hiatus).

- The epidural space can be entered anywhere in its length from the C3-4 interspace to the sacral hiatus at S4-5. Because the spinal cord ends at approximately the L1 level, most epidurals are performed in the lower lumbar region, and virtually all spinals are done in this region to avoid injury to the cord by an inadvertent puncture.

- Epidural analgesia may be contemplated in the emergency department (ED) for the following indications:
  - Multiple rib fractures: thoracic epidural.
  - Painful (noninfective) anorectal conditions: caudal block.
  - Lower limb crush and multiple fracture injuries: lumbar epidural.
  - Intractable renal colic: lumbar epidural.

- The following may mitigate for or against neuraxial analgesia:
  - Coagulopathy (against).
  - Desire to limit systemic opioids, but produce analgesia (for).
  - Systemic sepsis (against).
  - Hemodynamic instability (against).

This chapter is intended to introduce the topic of neuraxial analgesia to the nonanesthesia practitioner for the purpose of creating an understanding as to how neuraxial analgesia is employed in the management of acutely painful conditions, and the limitations of the techniques.

ANATOMY AND DEFINITIONS

The term *neuraxis* generally refers to those neural elements contained within the cranium and spinal canal (the brain, spinal cord, and spinal nerve roots [until they exit the spinal canal]). Blocks performed on the neuraxis include epidural, spinal, and caudal (an epidural block performed through the sacral hiatus).

The bony vertebral column consists of 24 individual vertebrae (7 cervical, 12 thoracic, and 5 lumbar), the sacrum comprised of five fused vertebrae, and the four fused coccygeal segments[1] (Fig. 24-1). The spinal canal is formed by the vertebral body, the pedicles, and laminae (Fig. 24-2). The spinal cord extends from the base of the skull, being continuous with the brain stem, to approximately the level of the L1 vertebral body in the adult. The dural sac ends at roughly S2, and so between L1 and S2 the subarachnoid space contains only nerve roots (cauda equina). Nerve roots traverse the epidural space to exit the spinal canal between vertebral bodies, or in the case of the sacrum, via neural foramina.

The neural elements within the spinal canal are surrounded by a series of membranes (Fig. 24-3):

- The dura mater (*tough mother*) is rather thick and continuous with the intracranial dura.

- The arachnoid mater adheres to the dura, so that puncture of the dura by a needle is ordinarily associated with penetration into the fluid-filled subarachnoid space.

- The pia mater is adherent to the spinal cord and of no consequence to this discussion.

Two spaces derive from this anatomy:

- The subarachnoid space filled with cerebrospinal fluid (CSF, an ultrafiltrate of plasma) and the

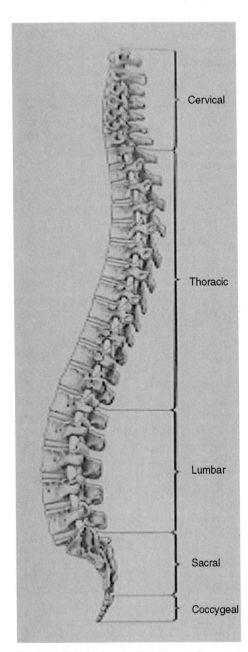

Fig. 24-1. Spinal column. Note the natural curvature of the various segments of the spinal column and the orientation of the spinous processes, from horizontal in the lumbar and cervical regions to a much more vertical orientation in the thoracic region. For this reason a paraspinous approach to neuraxial block is ordinarily employed in the thoracic region. (Reproduced from Scott DB. *Techniques of Regional Anesthesia.* Norwalk, CT: Appleton & Lange; 1989:163.)

location of injection of medications to produce spinal anesthesia (e.g., bupivicaine 0.5%) or analgesia (e.g., fentanyl and morphine). The average adult has between 120 and 150 mL of CSF, 25–35 mL of which is in the spinal subarachnoid space. On average, 500 mL of CSF is produced daily.[2]

- The epidural (or extradural) space. This space contains fatty tissue and blood vessels and surrounds the dural sac.

The epidural space can be entered anywhere in its length from the C3-4 interspace to the sacral hiatus at S4-5.[3] Because the spinal cord ends at approximately the L1 level, most epidurals are performed in the lower lumbar region, and virtually all spinals are done in this region to avoid injury to the cord by an inadvertent puncture.

A single shot of medication into either space is termed a *single shot* spinal or epidural. The placement of a small catheter into either space permits the intermittent and/or continuous infusion of medication and is termed a *continuous* spinal or epidural. Single shot techniques are usually employed in spinal anesthesia and continuous techniques in epidural anesthesia and analgesia. Continuous techniques tend to permit a more precise dermatomal limit of block than single shot techniques, and are slower to develop, mitigating the hypotension that is sometimes seen with extensive sympathetic blockade. The continuous technique, particularly with epidural placement, is much more the norm in managing pain.

Two terms merit description:

Neuraxial anesthesia:

- Typically involves the use of local anesthetic agents capable of rendering the body region inferior to the block insensitive to pain, and often-times immobile.

- The higher the concentration of local anesthetic agent employed, the more intense the block and the more likely that motor blockade will ensue.

Spinal anesthesia:

- Is typically induced with fairly concentrated solutions of preservative-free local anesthetic solutions (bupivicaine 0.75%, lidocaine 5%).

- Produces a block so intense that it appears to induce a 'chemical, though reversible, sectioning' of the spinal cord.

- May be hyperbaric or hypobaric in order that positioning can be employed to influence the extent of a block; isobaric solutions are also used.

1. Spinous process
2. Lamina
3. Spinal canal
4. Transverse process
5. Facet joint
6. Pedicle
7. Body

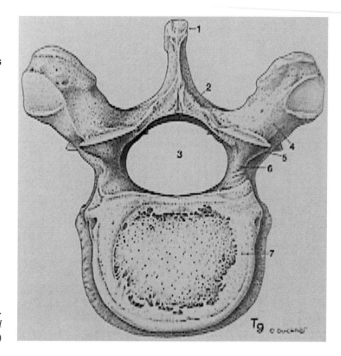

Fig. 24-2. Typical vertebra of the lumbar region. (Reproduced from Scott DB. *Techniques of Regional Anesthesia.* Norwalk, CT: Appleton & Lange; 1989:163.)

Epidural anesthesia employing concentrated solutions of local anesthetic agents produces profound sensory and motor blockade, in much the same way as a spinal anesthetic.

Neuraxial analgesia is employed in the management of acute and chronic pain syndromes.

Though Chapter 30 deals with the neurobiology of pain, a brief review serves to clarify the rationale behind neuraxial analgesia. The sensation of pain is mediated by complex neuronal pathways. Once activated, peripheral pain sensors transmit the neural impulse via peripheral pathways to the spinal cord, and then to the brain. The processing of a pain signal involves the following:

- Transduction: Noxious stimuli are transduced into electrical signals by nociceptors.
- Transmission: The pain signal is transmitted from the periphery to the cerebral cortex being relayed through the dorsal horn of the spinal cord and the thalamus.
- Modulation: The pain signal may be modulated by neural system elements and processes, the most important of which are descending supraspinal inhibitory influences activated by μ opioid receptors (Fig. 24-4).
- Perception: Pain is perceived as a subjective sensation by the cerebral cortex.

Pain signals are transmitted to the spinal cord by Aδ (mechanical and thermal stimuli) and C (mechanical, thermal, and chemical stimuli) fibers (see Chap. 27 for fiber type classification). Both fiber types synapse with second order neurons in the superficial dorsal horn of the spinal cord that relay the signal via the spinothalamic tracts to the thalamus, which in turn relays it to the somatosensory cortex (Fig. 24-5). Spinal cord dorsal root neurotransmission is mediated by substance P and glutamate, among others. Opioid receptors are found on both Aδ and C-fiber types. The binding of opioids to these opioid receptors (particularly the μ receptor) causes the nerve to become hyperpolarized and resistant to pain signal transmission. At least 70% of the μ receptors are located on the presynaptic Aδ and C-fibers; the rest are located on the postsynaptic second order neurons.

Four sites of opioid action have been identified, one supraspinal, two spinal, and one peripheral:

1. In the midbrain, disinhibiting descending modulation influences.
2. Second order neurons preventing ascending pain signal transmission.
3. C-fiber synapses in the dorsal horn.
4. At the peripheral terminals of the nociceptive C-fibers.

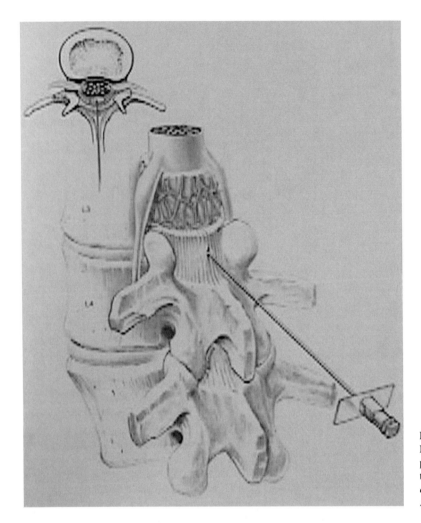

Fig. 24-3. Spaces of the neuraxis. Note how the epidural space is heavily populated with venous vascular structures. (Reproduced from Katz J. *Atlas of Regional Anesthesia.* Norwalk, CT: Appleton & Lange; 1985:179.)

Thus, at the level of the spinal cord, opioid analgesics are able to inhibit both primary afferent Aδ- and C-fibers transmission and the second order neurons inhibiting the transmission of pain signals. This explains the rationale for placing opioids in the epidural and spinal spaces in managing pain.

The goal in neuraxial analgesia is to relieve all, or substantially all, of the patient's pain while at the same time preserving touch, temperature, and proprioceptive sensation and motor power. Very small doses of opioids administered spinally are exceptionally effective analgesics. Ordinarily, the epidural administration of dilute local anesthetic solutions alone, coupled with opioids or opioids alone (termed epidural opioid analgesia [EOA]) are commonly used to manage pain syndromes and are exceptionally effective, particularly when used as a continuous infusion. As mentioned in Chapter 27 (*local anesthetics*), Aδ and C-fibers are lightly myelinated and nonmyelinated, respectively, and are therefore exquisitely sensitive to blockade by very dilute solutions of local anesthetic agent.

The addition of a patient-initiated demand bolus of medication to a background infusion is termed patient-controlled epidural analgesia (PCEA), and is now commonly employed in laboring parturients and for acute postoperative pain.

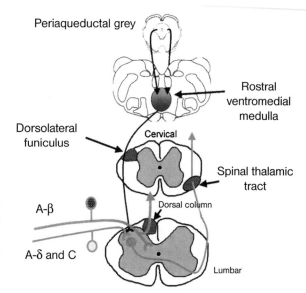

Fig. 24-4. Descending inhibitory modulation pathways. The afferent pain signal may be modulated by neural system elements and processes, the most important of which are descending supraspinal inhibitory influences activated by μ opioid receptors. (Reproduced from *Anesthesiology News. Special Report: Recent Developments in Epidural Opioid Analgesia.* McMahon Publishing Group; July 2004: Fig. 2.)

CLINICAL APPLICATIONS

With the advent of modern anesthesia, it is exceedingly uncommon in North America for non-anesthesia-certified practitioners to administer neuraxial analgesia or anesthesia, though there are some notable exceptions (e.g., obstetricians performing lumbar epidurals for labor analgesia and caudal blocks for delivery). So, for the most part, the acute care physician will be consulting with an anesthesia practitioner.

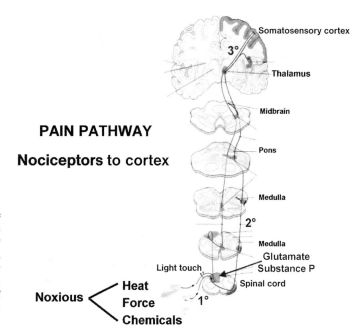

Fig. 24-5. Ascending pain pathways. Nerve cells in the superficial dorsal horn of the spinal cord relay the afferent signal from the periphery via the spinothalamic tracts to the thalamus, which in turn relays it to the somatosensory cortex. (Reproduced from *Anesthesiology News. Special Report: Recent Developments in Epidural Opioid Analgesia.* McMahon Publishing Group; July 2004: Fig. 1.)

It is unlikely that spinal techniques will find much use in the acute care setting, hence this discussion will deal only with epidural techniques.

INDICATIONS AND TECHNIQUES

- Multiple rib fractures: Thoracic epidural. This is probably the best example of a condition that responds well to EOA.[4–9] Patient comfort, the ability to cough and clear secretions, and avert endotracheal intubation are positive outcomes of EOA for patients suffering from multiple rib fractures.
- Painful (noninfective) anorectal conditions: caudal block (Fig. 24-6).
- Lower limb crush and multiple fracture injuries: lumbar epidural.
- Intractable renal colic: lumbar epidural.

Some of the issues that the acute care practitioner may want to consider when contemplating an anesthesia consult for epidural acute pain management include the following:

- Will the patient be admitted to hospital or kept for observation for a period of time sufficient to warrant the procedure? EOA is technically challenging and not without a defined incidence of complications (block failure, central nervous system [CNS] depression, epidural hematoma, and so forth). It would be inappropriate to undertake this method of acute pain management for insignificant, chronic, or brief duration indications.
- Is the source of the pain sufficiently discrete to lend itself to territorial neural blockade consistent with contiguous dermatomes (Fig. 24-7) amenable to epidural blockade?
- Is this pain syndrome likely to be self-limited in duration to 48–96 hours? Acute pain ought to diminish with time to permit the application of conventional methods of analgesia.
- Can the patient be positioned (seated or lateral decubitus) to enable the epidural to be placed?

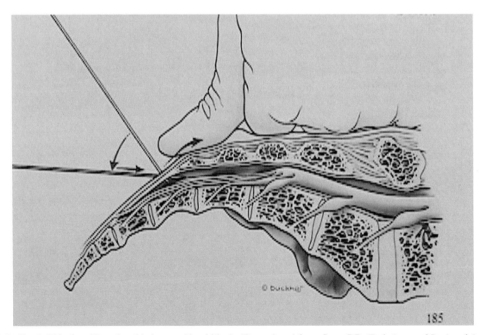

Fig. 24-6. Caudal block. Note that this is an epidural block. (Reproduced from Scott DB. *Techniques of Regional Anesthesia.* Norwalk, CT: Appleton & Lange; 1989:185.)

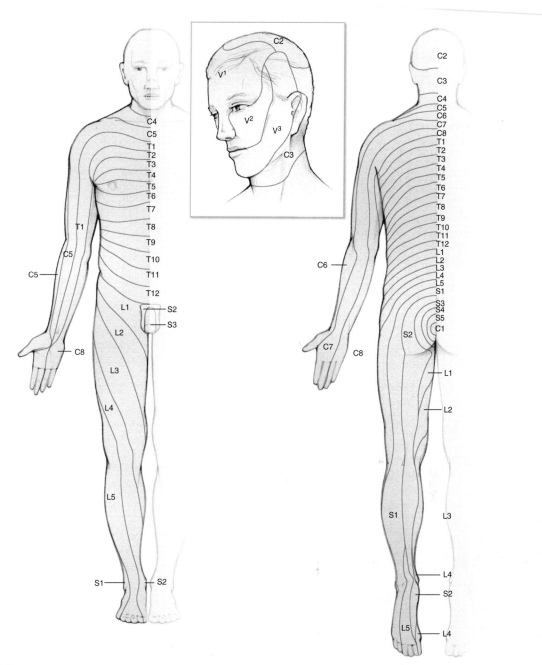

Fig. 24-7. Dermatome representation. Key truncal dermatome landmarks include the nipples at T4, the inferior costal margin at T6, the inferior borders of the scapulae at T8, the umbilicus at T10, and the inguinal ligaments at T12. (Reproduced from: White JS. *USMLE Road Map: Gross Anatomy*. New York: Lange/ McGraw-Hill, 2003: p. 16.)

- Is the patient hemodynamically stable? Unless the epidural will employ opioids alone, sympathetic blockade may be contraindicated in the hemodynamically unstable patient.

- Is the patient septic (fever, elevated white count)? This is a relative contraindication to epidural catheter placement as it has been associated with epidural abscess formation.[10–24]

- Is a coagulopathy present? An epidural hematoma may be precipitated.[25–31]

- Is there a need to limit systemic opioids? In which case, EOA may be desirable.

- Does the patient have sleep apnea? This may seem like an odd question, but the association or EOA and sudden, unheralded apnea in patients suffering from sleep apnea is well established.[32–34] It is uncertain whether the use of continuous positive airway pressure (CPAP) or bi-level pressure support mitigates this risk. In the event a patient with sleep apnea requires EOA continuous pulse oximetry monitoring and observation is indicated.

CONCLUSION

Neuraxial analgesia has become the standard of care in dealing with certain types of acute postoperative pain such as with post-thoracotomy and major laparotomy. This form of pain management is exceedingly effective in patients with multiple rib fractures and other acute pain syndromes in enhancing cough and secretion clearance and early mobilization. The early involvement of anesthesia providers in managing acute pain has the potential to greatly enhance patient satisfaction and outcome in certain pain syndromes.

REFERENCES

1. Katz J. Atlas of regional anesthesia. Norwalk, CT: Appleton-Century-Crofts; 1985:168–169.
2. Bridenbaugh PO, Greene NM, Brull SJ. Spinal (subarachnoid) neural blockade. In: Cousins MJ, Bridenbaugh PO. *Neural Blockade*. Philadelphia, PA: Lippincott-Raven; 1998:203–241.
3. Scott DB. *Techniques of Regional Anesthesia*. Norwalk, CT: Appleton & Lange/Mediglobe; 1989:161–199.
4. Bulger EM, Edwards T, Klotz P, et al. Epidural analgesia improves outcome after multiple rib fractures. *Surgery*. 2004; 136:426–430.
5. Karmakar MK, Ho AM. Acute pain management of patients with multiple fractured ribs. *J Trauma*. 2003;54:615–625.
6. Bulger EM, Arneson MA, Mock CN, et al. Rib fractures in the elderly. *J Trauma*. 2000;48:1040–1046.
7. Wu CL, Jani ND, Perkins FM, et al. Thoracic epidural analgesia versus intravenous patient-controlled analgesia for the treatment of rib fracture pain after motor vehicle crash. *J Trauma*. 1999;47:564–567.
8. Wisner DH. A stepwise logistic regression analysis of factors affecting morbidity and mortality after thoracic trauma: effect of epidural analgesia. *J Trauma*. 1990;30:799–804.
9. Ullman DA, Fortune JB, Greenhouse BB, et al. The treatment of patients with multiple rib fractures using continuous thoracic epidural narcotic infusion. *Reg Anesth*. 1989;14:43–47.
10. Moen V, Dahlgren N, Irestedt L. Severe neurological complications after central neuraxial blockades in Sweden 1990–1999. *Anesthesiology*. 2004;101:950–959.
11. Dhillon AR, Russell IF. Epidural abscess in association with obstetric epidural analgesia. *Int J Obstet Anesth*. 1997;6:118–121.
12. Hooten WM, Kinney MO, Huntoon MA. Epidural abscess and meningitis after epidural corticosteroid injection. *Mayo Clin Proc*. 2004;79:682–686.
13. Steffen P, Seeling W, Essig A, et al. Bacterial contamination of epidural catheters: microbiological examination of 502 epidural catheters used for postoperative analgesia. *J Clin Anesth*. 2004;16:92–97.
14. Schroeder TH, Krueger WA, Neeser E, et al. Spinal epidural abscess—a rare complication after epidural analgesia for labour and delivery. *Br J Anaesth*. 2004;92:896–898.
15. Ay B, Gercek A, Konya D, et al. Spinal abscess after epidural anesthesia: need for more vigilance and better patient advice. *J Neurosurg Anesthesiol*. 2004;16:184–185.
16. Veiga Sanchez AR. Vertebral osteomyelitis and epidural abscess after epidural anesthesia for a cesarean section. *Rev Esp Anesiol Reanim*. 2004;51:44–46.
17. Gosavi C, Bland D, Poddar R, et al. Epidural abscess complicating insertion of epidural catheters. *Br J Anaesth*. 2004;92:294.
18. Huang RC, Shapiro GS, Lim M, et al. Cervical epidural abscess after epidural steroid injection. *Spine*. 2004;29:E7–E9.
19. Hearn M. Epidural abscess complicating insertion of epidural catheters. *Br J Anaesth*. 2003;90:706–707.
20. Hernandez JM, Coyle FP, Wright CD, et al. Epidural abscess after epidural anesthesia and continuous epidural analgesia in a patient with gastric lymphoma. *J Clin Anesth*. 2003; 15:48–51.
21. Phillips JM, Stedeford JC, Hartsilver E, et al. Epidural abscess complicating insertion of epidural catheters. *Br J Anaesth*. 2002;89:778–782.
22. Tay SM, Lee R. Case report: catheter-related epidural abscess. *Ann Acad Med Singapore*. 2001;30:62–65.
23. Simpson J, Foinette KM, Lobo DN, et al. Spinal epidural abscess: adding insult to injury? *Injury*. 1999;30:504–508.
24. Nordstrom O, Sandin R. Delayed presentation of an extradural abscess in a patient with alcohol abuse. *Br J Anaesth*. 1993; 70:368–369.
25. Hemmerling TM, Olivier JF, Basile F, et al. Epidural hematoma after anticoagulation with a thoracic epidural

catheter in place: a mere coincidence? *Anesth Analg.* 2004; 99:1267–1268.

26. Horlocker TT. What's a nice patient like you doing with a complication like this? Diagnosis, prognosis and prevention of spinal hematoma. *Can J Anaesth.* 2004;51:527–534.

27. Guay J. Estimating the incidence of epidural hematoma—is there enough information? *Can J Anaesth.* 2004;51:514–515.

28. Horlocker TT, Wedel DJ, Benzon H, et al. American Society of Regional Anesthesia and Pain Medicine. Regional anesthesia in the anticoagulated patient: defining the risks. *Reg Anesth Pain Med.* 2004;29(suppl 2):1–12.

29. Abramovitz S, Beilin Y. Thrombocytopenia, low molecular weight heparin, and obstetric anesthesia. *Anesthesiol Clin North Am.* 2003;21:99–109.

30. Horlocker TT. Thromboprophylaxis and neuraxial anesthesia. *Orthopedics.* 2003;26(Suppl 2):s243–s249.

31. Persson J, Flisberg P, Lundberg J. Thoracic epidural anesthesia and epidural hematoma. *Acta Anaesthesiol Scand.* 2002;46: 1171–1174.

32. Rennotte MT, Baele P, Aubert G, et al. Epidural opioids and respiratory arrests. *Anesth Analg.* 1999;88:962.

33. Ostermeier AM, Roizen MF, Hautkappe M, et al. Three sudden postoperative respiratory arrests associated with epidural opioids in patients with sleep apnea. *Anesth Analg.* 1997;85:452–460.

34. Drummond GB. Effects of extradural sufentanil and morphine on ventilation. *Br J Anaesth.* 1995;74:492–493.

25

Regional Anesthesia: Nerve Blocks

Michael F. Murphy

HIGH YIELD FACTS

- Ordinarily, bupivacaine or lidocaine will be used. Mixing the two together in the same syringe (e.g., lidocaine 2% and bupivacaine 0.5%) will yield a block that has a rapid onset and a long duration.
- Skin wheals utilizing 25- or 27-gauge needles at skin puncture points will eliminate block needle entry pain and facilitate tactile appreciation of tissue resistance and the penetration through fascia and other tissue planes.
- The topical application of local anesthetic agent to mucous membranes at needle entry points will do likewise.
- When performing a nerve block, use lots of local anesthetic agent and use your knowledge of the anatomy to inject it near the nerve, not into it.
- Refer to an atlas of regional anesthesia to refresh your memory of the anatomy before performing it, especially if you do this particular block rarely.
- Establish venous access if the dose of local anesthetic may approach dosage maximums and remember to calculate the dose maximum on ideal not actual body weight.
- Generally, the needle used to do a block ought to be a 22-gauge needle. Where the distance to be traversed subcutaneously is substantial (e.g., supraorbital block), consider using a $3^1/_2$ in. spinal needle to reduce the number of cutaneous punctures.

DEFINITIONS

The placement of local anesthetic agents near sensory receptors and nerves is intended to disrupt neural transmission, specifically the transmission of painful stimuli.

This may be performed to either enable the painless performance of a procedure or to manage pain.

In clinical practice, this may take several forms:

1. Topical anesthesia
2. Local infiltration
3. Field block anesthesia
4. Nerve block
5. Intravenous (IV) regional anesthesia (*Bier block*)
6. Neuraxial anesthesia (epidural and spinal anesthesia)

Topical Anesthesia

Since intact skin serves as an effective barrier to the penetration of drugs, if one wished to gain access to the sensory nerve endings in the skin one would normally be required to infiltrate the medication subcutaneously. Even so, some success has been achieved with transdermal preparations such as EMLA, especially for simple procedures such as starting an IV or drawing blood in children. Similar results have been found with iontophoretic delivery systems. These are discussed in greater detail in Chapter 26. Local anesthetic agents are moderately effective when applied to open wounds and abraded dermis contributing to the popularity of such combination preparations as tetracaine adrenaline cocaine (TAC), lidocaine epinephrine tetracaine (LET), as well as single agents such as lidocaine (2–4% solutions). Mucous membranes are, for the most part, freely permeable to local anesthetic agents such that topical anesthesia of the cornea, gingiva, pharynx, larynx, trachea and conducting airways, esophagus, rectum, bladder, and so forth is readily achieved (see Chap. 47).

Local Infiltration

This is the usual method employed to render a wound insensitive for the purpose of repair. Injection of local anesthetic agent around a wound through intact skin is called a *field block* and is usually more painful than local infiltration through the wound.

Field Block

A field block is the infiltration of a wall of local anesthetic agent to surround an operative site (Fig. 25-1). For the most part, sensory nerves travel in the subcutaneous tissues to elaborate sensory nerve endings in the dermis. Injection into the subcutaneous tissue meets with less resistance and is less painful than injection into the dermis. Field blocks are useful for large cutaneous wounds (e.g., scalp) when minimal tissue distortion is desired (e.g., vermillion border

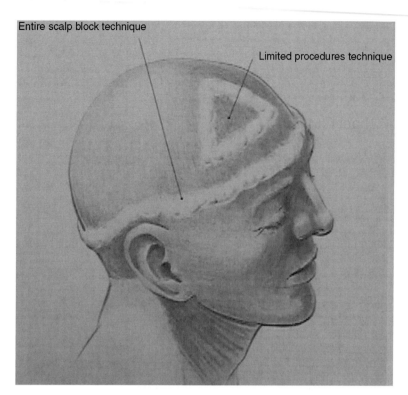

Entire scalp block technique

Limited procedures technique

Fig. 25-1. Field block. A wall of local anesthetic agent is raised in the subcutaneous tissue to surround a territory to be blocked. (Reproduced from Katz J. *Atlas of Regional Anesthesia*. Norwalk, CT: Appleton & Lange; 1985:3.)

or facial wounds), or for the incision and drainage of cutaneous and subcutaneous abscesses.

Nerve Block

Regional anesthesia achieved by the injection of local anesthetic agent near a nerve, nerves, or plexi supplying a particular area is called a nerve block. The region may be relatively circumscribed such as in an ankle or wrist block, or an entire limb as in a brachial plexus block (*major regional anesthesia*).

Intravenous Regional Anesthesia

Also dubbed Bier block after Augustus Bier, the man who first described the block, this block involves the direct injection of local anesthetic agent intravenously into a previously exsanguinated and tourniqueted arm or foot. This block provides excellent anesthesia for fracture reductions and minor procedures (e.g., laceration repair or foreign body removal). The duration of the block is usually limited by tourniquet pain to 45 minutes or so.

Neuraxial Anesthesia

Epidural or spinal anesthesia is referred to as major neuraxial anesthesia. These techniques are employed to facilitate an array of surgical procedures and in the management of a variety of painful conditions, and are discussed in more detail in Chapter 24.

AGENT SELECTION

The array of local anesthetic agents available for use would suggest that selecting an appropriate agent might be a difficult decision. Fortunately, such is not the case. No matter if one's goal is to manage procedural pain or an acute pain syndrome, depending on the duration of anesthesia desired, one need only be familiar with three preparations:

Plain Lidocaine (1 or 2%)

The average duration of anesthesia ranges from 60 to 120 minutes. These preparations are typically administered by infiltration, field, or nerve block and are adequate for most minor wound repairs. The usual preparations are 1%

(1 g/100 mL or 10 mg/mL) and 2% (20 mg/mL). Either provides an acceptable sensory block, though motor block (infrequently desirable in the setting of procedures and pain management) is more reliable with the higher concentration. The dosage maximum of 4 mg/kg often guides which strength is selected. Local infiltration with higher concentrations of lidocaine produces longer wound healing times than do lower concentrations, due to delayed fibroblastic activity. Since anesthesia is relatively unchanged with varying concentrations, use of the lowest concentration possible is therefore recommended for wound repair.

Multidose ampules contain methylparaben as a preservative which has been implicated in anaphylaxis. This also renders the preparation inappropriate for IV use. The multidose type of ampule can be recognized by the rubber stopper held in place by a nonremovable metal collar that requires perforation by hypodermic needle to access the medication. Multi-dose ampules have been identified as factors in disease transmission (e.g., hepatitis C) and for this reason unit dose vials are commonly recommended.[1]

Lidocaine (1, 1.5, 2%) with Epinephrine (1:100,000 or 1:200,000)

This preparation increases the duration of anesthesia by 1.2–2 times, and increases the dosage to a maximum of 7 mg/kg. Epinephrine-induced reduction in blood supply slows washout of the agent (increased duration) and attenuates the pace of rise (increased dose maximum) of the agent in the blood. Although for a long time this combination was felt to be inappropriate for use when vascular supply was questionable, or in end organs such as ear pinnae, digits, penis, and so forth, routine use of lidocaine with epinephrine by hand surgeons and podiatrists has shown this to be of minimal concern for anesthesia of a digit. The amount of epinephrine in commercial preparations is 1:100,000 (10 mcg/mL) or 1:200,000 (5 mcg/mL). Either preparation increases the dosage maximum and prolongs the duration of the block, though the 1:200,000 preparation may lead to a less intense systemic vasoconstrictor response (e.g., tachycardia, sense of anxiety, and angina). Again, methylparaben is used in the multidose ampules. Unit dose vials are available.

Bupivacaine (0.25, 0.5%)

The duration of action of this drug ranges from 120 to 240 minutes when infiltrated and 240–1440 minutes for peripheral nerve blocks.[2] It is thus an ideal drug for long procedures when lidocaine with epinephrine is contraindicated, and for acute pain management (e.g., rib or femoral nerve blocks). The duration of action of a local anesthetic agent is governed by the affinity of the drug

for protein. Bupivacaine has a high affinity for protein and thus has a long duration of action. The addition of epinephrine to bupivacaine solutions does little to affect the duration of block, unlike lidocaine, as the duration of block is unrelated to tissue blood flow. The 0.5% preparation contains 5 mg/mL bupivacaine and so is unlikely to challenge dosage maximum recommendations (3 mg/kg) in most patients.[2] When using this medication one must recall that the onset time may approach 20 minutes, particularly when used to perform nerve blocks. This shortcoming can be mitigated by mixing bupivacaine and lidocaine in the same syringe to achieve rapid onset and long duration (e.g., 5 mL of bupivacaine 0.5% plus 5 mL of lidocaine 2% in a 10 mL syringe gives 10 mL of bupivacaine 0.25% and lidocaine 1%).

PREPARATION AND TECHNIQUE

With the exception of IV regional anesthesia, none of the other techniques require special equipment. The following general comments regarding preparation and monitoring apply to all techniques:

- Aseptic handling of syringes, needles, and other equipment to be used is recommended, as is aseptic skin preparation. Unless sterile drapes obscure essential landmarks used in the performance of the block, they are also recommended.

- Skin wheals utilizing 25- or 27-gauge needles at skin puncture points will eliminate block needle entry pain and facilitate tactile appreciation of tissue resistance and the penetration through fascia and other tissue planes. The topical application of local anesthetic agent to mucous membranes at needle entry points will do likewise.

- Standard hypodermic needles have 60° sharpened bevels (cutting point). Regional anesthesia needles have 45° noncutting points designed to give tactile fidelity as tissue planes are penetrated. The author recommends that 22-gauge needles (either cutting or nerve block) be used to perform blocks where appreciation of transiting tissue planes is desirable (e.g., median, femoral, and other deep nerve blocks). There are two other important reasons for this recommendation:
  - *Aspiration for blood:* The intravascular injection of agent is undesirable as it leads to block failure and perhaps systemic toxicity. A larger gauge needle will often yield blood on aspiration where a smaller gauge (e.g., 25-gauge) may fail to do so.
  - *Intraneural injection:* Injection of the local anesthetic agent directly into nervous tissue (e.g., peripheral nerve) is undesirable as it may lead to pressure necrosis of the nerve. This event is

heralded by pain on injection and resistance to injection. With smaller needles (e.g., 25-gauge) *needle resistance* is difficult to discriminate from *tissue resistance*; needle resistance is mitigated by using a larger gauge of needle.

- *Elicitation of paresthesias:* The intent in performing a nerve block is to place the local anesthetic agent in close proximity to the nerve, not in it. Some authors have recommended the elicitation of paresthesias by intentionally "needling" the nerve as an indication that the tip of the needle is near where it needs to be. This author recognizes that this may occur inadvertently from time to time, but that to do so intentionally raises the specter of nerve fascicle damage that may be undesirable, particularly in very important sensory and motor nerves such as the median and ulnar nerves. Furthermore, the sudden elicitation of a paresthesia may provoke a sudden reflex withdrawal by the patient that may lead to injury or needle breakage. A thorough understanding of the anatomy ought to make this potentially hazardous practice unnecessary.

- *Intravenous line establishment:* An IV ought to be established prior to a procedure when:
  - Agent dosage maximums may be approached and toxicity is a consideration (e.g., femoral and multiple intercostal nerve blocks).
  - Adjuvant sedative or analgesic medications are to be given.
  - For all cases of IV regional anesthesia.

- Monitoring and resuscitation equipment must be available in any venue where local anesthetic agents are in use, particularly when intravascular injection is a possibility and when dosage maximums may be approached. Routine monitoring beyond these two situations is not recommended.

- *Ancillary medications:* Local anesthetic-induced seizures are usually self-limiting and require little in specific therapy beyond general supportive care such as airway maintenance, administration of oxygen, and positioning to prevent aspiration (i.e., left lateral decubitus, slightly head down [*tonsil* position]); however, should antiseizure medications be considered, dosing is as for other types of seizures. Should potent anesthetic induction drugs be considered, the initial doses are 10% of the induction dose of the drug, and titrated to effect.

- *Use of landmarks:* Bony landmarks are used extensively to aid in the location of nervous structures for blockade. Several of the blocks to be described are performed where arteries and nerves run together. This serves as a "caution caveat" with

respect to arterial damage as well as to the advisability of using epinephrine-containing solutions.

COMPLICATIONS

Some complications are specific to a particular block and will be discussed in the context of that block. Several complications are common to all techniques, including the following:

Needle breakage

This is an exceedingly uncommon event, being more common if small (25–30-gauge) and long (1.5 in.) needles are used or if needles are bent to perform blocks (e.g., posterior superior alveolar [PSA] block). Despite the sterile and inert nature of these needles (as opposed to acupuncture needles or those used by IV drug abusers), most recommend the retrieval of the broken fragment.[3–9]

Needle Damage to Nerves, Vessels, Viscera, and Other Structures (Pleura)

These complications are also exceedingly rare and are often technique associated. Detailed knowledge of the anatomy associated with the technique and attention to detail when performing the block are essential aspects in minimizing these complications.

Neurotoxicity

Local anesthetic agents and additives have been implicated as producing damage to nerve tissue in the past (e.g., chloroprocaine combined with sodium metabisulfite); however, none of the currently used agents have been associated with neurotoxicity.

Vascular complications

- Intra-arterial injection: Oftentimes a peripheral nerve travels in close proximity to an artery (e.g., ulnar and femoral nerves) raising the specter of an inadvertent intra-arterial injection of the local anesthetic agent. This is not ordinarily of significant consequence (aside from the mechanical issue of the arterial puncture), though one must recognize that the injected medication will shortly transit to the venous side of the circulation and produce systemic effects (see Chap. 27).

- Hematoma formation, of particular concern in patients on anticoagulants (Coumadin and heparin) and antiplatelet agents, may be an issue if the block is to be performed in a particularly vascular area (PSA block) or if the presence of an expanding hematoma in a confined space (e.g., median nerve block at the wrist) is undesirable. Otherwise, hematoma formation is not of particular concern.

Infection

Infection related to a peripheral nerve block is exceedingly uncommon. There are isolated reports of infection following dental blocks and others.[10–16] It is recommended that needles not traverse infected tissue when performing blocks, and that the benefit of the block be weighed against the benefit in patients exhibiting systemic signs of sepsis. This is more of an issue for epidural and spinal anesthesia than it is for peripheral neural blockade.

INDIVIDUAL BLOCKS

Unless otherwise stipulated, the block needle ought to be a 22-gauge needle. Where the distance to be traversed subcutaneously is substantial consider using a $3^1/_2$ in. spinal needle to reduce the number of cutaneous punctures. For each of these blocks assume that the area of the block is aseptically prepared and draped and that needle insertion points are preceded by the intradermal injection of 0.1–0.2 mL of local anesthetic agent to render insertion of the 22-gauge needle painless, or topical application where puncture points are through mucous membranes (e.g., dental blocks through the mouth). Generally speaking,

larger injected volumes result in higher success rates, though one needs to observe dosage maximums and be cautious to avoid creating such high intratissue pressures that venous or arterial blood flow becomes hindered (especially in end organs such as ears, flap lacerations, and digits). The author typically uses fully loaded 10-mL syringes when performing blocks, unless otherwise noted.

Head and Neck Blocks

Ear Block

Indications: This block is particularly useful for complex lacerations of the pinna of the ear where the infiltration of local anesthetic agent may distort tissues and hinder the anatomic reapproximation of tissues.

Anatomy and landmarks: This block is a field block. Sensation to the pinna of the ear is supplied by branches of the trigeminal (auriculotemporal branch of the mandibular n.) and by branches of the cervical plexus (great auricular n.). All of these nerves course onto the ear via the subcutaneous tissue (Fig. 25-2). The superior portion of the auditory canal is supplied by a branch of the auriculotemporal nerve, and the inferior portion by a branch of the vagus nerve (Alderman's nerve).

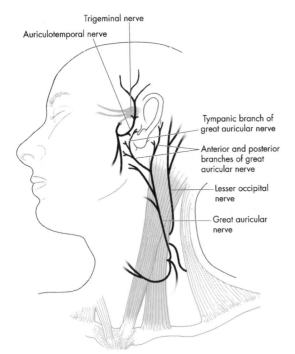

Trigeminal nerve

Auriculotemporal nerve

Tympanic branch of great auricular nerve

Anterior and posterior branches of great auricular nerve

Lesser occipital nerve

Great auricular nerve

Fig. 25-2. Sensory nerve supply of the ear. (Redrawn from: Katz J. *Atlas of Regional Anesthesia.* Norwalk, CT: Appleton & Lange, 1985: p. 37.)

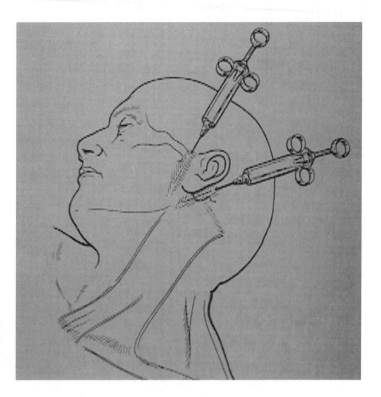

Fig. 25-3. Field block of the ear. (Reproduced with permission from Murphy TM. Somatic blockade of the head and neck. In: Cousins ML, ed. *Neural Blockade*. Philadelphia, PA: Lippincott-Raven; 1998:510.)

Technique: Block of the pinna is performed by raising a wall of local anesthetic agent around the ear (Fig. 25-3). Pass the block needle subcutaneously anteriorly and posteriorly, both from above (*upside-down V*) and below (*right-side up V*) injecting 5–7 mL in each limb of the block as the needle is withdrawn (Fig. 25-4). The auditory canal is blocked by infiltrating local anesthetic agent at the opening of the canal.

Complications: Compromised arterial flow or reduced venous drainage when large volumes are employed.

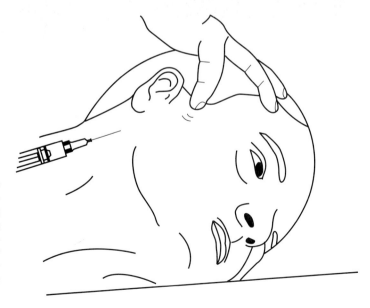

Fig. 25-4. Field block of the ear. Note how the index finger locates the temporal artery anterior to the ear to assist in avoiding arterial puncture and injection of agent. (Redrawn from Murphy MF. Regional anesthesia in the emergency department. In: Campbell W, ed. Airway Management and Anesthesia in the Emergency Department. *Emerg Med Clin North Am.* 1988;6: 783–810, with permission from Elsevier.)

Facial Blocks

Supraorbital Block

Indications: Extensive road rash of the forehead and large scalp lacerations in the brow to vertex territory.

Anatomy and landmarks: The supraorbital and supratrochlear nerves are terminal branches of the ophthalmic nerve (first division of the trigeminal nerve). Both emerge from the brow margin of the orbit to supply the forehead as far back as the vertex (Fig. 25-5).

Technique: This is a field block. A 22-gauge 3.5 in. spinal needle is advanced in subcutaneous tissue from the midline to the far lateral edge of the brow and 10 mL of solution is deposited as the needle is withdrawn slowly (Fig. 25-6). If necessary, the same procedure is repeated on the opposite side to anesthetize the entire forehead.

Complications: Provided the patient is cooperative, there are no particular complications. In an uncooperative patient, sudden movement may risk a globe puncture.

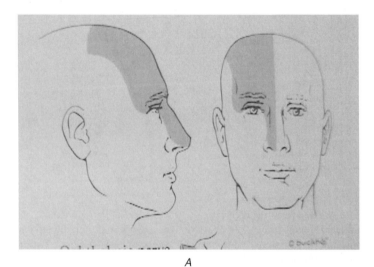

A

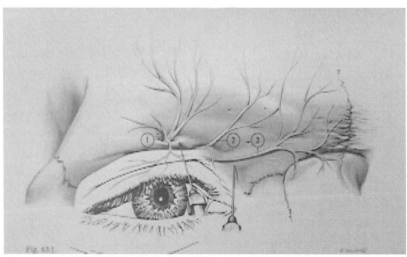

B

Fig. 25-5. Supraorbital nerve block: sensory nerves and area of unilateral block. (Reproduced from Scott DB. *Techniques of Regional Anesthesia.* Norwalk, CT: Appleton & Lange; 1989:63.)

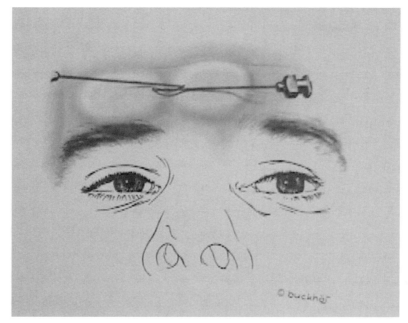

A

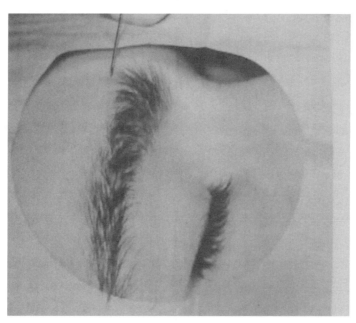

B

Fig. 25-6. Supraorbital nerve block: performance of the block. (Part *A* reproduced from Scott DB. *Techniques of Regional Anesthesia.* Norwalk, CT: Appleton & Lange; 1989:63. Part *B* reproduced from Murphy MF. Regional anesthesia in the emergency department. In: Campbell W, ed. Airway Management and Anesthesia in the Emergency Department. *Emerg Med Clin North Am.* 1988;6:783–810, with permission from Elsevier.)

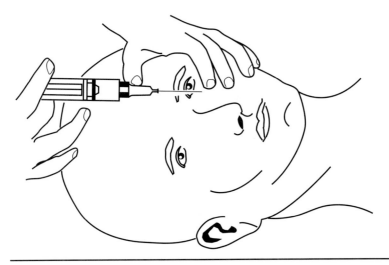

Fig. 25-7. Infraorbital nerve block: extraoral approach. Note that the index finger of the left hand is palpating the infraorbital foramen to assist in needle advancement and tip placement and also that the needle is directed in such a way as to avoid entry into the canal and pressure injury to the nerve on injection. (Redrawn from Murphy MF. Regional anesthesia in the emergency department. In: Campbell W, ed. Airway Management and Anesthesia in the Emergency Department. *Emerg Med Clin North Am* 1988;6:783–810, with permission from Elsevier.)

Infraorbital Nerve Block

Indications: Lacerations of the upper lip and nasal alae where anatomic approximation is desired; dental pain involving the upper incisors, canines, and premolar teeth.

Anatomy and landmarks: The maxillary branch (V2) of the trigeminal nerve provides sensation to the upper teeth: the molars (PSA nerve), the incisors, canines and premolars (middle superior alveolar [MSA] and anterior superior alveolar [ASA] nerves), together with the adjacent mucosa and gums. The ASA also provides sensation to the ipsilateral upper lip, a portion of the nasal ala, and a variable portion of the nasal cavity. The ASA and MSA emerge from the maxilla just below the orbital rim through the infraorbital foramen as a nerve called the infraorbital nerve. The PSA branches from V2 in the pterygopalatine fossa to supply the molars and adjacent gum and mucous membrane. The infraorbital foramen is palpable just nasal of the midline 0.5–1.0 cm below the inferior orbital rim.

Technique: The infraorbital nerve can be blocked by both intraoral and extraoral percutaneous approaches. In the percutaneous approach the patient is placed supine. Standing at the head of the bed, the infraorbital foramen is palpated and the block needle is inserted at a 45° angle to contact bone (Fig. 25-7) and then withdrawn 1–2 mm. About 5–7 mL of local anesthetic agent is deposited. The needle must not be inserted directly into the foramen to avoid pressure injury to the nerve. Alternatively, an oral approach may be used. For this approach the needle is inserted upward through the buccal sulcus just above the canine and directed superiorly to the foramen while palpating for the needle tip (Fig. 25-8).

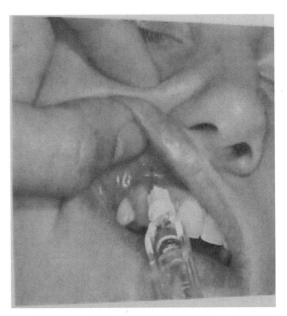

Fig. 25-8. Infraorbital nerve block: intraoral approach. Again the index finger palpates the infraorbital foramen to assist needle guidance. (Reproduced from Scott DB. *Techniques of Regional Anesthesia*. Norwalk, CT: Appleton & Lange; 1989:65.)

Complications: Pressure necrosis of the nerve, intraorbital injection producing optic nerve block, and ocular penetration.

Mental Nerve Block

Indications: Lacerations of the lower lip where anatomic approximation is desired.

Anatomy and landmarks: The mental nerve is the terminal branch of the mandibular nerve branch (V3) emerging from the mental foramen of the mandible directly inferior to the mandibular canine. Importantly, and contrary to what might be expected, the mental foramen travels obliquely in a posterior direction through the anterior cortex of the mandible. The positions of the supraorbital notch, the infraorbital foramen, and the mental foramen can be approximated by recalling that they lie on a straight line that passes vertically through the pupil and the corner of the mouth (Fig. 25-9).

Technique: Like the infraorbital nerve, the mental nerve can be approached percutaneously or intraorally (Fig. 25-10

and 25-11, respectively). The mental foramen is easily palpated in the buccal sulcus below the mandibular canines guiding the location of deposit of local anesthetic solution.

Complications: Recalling the orientation of the mental foramen, it is important to avoid intraforamen injection to avoid pressure injury to the nerve.

Dental Blocks

Posterior Superior Alveolar (PSA) Nerve Block

Indications: Dental pain involving the maxillary molar teeth.

Anatomy and landmarks: This nerve is blocked in the pterygopalatine space.

Technique: Apply topical local anesthetic agent to the maxillary buccal sulcus opposite the second molar. Access to the PSA nerve is achieved by bending a 5/8 in. needle to a 45° angle (Fig. 25-12) and then inserting it to the hilt obliquely upward through the buccal sulcus at the posterior border of the second molar (Fig. 25-13).

Complications: The pterygopalatine space is intensely vascular. Gentle technique and meticulous aspiration is recommended to prevent hematoma formation which is not dangerous but may be quite painful. Needle fracture.

Mandibular Nerve Block

Indications: Dental pain mandibular teeth; lacerations anterior two-thirds of the tongue.

Anatomy and landmarks: The mandibular branch of the trigeminal nerve (V3) divides into several branches below the foramen ovale. The lingual and inferior alveolar branches descend on the medial side of the mandibular ramus (Fig. 25-14). The inferior alveolar branch enters the substance of the mandible through the mandibular foramen just above the last molar to supply sensation to the mandibular molar teeth and emerge from the mental foramen as the mental nerve. The lingual branches course through the lingual sulci on either side to supply sensation to the anterior two-thirds of the tongue.

Technique: This block is performed with the patient seated and the mucosa prepared with topical local anesthetic. To block the patient's right side, the operator inserts a gloved left thumb to the anterior border of the ramus of the mandible (Fig. 25-15). The block needle is advanced along the dorsal surface of the thumb to contact bone on the medial surface of the mandibular ramus (Fig. 25-16). The needle/syringe is rotated in a horizontal plane to the opposite side of the mouth (Fig. 25-17) maintaining contact with bone. Once in position the local anesthetic agent is injected.

Complications: None specific.

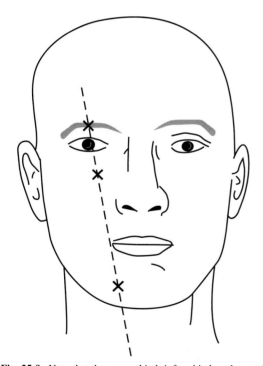

Fig. 25-9. Note that the supraorbital, infraorbital, and mental foramina all lie along a vertical line connecting the midportion of the pupil with the corner of the mouth. (Redrawn from Murphy MF. Regional anesthesia in the emergency department. In: Campbell W, ed. Airway Management and Anesthesia in the Emergency Department. *Emerg Med Clin North Am.* 1988;6: 783–810, with permission from Elsevier.)

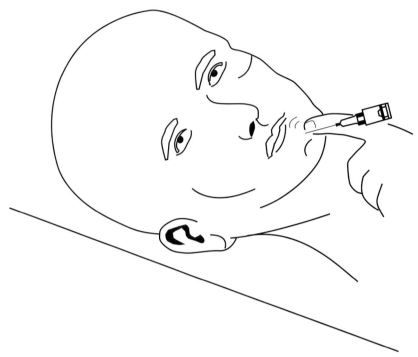

Fig. 25-10. Infraorbital nerve block: extraoral approach. (Redrawn from Murphy MF. Regional anesthesia in the emergency department. In: Campbell W, ed. Airway Management and Anesthesia in the Emergency Department. *Emerg Med Clin North Am.* 1988;6:783–810, with permission from Elsevier.)

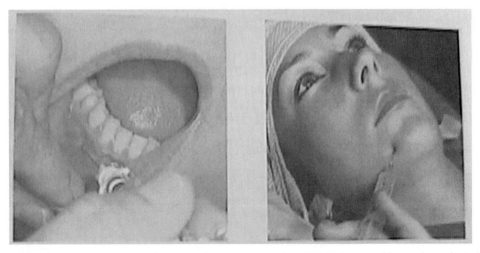

Fig. 25-11. Infraorbital nerve block: intraoral approach. (Reproduced from Scott DB. *Techniques of Regional Anesthesia.* Norwalk, CT: Appleton & Lange; 1989:71.)

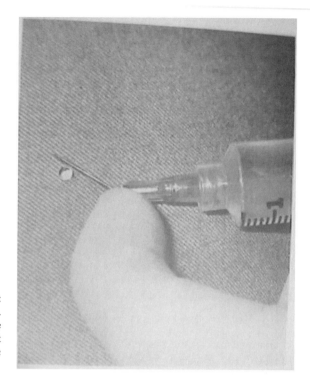

Fig. 25-12. Posterior superior alveolar (PSA) nerve block: bending the needle to achieve the optimal angle of approach. (Reproduced from Murphy MF. Regional anesthesia in the emergency department. In: Campbell W, ed. Airway Management and Anesthesia in the Emergency Department. *Emerg Med Clin North Am.* 1988;6:783–810, with permission from Elsevier.)

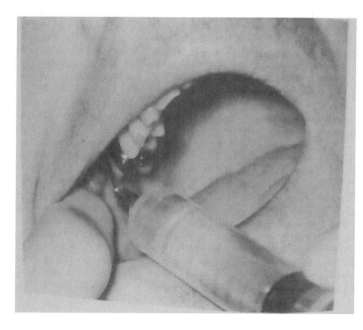

Fig. 25-13. Posterior superior alveolar (PSA) nerve block. Note the entry point in the buccal sulcus opposite the second molar. (Reproduced from Murphy MF. Regional anesthesia in the emergency department. In: Campbell W, ed. Airway Management and Anesthesia in the Emergency Department. *Emerg Med Clin North Am.* 1988;6:783–810, with permission from Elsevier.)

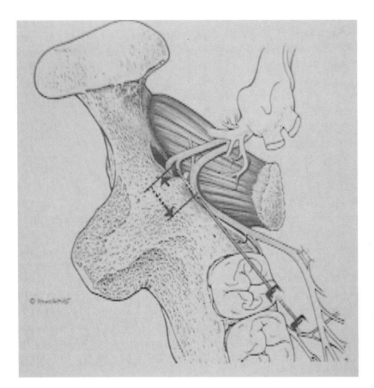

Fig. 25-14. Mandibular nerve block: anatomy of the lingual and mandibular nerves. (Reproduced from Scott DB. *Techniques of Regional Anesthesia.* Norwalk, CT: Appleton & Lange; 1989:69.)

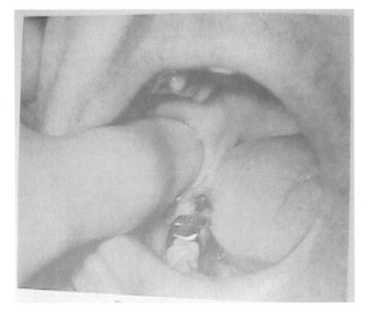

Fig. 25-15. Mandibular nerve block: thumb position on the anterior border of the mandibular ramus. (Reproduced from Murphy MF. Regional anesthesia in the emergency department. In: Campbell W, ed. Airway Management and Anesthesia in the Emergency Department. *Emerg Med Clin North Am.* 1988;6:783–810, with permission from Elsevier.)

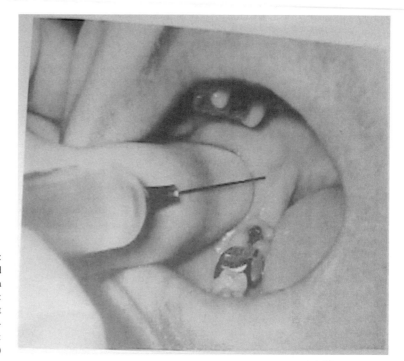

Fig. 25-16. Mandibular nerve block: Initial needle approach. (Reproduced from Murphy MF. Regional anesthesia in the emergency department. In: Campbell W, ed. Airway Management and Anesthesia in the Emergency Department. *Emerg Med Clin North Am.* 1988;6: 783–810, with permission from Elsevier.)

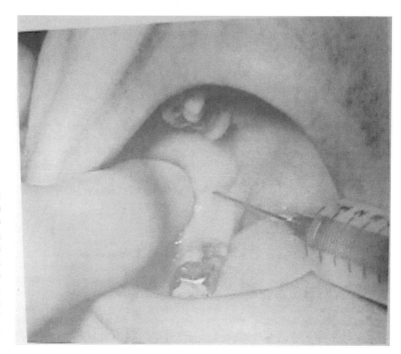

Fig. 25-17. Mandibular nerve block: Note that the syringe and needle are rotated to the opposite side of the mouth to permit needle tip positioning on the anteromedial aspect of the ramus closer to the nerves. (Reproduced from Murphy MF. Regional anesthesia in the emergency department. In: Campbell W, ed. Airway Management and Anesthesia in the Emergency Department. *Emerg Med Clin North Am.* 1988;6:783–810, with permission from Elsevier.)

Nerve Blocks at the Wrist

Ulnar Nerve Block

Indications: Laceration repair; metacarpal fracture reduction, particularly when combined with median and/or radial nerve blocks.

Anatomy and landmarks: The ulnar nerve at the wrist lies between the flexor carpi ulnaris (FCU) tendon and the ulnar artery just deep to the superficial fascia (Fig. 25-18). It enters the palmar aspect of the hand through a fibro-osseous tunnel (Guyon's canal). The dorsal cutaneous branch of the ulnar nerve comes off proximal to the ulnar styloid and passes subcutaneously onto the dorsoulnar aspect of the hand.

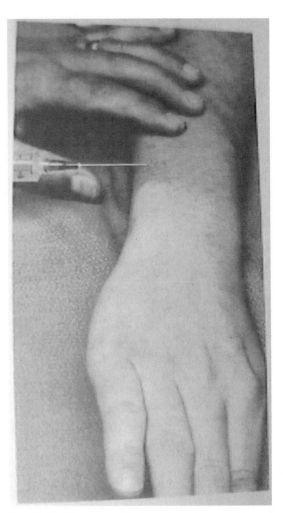

Fig. 25-19. Ulnar nerve block at the wrist: dorsal branch (Reproduced from Murphy MF. Regional anesthesia in the emergency department. In: Campbell W, ed. Airway Management and Anesthesia in the Emergency Department. *Emerg Med Clin North Am.* 1988;6: 783–810, with permission from Elsevier.)

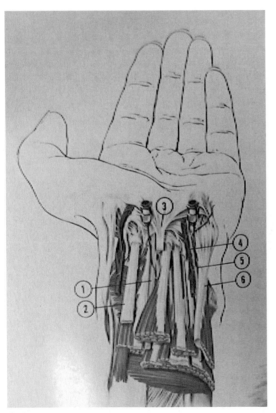

1. Median nerve
2. Flexor carpi radialis tendon
3. Palmaris longus tendon
4. Ulnar artery
5. Ulnar nerve
6. Flexor carpi ulnaris tendon

Fig. 25-18. Median, and ulnar nerves at the wrist. (Reproduced from Scott DB. *Techniques of Regional Anesthesia.* Norwalk, CT: Appleton & Lange; 1989:113.)

Technique: Approach the ulnar nerve from the medial side of the wrist at the level of the proximal wrist crease. Insert the block needle beneath the FCU tendon and inject very slowly to ensure the needle is not in the nerve. Withdraw the needle to skin, but not out and advance it subcutaneously around the dorsum of the wrist just proximal to the ulnar styloid (Fig. 25-19). Inject as the needle is withdrawn to block the dorsal cutaneous branch.

Complications: The ulnar nerve is an exceedingly important sensory and motor nerve. Eliciting paresthesias by "needling" the nerve is not recommended. Injection into Guyon's canal may produce pressure injury to the nerve.

Median Nerve Block

Indications: Laceration repair; metacarpal fracture reduction, particularly when combined with ulnar and/or radial nerve blocks.

Anatomy and landmarks: The median nerve is located just below and slightly radial to the palmaris longus (PL) tendon (Fig. 25-18). With the wrist slightly dorsiflexed, the nerve can be easily balloted. It gives off a small palmar branch immediately before entering the carpal tunnel at the level of the proximal wrist crease.

Technique: Have patients touch the tips of their fingers together and flex the wrist slightly to raise the PL tendon. Insert the block needle perpendicular to skin at the level of the proximal wrist crease (Fig. 25-20). Take note as the needle pops through the skin stopping abruptly when it pops through the deep fascia. Inject very slowly to ensure the needle is not in the nerve. Deposit 2–3 mL in the subcutaneous tissue to get the palmar branch.

Complications: The median nerve is an exceedingly important sensory and motor nerve. Eliciting paresthesias by "needling" the nerve is not recommended. Injection into the carpal tunnel may produce pressure injury to the nerve.

Radial Nerve Block

Indications: Laceration repair; metacarpal fracture reduction, particularly when combined with ulnar and/or median nerve blocks.

Anatomy and landmarks: The radial nerve is not a single nerve, but a series of nervelets at the level of the wrist. These nervelets sweep into the dorsum of the hand in the subcutaneous tissue around the radial styloid.

Technique: This block is a field block. Insert the block needle subcutaneously just proximal to the radial styloid and deposit local anesthetic agent into the subcutaneous tissue (Fig. 25-21).

Complications: None unique to the block.

Hand Blocks

Digital Nerve Block

Indications: Laceration repair, fracture reduction, and foreign body removal.

Anatomy and landmarks: The digital nerves are terminal branches of the ulnar and median nerves, and travel with the digital arteries into the digits along their volar surfaces (Fig. 25-22).

Technique: The hand is turned upright. The block needle is inserted at the volar base of each side of the digit and local anesthetic agent injected.

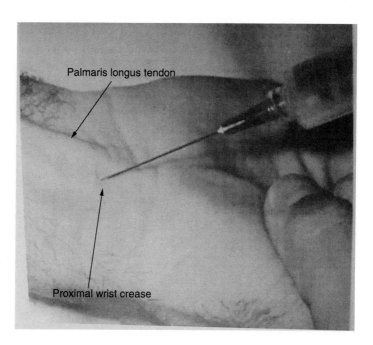

Palmaris longus tendon

Proximal wrist crease

Fig. 25-20. Median nerve block at the wrist. (Reproduced from Murphy MF. Regional anesthesia in the emergency department. In: Campbell W, ed. Airway Management and Anesthesia in the Emergency Department. *Emerg Med Clin North Am.* 1988;6:783–810, with permission from Elsevier.)

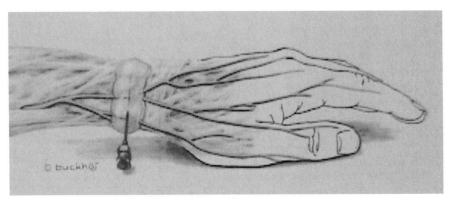

Fig. 25-21. Radial nerve anatomy at the wrist. (Reproduced from Scott DB. *Techniques of Regional Anesthesia*. Norwalk, CT: Appleton & Lange; 1989:113.)

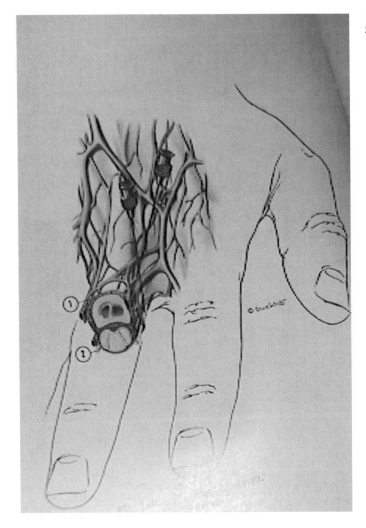

1. Dorsal branch digital nerve
2. Rolar branch digital nerve

Fig. 25-22. Digital nerve anatomy. (Reproduced from Scott DB. *Techniques of Regional Anesthesia*. Norwalk, CT: Appleton & Lange; 1989:114.)

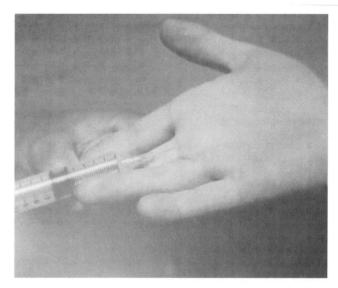

Fig. 25-23. Metacarpal nerve block: Volar approach. (Reproduced from Murphy MF. Regional anesthesia in the emergency department. In: Campbell W, ed. Airway Management and Anesthesia in the Emergency Department. *Emerg Med Clin North Am.* 1988;6: 783–810, with permission from Elsevier.)

Complications: Large amounts of injected solution run the risk of pressure damage to the nerve.

Metacarpal Block

Indications: Laceration repair; fracture reduction; foreign body removal, particularly when the arterial supply to the digit is of concern.

Anatomy and landmarks: The arterial supply to each digit consists of ulnar and radial digital arteries at the level of the base of the digit. These digital arteries are formed just proximal to the metacarpal heads by anastomosing contributions from both the superficial (radial artery) and deep (ulnar artery) palmar arterial arches. Thus, at this

level there are four arterial contributors to each digit; at the base of the digit there are two: ulnar and radial. A block performed just proximal to the metacarpal heads is less likely to interrupt four contributors than a digital block at the base of the digit. The digital nerves are just deep to the palmar fascia and travel in straight lines from the entry point of the ulnar or median nerves into the palm making it possible to estimate their approximate location.

Technique: Several techniques have been described. With the palm up, hyperextend the digit to be blocked and insert a 25-gauge 5/8 in. needle to the hilt in the direction of the digital nerve (Fig. 25-23). The dorsal contributors are blocked by subcutaneous infiltration (Fig. 25-24). Alternatively, dorsal subcutaneous infiltration

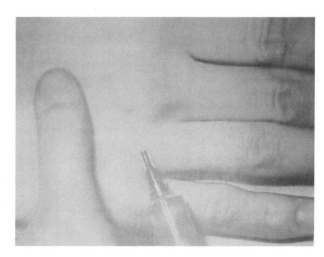

Fig. 25-24. Digital block: Dorsal branches. (Reproduced from Murphy MF. Regional anesthesia in the emergency department. In: Campbell W, ed. Airway Management and Anesthesia in the Emergency Department. Emerg Med Clin North Am. 1988;6:783–810, with permission from Elsevier.)

can be followed by the vertical insertion of a block needle through the infiltrated area while palpating for the tip volarly just proximal to the metacarpal head.

Complications: None unique to the block.

Trunk Blocks

Intercostal Nerve Block (Rib Block)

Indications: Multiple rib fractures.

Anatomy and landmarks: The intercostal neurovascular bundles run in grooves on the inferior, inner aspect of each rib, oriented vein-artery-nerve superiorly to inferiorly (Fig. 25-25). The ribs are most easily palpated at the *rib angle* located posterolaterally, just lateral to the paraspinal muscle mass. With the patient seated and the ipsilateral arm raised over the head the highest rib angle that can be palpated is that of the fifth rib (Fig. 25-26).

Technique: In the above position, the ribs to be blocked are identified and marked at the angle with an intradermal wheal. While palpating the inferior border of each rib the block needle is advanced at right angles to the rib to contact the inferior border of the rib (Fig. 25-27). It is then "walked off" the inferior border of the rib to access the intercostal nerve (Fig. 25-28). Often a "pop" is appreciated as the neurovascular space is entered. Aspiration for air or blood is performed.

Complications: Pneumothorax is the most feared complication and is fairly common. An expiratory chest x-ray 1 hour postblock is mandatory.

Penile Block

Indications: Reduction of a paraphimosis, postcircumcision pain, lacerations, or other acutely painful penile lesions.

Anatomy and landmarks: The dorsal nerve of the penis, a branch of the pudendal nerve, lies just deep to Buck's fascia, and is the major sensory supply to the penis (Fig. 25-29).

Technique: This nerve is easily blocked by fanning an injection just deep to Buck's fascia (Fig. 25-30).

Complications: None unique to the block.

Femoral Nerve Block

Indications: Femoral shaft fracture pain. This block is of less value in managing the pain of hip fractures and femur fractures in the region of the knee.

Anatomy and landmarks: The femoral nerve emerges below the midportion of the inguinal ligament, just lateral to the femoral artery and deep to fascia (Fig. 25-31).

Technique: Palpate the femoral arterial pulse with one finger and insert the block needle just lateral to the pulsation. Pop through the fascia, aspirate, and inject 20 mL of solution.

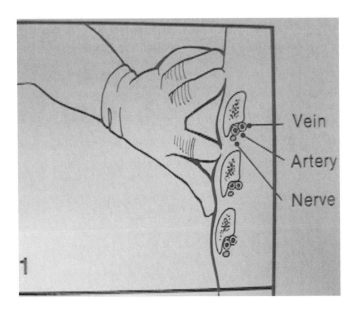

Fig. 25-25. Intercostal nerve block: Note the location of the neurovascular bundle at the inferior rib margin. (Reproduced from Katz J. *Atlas of Regional Anesthesia.* Norwalk, CT: Appleton & Lange; 1985:101.)

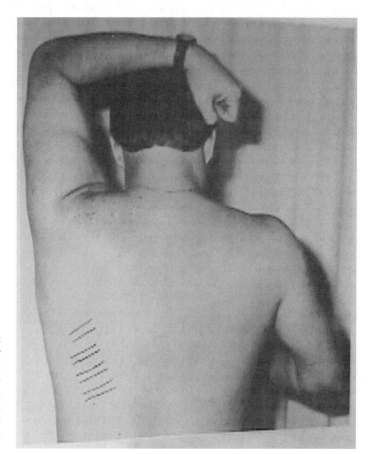

Fig. 25-26. Intercostal nerve block: Patient positioning to gain access to the greatest number of rib angles by rotating the scapula laterally. (Reproduced from Murphy MF. Regional anesthesia in the emergency department. In: Campbell W, ed. Airway Management and Anesthesia in the Emergency Department. *Emerg Med Clin North Am.* 1988;6:783–810, with permission from Elsevier.)

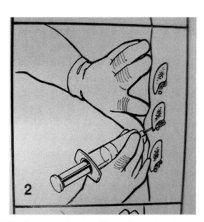

Fig. 25-27. Intercostal nerve block: Locating the inferior rib border. (Reproduced from Katz J. *Atlas of Regional Anesthesia.* Norwalk, CT: Appleton & Lange; 1985:101.)

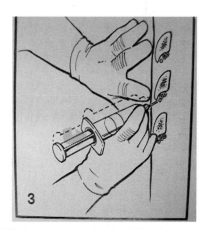

Fig. 25-28. Intercostal nerve block: "Walking" the needle off the inferior border of the rib. (Reproduced from Katz J. *Atlas of Regional Anesthesia.* Norwalk, CT: Appleton & Lange; 1985:101.)

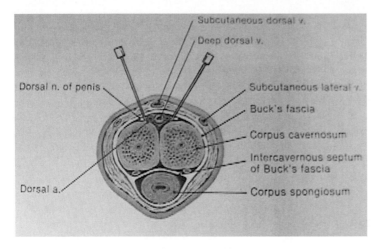

Fig. 25-29. Penile nerves. (Reproduced from Katz J. *Atlas of Regional Anesthesia.* Norwalk, CT: Appleton & Lange; 1985:139.)

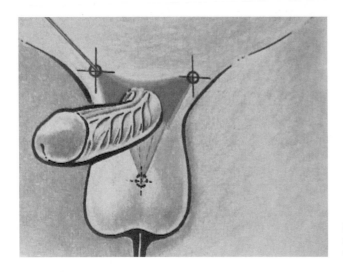

Fig. 25-30. Field block of the penis. (Reproduced from Katz J. *Atlas of Regional Anesthesia.* Norwalk, CT: Appleton & Lange; 1985:139.)

1. Lateral femoral certaneous nerve
2. Femoral nerve

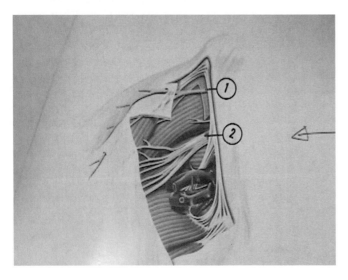

Fig. 25-31. Femoral nerve anatomy at the inguinal ligament. Note the arrangement: vein, artery, and then nerve, medial to lateral. (Reproduced from Scott DB. *Techniques of Regional Anesthesia.* Norwalk, CT: Appleton & Lange; 1989:127.)

Complications: The proximal spread of agent may reach the nerve root level and block contributors to the sciatic nerve as well as the femoral nerve. Ensure that as much as possible a neurologic examination is performed and recorded prior to the block to ensure that these important nerves are intact postfracture. Remember to inform subsequent caregivers that the block has been performed.

Ankle Blocks

Anterior Ankle Block

Indications: Laceration repair; metatarsal fracture reduction, particularly when combined with a posterior ankle block.

Anatomy and landmarks: Three nerves supply the dorsum of the foot: the superficial and deep peroneal nerves (branches of the sciatic nerve) and the saphenous nerve (a branch of the femoral nerve) (Fig. 25-32A–B). The superficial peroneal nerves fan subcutaneously onto the dorsum of the foot between the midline and the lateral malleolus at the level of the lateral malleolus. The deep peroneal nerve runs deep to fascia between the tibialis anterior (TA) and extensor hallucis longus (EHL) tendons. More distally, it runs subcutaneously beside the dorsalis pedis pulse in the first webspace. The saphenous nerve runs in close proximity to the long saphenous vein anterior to the medial malleolus.

Technique: With the patient lying supine, subcutaneous infiltration anteriorly to the top of each malleolus from the midline will anesthetize the saphenous and superficial peroneal nerves (Fig. 25-33). The deep peroneal nerve can

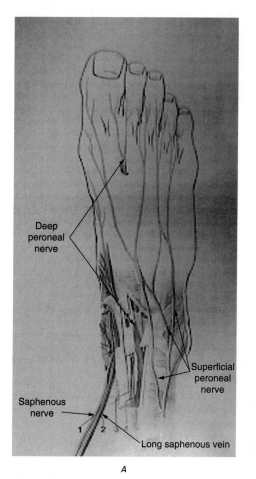

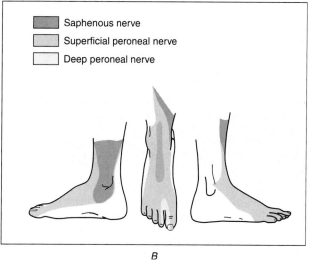

A   *B*

Fig. 25-32. Sensory anatomy and supply at the level of the anterior ankle. (Reproduced from Scott DB. *Techniques of Regional Anesthesia.* Norwalk, CT: Appleton & Lange; 1989:135.)

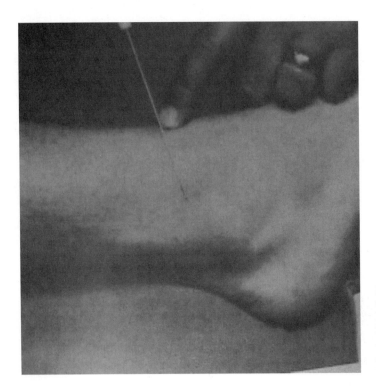

Fig. 25-33. Anterior ankle block: Approach to the block. (Reproduced from Murphy MF. Regional anesthesia in the emergency department. In: Campbell W, ed. Airway Management and Anesthesia in the Emergency Department. *Emerg Med Clin North Am.* 1988;6:783–810, with permission from Elsevier.)

be blocked between the TA and EHL tendons, though it is easier to do so by injecting around the dorsalis pedis pulse.

Complications: None unique to the block.

Posterior Ankle Block

Indications: Laceration repair; metatarsal fracture reduction, particularly when combined with an anterior ankle block; and foreign body removal.

Anatomy and landmarks: The sole of the foot is supplied by two nerves: the sural and posterior tibial (or simply tibial), both terminal branches of the sciatic. The sural nerve is immediately posterior to the lateral malleolus. The tibial nerve runs with the posterior tibial artery deep to fascia posterior to the medial malleolus (Fig. 25-34A–B).

Technique: With the patient lying prone have the foot hang over the end of the stretcher. Dorsiflex the foot slightly. Inject subcutaneously from the midline of the Achilles tendon to the top of the lateral malleolus to block the sural nerve. Palpate the posterior tibial pulse and insert the block needle immediately below your palpating finger until bone is contacted (Fig. 25-35). Withdraw slightly and inject.

Complications: The tibial nerve and posterior tibial artery travel in a fibroosseous tunnel. The injection of very large volumes of solution may compress and injure these structures.

Intravenous Regional Anesthesia (Bier Block)

Indications: Fracture reductions of the forearm, or ankle and foot. Always start an IV in an uninjured limb in the event resuscitation medications are required.

Technique: This block may be performed on the arm (cuff on the upper arm) (Fig. 25-36A) or the lower leg (cuff on the calf) (Fig. 25-36B). In either case, 40 mL of lidocaine 0.5% (200 mg) without preservative or epinephrine is usually used in adults. Thirty milliliters may be employed in smaller adult limbs. Place an IV cannula in the limb to be blocked, tape it in place, and cap it (Fig. 25-36C). Place a tourniquet on the limb. Exsanguination of an acutely injured limb is ordinarily accomplished by elevating the limb for several minutes (Fig. 25-36D), otherwise an Esmarch elastic bandage is used (Fig. 25-36E). Once exsanguination is accomplished, inflate the tourniquet 100 mmHg above systolic pressure.

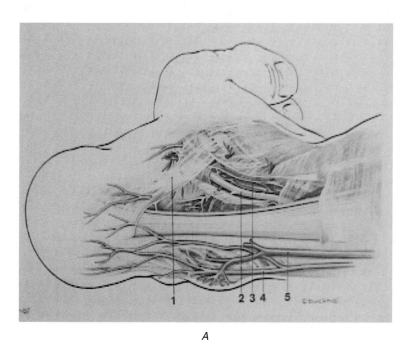

1. Deep fascia
2. Tibial nerve
3. Tibial artery
4. Sural nerve
5. Short saphenous vein

A

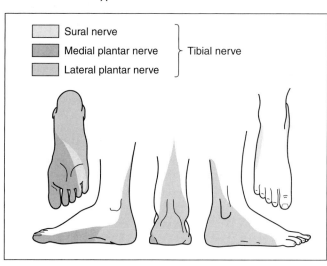

B

Fig. 25-34. Sensory anatomy and supply at the level of the posterior ankle. (Reproduced from Scott DB. *Techniques of Regional Anesthesia.* Norwalk, CT: Appleton & Lange; 1989:135.)

Inject the lidocaine slowly to prevent an excessive rise in pressure overcoming the cuff occlusion pressure (Fig. 25-36*F*).

Complications: Patients will ordinarily complain of a burning dysesthesia on injection of the lidocaine. Moderate-to-severe ischemic pain will ensue after 35–45 minutes of cuff inflation. Do not deflate the cuff less than 30 minutes following injection. Deflate initially for 30 seconds and wait 60 seconds. Note signs of toxicity, ordinarily tinnitus, buzzing in the ears, or drowsiness. Repeat this cycle two more times to prevent excessive blood levels of lidocaine and lidocaine-induced seizures. The block will recede rapidly once the cuff is deflated, so be prepared to manage pain.

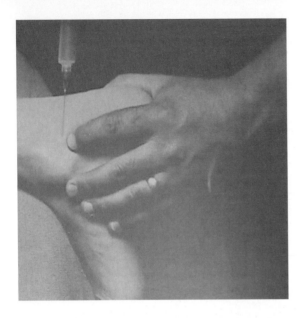

Fig. 25-35. Posterior ankle block: Approach to the block. (Reproduced from Murphy MF. Regional anesthesia in the emergency department. In: Campbell W, ed. Airway Management and Anesthesia in the Emergency Department. *Emerg Med Clin North Am.* 1988;6:783–810, with permission from Elsevier.)

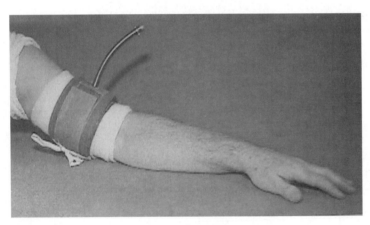

A

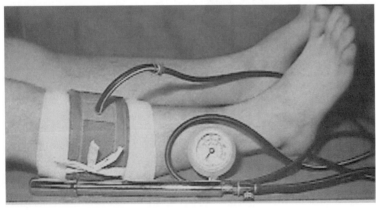

B

Fig. 25-36. Intravenous regional anesthesia (Bier block): *A.* upper limb tourniquet placement. *B.* Lower limb tourniquet placement. *C.* Insertion of IV. *D.* Exsanguination of the limb by elevation. *E.* Exsanguination of the limb employing an elastic bandage (e.g., Esmarch) followed by inflation of the tourniquet. *F.* Injection of the local anesthetic agent. (Reproduced from Scott DB. *Techniques of Regional Anesthesia.* Norwalk, CT: Appleton & Lange; 1989:51.)

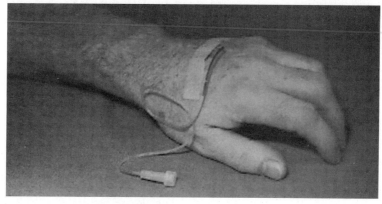

C

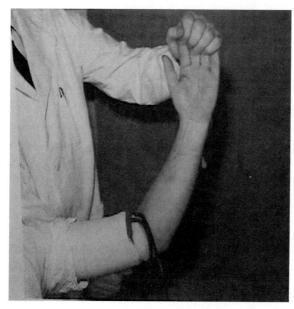

D

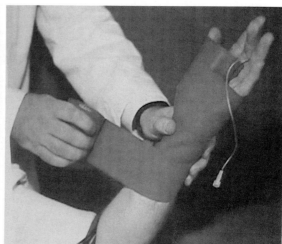

E

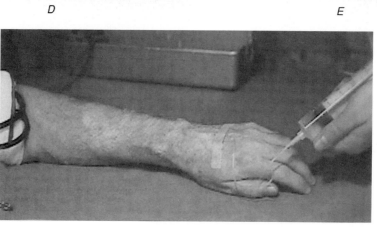

F

Fig. 25-36. (*Continued*)

REFERENCES

1. Centers for Disease Control and Prevention (CDC). Transmission of hepatitis B and C viruses in outpatient settings—New York, Oklahoma, and Nebraska, 2000–2002. *MMWR Morb Mortal Wkly Rep.* 2003;52(38):901–906.
2. Covino BG, Wildsmith JAW. Clinical pharmacology of local anesthetic agents. In: Cousins MJ, Bridenbaugh PO, eds. *Neural Blockade.* Philadelphia, PA: Lippincott-Raven; 1998:97–128.
3. Bedrock RD, Skigen A, Dolwick MF. Retrieval of a broken needle in the pterygomandibular space. *J Am Dent Assoc.* 1999;130(5):685–687.
4. Bhatia S, Bounds G. A broken needle in the pterygomandibular space: report of a case and review of the literature. *Dent Update.* 1998;25:35–37.
5. Teh J. Breakage of Whitacre 27 gauge needle during performance of spinal anaesthesia for caesarean section. *Anaesth Intensive Care.* 1997;25:96.
6. Williams MF, Eisele DW, Wyatt SH. Neck needle foreign bodies in intravenous drug abusers. *Laryngoscope.* 1993; 103:59–63.
7. Zeltser R, Cohen C, Casap N. The implications of a broken needle in the pterygomandibular space: clinical guidelines for prevention and retrieval. *Pediatr Dent.* 2002;24(2):153–156.
8. Yamashita H, Tsukayama H, White AR, et al. Systematic review of adverse events following acupuncture: the Japanese literature. *Complement Ther Med.* 2001;9:98–104.
9. Sood A, Miglani S, Moorthy D. Breakage of insulin syringe needle in subcutaneous tissue. *J Pediatr Endocrinol Metab.* 2001;14:101–102.
10. Nish IA, Pynn BR, Holmes HI, et al. Maxillary nerve block: a case report and review of the intraoral technique. *J Can Dent Assoc.* 1995;61:305–310.
11. Nseir S, Pronnier P, Soubrier S, et al. Fatal streptococcal necrotizing fasciitis as a complication of axillary brachial plexus block. *Br J Anaesth.* 2004;92:427–429.
12. Adam F, Jaziri S, Chauvin M. Psoas abscess complicating femoral nerve block catheter. *Anesthesiology.* 2003; 99: 230–231.
13. Basu A, Bhalaik V, Stanislas M, et al. Osteomyelitis following a haematoma block. *Injury.* 2003;34:79–82.
14. Wachter R, Otten JE, Buitrago-Tellez C, et al. Mandibular osteomyelitis after mandibular conduction anesthesia. *Mund Kiefer Gesichtschir.* 1998;2:39–41.
15. Weinand FS, Pavlovic S, Dick B. Endophthalmitis after intra-oral block of the infraorbital nerve. *Klin Monatsbl Augenheilkd.* 1997;210:402–4.
16. Kitay D, Ferraro N, Sonis ST. Lateral pharyngeal space abscess as a consequence of regional anesthesia. *J Am Dent Assoc.* 1991;122:56–59.

26

Topical Anesthesia

Sharon E. Mace

HIGH YIELD FACTS

- Widespread clinical uses: Prevents the pain associated with laceration repair, venipuncture, lumbar puncture, abscess drainage, minor surgical procedures, and other procedures.

- Advantages include: Painless application, avoids use of a needle, no tissue distortion, and often as effective as infiltrative anesthesia.

- Vasoconstrictors increase anesthetic effectiveness but must avoid using them on surfaces with end-arteriolar blood supply.

- Can be absorbed systemically, produce detectable blood levels, and systemic effects so do not exceed recommended dose to prevent toxicity.

- Topical anesthetics without cocaine (lidocaine epinephrine tetracaine [LET]) are preferred over cocaine-containing combination anesthetics (e.g., cocaine, and tetracaine adrenaline cocaine [TAC]) to avoid cocaine toxicity.

- Can be used on broken skin (e.g., lacerations/abrasions), intact skin, and mucosal surfaces.

- Iontophoresis and phonophoresis may enhance speed of onset.

INTRODUCTION

Topical anesthesia is the direct application of local anesthetic agents to surface tissues in order to produce anesthesia.[1] It is a safe and effective method of eliminating or minimizing pain and the accompanying anxiety and fear experienced by patients of all ages who are undergoing various procedures in many different clinical situations. The judicious use of topical anesthetics can provide effective cutaneous anesthesia for minor procedures, suturing lacerations, and can eliminate or minimize the pain associated with the injection of local anesthetics, perhaps decreasing or avoiding the need for systemic sedation or analgesia.[2-4]

Local anesthesia is the loss of sensation in a specific part of the body without losing consciousness and without affecting the central control of vital functions.[1] Topical anesthesia is one technique of administering local anesthesia. Other techniques of administration of local anesthesia include infiltration anesthesia, field-block anesthesia, nerve block anesthesia, Bier block (intravenous [IV] regional anesthesia), spinal anesthesia, and epidural anesthesia.[1,5] These will be discussed in other chapters.

The application of topical anesthetics to the intact skin, lacerations, and mucosal surfaces produces local analgesia and the elimination of pain.[2-5] It also has a significant psychological benefit.[6,7] Research has shown that patients who are informed they will be receiving a topical anesthetic anticipate less injection pain than patients who are not informed.[8] Much of the pain, anxiety, and fear experienced by children (and adults) prior to a medical or dental procedure is the sight of a needle and the discomfort/pain associated with the first injection.[6,7,9,10] One of the most widely used types of pain control, local infiltration anesthesia, can create pain and anxiety because of the injection.[6,7,9-11] Effective topical anesthesia can reduce or even abolish the pain and anxiety associated with local injection.[6,7,9-11] In pediatrics, the anticipation of a local injection prior to an upcoming procedure can create chaos by turning a quiet cooperative youngster into an anxious, frightened, screaming, and uncooperative child.[7] There has been much research and an expanding pharmacopia of topical anesthetics available to the practitioner for use in patients of all ages in a myriad of settings.[12-15]

With the advent of topical anesthesia,[1] a myriad of procedures (Table 26-1) can be performed in children without *brutane* or major restraints, and in adults without the risks of general anesthesia or procedural sedation.[16-20]

Topical anesthetics are available in many forms: solutions, gels, pastes, patches, powders, lozenges, tablets, ointments, and aerosols. Specialized techniques for the application of topical anesthetics, such as impregnated patches and the inclusion of anesthetics into liposomes are being developed.[21] Unique delivery systems such as iontophoresis have been devised.[22-24]

Topical anesthetics can be effectively employed virtually on any body surface including the epidermis (whether broken or intact), ear canal, cornea, and the mucosal surfaces of the airway, nasal passages, oropharynx, gastrointestinal, genital, or urinary tract.[5,17-20]

Advantages of topical anesthesia when compared to local infiltration include the following:

- Painless application.
- Avoids use of a needle.

Table 26-1. Indications (Uses) for Topical Anesthesia*

Adjunctive medication (premedication) prior to local infiltration anesthesia to decrease or eliminate injection pain/anxiety
Laceration repair
Symptomatic treatment:
   For painful oral mucosal lesions (such as ulcerations)
   For otitis externa
   For painful rashes/skin lesions
   Skin abrasions
Procedures
   Airway procedures: Intubations, laryngoscopy, and bronchoscopy
   Head, eyes, ears, nose, throat (HEENT) procedures:
      Ophthalmology: slit lamp examination, foreign body (FB) removal
      Otolaryngology: Nasal packing, FB removal
   Gastroenterology: Nasogastric/orogastric tube placement
   Urology: Foley catheter placement
   Neurologic: Lumbar punctures
   Hematologic/oncologic: Venipuncture, bone marrow aspiration
   Vascular: Peripheral or central venous or arterial line placement, arterial blood gas sampling
   Infectious: Incision and drainage of abscesses
   Dermatology: Removal of skin lesions
   Dental: Tooth extraction/implantation, other procedures involving gums/gingiva/teeth

*This list is not meant to be an all-inclusive list but lists some of the common uses of topical anesthetics.

- No distortion of the wound edges of the laceration.
- If a vasoconstrictor is used, improved hemostasis and longer duration of anesthesia.[25]

The main disadvantage of topical anesthesia versus local infiltration is a slower onset.[25]

Topical anesthetics tend to work better on the head and neck than on the extremities, probably because of the increased vascularity of the head and neck.[26,27] In most studies, topical anesthetics are as effective as local infiltration.[28,29] A few studies indicated that topical anesthetics were somewhat less effective than local infiltration, although the difference may not be clinically significant.[30,31]

PHARMACOLOGY

A detailed discussion of the pharmacology and the neuropharmacology of local anesthetic-induced neural blockade is discussed in Chapter 27.

TOPICAL ANESTHETICS FOR LACERATION REPAIR

One of the commonest uses of topical anesthetics is for repair of skin lacerations.[5] Preparations employed for this indication typically consist of several components: a single local anesthetic agent or combinations of local anesthetic agents (amides or esters) and a vasoconstrictor.[28,32–34] The most commonly used local anesthetics are lidocaine (the amide in LET) and tetracaine (an ester, in both LET and TAC).[5,31] Other amide and ester local anesthetics have been used including amides: mepivacaine, bupivacaine, prilocaine, etidocaine and the ester; procaine.[28,31,33,34] None of the other local anesthetic combinations have been shown to have any significant advantage over LET, though they may be more expensive than LET, and less costly than TAC.[28,34,35] Because of the serious side effects, including death, associated with cocaine toxicity from topical anesthetics, LET has replaced TAC as the topical anesthetic of choice for the repair of skin lacerations.[36,37]

Vasoconstrictors are a critical component of such topical anesthetic preparations.[38,39] Vasoconstrictors (e.g., epinephrine) increase the duration of the topical block by inducing local vasoconstriction and slowing the elimination of the local anesthetic agents.[40,41] Failure to use a vasoconstrictor with the topical local anesthetic may lead to inadequate anesthesia. In addition to increasing the quality and duration of anesthesia, vasoconstrictors also assist in hemostasis and decrease the toxicity of the local anesthetic.[40] Other vasoconstrictors, specifically, norephinephrine and phenylephrine, have been used by some because of their greater alpha-receptor selectivity, though the clinical superiority of one vasoconstrictor over another has not been demonstrated.[28,30,31,32]

Tetracaine Adrenaline Cocaine (TAC)

TAC, introduced in 1980, was the first combination topical solution for achieving local anesthesia for laceration repair.[42] TAC consists of tetracaine, adrenaline, and cocaine. The original TAC formulation contains tetracaine 0.5% (5 mg/mL), adrenaline 0.05% (500 mcg/mL), and cocaine 11.8% (118 mg/mL). TAC is also known as TEC (tetracaine, epinephrine, cocaine).[42]

TAC, LET, or any other topical anesthetic combination containing a vasoconstrictor should not be applied to any site that receives an end-arteriolar blood supply (e.g., nose, ear, fingers, toes, and penis) because of the risk of excessive vasoconstriction leading to ischemia and tissue necrosis.[5,25]

To avoid the complications that have occurred with TAC, it should never be placed on or near a mucosal surface (e.g., mouth or nares), or the conjunctiva.[43,44] TAC is ineffective through intact skin but is quickly absorbed from mucosal surfaces. The adverse effects of TAC are secondary to the inadvertent systemic absorption of cocaine leading to cocaine toxicity including agitation, seizures, respiratory arrest, and death.[43–45] These complications led to a revised formulation of TAC. The modified solution contains cocaine 4% (40 mg/mL) instead of the original 11.8% concentration. The recommended maximum dose of 11.8% cocaine TAC in otherwise healthy individuals is 3–4 mL in an adult and 1–3 mL in children. With the preferred 4% cocaine TAC solution, the maximum is 0.15 mL/kg, with a maximum total dose of cocaine being 150 mg.[1,38] TAC has other disadvantages including the following:

- Cost (relatively more expensive than LET and other solutions).
- Refrigeration is needed to prolong its shelf life.
- Additional paperwork is required because it is a controlled drug (schedule II in the United States).

Lidocaine Epinephrine Tetracaine (LET)

Due to the problems associated with TAC, other topical anesthetic solutions have been developed. The composition of LET, also referred to as LAT or TLE, is lidocaine 1–4% (10–40 mg/mL), epinephrine 1:2000–1:1000 (500–1000 mcg/mL), and tetracaine 0.5–2.0% (5–20 mg/mL). LET provides local anesthesia equivalent to TAC but without the risks, and has replaced TAC as the topical solution of choice for laceration repair.[36,37] The usual LET formulation is 4% lidocaine, 0.1% epinephrine, and 0.5% tetracaine, and it is prepared in single-use 5-mL vials.[46,47]

The recommended technique for administering LET (and other combination local anesthetic solutions) is to drip some of the solution directly onto the wound from a syringe, and then apply the remainder to a cotton ball or sterile gauze.

The soaked cotton ball or gauze is placed into the wound and covered with a semiocclusive dressing (such as tegaderm), or held in place by a third person (e.g., parent). The parent wears gloves to prevent them from absorbing any of the local anesthetic, LET must be left in place for 20–30 minutes in order to attain adequate anesthesia. A gel form of LET is made by adding methylcellulose to the LET solution. A gel form of TAC is also available.[46,47] The gel can be applied directly to the wound using a sterile cotton swab. The advantages of the gel are the following[29,46,47]:

- Greater probability of the preparation staying in the wound.
- Less chance of the agents dripping onto a mucous membrane so it can be used with caution near the mouth, eyes, or nose.
- Perhaps, greater anesthetic effect.

In general, topical anesthetic preparations (TAC, LET, and others) produce better anesthetic effect in face and scalp wounds than in extremity or truncal wounds.[26,27] This is probably related to the richer vascular supply of the face and scalp.

Other local anesthetic combination solutions are available, have no real advantage over LET, but can be used in certain situations such as a true allergy to lidocaine.

TOPICAL ANESTHETICS FOR MUCOSAL SURFACES

Lidocaine

Lidocaine is the most commonly used local anesthetic agent.[4,36,48] It may be used in combination with other agents or by itself to induce topical anesthesia. It is available in different concentrations (0.5–30%) and in various preparations (solution, ointment, cream, or jelly).[49,34,39] Atomized lidocaine spray (4%) and lidocaine gel (2%) have been used for topical analgesia before the insertion of a nasogastric tube, while the 10% lidocaine spray (though recently withdrawn from the market by the manufacturer) with a long delivery arm is used for anesthetizing the upper airway prior to various airway procedures.[50,51] Viscous 2% lidocaine is prescribed for painful ulcers and other lesions of the mouth, is a component of the *GI cocktail*, is used to facilitate the cleansing of skin abrasions, and is used for topical anesthesia (2–4%) prior to endoscopic procedures (e.g., placement of nasogastric or lavage tubes).[7,36,50,51] Urethral anesthesia can be obtained by injecting 2% lidocaine jelly via a catheter tip syringe and leaving the jelly in contact with the urethral mucosal for 5–20 minutes.

Studies employing the topical application of plain 1% or 2% lidocaine solution as local anesthesia for suturing lacerations have demonstrated no anesthetic effect.[48]

Cocaine

Cocaine is the only local anesthetic agent with vasoconstricting properties due to its inhibition of norepinephrine reuptake locally.[52] It has been used in otolaryngology as a topical anesthetic and local vasoconstrictor.[53] As with the use of TAC for laceration repair, adverse events including myocardial infarction, seizures, dysrhythmias, survivable cardiac arrest, and deaths have been reported with the topical application of cocaine for otolaryngology or airway procedures.[54,55] Because of these complications, other topical anesthetics are replacing the use of cocaine during otolaryngologic procedures.[55,56] There is some evidence that other topical anesthetics are more effective than cocaine when used as topical anesthetic for procedures involving the nasopharynx.[51,57]

Benzocaine

Benzocaine is supplied in a variety of concentrations up to 20% as a liquid, gel, or spray formulation and is often employed to produce mucosal anesthesia. It can be applied to mouth ulcers/lesions and open wounds for pain relief. It is used as topical anesthesia prior to endoscopic procedures, for example, insertion of nasogastric tubes. An otic preparation of benzocaine and antipyrine is prescribed for pain relief with otitis externa. Benzocaine has several disadvantages:

- As an ester there is an increased risk of an allergic reaction.
- The potential for methemoglobinemia (see Chap 27).[58]

TOPICAL ANESTHETICS FOR INTACT SKIN

Eutectic Mixture of Local Anesthetic (EMLA) Agents

EMLA cream is a eutectic mixture of local anesthetics. It consists of an emulsification of 2.5% lidocaine and 2.5% prilocaine in a 1:1 ratio. EMLA is a topical anesthetic applied to intact skin that has been successful in eliminating or decreasing the pain associated with various procedures.[59–64] Such procedures include venipuncture, arterial puncture, lumbar puncture, arthrocentesis, bone marrow biopsy, superficial skin procedures, immunizations, and even circumcision.[59–64] EMLA, however, did not decrease the pain from heel lancing.[63] EMLA is currently suggested only for use on intact skin, although studies

using EMLA for topical anesthesia in open wounds indicate that it is effective.[65,66]

A thick layer of EMLA cream is applied to intact skin and then covered with a semiocclusive dressing. The application should not be massaged or rubbed into the skin and should be left in a thick layer. Adequate analgesia occurs in 1 hour with a peak effect in 2 hours, and lasts for 1 hour after removal. Animal studies suggested a greater wound infection rate and delayed healing but this has not been seen in clinical studies.[37]

A major concern with EMLA cream is methemoglobinemia,[38,39,67] which is due to the prilocaine component. Infants have a relatively immature nicotinamide adenine dinucleotide (NADH) reductase enzyme system which theoretically increases the risk of methemoglobinemia.[39] Therefore, EMLA ought to be used with caution in infants <3 months old (maximum dose = 1 g for 1 hour) and not used in patients prone to methemoglobinemia. Patients at risk for methemoglobinemia include those on sulfonamides, nitrates, primaquine, and other drugs that can also lead to methemoglobinemia.[39]

Reactions to EMLA are rare with minor skin irritation (redness, blanching, and rash) being the most common. The usual dose in school age children is 2.5–5 g applied 1 hour prior to the procedure.[69] A more rapid onset (15 minutes) and shorter duration of anesthesia is associated with EMLA use over atopic or psoriatic skin. The maximum total dose of EMLA by weight and age is: (1) 0–3 months or <5 kg, 1 g; (2) 3–12 months or >5 kg, 2 g; (3) 1–6 years and >10 kg, 10 g; and (4) 7–12 years and >20 kg, 20 g. The maximum time of application is 1 hour for the age of 0–3 months and 4 hours for all other ages. However, less can be used.

EMLA

- Should not be ingested.
- Is contraindicated in infants <1 month of age or infants <1 year if susceptible to methemoglobinemia.
- When used in children <20 kg, the size of application and the duration of contact should be limited.
- Is not indicated for ophthalmic use.
- Should be used with caution in those taking class I antiarrhythmics (same precaution as for injectable local anesthetics).
- Maximum total dose is by weight and age. Less than the maximum dose can be used.

Liposomal Encapsulated Preparations

L-M-X-4, previously known as ELA Max, is a topical anesthetic cream containing 4% lidocaine cream in a liposomal delivery system. It is applied to intact skin 30 minutes prior to a procedure such as venipuncture.[68,69] The manufacturer has no written guidelines for L-M-X-4 and suggests using EMLA guidelines. L-M-X-4 contains 4% lidocaine cream so adhering to the lidocaine maximum dosage (without a vasoconstriction) or 4 mg/kg seems prudent. The usual pediatric dose in several studies was 2.5 g.[68,69] It is applied in a similar fashion as for EMLA cream using an semiocclusive dressing.[68,69] An advantage of L-M-X-4 over EMLA cream is that it has a faster onset. Adequate anesthesia occurs in 30 minutes instead of 1 hour. It also has a longer duration of anesthesia, is less expensive than EMLA cream, and avoids the risk of methemoglobinemia. Indications for the use of L-M-X-4 are similar to that for EMLA cream such as for IV insertion, lumbar puncture, and venipuncture. Studies indicate that subcutaneous buffered lidocaine and topical L-M-X-4 resulted in equivalent reductions in pain and anxiety during peripheral IV catheter insertion.[70]

Tetracaine

Tetracaine (Amethocaine), available as a 4% gel, is applied in a 1 g dose to intact skin under a semiocclusive dressing for 30–40 minutes. It provides effective topical anesthesia to 85% of pediatric patients prior to venipuncture and the success of venipuncture was not affected.[71] Tetracaine gel is reported to be as effective as EMLA cream but provides local anesthesia in 30 minutes while EMLA takes 60 minutes.[72] Side effects of the tetracaine gel are similar to those with other topicals like EMLA and L-M-X-4, and include transient skin reactions such as local edema, erythema, and pruritus.

Refrigerant Anesthetic Sprays (Vapocoolants)

Vapocoolants or skin refrigerants are not local anesthetics. The two commonly used vapocoolant sprays are ethyl chloride (chloromethane) and fluori-methane (dichlorodifluoromethane and dichloromonofluoromethane). They produce topical anesthesia by desensitizing the peripheral nerves. When the vapocoolant touches the skin, it vaporizes. This results in a temporary decrease to a temperature of −20°C, which momentarily freezes the skin turning the affected skin white.[25] Vapocoolants have been used to provide topical anesthesia for procedures like injections, venipuncture, and the incision and drainage of small abscesses.[73,74] They have also been used to alleviate muscle pain, myofascial pain, and pain from athletic injuries.

The procedure for applying the vapocoolant is to hold the sprayer bottle upside down at a 10–30-cm distance from the skin and spray for 3–7 seconds. The anesthetic effect of vapocoolants is almost instantaneous but very brief, lasting only 30–60 seconds. They should not be used on mucosal surfaces.

Advantages of refrigerant anesthetic sprays are an easy and instantaneous method for achieving topical anesthesia without using a needle.

Disadvantages include the following:

- The short duration of anesthesia.
- Possible skin ulceration and/or frostbite from prolonged spraying.
- Ethyl chloride is highly flammable and should not be used near electric cautery or open flames.[36] Fluori-methane is not flammable.[39]
- Inhalation of the vapocoolant sprays should be avoided since methyl chloride has opioid and general anesthetic properties with the potential for a drug of abuse.
- Occasional discomfort when the anesthetized skin thaws.
- The theoretical possibility of delayed skin healing and/or decreased resistance to infection.

TOPICAL ANESTHESIA: AUGMENTING DERMAL PENETRATION

The epidermis provides an effective barrier to the penetration of substances including medications. Two methods of delivering medications are employed to augment the penetration of local anesthetic agents through intact skin: iontophoresis and phonophoresis.[75] Iontophoresis is the technique of delivering medications topically utilizing an electric current. When a constant direct current is applied, ions (charged particles) will move toward oppositely charged (positive and negative) poles. Most local anesthetic agents are weak bases and thus are positively charged in an acidic environment, rendering them amenable to iontophoretic techniques.

The procedure involves the application of a local anesthetic agent under electrodes applied to the skin, and then passing a DC current through the electrodes. The ions gravitate to the opposite charge.

The advantage of iontophoresis is that it generates a faster onset (10 minutes) than with the topical anesthetic creams (L-M-X-4 or EMLA) or tetracaine gel.

Negative aspects of iontophoresis include the following:

- Only a small surface area can be anesthetized due to the limited surface area of the conducting pad/electrode.
- A limited number of sites where it can be used due to its bulky apparatus and inability to fit over certain body surfaces, specifically, the face and the fingers.

- Some patients complain of stinging, warmth or cold, and burning at the site, a side effect that could frighten a small child.
- A potential hazard is burning of tissue exposed to the DC current. Limiting the current density to 1 mA/cm^2 is recommended to avoid this possibility.

The technical design of the gel electrode has been improved creating a less cumbersome, more malleable form that can anesthetize a larger surface area and be applied to other parts of the body. Multiple studies have documented the effectiveness of iontophoresis in achieving topical anesthesia in children and adults prior to a variety of procedures including IV line placement, venipuncture, radial artery cannulation, and minor surgical procedures such as skin biopsy, excision of skin lesions, drainage of abscess, paracentesis, and removal of a FB.[76–81] With further technical advances, iontophoresis may become a more popular method of providing topical anesthesia.

Phonophoresis is a technique that employs ultrasonic sound waves to enhance the dermal penetration of topically administered local anesthetic agents.[9,75] Use of a coupling agent (typically, a gel or water) permits the transference of the sound waves to and through the skin surface. Although the exact mechanism has yet to be determined, ultrasound is believed to increase the delivery of medication by fostering a combination of mechanical, thermal, and even chemical changes in the dermal tissues.[9] The effectiveness of phonophoresis in achieving local anesthesia is currently being tested.[82] Future technology may allow for the successful development of this method.

SUMMARY

Topical anesthetics enjoy wide usage in clinical practice. Topical anesthetics are anesthetics applied directly to surface tissue to produce local anesthesia. They can be applied to intact skin, broken skin, and mucosal surfaces. Topical anesthesia can be as effective as infiltrative anesthesia and has several advantages over infiltrative anesthesia. These advantages include: painless application, avoiding use of a needle, and no distortion of the wound edges. In addition, if a vasoconstrictor is used, there is improved hemostasis and a longer duration of anesthesia. One disadvantage of topical anesthetics is a slower onset. Topical anesthetics tend to work better on the head and neck than on the extremities. There has been much research involving topical anesthesia and it is likely new drugs and better methods of drug delivery will be available in the future.

REFERENCES

1. Catterall W, Mackie K. Local anesthetics. In: Hardman JG, Limbird L, Gilman AG, eds. *Goodman and Gilman's The Pharmacological Basis of Therapeutics*. New York: McGraw-Hill; 2001:367–384.
2. McGee D. Local and topical anesthesia. In: Roberts JR, Hedges JR, Chanmergan AS, eds. *Clinical Procedures in Emergency Medicine*. Philadelphia, PA: W.B. Saunders; 2004:533–551.
3. Liu SS, Hodgson PS. Local anesthetics. In: Barash PG, Cullen BF, Stoelting RK, eds. *Clinical Anesthesia*. Philadelphia, PA: Lippincott Williams & Wilkins; 1997:449–469.
4. Strichartz GR, Berde CB. Local anesthetics. In: Miller RD, ed. *Miller's Anesthesia*. Philadelphia, PA: Elsevier; 2005: 573–603.
5. Houck C. Local analgesia. In: Krauss B, Brustowicz RM, eds. *Pediatric Procedural Sedation and Analgesia*. Philadelphia, PA: Lippincott Williams & Wilkins; 1999:59–65.
6. Meecham JG. Effective topical anesthetic agents and techniques. *Dent Clin North Am*. 2002;46:759–766.
7. Shannon M. Topical analgesia. In: Krauss B, Brustowicz RM, eds. *Pediatric Procedural Sedation and Analgesia*. Philadelphia, PA: Lippincott Williams & Wilkins; 1999:67–71.
8. Martin MD, Ramsay DS, Whitney C, et al. Topical anesthesia: differentiating the pharmacological and psychological contributions to efficacy. *Anesth Prog*. 1994;41:40–47.
9. Lerner EV, Bucalo BD, Kist DA, et al. Topical anesthetic agents in dermatologic surgery. *Dermatol Surg*. 1997;23:673–683.
10. Ram D, Peretz B. Administering local anesthesia to pediatric dental patients current status and prospects for the future. *Int J Paediatr Dent*. 2002;12:80–89.
11. Maurice SC, O'Donnell JJ, Beattie TF. Emergency analgesia in the pediatric population. Part II Pharmalogical methods of pain relief. *Emerg Med J*. 2002;19:101–105.
12. Knapp JF. An update of current clinical practices in pediatric emergency medicine. *Pediatr Rev*. 1997;18:424–428.
13. Ruetsch YA, Boni T, Borgest A. From cocaine to ropivacaine. The history of local anesthetic drugs. *Curr Top Med Chem*. 2001;1:175–182.
14. Chen BK, Cunningham B. Topical anesthetics in children, agents and techniques that equally comfort patients, parents, and clinicians. *Curr Opin Pediatr*. 201;13:324–330.
15. Berde C. Local anesthetics in infants and children. *Pediatr Anesth*. 2004;14:387–393.
16. Hollander JE, Shuger AJ. Laceration management. *Ann Emerg Med*. 1999;34:356–367.
17. Glauser J, Cullinson B. Procedural sedation. Part II: Specific scenarios, topical agents, and establishment of procedural sedation policy within the emergency department. *Emerg Med Rep*. 2002;23:263–273.
18. Stewart GM, Rosenberg N. Use of topical lidocaine in pediatric laceration repair: a review of topical anesthetics. *Pediatr Emerg Care*. 1998;14:419–423.
19. Zilbert A. Topical anesthesia for minor gynecological procedures: a review. *Obstet Gynecol Surv*. 2002;57:171–178.

20. Kennedy RM, Luhmann JD. Pharmacological management of pain and anxiety during emergency procedures in children. *Pediatr Drugs*. 2001;3:337–354.

21. Grant SA. The holy grail: long acting local anaesthetics and liposomes. *Best Pract Res Clin Anaesthesiol*. 2003;17:111–136.

22. Kalia YN, Merino V, Guy RH. Transdermal drug delivery. *Dermatol Clin*. 1998;16:289–299.

23. Zempsky WT, Ashburn MA. Iontophoresis: noninvasive drug delivery. *Am J Anesthesiol*. 1998;25:158–162.

24. Panchagnula R, Pillai O, Nair VB, et al. Transdermal iontophoresis revisited. *Curr Opin Chem Biol*. 2000;4:468–473.

25. Higginbotham E, Vissers RJ. Local and regional anesthesia. In: Tintinalli JE, Kelen GD, Stapczynski JS, eds. *Emergency Medicine A Comprehensive Study Guide*. New York: McGraw-Hill; 2004:264–275.

26. Bonadio WA, Wagner V. Efficacy of TAC topical anesthetic for repair of pediatric lacerations. *Am J Dis Child*. 1988;142:203–205.

27. Hegenbarth MA, Alteri Mf, Hawk WH, et al. Comparison of topical tetracaine adrenaline and cocaine (TAC) versus lidocaine epinephrine and tetracaine (LET) for anesthesia lacerations in children. *Ann Emerg Med*. 1995;25:203–208.

28. Smith GA, Strausbaugh SD, Harbeck-Weber C, et al. Comparison of topical anesthetics with lidocaine infiltration during laceration repair in children. *Clin Pediatr*. 1997;36:17–23.

29. Ernst AA, Marves-Valls E, Nick TG, et al. Topical lidocaine adrenaline tetracaine (LET gel) versus injectable buffered lidocaine for local anesthesia in laceration repair. *West J Med*. 1997;167:79–81.

30. Smith GA, Strausbaugh GA, Harbeck-Weber C, et al. Tetracaine-lidocaine-phenylephrine topical anesthesia compared with lidocaine infiltration during repair of mucous membrane lacerations in children. *Clin Pediatr*. 1998;37:405–412.

31. Smith GA, Strausbaugh SD, Harbeck-Weber C, et al. Prilocaine-phenylephrine topical anesthesia for repair of mucous membrane lacerations. *Pediatr Emerg Care*. 1998;14:324–328.

32. Smith GA, Strausbaugh SD, Harbeck-Weber C, et al. New non-cocaine containing topical anesthetics compared with tetracaine—adrenaline-cocaine during repair of lacerations. *Pediatrics*. 1997;100:825–830.

33. Kunn M, Rossi SOP, Plummer JL, et al. Topical anaesthesia for minor lacerations: MAC verses TAC. *Med J Aust*. 1996;164:277–280.

34. Smith GA, Strausbaugh SD, Harbeck-Weber C, et al. Comparison of topical anesthetics without cocaine to tetracaine-adrenaline-cocaine and lidocaine infiltration during repair of lacerations: bupivacaine-norepinephrine is an effective new topical anesthetic agent. *Pediatrics*. 1996;97:301–307.

35. Schilling CG, Bank DE, Borchert BA, et al. Tetracaine, epinephrine (adrenalin), and cocaine (TAC) versus lidocaine, epinephrine, and tetracaine (LET) for anesthesia of lacerations in children. *Ann Emerg Med*. 1995;25:203–208.

36. Simon B, Hern HG Jr. Wound management principles. In: Marx JA, Hockberger RS, Walls RM, et al, eds. *Rosen's Emergency Medicine*. St. Louis, MO: Mosby; 2002:737–751.

37. Paris PM, Yealy DM. Pain management. In: Marx JA, Hockberger RS, Walls RM, et al. *Rosen's Emergency Medicine Concepts and Clinical Practice*. St. Louis, MO: Mosby; 2002:2555–2577.

38. Proudfoot J. Analgesia, anesthesia, and conscious sedation. *Emerg Med Clin N Am*. 1995;13:357–379.

39. Rodriquez E, Jordan R. Contemporary trends in pediatric sedation and analgesia. *Emerg Med Clin North Am*. 2002;20:199–222.

40. Naftalin LW, Yagiela JA. Vasoconstrictors: indications and precautions. *Dent Clin North Am*. 2002;46:733–746.

41. Neal JM. Effects of epinephrine in local anesthetics on the central and peripheral nervous systems: neurotoxicity and neural blood flow. *Reg Anesth Pain Med*. 2003;28:124–134.

42. Pryor GJ, Kilpatrick WR, Opp DR. Local anesthesia in minor lacerations: topical TAC versus lidocaine infiltration. *Ann Emerg Med*. 1980;9:568–571.

43. Dailey RH. Fatality secondary to misuse of TAC solution. *Ann Emerg Med*. 1988;17:159–160.

44. Daya MR, Burton BT, Schleiss MR, et al. Recurrent seizures following mucosal application of TAC. *Ann Emerg Med*. 1988;17:646–648.

45. Schubert CJ, Wason S. Cocaine toxicity in an infant following intranasal instillation of a four percent cocaine solution. *Pediatr Emerg Care*. 1992;8:82–84.

46. Ernst AA, Marvez E, Nick TG, et al. Lidocaine adrenaline tetracaine gel versus tetracaine adrenaline cocaine gel for topical anesthesia in linear scalp and facial lacerations in children aged 5 to 17 years. *Pediatrics*. 1995;95:255–258.

47. Resch K, Schilling C, Borchert BD, et al. Topical anesthesia for pediatric lacerations: a randomized trial of lidocaine-epinephrine-tetracaine solution versus gel. *Ann Emerg Med*. 1998;32:693–697.

48. Stewart GM, Simpson P, Rosenberg NM. Use of topical lidocaine in pediatric laceration repair: a review of topical anesthetics. *Pediatr Emerg Care*. 1998;14:419–423.

49. Scholz A. Mechanisms of (local) anesthetics on voltage-gated sodium and other ion channels. *Br J Anaesth*. 2002;89:52–61.

50. Wolfe TR, Fosnocht DE, Linscott MS. Atomized lidocaine as topical anesthesia for nasogastric tube placement: a randomized double-blind placebo-controlled trial. *Ann Emerg Med*. 2000;35:421–425.

51. Ducharme J, Matheson K. What is the best topical anesthetic for nasogastric insertion? A comparison of lidocaine gel, lidocaine spray, and atomized cocaine. *J Emerg Nurs*. 2003;29:427–430.

52. Cox B, Durieux ME, Marcus MAE. Toxicity of local anaesthetics. *Best Pract Res Clin Anaesthesiol*. 2003;17:111–136.

53. De R, Uppal HS, Shehab ZP, et al. Current practices of cocaine administration by UK otorhinolaryngologists. *J Laryngol Otol*. 2003;117:109–112.

54. Osula S, Stockton P, Abdelaziz MM, et al. Intratracheal cocaine induced myocardial infarction: an unusual complication of fiberoptic bronchoscopy. *Thorax.* 2003;58:733–734.

55. Long H, Greller H, Mercurio-Zappala M, et al. Medical use of cocaine: a shifting paradigm over 25 years. *Laryngoscope.* 2004;14:1625–1629.

56. Smith JC, Rockley TJ. A comparison of cocaine and 'co-phenlcaine' local anaesthesia in flexible nasendoscopy. *Clin Otolaryngol.* 2002;27:192–196.

57. Cara DM, Norris AM, Neale LJ. Pain during awake nasal intubation after topical cocaine or phenylephrine/lidocaine spray. *Anaesthesia.* 2003;58:775–803.

58. Cooper HA. Methemoglobinemia caused by benzocaine topical spray. *South Med J.* 1997;90:946–948.

59. Yamamoto LG, Boychuk RB. A blinded randomized paired placebo-controlled trial of 20-minute EMLA cream to reduce the pain of peripheral IV cannulation in the ED. *Am J Emerg Med.* 1998;16:634–636.

60. Halperin DL. Topical skin anesthesia for venous, subcutaneous drug reservoir and lumbar puncture in children. *Pediatrics.* 1989;84:281–284.

61. Robieux I, Kumar R, Radhakrishman S, et al. Assessing pain and analgesia with a lidocaine-prilocaine emulsion in infants and toddlers during venipuncture. *J Pediatr.* 1991;118:971–973.

62. Uhari M. A eutectic mixture of lidocaine and prilocaine for alleviating vaccination pain in infants. *Pediatrics.* 1993;92:719–721.

63. Taddio A, Ohlsson A, Einarson TR, et al. A systematic review of lidocaine-prilocaine cream (EMLA) in the treatment of acute pain in neonates. *Pediatrics.* 1998;101(2):e1,299.

64. Taddio A, Stevens B, Craig K, et al. Efficacy and safety of lidocaine-prilocaine cream for pain during circumcision. *N Engl J Med.* 1997;336:1197–1201.

65. Zempsky WT, Karasic RB. EMLA versus TAC for topical anesthesia of extremity wounds in children. *Ann Emerg Med.* 1997;30:163–166.

66. Singer AJ, Stark MJ. LET versus EMLA for pretreating lacerations: a randomized trial. *Acad Emerg Med.* 2001;8:223–230.

67. Brisman M, Llung BML, Otterbom I, et al. Methaemoglobin formation after the use of EMLA cream in term neonates. *Acta Paediatr.* 1998;87:1191–1194.

68. Eichenfield LF, Funk A, Fallon-Friedlander S, et al. A clinical study to evaluate the efficacy of ELA-May (4% liposomal lidocaine) as compared with eutectic mixture of local anesthetics cream for pain reduction of venipuncture in children. *Pediatrics.* 2002;109:1093–1099.

69. Kleiber C, Sorenson M, Whiteside K, et al. Topical anesthetics for intravenous insertion in children: a randomized equivalency study. *Pediatrics.* 2002;110:758–761.

70. Luhmann J, et al. A comparison of buffered lidocaine vs ELA-Max before peripheral intravenous catheter insertions in children. *Pediatrics.* 2004;113:217.

71. Lawson RA, Smart NG, Gudgeon AC, et al. Evaluation of an amethocaine (tetracaine) gel preparation for percutaneous analgesia before venous cannulation in children. *Br J Anaesth.* 1995;75:282–285.

72. Taddio A, Gurguis MGX, Karen G. Lidocaine prilocaine cream versus tetracaine gel for procedural pain in children. *Ann Pharmacother.* 2002;36:687–692.

73. Ramsook C, Kozinetz CA, Moro-Sutherland D. Efficacy of ethyl chloride as a local anesthetic for venipuncture and intravenous cannula insertion in a pediatric emergency department. *Pediatr Emerg Care.* 2001;17:341–343.

74. Cohen-Reis E, Holubkov R. Vapocoolant spray is equally effective as EMLA cream in reducing immunization pain in school-aged children. *Pediatrics.* 1997;100:1–6.

75. Kasan DG, Lynch AM, Stiller MJ. Physical enhancement of dermatologic drug delivery: iontophoresis and phonophoresis. *J Am Acad Dermatol.* 1996;34:657–666.

76. Zempsky WT, Anand KJS, Sullivan KM, et al. Lidocaine iontophoresis for topical anesthesia before intravenous line placement in children. *J Pediatr.* 1998;132:1061–1063.

77. Kim MK, Kini NM, Troshynski TJ, et al. A randomized clinical trial of dermal anesthesia by iontophoresis for peripheral intravenous catheter placement in children. *Ann Emerg Med.* 1999;33:395–399.

78. Zempsky WT, Parkinson TM. Lidocaine iontophoresis for local anesthesia before shave biopsy. *Dermatol Surg.* 2003;29:627–630.

79. De Cou JM, Abrams RS, Hammond JH, et al. Iontophoresis: a needle-free electrical system of local anesthesia delivery for pediatric surgical office procedures. *J Pediatr Surg.* 1999;34:946–949.

80. Sherwin J, Awad IT, Sadler PJ, et al. Analgesia during radial artery cannulation. *Anaesthesia.* 2003;58:471–479.

81. Schultz AA, Strout TD, Jordan P, et al. Safety, tolerability, and efficacy of iontophoresis with lidocaine for dermal anesthesia in ED pediatric patients. *J Emerg Nurs.* 2002;28:289–296.

82. Katz NP, Shapiro DE, Herrman TE, et al. Rapid onset of cutaneous anesthesia with EMLA cream after pretreatment with a new ultrasound-emitting device. *Anesth Analg.* 2004;98:371–376.

27

Local Anesthesia

Michael F. Murphy
Orlando Hung

HIGH YIELD FACTS

- A 1% solution contains 1 g of a substance per 100 mL of solution, or 10 mg/mL. When using large volumes of local anesthetic agent (e.g., Bier block and multiple rib blocks) calculate the dose of drug administered to avoid toxicity.

- The duration of a block is related to how tightly protein bound the agent is; potency is related to lipid solubility. Highly protein bound and highly lipid soluble local anesthetics such as tetracaine when employed topically (say, in the nose) produce prolonged insensitivity to even powerful noxious stimuli such as NG tube insertion.

- IgE-mediated anaphylaxis to amide-type local anesthetic agents is so rare as to be almost unheard of; the same cannot be said of the ester types, but they are rarely used in emergency practice nowadays.

- Know bupivacaine and lidocaine well. They are the most commonly used and may be the only two local anesthetic agents in an emergency department (ED).

- Be cautious with benzocaine (Hurricaine, Cetacaine) . . . it produced blue people (methemoglobinemia).

Local anesthetics are agents that *reversibly* block nerve conduction when applied to nervous tissue (central and peripheral) in an appropriate manner and concentration. It is this reversibility that makes them useful in day-to-day clinical practice. This chapter will briefly review the history of local anesthetic agents, the relevant pharmacology and toxicology of commonly used agents, the neuropharmacology of local anesthetic-induced block, as well as the clinical applications of these agents.

HISTORY

Niemann was the first to describe the local anesthetic properties of cocaine in Europe in the 1860s. This alkaloid, derived from the Andean shrub *Erythroxylon coca*, had been used for centuries by the inhabitants of the Peruvian Andes to produce a sense of well-being. Niemann noted that it had a bitter taste and that it made the tongue numb. Subsequently in 1880, Von Anrep injected a liquid derived from the coca leaves subcutaneously and discovered that it produced local anesthesia.[1] Koller and Freud are credited for introducing cocaine into clinical practice later in the 1880s. Freud also took advantage of the central effects of the agent to wean a colleague from a morphine addiction and in the process produced a cocaine addict! Freud himself is reputed to have suffered from morphine and cocaine addictions.[2] Koller used the drug to produce topical ophthalmic anesthesia. Corning used it to produce spinal anesthesia in dogs.[1]

The toxicity of cocaine motivated investigators to synthesize the ester (amino ester) derivative of paraaminobenzoic acid (PABA), procaine (Novocain) in 1904. Manipulations of this ester type, PABA-derived chemical structure led to the development of numerous other compounds including tetracaine (Pontocaine), benzocaine (Hurricaine and Cetacaine), proparacaine (Ophthaine and Ocucaine) and chloroprocaine (Nesacaine). Thus, these agents are collectively referred to as the *ester derivative* class of local anesthetic agents.

In 1943, Lofgren synthesized an amide (aminoamide) derivative of diethylaminoacetic acid dubbed lidocaine (Xylocaine). Additional amide derivatives include commonly used agents such as mepivicaine (Carbocaine and Polocaine), bupivicaine (Marcaine and Sensorcaine), prilocaine (Citanest), etidocaine (Duranest), dibucaine (Nupercaine), and ropivacaine (Naropin)

PHARMACOLOGY

The ideal local anesthetic agent should avoid tissue irritation and nerve damage. It should not be toxic at usual clinical doses. In addition, it ought to display the following properties:

- Have a finite duration of action.
- Demonstrate a rapid onset.
- Be reasonably priced.

All of the agents in clinical use today meet these requirements. The practicing clinician is interested in the specifics of the pharmacologic properties only in as much as they influence the clinical behavior of the agent.

Specifically, how potent the agent is in producing sensory or motor block, how quickly the block comes on, and how long it will last. Subsidiary concerns relate to the susceptibility of an individual patient to the side effects and potential toxicity of a particular agent.

Table 27-1 presents the physicochemical and biologic properties of local anesthetic agents to be discussed in the following paragraphs.

Potency

Potency relates to the degree to which individual agents block transmission in neural tissue. For example, tetracaine applied topically in the nose produces a more profound sensory block than an equivalent dose of procaine. The nerve cell membrane is essentially a lipoprotein matrix, so local anesthetic agents that are more lipid soluble (e.g., tetracaine and etidocaine) are more potent than those that are less lipid soluble (e.g., procaine and lidocaine).

Duration of Block

Local anesthetic agents interrupt neural impulse transmission by occluding sodium channels along the axon membrane. The local anesthetic agent binds to a protein receptor in that sodium channel producing blockade. Local anesthetic agents that are tightly protein bound (e.g., bupiviacine, etidocaine, and tetracaine) produce a block of longer duration than those that are less tightly bound (e.g., procaine and prilocaine). The duration of the block is also related to the concentration of local anesthetic agent used.

Speed of Onset

The speed with which the block commences is directly related to the rapidity with which the agent is able to diffuse through the nervous tissue membrane to the protein receptor in the sodium channel. This, in turn, is related to the concentration gradient (e.g., 1% vs. 2% lidocaine) between the site of injection and the site of action, and the amount of drug in the nonionized form, as it is the latter that moves most quickly through tissues and across lipid membranes. Local anesthetic agents are weak bases (proton receptors) that tend to become positively charged (ionized) as the pH of the environment falls (e.g., infected tissue), thereby reducing movement through tissues and lipid membranes and delaying the onset of the block.

The pKa of a substance is the pH at which 50% of the agent is ionized and 50% is nonionized. The pKa values of local anesthetic agents vary from 7.6 (mepivicaine) to 8.9 (procaine). Accordingly, at physiologic pH (7.4) procaine is almost totally ionized with a slow onset time while mepivicaine is a little more than 50% ionized allowing a more rapid onset. The pKa of local anesthetic agents may be relevant to some aspects of the their clinical use. A common strategy to obtain a rapid-onset block with a long duration of action is to mix a low pKa agent (e.g., lidocaine) with a highly protein-bound agent (e.g., bupivicaine). Clinicians are usually taught that local anesthetic agents are not particularly effective at producing adequate local anesthesia when injected into infected tissues. Low tissue pH results in relatively more of the

Table 27-1. Physicochemical and Biologic Properties of Local Anesthetic Agents

Agent	Lipid Solubility	Potency	Protein Binding (%)	Average Duration (min)	pKa (25°C)	Onset (min)	Maximum Dose (mg/kg)
			Esters				
Procaine	Low	1	6	40	8.9	18	7
Chloroprocaine	Low	1	–	45	8.7	5	8
Tetracaine	High	8	76	200	8.5	15	1.5
			Amides				
Bupivacaine	High	8	96	200	8.1	10	3
Lidocaine	Medium	2	64	100	7.9	5	4
Prilocaine	Medium	2	55	100	7.9	5	5
Etidocaine	High	6	94	200	7.7	3	3
Mepivicaine	Low	2	78	100	7.6	3	4

Source: From Savarese JJ, Covino BG. In: Miller RD, ed. *Anesthesia.* New York: Churchill Livingstone; 1986:985–1013; and Tucker GT. Pharmacokinetics of local anesthetics. *Br J Anaesth.* 1986;58:717–731.

agent being ionized, leading to poor tissue penetration. To some extent this can be mitigated by increasing the concentration of the local anesthetic agent used, or buffering it with bicarbonate.[3]

Biotransformation and Elimination

As with all drugs, the balance between the rate of absorption and the rate of elimination influences the toxicity of local anesthetic agents. Generally, the more concentrated the local anesthetic solution, the higher the blood level and the greater the risk of adverse reactions. This has led to the practice of using the lowest concentration of agent consistent with achieving a satisfactory block.[4]

The rate of absorption of a local anesthetic depends on the route of delivery, and the vascularity of the area where it is deposited, particularly in the case of local anesthesia achieved by infiltration and nerve block. As one might expect, intravenous, pulmonary, and mucosal routes more rapidly achieve peak blood levels than subcutaneous and intramuscular routes, with epidural routes being of intermediate speed. The addition of vasoconstrictor agents (e.g., epinephrine and phenylephrine) to the local anesthetic solution reduces the vascularity to the site of drug administration, enhancing the duration of some agents (decreasing "washout") and increasing the maximum dose allowable.

Typically, agents of the ester class are degraded rather rapidly by liver and plasma esterases limiting their potential for toxicity, though the hydrolysis of tetracaine may be up to five times slower than that of procaine.[5] The amide class of local anesthetic agents are more resistant to hydrolysis and for the most part are metabolized somewhat more slowly by mixed function oxidases in the liver.[6] This contributes to the generally increased toxicity of amide class.

Dosage

Table 27-1 lists the maximum dosage guidelines on a per kilogram of *ideal body weight* basis. The clinical situations where one may inadvertently exceed these maximums are the following:

- *Pediatrics:* In the very young, the ratio of lean to total body weight is lower; small errors in calculation may lead to substantial overdoses.
- Obese patients.
- Nerve block anesthesia: Higher cumulative doses may be required for multiple intercostal blocks for rib fracture pain management or for topical or infiltration local anesthetic agents for large areas of "road rash."

In addition, toxicity may occur rapidly when slow diffusion out of tissues does not occur due to the following:

- The inadvertent intravascular injection of an agent, or the injection of large doses of medication into a very vascular area (e.g., pterygopalatine fossa and inflamed tissue).
- Use of an agent topically on a vascular and mucous membrane (e.g., nasal, oral, or tracheal mucosa).

Additives

Three substances are commonly added to local anesthetic solutions: Vasoconstrictors, antibacterial agents, and buffering solutions. The addition of vasoconstricting agents (e.g., epinephrine and phenylephrine) to infiltrated local anesthetic agents reduces regional blood flow and retards the pace of absorption of the local anesthetic agent. This leads to:

- Reduced blood loss.
- Prolonged duration of the block, particularly for the shorter acting agents like lidocaine.
- Attenuation of the rate of rise, and peak level of the agent in the blood serving to increase the maximum tolerable dose.

Lidocaine solution with 1:100,000 epinephrine contains 10 mcg/mL of epinephrine; 1:200,000 contains 5 mcg/mL. The addition of a vasoconstrictor agent limits the use of these agents in situations where ischemia may occur (flaps and end organs and digits) and in patients where systemic absorption of the vasoconstrictor may produce untoward effects (e.g., coronary artery disease and hypertension).

Preservative agents are so dubbed because they "preserve the sterility" of the solution in multidose vials. EDTA and sodium bisulfite have been used in some local anesthetic preparations in the past as antioxidants (*stabilizers*), though they have been abandoned for the most part. Methylparaben is often added to multidose vials as an antibacterial agent. While useful in preserving the sterility of multidose vials with respect to the most commonly found bacteria and fungi, methylparaben is not effective against viruses. This led directly to the recommendation in the early 1990s that health care providers confine their use of local anesthetic agents to those drawn from unit dose vials. In addition, methylparaben is metabolized to a PABA derivative and has been implicated in the vast majority of IgE-mediated anaphylactic reactions to amide class local anesthetic agents (rather than the local anesthetic agent itself).

Buffering local anesthetic agents with bicarbonate or THAM serves to reduce pain on injection, improve the performance of the agent in acidic environments, and improve the penetration of topically applied agents, particularly when applied to mucous membranes.[7]

NEUROPHARMACOLOGY OF NEURAL BLOCKADE

The capacity of a local anesthetic agent to induce blockade of neural transmission in the peripheral nervous system is related to the structure of the peripheral nerve. The peripheral nervous system is composed of the roots, rami and branches of cranial and spinal nerves, and the elements of the autonomic nervous system that accompany them.

Structurally, a mixed peripheral nerve contains multiple small bundles of nerve fibers called *fascicles* bound together by a fibrous *endoneurium*. The fascicle is surrounded by fibrous *perineurium* and multiple fascicles are assembled into a peripheral nerve and wrapped in *epineurium.* These connective tissue elements organize and protect the nervous tissue and provide a conduit for lymphatics and blood vessels. At the same time, these elements impede the diffusion of local anesthetic agents to their intended sites of action. In addition, their fibrous and unelastic nature contributes to pressure-induced nerve damage when substances are injected directly into nerves.

Individual nerve fibers vary in their degree of myelinization, speed of conduction, and susceptibility to blockade. A-alpha and A-beta fibers are heavily myelinated, rapidly conducting fiber types subserving motor and proprioceptive functions (Table 27-2). This degree of myelinization insulates these fibers from local anesthetic agents and prevents blockade by weak solutions of local anesthetic agents. A-delta and C-fibers are afferent sensory fibers conducting pain, temperature, and touch sensations. They are the least myelinated fibers and the easiest to block, even with weak solutions of local anesthetic agents. B fibers,

preganglionic sympathetic fibers, are lightly myelinated. This explains why vasodilation (sympathetic block) and sensory block occur quickly, followed by a variable amount of motor block following the injection of a local anesthetic agent near a mixed peripheral nerve (nerve block).

The ability to deliberately vary the concentration of local anesthetic agent to block some nerve fibers and not others is called *differential neural blockade*. The goal is to preserve motor function and proprioception but obliterate pain. The best clinical example of how this property of local anesthetic agents is employed is the use of continuous epidural infusions of local anesthetic agents (bupivicaine 0.0625–0.125%) and opioids (fentanyl 2–5 mcg/mL) to control acute postoperative pain (e.g., thoracotomy and large abdominal incisions) and the pain of labor ("walking" epidural). It is also used diagnostically by chronic pain specialists to determine which fiber type is responsible for pain transmission in a particular pain syndrome with a view to planning more effective long-term pain management strategies.

TOXICITY AND ADVERSE REACTIONS

Adverse reactions and responses to local anesthetic agents are fairly common. They typically take one of six forms:

1. Vasoconstrictor reactions
2. Agent toxicity (particularly neurologic and cardiac)
3. IgE-mediated anaphylaxis
4. Methemoglobinemia
5. Injection pain
6. Vasovagal reactions (presyncope and syncope)

Vasoconstrictor Reaction

This is perhaps the most common adverse reaction reported. The setting is often the dental chair when shortly after the injection of local anesthetic agent with epinephrine into a

Table 27-2. Classification and Function of Peripheral Nerve Fibers

Class	Subclass	Myelin	Function
A	Alpha (α)	+++	Motor, proprioception
	Beta (α)	+++	Motor, touch, pressure
	Gamma (γ)	++	Muscle spindle, reflex
	Delta (δ)	+	Pain, temperature, nociception
B		+	Preganglionic autonomic
C		0	Pain, temperature, nociception

Source: After Refs. 1 and 2.

particularly vascular space (e.g., the pterygopalatine space for a posterior superior alveolar block), the patient complains of suddenly feeling apprehensive and panicky and senses rapid heart action. The event abates rapidly. The patient will often relate this reaction as an *allergic* reaction to subsequent health care providers.

Agent Toxicity

The major manifestations of local anesthetic toxicity relate to the central nervous system (CNS) and the cardiovascular system (CVS). The direct intravascular injection of a moderately large dose of local anesthetic agent (e.g., lidocaine 100 mg: 5 mL of 2%, or 10 mL of 1%) will produce numbness and tingling of the lips, a metallic taste and the sensation that hearing is muffled or even tinnitus. It is sometimes said that "… if the patient hears sirens and you don't … prepare to manage a local anesthetic seizure." Drowsiness (even coma) and tonic clonic seizures may also result. The latter tend to be self-limited and benign, requiring little specific therapy.

Less often, the toxicity is related to the continuous absorption of agent from a large depot injection (e.g., multiple intercostal nerve blocks) or the injection of a moderately large dose of medication in a very vascular area (e.g., caudal epidural block). Drowsiness and perhaps continuous seizure activity may result, requiring aggressive antiseizure management.

The CVS is four to seven times less susceptible than the CNS to the toxic effects of local anesthetic agents though there is some variability between different local anesthetic agents. Direct myocardial depression and pump failure may be seen, particularly if the patient is also on beta-blockers or calcium channel blockers. Toxicity of the agents can lead to conduction disturbances up to and including heart block and asystole. It is generally recommended that if the etiology of a cardiac arrest is suspected to be due to a local anesthetic agent, then resuscitative efforts should continue for a prolonged period allowing termination of action of the agent in the cardiac conduction system.

IgE-Mediated Anaphylaxis

Anaphylaxis to local anesthetic agents is very rare, particularly to the amide class.[8] Case reports of anaphylaxis to amide agents are exceedingly rare, so much so that an incidence cannot be computed. Even at that, the methylparaben added to multidose vials as a preservative is often implicated as the culprit more so than the amide local anesthetic. Metabolism of ester class agents to PABA derivatives has been credited with the potential for this class of agent to produce anaphylaxis.

The investigation of a reported allergic reaction to local anesthetic agents ought to begin with an exhaustive history looking especially for symptoms consistent with vasoconstrictor reactions, agent toxicity, or vasovagal type reactions. The patient is rarely aware of the name of the specific local anesthetic agent. Retrieval of the specific event record is often very difficult. If anaphylaxis remains a possibility, intradermal testing (1 mm skin wheal) utilizing progressively less dilute solutions (beginning at 1:10,000) of the local anesthetic agent one wishes to use has been recommended by some.[8,9]

Benzyl alcohol 0.9% and diphenhydramine 0.5–1.0% have also been used to produce local anesthesia when the clinician has wished to avoid the issue of local anesthetic allergy all together. The duration of action of both agents is somewhat less than lidocaine with both tending to produce more pain on injection.[10–14] A 1% concentration of diphenhydramine is more effective at producing local anesthesia than the 0.5% solution.

Methemoglobinemia

Hemoglobin is continuously oxidized to methemoglobin, its ferric state, in the red cell rendering it incapable of combining with oxygen. Ordinarily, this methemoglobin is continuously reduced back to its ferrous state by enzymes such as methemoglobin reductase to maintain *normal* levels of methemoglobin of about 1% (higher in smokers).[15] Though other local anesthetic agents interfere with methemoglobin reductase to some extent (e.g., lidocaine), prilocaine and benzocaine are particularly problematic. This surfaces in day-to-day practice most often with the use of benzocaine sprays (Hurricaine and Cetacaine) on mucosal surfaces. Methemoglobinemia has also been reported in patients following the application of eutectic mixture of local anesthetic (EMLA) cream for topical anesthesia for circumcision and laser epilation therapy of the legs.[16,17]

Injection Pain

All of the following techniques have been found to reduce the pain associated with the infiltration of local anesthetic agents[18–22]:

1. Using buffered solutions: Buffering is usually accomplished by mixing 1% lidocaine with 8.4% sodium bicarbonate in a 9:1 ratio.
2. Using solutions warmed to 37–39°C (98.6–102°F).
3. Preapplication of a topical agent.
4. Using small needles.
5. Minimizing the number of punctures.

6. Injecting into the subcutaneous space as opposed to the dermis.

7. Injecting slowly.

CLINICAL USE

In clinical practice. local anesthetic agents are used to induce neural blockade in several ways:

1. Topical anesthesia
2. Local infiltration
3. Field block anesthesia
4. Nerve block
5. Neuraxial anesthesia (epidural and spinal anesthesia): see Chapter 24

Topical Anesthesia

This section provides a brief overview of topical anesthesia. A more complete discussion is provided in Chapter 26.

Intact skin serves as an effective barrier to the penetration of drugs meaning that, for the most part, if one wishes to gain access to the sensory nerve endings in the skin, one must infiltrate the medication subcutaneously. There are, however, innovative ways in which this relatively impenetrable barrier can be attenuated and broached. The mixing of 2.5% solid lidocaine base with 2.5% solid prilocaine base produces an oily substance (a *eutectic mixture* of local anesthetic agents or EMLA) at room temperature that when mixed with an inert vehicle produces a cream containing local anesthetic agent. The lidocaine and prilocaine-free base (nonionized) penetrate intact skin slowly to anesthetize dermal and subcutaneous sensory nerve endings to a depth of roughly 5 mm.[23] Peak blood levels of both agents remain well below toxic limits, provided the mixture is used on intact skin and not on abraded integument or mucous membranes.

ELA-max is a 4% liposomal encapsulated lidocaine cream that has been demonstrated to be as effective as EMLA for similar indications.[24,25] Liposomes are microscopic phospholipid bilayer vesicles which act as permeable barriers to entrap either hydrophilic or lipophilic drug molecules. In addition to being effective drug carriers, liposomes can enhance drug delivery to the dermis by increasing the rate of dermal penetration of drugs.[26] Liposome-encapsulated tetracaine (5%) has been shown to provide more effective topical anaesthesia than EMLA for intravenous catheter placement a after 60-min application.[27]

The dermis can be made more permeable to local anesthetic agents by applying a direct current through a lidocaine-soaked pad on the skin. This *electrophoresis* causes the transport of sufficient amounts of lidocaine to afford anesthesia. The procedure is time consuming and awkward in clinical practice and has not gained widespread popularity.

Local anesthetic agents are moderately effective when applied to open wounds and abraded dermis contributing to the popularity of such substances as TAC (tetracaine adrenaline cocaine), LET (lidocaine epinephrine tetracaine), and viscous lidocaine (2–4% solutions). Gel or ointment formulations of TAC and LET are somewhat easier to contain in a particular location than their aqueous counterparts.

Mucous membranes, on the other hand are for the most part freely permeable to local anesthetic agents such that topical anesthesia of the cornea, gingiva, pharynx, larynx, trachea and conducting airways, esophagus, rectum, bladder, and so forth is readily achieved. Due to high absorption and bioavailability of the agents when applied to mucosal surfaces or abraded skin there exists a greater risk of systemic toxicity in the event that recommended dose maximums are exceeded.

The local anesthetic agent is typically applied directly to the mucosal surface in an aqueous, gel (viscous), or cream base format. Nebulization may be employed to topically anesthetize the upper or lower airway. The encapsulation of nebulized local anesthetic agents in liposomes has been employed to enhance penetration and prolong the duration of the block.

Local Infiltration

This is the usual method employed to render a wound insensitive for the purpose of surgical repair. As mentioned previously, buffered solutions of local anesthetic agent are less painful on infiltration as is the subcutaneous infiltration of agent as opposed to the injection directly into the dermis. Injection of a local anesthetic agent around a wound through intact skin is called a field block and is usually more painful than local infiltration through the wound.

Field Block

A field block is the infiltration of a wall of local anesthetic agent to surround an operative site. For the most part, sensory nerves travel in the subcutaneous tissues to elaborate sensory nerve endings in the dermis. Injection into the subcutaneous tissue meets with less resistance and is less painful than injection into the dermis. Field blocks are useful for large cutaneous wounds (e.g., scalp), when minimal tissue distortion is desired (e.g., vermillion border or facial wounds) or for the incision and drainage of cutaneous and subcutaneous abscesses.

Nerve Block

Regional anesthesia that is achieved by injecting a local anesthetic near a nerve, nerves, or plexi innervating that particular area is called a nerve block. The region may be relatively circumscribed such as in an ankle or wrist block, an entire limb as in a brachial plexus block (*major regional anesthesia*) or half the body such as in an epidural or spinal anesthetic (*major neuraxial anesthesia*). These blocks are used to facilitate an array of surgical procedures and in the management of a variety of painful conditions.

SUMMARY

Local anesthetic agents are employed in many ways to enhance the quality of care delivered in managing acute and chronic pain, minor surgical procedures, and wounds. Clinicians employing these agents need to have a firm grasp of their dosage limits, toxicity, and routes of administration to best use them safely.

REFERENCES

1. Murphy MF. Local anesthetic agents. *Emerg Med Clin North Am.* 1988;6:769–776.
2. deJong RH. *Local Anesthetics.* St Louis, MO: Mosby; 1994:4.
3. deJong RH. *Local Anesthetics.* St Louis, MO: Mosby; 1994:110–111.
4. deJong RH. *Local Anesthetics.* St Louis, MO: Mosby; 1994:147.
5. deJong RH. *Local Anesthetics.* St Louis, MO: Mosby; 1994:177.
6. deJong RH. *Local Anesthetics.* St Louis, MO: Mosby; 1994:188, 193.
7. deJong RH. *Local Anesthetics.* St Louis, MO: Mosby; 1994:112.
8. Fisher MM, Bowey CJ. Alleged allergy to local anaesthetics. *Anaesth Intensive Care.* 1997;25:611–614.
9. Lu DP. Managing patients with local anesthetic complications using alternative methods. *Pa Dent J.* (Harrisb). 2002;69:22–29.
10. Bartfield JM, Jandreau SW, Raccio-Robak N. Randomized trial of diphenhydramine versus benzyl alcohol with epinephrine as an alternative to lidocaine local anesthesia. *Ann Emerg Med.* 1998;32:650–654.
11. Ernst AA, Marvez-Valls E, Nick TG, et al. Comparison trial of four injectable anesthetics for laceration repair. *Acad Emerg Med.* 1996;3:228–233.
12. Ernst AA, Marvez-Valls E, Mall G, et al. 1% lidocaine versus 0.5% diphenhydramine for local anesthesia in minor laceration repair. *Ann Emerg Med.* 1994;23:1328–1332.
13. Green SM, Rothrock SG, Gorchynski J. Validation of diphenhydramine as a dermal local anesthetic. *Ann Emerg Med.* 1994;23:1284–1289.
14. Dire DJ, Hogan DE. Double-blinded comparison of diphenhydramine versus lidocaine as a local anesthetic. *Ann Emerg Med.* 1993;22:1419–1422.
15. deJong RH. Local *Anesthetics.* St Louis, MO: Mosby; 1994:365.
16. Couper RT. Methaemoglobinaemia secondary to topical lignocaine/ prilocaine in a circumcised neonate. *J Paediatr Child Health.* 2000;36:406–407.
17. Hahn IH, Hoffman RS, Nelson LS. EMLA-induced methemoglobinemia and systemic topical anesthetic toxicity. *J Emerg Med.* 2004;26:85–88.
18. Davies RJ. Buffering the pain of local anaesthetics: a systematic review. *Emerg Med* (Fremantle). 2003;15:81–88.
19. Christoph RA, Buchanan L, Begalla K, et al. Pain reduction in local anesthetic administration through pH buffering. *Ann Emerg Med.* 1988;17:117–120.
20. Bartfield JM, Crisafulli KM, Raccio-Robak N, et al. The effects of warming and buffering on pain of infiltration of lidocaine. *Acad Emerg Med.* 1995;2:254–258.
21. Schooff M. Lessening the pain of lidocaine injection. *J Fam Pract.* 1998;46:279.
22. Scarfone RJ, Jasani M, Gracely EJ. Pain of local anesthetics: rate of administration and buffering. *Ann Emerg Med.* 1998;31:36–40.
23. Broadman LM, Rice LJ. Neural blockade for pediatric surgery. In: Cousins MJ, Bridenbaugh PO, eds. *Neural Blockade, in Clinical Anesthesia and Management of Pain.* Philadelphia, PA: Lippincott-Raven; 1998:633.
24. Eichenfield LF, Funk A, Fallon-Friedlander S, et al. A clinical study to evaluate the efficacy of ELA-Max (4% liposomal lidocaine) as compared with eutectic mixture of local anesthetics cream for pain reduction of venipuncture in children. *Pediatrics.* 2002;109:1093–1099.
25. Tang MB, Goon AT, Goh CL. Study on the efficacy of ELA-Max (4% liposomal lidocaine) compared with EMLA cream (eutectic mixture of local anesthetics) using thermosensory threshold analysis in adult volunteers. *J Dermatolog Treat.* 2004;15:84–87.
26. Foldvari M, Gesztes A, Mezei M. Dermal drug delivery by liposome encapsulation: clinical and electron microscopic studies. *J Microencapsul.* 1990;7:479–489.
27. Hung OR, Comeau L, Riley M, et al. Comparative topical anesthesia of EMLA and liposome-encapsulated tetracaine. *Can J Anaesth.* 1997;44:707–711.

28

Rapid Sequence Intubation (RSI)

Michael F. Murphy
Ron M. Walls

Emergency airway management is a crucially important part of the resuscitation of a critically ill or injured patient and the difficulties and variations presented can challenge the provider to the extremes of resourcefulness, judgment, and skill. From the patient's perspective, endotracheal intubation is associated with substantial stimulation and physiologic responses. Attenuating the aggression of these responses to intubation, maintaining adequate oxygen saturations during the procedure, and protecting the airway from aspiration are integral to the procedure. In the absence of an identified difficult airway, rapid sequence intubation (RSI) is the method of choice for emergency airway management. Even in some difficult airways, RSI, often with a "double setup" is still the preferred method. RSI can be considered at the "deep" end of the spectrum of procedural sedation, in which general anesthesia is induced for the purpose of securing the airway. In other words, RSI is a special method of deep (general anesthesia) sedation that facilitates the procedure of emergency intubation.

RAPID SEQUENCE INTUBATION (RSI)

RSI is defined as the virtually simultaneous administration of an induction agent and a neuromuscular blocking agent to facilitate endotracheal intubation.[1] RSI consists of several logical and sequential steps that are intended to:

- Render a patient amnestic for the event.
- Ensure that oxygenation is maintained through the procedure.

HIGH YIELD FACTS

- Rapid sequence intubation (RSI) is the virtually simultaneous administration of an induction agent and a neuromuscular blocking agent to facilitate endotracheal intubation.

- The goals of RSI are to maintain oxygenation, minimize aspiration risk, modulate the physiologic responses, ensure tube placement, patient amnestic for procedure.

- Physiologic responses to intubation are ↑ intracranial pressure (ICP), ↑ airways resistance, ↑ adrenergic activity, ↑ cholinergic response.

- ↑ adrenergic activity causes ↑ systolic/diastolic blood pressure (BP), ↑ heart rate (HR), ↑ MVO_2, ventricular dysrhythmias, ↓ gastric emptying, ileus.

- ↑ cholinergic response causes bronchoconstriction, bronchorrhea; rarely bradycardia except in children/infants (especially if hypoxemic).

- At-risk patients include patients with reactive airway disease, aorta/major vessel rupture, ischemia/valvular heart disease, heart failure, L → R shunts, corpulmonale, ↑ ICP.

- Seven Ps of RSI: preparation, preoxygenation, pretreatment, paralysis with induction, protection/positioning, pass the tube, and postintubation management.

- Nonpharmacologic methods to limit adverse physiologic responses: limit laryngoscopy time, preoxygenate, hyperventilate, use a less stimulating technique, atraumatic passing of tube, and keep tube off carina.

- Pretreatment drugs: lidocaine 1–1.5 mg/kg, fentanyl 2–3 mcg/kg, atropine (if ≤10 years old, bradycardic, or asystole) 0.01–0.02 mg/kg (minimum 0.1 mg, maximum 0.5 mg).

- Ensure that the risk of pulmonary aspiration is minimized.
- Mitigate the intensity of physiologic responses that may threaten the integrity of vital organs.
- Ensure that the tube is placed correctly within the trachea.

Employing RSI medications assumes that one is highly competent in the following:

1. Bag and mask ventilation.
2. Evaluation of the airway for possible difficult intubation or bag/mask ventilation.
3. The use of rescue devices and the performance of a surgical airway.

PROCEDURAL EFFECTS

The larynx is the most heavily innervated sensory structure in the body.[2] Laryngoscopy and endotracheal intubation stimulate sensory nerve endings in the upper airway to produce intense physiologic responses that can produce serious results in some patients if not attenuated.

Patients with limited cardiopulmonary and central nervous system (CNS) reserve present an additional challenge when it comes to endotracheal intubation. The individual performing the intubation must *assess the reserve* of each of these organ systems, evaluate how the act of intubation might affect them, and then select adjunctive medications and a technique to mitigate these adverse effects.

The intensity of these physiologic responses is related to the intensity of stimulation, which in turn depends on[3]:

- The duration of laryngoscopy.
- The aggressiveness of laryngoscopy.
- The degree of attendant hypoxemia/hypercarbia.
- Stimulation of the carina by the endotracheal tube.
- The use of alternative placement techniques (e.g., lighted stylet) that produce less stimulation.

The three most important organ systems impacted by endotracheal intubation are the brain, the heart, and the lungs. Depending on the patient, the following organ system responses to endotracheal intubation may be the most important to consider:

- Increased intracranial pressure (ICP) and cerebral blood flow, particularly if autoregulation is disturbed.
- The upper airway and respiratory system.
  - Increased airways resistance, e.g., in reactive airways disease.

- The autonomic nervous system: (a) *Adrenergic responses*: Endotracheal intubation causes increased adrenergic activity with activation of the sympathetic nervous system and elevated circulating catecholamines. This in turn results in the following:
  - An increased systolic blood pressure (SBP) and mean arterial blood pressure (MAP) (up to two times normal).
  - Increased diastolic blood pressure (DBP) (up to 50% increase).
  - Increased heart rate (HR) (up to 50% increase).
  - Overall increased cardiac work and myocardial oxygen consumption (MVO_2).
  - Increased rate/pressure product (increased intravascular *shear* pressure).
  - Ventricular dysrhythmias (increased automaticity/irritability due to increased circulating catecholamines and increased BP).
  - Decreased gastric emptying (increased gastric volume and risk of aspiration).

Cholinergic responses:

- Bronchoconstriction and bronchorrhea.
- Bradycardia: Rarely but occasionally in children and infants, especially if hypoxemic.

PATIENTS AT RISK

All patients should be considered as potentially at risk from the adverse cardiovascular and pulmonary responses to endotracheal intubation; however, patients with the following underlying conditions may be at *particular risk:*

The upper airway and respiratory system

- Reactive airways disease.

The cardiovascular system

- Major vessel aneurysm rupture (congenital, traumatic, or atherosclerotic).
- Aortic or major vessel dissection.
- Ischemic heart disease (IHD).
- Left ventricular systolic or diastolic dysfunction (failure) due to any etiology (e.g., ischemic, hypertensive, and congestive).
- Valvular heart disease: Stenotic lesions limit the heart's ability to provide an adequate cardiac output to meet the needs of the body; regurgitant lesions may see increased regurgitant flow in the face of increased systemic vascular resistance (SVR).

- Left to right shunts (e.g., ventricular septal defect ([VSD]) will increase as SVR and LV systolic pressures increase.

- Cor pulmonale: The stress of intubation increases pulmonary vascular resistance (PVR) and in the face of cor pulmonale, may produce acute right heart failure.

- Cardiomyopathy, IHD, metabolic disturbance (especially acidosis, hyperkalemia, and hypokalemia), or hypoxemia: ventricular and atrial arrhythmias may be induced.

The brain

- Patients with intracranial hypertension or increased ICP.
- Patients with intracranial hemorrhage.

RSI: THE PROCEDURE

RSI can be thought of as a series of steps; the *seven Ps of RSI*.[4] It is a useful framework for discussing the procedure:

1. Preparation

2. Preoxygenation

This is a crucial step permitting oxygen saturations to remain acceptable during the period of apnea as the neuromuscular blocking agent becomes fully effective. The goal is to replace the nitrogen in the patient's functional residual capacity (FRC; normally 30 mL/kg) with oxygen. The ability to do so varies with the time available, the ability of the oxygen delivery apparatus to deliver high concentrations oxygen used, and the patient's condition.

3. Pretreatment

The goal of pretreatment is to attenuate the adverse responses to intubation, particularly the surges in HR, BP, ICP, and airways resistance. Ideally, the pretreatment medications ought to precede the induction agent by 3 minutes to be optimally effective. Not all patients are equally at risk from these responses. Based on the best available evidence and expert recommendations at least, the following patients should be considered for pretreatment:

- Those suspected to have elevated ICP and imperfect autoregulation: lidocaine 1.5 mg/kg and fentanyl 3–13 mcg/kg (ordinarily 3–5 mcg/kg).[5–9]

- Those with significant IHD, or major vessel dissection or rupture: fentanyl 3–13 mcg/kg (ordinarily 3–5 mcg/kg).[10–13] Caution ought to be exercised in administering fentanyl to patients with compensated or uncompensated shock, who are dependent on sympathetic drive.

- Adults with significant existing reactive airways disease: lidocaine 1.5 mg/kg.[14–22]

- Children up to the age of 10, or any patient with potentially hemodynamically significant bradycardia where succinylcholine is to be used: atropine 0.02 mg/kg (minimum 0.1 mg, maximum 0.5 mg).

4. Paralysis with induction

Both the induction agent and the neuromuscular blocking agent (usually succinylcholine) are administered by rapid intravenous (IV) push. Induction agents have profound effects on all three vital organ systems: the CNS, cardiovascular system, and ventilation. These effects depend on the particular drug, the patient's underlying physiologic condition, and the dose and speed of injection of the drug. Because RSI requires rapid administration of the sedative/induction agent, the choice of drug and the dose *must be tailored* to capitalize on desired effects, while minimizing those that might adversely affect the patient. In highly compromised patients with minimal or no cardiovascular reserve, an amnestic dose may be selected, rather an induction dose. While the sedative/induction dose might be tailored, the dose of the neuromuscular blocking agent is not. (e.g., succinylcholine 1.5 mg/kg and rocuronium 1 mg/kg).

5. Protection and positioning

Cricoid pressure is maintained to prevent regurgitation and aspiration until proper placement of the endotracheal tube is confirmed. Premature release of cricoid pressure is a common error, and places the patient at risk of aspiration, particularly if an inadvertent esophageal intubation has occurred. It has been recommended that cricoid pressure be released immediately should active vomiting occur to avoid the possibility of esophageal rupture, but there is no evidence in support of this, and fortunately, active vomiting is not possible with neuromuscular blockade. Most experts on airway management agree that positioning the head and neck is an important step in gaining the best view of the larynx with conventional laryngoscopy. It has long been taught that the "sniffing the morning air" or "sipping English tea" positioning of the head and neck, when possible, is best. Recent studies have shown that simple extension of the neck appears to facilitate the same glottic view as does extension accompanied by elevation (the two motions that achieve the "sniffing" position.) Most providers, however, still prefer the sniffing position, absent any contraindications (e.g., potential cervical spine injury).

6. Placement (of the tube into the trachea)

7. Postintubation management

MITIGATING AND PREVENTING THE ADVERSE PHYSIOLOGIC RESPONSES TO INTUBATION

Nonpharmacologic Methods

Increased stimulation of the larynx proportionately increases the adrenergic and ICP responses to intubation. Therefore, limiting the duration and aggression of laryngoscopy mitigates the degree of the physiologic response. Preoxygenation minimizes the possibility of hypoxemia during intubation, and the adrenergic response that it generates.

In summary, the nonpharmacologic methods of limiting the adverse physiologic responses to intubation include the following:

- Limit the time of laryngoscopy.
- Preoxygenate and use a pulse oximeter.
- Hyperventilate modestly by bag and mask (decrease $PaCO_2$), if increased ICP or impaired autoregulation is suspected.
- Use an alternative technique that is associated with less stimulation, if reasonable (e.g., lighted stylet).
- Pass the endotracheal tube in an atraumatic way.
- Keep the tube off the carina.

Pharmacologic Methods

When using medications to attenuate the physiologic responses to intubation one must balance the need to control the response against the capacity of the patient to respond to the stimulus. Consider the following:

- The additive or potentiating effects of one technique or drug on another (e.g., patients with total upper-airway anesthesia may require less induction agent, intoxicated patients need less induction agent, and the patient with borderline hypotension may be worsened by the synergistic effects of fentanyl and the induction agent).
- The patient's physiologic reserve: Patients who have reduced cardiac reserve (ventricular systolic or diastolic dysfunction or valvular heart disease) are more sensitive to myocardial depressants such as induction agents, as are patients who are hypovolemic, such as those with uncontrolled hypertension, blood loss, or dehydration.
- The potential of an adverse outcome is related to the physiologic response to intubation: The physiologic response to intubation may be especially detrimental in patients with moderate-to-severe asthma, IHD, elevated ICP, intracranial hemorrhage, or rupturing or major vessel dissection.
- Underlying sympathetic tone: If the sympathetic nervous system is already maximally stimulated (e.g., hemorrhagic shock) and the patient is barely compensated, one must be cautious with any drug that can reduce sympathetic tone. This includes all sedative hypnotic agents, neuroleptics, opioids, lidocaine, and histamine releasers. Etomidate (perhaps in a reduced dose), ketamine, succinylcholine, and pancuronium are the best choices.

RSI MEDICATIONS

Induction Agents

Anesthetic induction agents are all potent drugs possessing profound effects on the three major vital organ systems: the heart, the brain, and the lungs. All have the potential of producing hypotension and apnea. The degree to which these drugs produce hypotension and apnea depends on the particular drug, the patient's underlying physiologic condition, and the dose and speed of injection of the drug. The faster rates of administration and higher doses are generally associated with more pronounced effects. Because RSI requires rapid administration of the sedative/induction agent, the choice of drug and the dose must be individualized to capitalize on desired effects, while minimizing those that might adversely affect the patient.

When using medications to mitigate the adverse physiologic responses to intubation in patients with marginal pulmonary or cardiovascular reserve (e.g., those that are critically ill), administer conservative doses and err on the side of "too little" rather than "too much" choosing amnesia rather than anesthesia. If postintubation hypertension and tachycardia occur, they can be managed by administering small doses of some induction agents (e.g., propofol and pentothal) or by titrating an opioid such as fentanyl.

All of the induction agents discussed in "RSI: The Procedure" may be used in RSI. Dosing of induction agents in normal sized and obese adults should be based on ideal body weight in kilograms. This can be estimated by subtracting 100 from the patient's height in centimeters, i.e., 6 ft 4 in. = 76 in. × 2.54 cm/in. = 193 cm − 100 = 93 kg.[23] This provides a very acceptable estimate of ideal body weight and the administered induction dose can then be adjusted based on the clinical status of the patient.

Etomidate is generally considered the induction agent of choice in RSI in an emergency, particularly when hemodynamic stability is questioned. Etomidate is somewhat less effective than some of the other induction agents with respect to mitigating the rise in BP that attends intubation, perhaps an undesirable event in some conditions (e.g., elevated ICP, ischemic coronary disease, and major vessel dissection). In such cases, pretreatment with fentanyl (3–5 mcg/kg) is recommended to minimize this adverse effect.

Ketamine is the RSI induction agent of choice for patients with reactive airways disease, and is the most hemodynamically stable of the induction agents, making it also a desirable induction agent for patients who are hypovolemic or hypotensive. Ketamine's associated catecholamine release may increase myocardial oxygen demand in patients with IHD. The use of ketamine in patients with elevated ICP remains controversial, and literature has been conflicting with respect to ketamine's ability (or lack of ability) to elevate ICP. The ability of ketamine to preserve central respiratory drive makes it an appealing choice for awake intubation and diagnostic work around the upper airway.

Propofol is an excellent induction agent in stable patients. Its potential to induce hypotension and reduced cerebral perfusion may limit its use in an emergency, though it does have the advantage over etomidate and ketamine of more effectively attenuating rises in BP that may be undesirable in some patients.

Pretreatment Agents

Lidocaine is recommended as a pretreatment agent in a variety of circumstances. It has been shown unequivocally that 1.5 mg/kg of lidocaine IV 3 minutes before intubation suppresses the cough reflex and attenuates the increase in airway resistance that attends stimulation of the tracheal mucosa by the placement of an endotracheal tube. There is also compelling evidence that lidocaine mitigates the rise in ICP seen with intubation at the same dosage level and timing before intubation. The evidence with respect to the ability of lidocaine to attenuate the sympathetic response to laryngoscopy is conflicting and lidocaine cannot be recommended for this purpose.[24–31]

All the opioids have been demonstrated to be effective in attenuating the sympathetic response to laryngoscopy. Fentanyl is the opioid selected by most for pretreatment, having been demonstrated to partially attenuate the reflex sympathetic response to laryngoscopy at doses as low as 2 mcg/kg, moderately attenuate at 6 mcg/kg, and almost totally obliterate it at 11–15 µg/kg. Unlike some opioids, such as morphine, fentanyl does not release histamine (hypotension) and has no direct effect on the pulmonary response to laryngoscopy and intubation. Although fentanyl has no direct effect on ICP, increasing doses of any of the opioids may suppress ventilation, resulting in hypercarbia, cerebral vasodilation, and subsequent increases in ICP. It is generally recommended that fentanyl 2–3 µg/kg be given as a pretreatment agent to patients with imperfect ICP control and those at risk of surges in BP or pulse rate (e.g., IHD, aortic dissection, and intracranial hemorrhage). Fentanyl should be administered over an interval of 30–60 seconds, as the last of the pretreatment drugs if more than one is to be given and avoided in patients who already have maximally activated their sympathetic nervous systems to maintain vital organ perfusion. Muscular rigidity is a unique and idiosyncratic response to opioids that is related to the dose and speed of opioid administration, the concomitant use of nitrous oxide, and the presence or absence of muscle relaxants. It is not reversible with naloxone (Narcan). Rigidity is rarely seen, and usually occurs only with fentanyl doses well in excess of 500 mcg. It primarily affects the chest and abdominal wall musculature. This rigidity has rarely been reported in conscious patients. This rigidity can be mitigated by the use of defasciculating doses of a nondepolarizing muscle relaxant, and rectified by the administration of a paralyzing dose of succinylcholine.

Atropine is advocated as a pretreatment drug for children 10 years of age and below. This recommendation may be modified if the patient is already excessively tachycardic. In adults, atropine may be indicated in the event that brady-cardia or asystole occurs with a repeat dose of succinylcholine.

The administration of succinylcholine may be associated with a significant rise in ICP when given to patients who already have imperfect ICP control. This rise in ICP can be abolished completely by prior administration of a full dose of a competitive (nondepolarizing) neuromuscular blocking agent, and substantially mitigated by the administration of a defasciculating dose of the same competitive agent. Vecuronium, pancuronium, and rocuronium are the nondepolarizing agents commonly used when succinylcholine is to be employed in these patients. The dose administered is 10% of the paralyzing dose of the same drug, 3 minutes prior to the administration of succinylcholine (i.e., 0.01 mg/kg of vecuronium or pancuronium and 0.06 mg/kg of rocuronium).

Muscle Relaxants

Succinylcholine remains the neuromuscular blocking agent of choice for RSI due to its rapid onset and relatively brief duration of action. The usual dose is 1.5 mg/kg of actual body weight. Succinylcholine has a few important contraindications, related to its propensity to cause severe, acute hyperkalemia in patients with certain myopathic conditions (e.g., muscular dystrophy), or receptor upregulation on muscle membranes (e.g., denervation syndromes, burns, and intra-abdominal sepsis). It is also contraindicated in patients with a personal or family history of malignant hyperthermia. In such cases, or by operator preference, a nondepolarizing neuromuscular blocking agent, such as rocuronium (1.0 mg/kg of ideal body weight) or vecuronium (0.01 mg/kg to *prime* then 0.15 mg/kg of ideal body weight 3 minutes later) may be substituted.

A detailed discussion of the use of neuromuscular blocking agents for emergency RSI can be found in Ref. 32.

REFERENCES

1. Walls RM. Rapid sequence intubation. In: Walls RM, Murphy MF, Luten RC, Schneider RE, eds. *Manual of Emergency Airway Management.* 2nd ed. Philadelphia, PA: Lippincott Williams & Wilkins; 2004:22.

2. Murphy MF. Applied functional anatomy of the airway. In: Walls RM, Murphy MF, Luten RC, Schneider RE, eds. *Manual of Emergency Airway Management.* 2nd ed. Philadelphia, PA: Lippincott Williams & Wilkins; 2004:38.

3. Murphy MF. The Critically ill patient. In: Walls RM, Murphy MF, Luten RC, Schneider RE, eds. *Manual of Emergency Airway Management.* 2nd ed. Philadelphia, PA: Lippincott Williams & Wilkins; 2004:281.

4. Walls RM. Rapid sequence intubation. In: Walls RM, Murphy MF, Luten RC, Schneider RE, eds. *Manual of Emergency Airway Management.* 2nd ed. Philadelphia, PA: Lippincott Williams & Wilkins; 2004:23.

5. Tam S. Intravenous lidocaine: optimal time of injection before tracheal intubation. *Anesth Analg.* 1987;66:1036–1038.

6. Donegan MF, Bedford RF. Intravenously administered lidocaine prevents intracranial hypertension during endotracheal suctioning. *Anesthesiology.* 1980;52:516–518.

7. Yano M, Nishiyama H, Yokota H, et al. Effect of lidocaine on ICP response to endotracheal suctioning. *Anesthesiology.* 1986;64:651–653.

8. Robinson N, Clancy M. In patients with head injury undergoing rapid sequence intubation, does pretreatment with intravenous lignocaine/lidocaine lead to an improved neurological outcome? A review of the literature. *Emerg Med J.* 2001;18:453–457.

9. Grover VK, Reddy GM, Kak VK, et al. Intracranial pressure changes with different doses of lignocaine under general anaesthesia. *Neurol India.* 1999;47:118–121.

10. Horak J, Weiss S. Emergent management of the airway. New pharmacology and the control of comorbidities in cardiac disease, ischemia, and valvular heart disease. *Crit Care Clin.* 2000;16:411–427.

11. Bruder N, Ortega D, Granthil C. Consequences and prevention methods of hemodynamic changes during laryngoscopy and intratracheal intubation *Ann Fr Anesth Reanim.* 1992;11:57–71.

12. Kovac AL. Controlling the hemodynamic response to laryngoscopy and endotracheal intubation. *J Clin Anesth.* 1996; 8:63–79.

13. Adachi YU, Satomoto M, Higuchi H, et al. Fentanyl attenuates the hemodynamic response to endotracheal intubation more than the response to laryngoscopy. *Anesth Analg.* 2002;95: 233–237.

14. Nishino T, Hiraga K, Sugimori K. Effects of i.v. lignocaine on airway reflexes elicited by irritation of the tracheal mucosa in humans anaesthetized with enflurane. *Br J Anaesth.* 1990;64:682–687.

15. Groeben H, Silvanus MT, Beste M, et al. Combined intravenous lidocaine and inhaled salbutamol protect against bronchial hyperreactivity more effectively than lidocaine or salbutamol alone. *Anesthesiology.* 1998;89:862–868.

16. Groeben H, Foster WM, Brown RH. Intravenous lidocaine and oral mexiletine block reflex bronchoconstriction in asthmatic subjects. *Am J Respir Crit Care Med.* 1996;154:885–888.

17. Maslow AD, Regan MM, Israel E, et al. Inhaled albuterol, but not intravenous lidocaine, protects against intubation induced bronchoconstriction in asthma. *Anesthesiology.* 2000;93:1198–2204.

18. Groeben H, Schlicht M, Stieglitz S, et al. Both local anesthetics and salbutamol pretreatment affect reflex bronchoconstriction in volunteers with asthma undergoing awake fiberoptic intubation. *Anesthesiology.* 2002;97:1445–1450.

19. Udezue E. Lidocaine inhalation for cough suppression. *Am J Emerg Med.* 2001;19:206–207.

20. Groeben H, Silvanus MT, Beste M, et al. Combined lidocaine and salbutamol inhalation for airway anesthesia markedly protects against reflex bronchoconstriction. *Chest.* 2000;118: 509–515.

21. Groeben H, Silvanus MT, Beste M, et al. Both intravenous and inhaled lidocaine attenuate reflex bronchoconstriction but at different plasma concentrations. *Am J Respir Crit Care Med.* 1999;159:530–535.

22. Groeben H, Grosswendt T, Silvanus M, et al. Lidocaine inhalation for local anaesthesia and attenuation of bronchial hyper-reactivity with least airway irritation. Effect of three different dose regimens. *Eur J Anaesthesiol.* 2000;17: 672–679.

23. Schneider RE, Caro DA. Sedative and induction agents. In: Walls RM, Murphy MF, Luten RC, Schneider RE, eds. *Manual of Emergency Airway Management* 2nd ed. Philadelphia, PA: Lippincott Williams & Wilkins; 2004:190.

24. Miller CD, Warren SJ. IV lignocaine fails to attenuate the cardiovascular response to laryngoscopy and tracheal intubation. *Br J Anaesth.* 1990;65:216–219.

25. Pathak D, Slater RM, Ping SS, et al. Effects of alfentanil and lidocaine on the hemodynamic responses to laryngoscopy and tracheal intubation. *J Clin Anesth.* 1990;2:81–85.

26. Helfman SM, Gold MI, DeLisser EA, et al. Which drug prevents tachycardia and hypertension associated with tracheal intubation: lidocaine, fentanyl, or esmolol? *Anesth Analg.* 1991;72:482–486.

27. Splinter WM, Cervenko F. Haemodynamic responses to laryngoscopy and tracheal intubation in geriatric patients: effects of fentanyl, lidocaine and thiopentone. *Can J Anaesth.* 1989;36:370–376.

28. Chraemmer-Jorgensen B, Hoilund-Carlsen PF, Marving J, et al. Lack of effect of intravenous lidocaine on hemodynamic responses to rapid sequence induction of general anesthesia: a double-blind controlled clinical trial. *Anesth Analg.* 1986;65: 1037–1041.

29. Payne KA, Murray WB, Oosthuizen JH. Obtunding the sympathetic response to intubation. Experience at 2 minutes after administration of the test agent in patients with cerebral aneurysms. *S Afr Med J.* 1988;73:584–586.

30. Singh H, Vichitvejpaisal P. Comparative effects of lidocaine, esmolol, and nitroglycerin in modifying the hemodynamic response to laryngoscopy and intubation. *J Clin Anesth.* 1995;7:5–8.

31. Feng CK, Chan KH, Liu KN, et al. A comparison of lidocaine, fentanyl, and esmolol for attenuation of cardiovascular response to laryngoscopy and tracheal intubation. *Acta Anaesthesiol Sin.* 1996;34:61–67.

32. Schneider RE, Caro DA. Neuromuscular blocking agents In: Walls RM, Murphy MF, Luten RC, Schneider RE, eds. *Manual of Emergency Airway Management.* 2nd ed. Philadelphia, PA: Lippincott Williams & Wilkins; 2004:200–211.

Part 1: PAIN MANAGEMENT

29

Defining Acute versus Chronic Pain

Knox H. Todd

HIGH YIELD FACTS

- All chronic pain begins as acute pain.

- Acute pain can be defined in terms of duration: characteristically it is of recent onset and lasts no more than a few days to several weeks.

- Chronic pain is best considered as pain lasting longer than the usual time period expected for a particular condition or injury and serves no adaptive purpose.

- The disparity between observed patient behaviors and physician expectations of such behaviors in the setting of chronic pain may lead to undertreatment of pain.

- Prompt treatment of acute pain may prevent both short- and long-term deleterious consequences and resultant chronic pain syndromes.

- Emergency department (ED)-based early and aggressive therapy for acute pain holds the promise of preventing or ameliorating physiologic changes that may set the stage for prolonged or chronic pain states.

- A mechanistic approach to analgesia offers more in chronic pain than a symptom-based approach.

INTRODUCTION

All chronic pain begins as acute pain. Despite this seemingly obvious statement, very little is known with respect to how acute pain becomes chronic. Multiple patients suffer from acute low back strain, yet only a minority develops chronic back pain. We have as of yet not identified factors that will allow us to predict which individuals will go on to develop chronic symptoms. The transition from acute to chronic pain syndromes results from complex physiologic and psychosocial transitions that we are only beginning to understand more completely. The importance of emergency medicine in understanding more about chronic pain is twofold. First, a surprisingly large proportion of patients who present to the emergency department (ED) with pain have underlying chronic pain syndromes. Preliminary results from the Pain and Emergency Medicine Initiative multicenter study indicate that as many as 44% of patients discharged from the ED after presenting with pain suffer from chronic pain. For approximately one-half of these patients the chronic pain syndrome, or an exacerbation of this condition, was the primary reason for their ED visit.[1] Second, we may be able to better intervene in acute pain in order to prevent the development of chronic pain syndromes. This opportunity represents an exciting new perspective on what proactive ED acute pain management might offer our patients in the longer term.

DEFINITIONS

Acute Pain

Acute pain can be defined in terms of duration: characteristically it is of recent onset and lasts no more than a few days to several weeks. It usually occurs in response to tissue injury and disappears when the injury heals. Acute pain serves an adaptive purpose in that it is associated with protective reflexes, such as withdrawal responses to remove a limb from danger, or muscle spasms that serve to immobilize an extremity. It appears that nociceptor stimulation results in release of vasoactive substances, increasing blood flow to the injured area to accelerate healing. Some responses associated with acute pain may be maladaptive; however, leading to impaired immune responses, elevated myocardial oxygen demands, hypercoagulation, and atelectasis.

Chronic Pain

In the past, chronic pain has been defined as pain that lasts for more than 3–6 months. It is probably better considered as pain lasting longer than the usual time period expected for a particular condition or injury. At present this definition may have practical limitations, for relatively little data exists defining normal duration and severity of pain for many conditions. Given our present understanding of pain-related pathology, chronic pain syndromes are often associated with low levels of identifiable pathology; however, as we better understand the biologic mechanisms underpinning chronic pain, this may change. Chronic pain serves no adaptive purpose.

Recurrent Pain

Recurrent pain may be considered a subset of chronic pain. Most patients with chronic pain experience acute exacerbations of their condition (e.g., low back pain), while patients with sickle cell disease, migraine, or inflammatory bowel disease may experience few symptoms between painful episodes.

Affective Differences between Acute and Chronic Pain

Of particular importance to the assessment of pain, we should note that acute and chronic pain may be associated with markedly different pain-related behaviors. The affective component of chronic pain is an important factor in lowering quality of life and worsening pain. It underlines the essential role of multidimensional pain scales when assessing chronic pain. When multidimensional scales were used in the acute pain setting, the affective component of pain appeared to be minimal. When present, it is usually related to loss of control and anxiety. These latter signs are usually more obvious than the more subtle affective aspects of chronic pain. Depression, resignation, and fatalism are difficult to identify in the cursory assessment possible in the ED. While acute pain is usually associated with objective signs of sympathetic nervous system activation and overt signs of physical suffering, patients with chronic pain may not exhibit such typical behaviors and signs of autonomic nervous system overactivity. Further, patients with chronic pain must still "carry on" with daily activities. Activities such as watching television and eating are often used as distracting activities by patients with chronic pain, yet are often considered by ED personnel as evidence of patients *not* being in pain, or exaggerating their degree of pain in an attempt to be seen more quickly. This disparity between observed patient behaviors and physician expectations of such behaviors in the setting of chronic pain may lead to inaccurate underestimation of pain intensity and ultimately undertreatment of pain.

PHYSIOLOGY

As discussed in Chapter 30, hyperalgesia (an exaggerated response to painful stimuli) and allodynia (pain elicited by innocuous stimuli) develop as a result of both peripheral and central nervous system sensitization. Peripheral sensitization involves a complex array of inflammatory mediators resulting from tissue injury. A multitude of inflammatory mediators have been described, including potassium and hydrogen ions, bradykinin, prostaglandins, leukotrienes, and serotonin, among others. This "inflammatory soup" serves to sensitize peripheral nociceptors, making them more responsive to mild and innocuous stimuli (hyperalgesia and allodynia). We experience this peripheral sensitization as tenderness of the skin to light touch, and an aching sensation in muscles and tendons.

Central sensitization involves amplification of nociceptive signals at the level of the dorsal root ganglion, mediated again by multiple agents, including substance P, nitric oxide, glutamate, aspartate, prostaglandins, and leukotrienes. Activation of the glutamate receptor, or NMDA (*N*-methyl-D-aspartate) receptor, is a key trigger to central sensitization, and is a target for the development of new analgesics.[2] Importantly, central sensitization affects the normal function of touch-sensitive A beta fibers. While normally mediating only touch and vibration, A beta fiber-invoked pain results from the sensitization process and underlies mechanical allodynia, where normally nonnoxious stroking of the skin is perceived as painful by the brain.[3,4]

LONG-TERM EFFECTS OF UNDERTREATED PAIN

Although we know that acute pain is accompanied by multiple deleterious neurohormonal effects, there are other reasons to pursue aggressive pain control. Although much remains to be understood in this regard, evidence is accumulating that acute pain causes rapid and marked "plastic" changes in normal neurophysiology. These changes may occur within minutes. Prompt treatment of acute pain holds the promise of preventing a cascade of physiologic events that promote both short- and long-term deleterious consequences and resultant chronic pain syndromes.

Much of the evidence supporting the impact of acute pain on future pain responses comes from the pediatric literature.

Given the rapid development of the central nervous system around the time of birth, it is possible that the neonatal period is a particularly receptive time for neuroplastic changes resulting from painful experiences that lead to long-term observable effects on exposure to noxious stimuli.

Taddio et al. reported in 1997 that infants undergoing circumcision without anesthesia displayed increased pain responses on subsequent vaccinations 4–6 months after circumcision. Blinded observers assigned higher facial action, cry duration, and visual analog pain scores to infants undergoing routine 4–6-month vaccinations who had previously undergone neonatal circumcision using a placebo anesthetic as compared to those circumcised using EMLA or uncircumcised infants.[5] Similarly, Fitzgerald et al. found that premature infants between 27 and 32 weeks of gestational age undergoing heel sticks exhibit hyperalgesic responses to subsequent heel sticks, and that eutectic mixture of local anesthetic (EMLA) administration could prevent such changes.[6]

In adults, evidence for the importance of aggressive acute pain control, if not preemptive analgesia, comes from studies of subjects undergoing abdominal surgery. Gottschalk et al. studied patients undergoing radical retropubic prostatectomy, who were randomized to receive preoperative epidural bupivacaine or fentanyl versus controls, followed by aggressive postoperative epidural analgesia for all patients. Visual analog pain scores during the intrahospital postoperative period were significantly lower for those receiving preemptive epidural therapies. Patients with active treatment also reported long-term decreases in postoperative pain and earlier resumption of normal activities, as compared to controls, despite aggressive postoperative epidural analgesic regimens provided to all subjects.[7]

Although clinical evidence is merely suggestive at this point, ED-based early and aggressive therapy for acute pain holds the promise of preventing or ameliorating physiologic changes that may set the stage for prolonged or chronic pain states. A great deal of work remains to be done in this area and despite these considerations, the treatment of acute pain and suffering is justified in and of itself.

MEDICATIONS USED FOR CHRONIC PAIN

In addition to opioids and nonsteroidal anti-inflammatory drugs, a wide variety of pharmacotherapeutic agents have been used as primary or adjunctive treatment for chronic pain states. These agents include antidepressants, anticonvulsants, neuroleptics, systemic local anesthetics, calcium channel blockers, NMDA receptor antagonists, corticosteroids, capsaicin, and others. We will comment on a few of the more common agents used by patients with chronic pain.

Antidepressants

Tricyclic antidepressants, atypical antidepressants, and selective serotonin reuptake inhibitors have been used to treat a variety of chronic pain states. It appears that the analgesic activity of antidepressants is independent of their mood effects and the mechanism of action has been attributed to a variety of postulated effects.[8] The efficacy of first-generation tricyclics is best supported by available evidence. In the mid-1960s, a randomized, controlled trial of amitriptyline for headaches provided the first evidence of a role for tricyclic agents in pain therapies.[9] One meta-analysis of 39 placebo-controlled studies found tricyclics to be efficacious in a variety of chronic nonmalignant pain syndromes.[10] In general, tricyclics are most effective for treatment of chronic neuropathic or central pain syndromes, including diabetic neuropathy, postherpetic neuralgia, and cancer pain. Their action is probably due to modification of sodium channels in afferent C-fibers.

Anticonvulsants

Phenytoin, carbamazepine, valproic acid, and gabapentin are the anticonvulsants most commonly employed to treat chronic pain, particularly neuropathic pain characterized by lancinating and burning qualities.[11] Given that neuropathic pain may involve pathologic spontaneous electrical activity of neurons, the stabilizing of neural membranes associated with anticonvulsants may be responsible for their analgesic activity. Carbamazepine is perhaps the most commonly used agent and has been used to treat trigeminal neuralgia, postherpetic neuralgia, and pain associated with diabetic neuropathy. Although expensive, gabapentin has been used to treat a wide variety of pain syndromes, including com-plex regional pain syndrome, migraine headache, and various painful neuropathies. Its action appears to be due to a novel method of pain control: modification of calcium channels in afferent pain fibers. Two randomized, controlled trials support its use in diabetic neuropathy and postherpetic neuralgia.[12,13]

NMDA Receptor Antagonists

As discussed previously, activation of the glutamate receptor, or NMDA receptor, appears to be a key trigger to central sensitization, with a likely role in the development of neuropathic pain.[2] NMDA receptor antagonists, such as dextromethorphan, amantadine, and ketamine, are felt to be promising agents in the prevention and treatment of such conditions. The role of these agents in the treatment of pain is being actively investigated.

CONCLUSIONS

Emergency physicians tend to view all pain presenting to the ED within the limited framework of acute pain. Certainly, much of the pain we see is self-limited, and carries the expectation that pain will last for only a brief period of time, until the underlying condition resolves or injury heals. As we learn more about the nature of pain presentations to our departments, we may find that chronic pain is a much more common presenting problem than we realize. We need to investigate further how aggressive intervention for acute pain may well prevent progression to chronic pain. Certainly, we see a large number of patients with recurrent pain presentations (e.g., low back pain) where simply treating acute pain addresses only part of a much more complex problem. Perhaps we will begin to view pain as neither acute nor chronic for many of our patients, but as an ongoing condition that waxes and wanes, or is silent with recurrent flares. Many patients have long standing symptoms with an uncertain pathologic underpinning, and will perhaps be best served by management approaches more akin to those used for diabetes, or other chronic diseases, than our current single-shot therapies. These newer approaches are likely to involve active case management strategies, with more attention given to follow-up and prevention, than is currently the case.

REFERENCES

1. Todd KH, Ducharme J, Choiniere M, et al. Pain and pain-related functional interference among discharged emergency department patients, *Ann Emerg Med.* 2004;44(suppl 4):S86.
2. Mao J, Price DD, Hayes RL, et al. Intrathecal treatment with dextrorphan or ketamine potently reduces pain-related behaviors in a rat model of peripheral mononeuropathy. *Brain Res.* 1993;605(1):164–168.
3. Torebjork HE, Lundbert LER, LaMotte RH. Central changes in processing of mechanoreceptive input in capsaicin-induced secondary hyperalgesia in humans. *J Physiol.* 1992;448: 765–780.
4. Koltzenburg M, Torebjork HE, Wahren LK. Nociceptor modulated central sensitization causes mechanical hyperalgesia in acute chemogenic and chronic neuropathic pain. *Brain.* 1994;117:579–591.
5. Taddio A, Katz J, Ilersich AL, et al. Effect of neonatal circumcision on pain response during subsequent routine vaccination. *Lancet.* 1997;349:599–603.
6. Fitzgerald M, Millard C, McIntosh N. Cutaneous hypersensitivity following peripheral tissue damage in newborn infants and its reversal with topical anaesthesia. *Pain.* 1989;39: 31–36.
7. Gottschalk A, Smith DS, Jobes DR, et al. Preemptive epidural analgesia and recovery from radical prostatectomy. *JAMA.* 1998;279(14):1976–1982.
8. Watson CP. Antidepressant drugs as adjuvant analgesics. *J Pain Symptom Manage.* 1994;9(6):392–405.
9. Lance JW, Curran DA. Treatment of chronic tension headache. *Lancet.* 1964;1:1235–1238.
10. Onghena P, Van Houdenhove B. Antidepressant-induced analgesia in chronic non-malignant pain: a meta-analysis of 39 placebo-controlled studies. Pain. 1992;49(2):205–219.
11. McQuay H, Carroll D, Jadad AR, et al. Anticonvulsant drugs for management of pain: a systematic review. *BMJ.* 1047; 311(7012):1047–1052.
12. Backonja M, Beydoun A, Edwards KR, et al. Gabapentin for the symptomatic treatment of painful neuropathy in patients with diabetes mellitus: a randomized controlled trial. *JAMA.* 1998;280(21):1831–1836.
13. Rowbotham M, Harden N, Stacey B, et al. Gabapentin for the treatment of postherpetic neuralgia: a randomized controlled trial. *JAMA.* 1998;280(21):1837–1842.

30

Neurobiology of Pain

James Ducharme

HIGH YIELD FACTS

- There needs to be a mechanism—specific approach, whereby pharmacologic and psychologic management target specific receptors and mediators.
- Prostanoids and interleukins are liberated into the circulation after injury, inducing cyclooxygenase (COX-2) sites hours after the injury.
- An inflammatory soup of mediators is required to depolarize pain fibers—single mediators are normally insufficient.
- Activation of *N*-methyl-D-aspartate (NMDA) and alpha-amino-3-hydroxy-5-methyl-4-isoxazolepropionic acid (AMPA) in the dorsal horn leads to windup and hyperalgesic states within a few hours of injury—the therapeutic window to prevent windup is thus small.
- Pain perception can be modified by signals coming downward from the cortex or thalamus.
- Cannabinoid receptors are probably responsible for most addictive behavior associated with opioid misuse.
- Neuropathic pain requires negation of impulses along nociceptive sodium or calcium channels—opioids are rarely if ever effective.

INTRODUCTION

The physiologic response to a nociceptive stimulus is more complex than initially proposed by Melzack and Wall in their gate theory of pain. This complexity mandates a paradigm shift by physicians in their approach to pain management. Rather than limiting control of pain to nonspecific analgesics such as opioids, there increasingly needs to be a mechanism—specific approach, whereby pharmacologic and psychologic management target specific receptors and mediators. Directed combination therapy, especially with respect to chronic pain, is becoming the norm. This approach improves pain control while minimizing adverse effects due to the possibility of reducing doses of each medication. Physicians should recognize that a single-medication approach to severe or chronic pain is rarely justified. Improved understanding of the neurobiologic systems involved will permit optimal treatment plans for all patients.

Why does pain perception exist? In order to prevent tissue damage, we have learned to associate certain categories of stimuli with danger that must be avoided.[1] Pain also encourages healing by discouraging use of an injured body part. In the modern era, pain serves as a signal for the patient to seek out care for the cause of the pain. Once under medical care, a patient no longer has a physiologic requirement for pain. It is *not* the physician's mandate to remove pain and pain sensitivity, but to control the degree of pain, while returning the heightened sensitivity to normal. In the following discussion we will attempt to describe the neurobiologic response to a painful stimulus, with the goal of offering therapeutic options of pain control based on this greater understanding of the mechanisms of pain.

PERIPHERAL RESPONSE

Table 30-1 lists relevant terms and their definitions.

A painful stimulus induces local cellular, neuronal, and circulatory system responses. With tissue damage, there is a stimulation of both the cyclooxygenase (COX) and lipoxygenase pathways. Resultant prostanoids and interleukins are transported through the circulation to the spinal cord where they induce the development of COX-2 receptors. Anti-inflammatory analgesics cannot control acute pain until these receptors are induced, which normally requires several hours. In persistent inflammatory states such as rheumatoid arthritis, COX-2 receptors are chronically present. It is the presence of interleukins in the circulation that also leads to the systemic symptoms associated with pain: nausea, tiredness, and decreased appetite.

Nociceptive neuronal fibers are essentially exposed nerve endings adjacent to capillaries and mast cells. Destructive stimuli such as heat, cold, mechanical force, ischemia, and chemical irritants damage tissue, including local mast cells and nociceptive fibers. Chemical mediators (histamine, bradykinin, and prostaglandins) are released from mast cells creating an inflammatory soup. This leads to capillary leakage, platelet aggregation, and release of serotonin. Leukotrienes from mast cells generate superoxides, activating additional inflammatory cells. It is this soup that initiates neuronal electrical activity. It is a combination of

Table 30-1. Definitions

Transduction	Conversion of a noxious thermal, mechanical, or chemical stimulus into electrical activity
Conduction	Passage of action potentials from peripheral nociceptor to terminals in the spinal cord and CNS
Transmission	Synaptic transfer and modulation of input from one nerve to another
Inflammatory pain	Response to injury by release of active substances leading to sensitization
Maladaptive/ functional pain	Abnormal responsiveness or function of the nervous system, resulting in presence of pain in clinical situations that are not normally painful (e.g., fibromyalgia)

CNS: central nervous system.

mediators that transduces injury into neuronal depolarization, for a single mediator normally does not provide enough stimulus except in secondary hyperalgesic states.

Damaged cells also release potassium and hydrogen ions, cytokines, and growth factors. The cations and adenosine triphosphate (ATP) stimulate the neuron directly, whereas prostaglandin E_2, nerve growth factor, and bradykinin sensitize the neuron, allowing it to be activated by lower level input.[2] Blocking production of any one of these agents will not eliminate sensitization. As a result, it is difficult to develop novel analgesics with peripheral action, for multiple actions would be required to achieve effective blockade of transduction.

Nociceptive fibers are not only C-fiber neurons. Initial pain is conducted by alpha-delta fibers, producing the initial sharp pain. C-fibers take longer to respond, producing the aching or throbbing pain that occurs shortly thereafter. The local consequences of activation of these fibers are the release of neuropeptides such as calcitonin gene-related peptide (CGRP), leading to further vasodilation, edema, and inflammation.[3] Depolarization and conduction along the pain fibers stimulates release of excitatory amino acids (glutamate and aspartate) and neuropeptides (substance P) at the synaptic junction in the dorsal root ganglion (DRG) (Fig. 30-1).

DRG AND SPINAL CORD STIMULATION

Within seconds of an injury, sensory spinal cord neurons in the dorsal horn become hyperresponsive. Inputs that would normally have been undetectable now evoke outputs. Normally innocuous stimuli elicit pain (allodynia), while painful stimulus creates an exaggerated response (hyperalgesia).

Action potentials arriving at the DRG synapse initiate the release of glutamate and substance P. Initial glutamate stimulates and activates AMPA receptors. As the painful stimulus persists, the corelease of substance P and glutamate remove magnesium from the N-methyl-D-aspartate (NMDA) receptor, allowing this pathway to also be activated. NMDA activation initiates intracellular calcium release, stimulating nitric oxide and protein kinase C. Cephalad transmission occurs via the spinothalamic tract. Both γ-aminobutyric acid (GABA) and glycine are able to inhibit AMPA and glutamate. This may mean that agents with GABA-blocking ability such as benzodiazepines have the potential to prevent additional recruitment or windup. In addition, mu receptors are present both pre and postsynaptically—beta-endorphins or opioids are often effective in controlling pain at this level. NMDA antagonists, such as ketamine or dextromethorphan, are also able to attenuate the pain response. Due to the widespread presence of NMDA receptors throughout the central nervous system (CNS), use of NMDA antagonists often leads to the recognized adverse effects of dissociation, dysphoria, and sedation before attaining pain control. Combination of low-dose ketamine with opioids appears to produce excellent analgesia while minimizing adverse effects from both agents.[4]

Downward Modulation

We have all witnessed an athlete overcome pain from injury to go on to victory. Similarly we are aware of the placebo effect in clinical analgesia trials. It is evident that the CNS is able to modify or even eliminate pain under certain circumstances. Acupuncture and its ritualistic behavior probably achieve most of its effect through similar mechanisms, explaining the inconsistency of clinical trial results.[5] The "fight or flight" response to perceived danger is considered a priority for survival, superceding pain sensation. How does such pain modulation occur, and is there a way to apply this understanding into clinical practice?

Although initially it was thought any modulation could only be inhibitory, it is now accepted that there is a parallel facilitatory mechanism.[6] Norepinephrine, serotonin, and

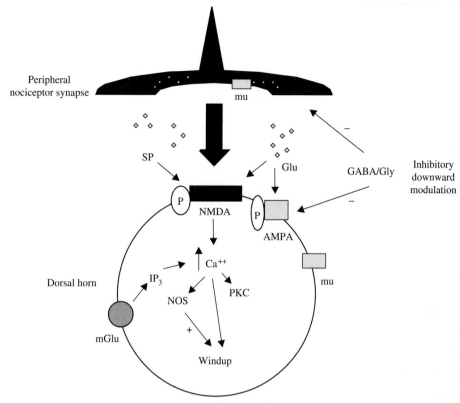

Fig. 30-1. Interaction at level of dorsal horn. (Modified from Bolay H, Moskowitz MA: Mechanisms of pain modulation in chronic syndromes. *Neurology* 2002;59(Suppl 2):S2–S7).

glutamate all produce facilitation, while endorphins, glycine, and GABA are inhibitory for pain sensation. Since both systems are active, it is the equilibrium between the two systems that is modifiable. It may be that in severe persistent pain or maladaptive pain the facilitatory system overrides the inhibition, resulting in normally nonpainful stimuli causing pain.[7] This has been supported by demonstrating that midazolam, a GABA-mimetic, can reduce neuropathic pain.

In acute injury, the inhibitory modulation is enhanced, so that by day 3 pain diminishes even in the presence of ongoing inflammation. As a result of downward inhibition both NMDA and AMPA dose-response curves shift, resulting in the dorsal horn responding less to ongoing peripheral stimulation. Further inhibition can be achieved by increasing endorphins with calcitonin or with the use of extrinsic opioids, GABA-mimetics, or NMDA antagonists. Again, use of these agents may be limited because of unacceptable adverse effects.

CENTRAL NERVOUS SYSTEM

Most cephalad transmission leads to the thalamus, with approximately 10% continuing to the somatosensory cortex. The anterior cingulate cortex is the most active area in imaging studies of pain.[8,9] Cortical involvement appears to be responsible for pain affect: attitudes, such as the unpleasantness (or pleasure) of pain; anticipation; and other negative emotions. Further thalamocortical transmission leads to cognitive evaluation of pain, response priorities, and directing attention or inattention to the painful stimulus.[10] It is cortical stimulation from recurring painful conditions that defines our interpretation and response to subsequent painful events.

Cortical response has been found to be related in part to anandamide, a cannabinoid endogenous ligand.[11] Cannabinoid 1 (CB₁) receptors appear to not only contribute to pain control, but also impact on cortical response. It is now recognized that most addictive behavior is through the

CB$_1$ receptors in the cortex, not mu receptors. Animal studies suggest that a combination of a CB$_1$ antagonist with an opioid would permit pain control without the negative affective behavior.[12,13] Although mu receptors are found from the DRG to the thalamus and up to the somatosensory cortex, most μ receptors are quiescent until induced by painful input—abrupt severe pain may initially be more difficult to control after even a few hours. As opioid receptors "come on line," they allow a greater response to exogenous opioids and better pain control even with windup producing hyperresponsiveness and secondary hyperalgesia.

NEUROPATHIC PAIN

In most cases of neuropathic pain there has been no concomitant tissue injury. Peripheral nerve damage has usually occurred either by transection (as during surgery), inflammatory destruction (postherpetic neuropathy), or degeneration (diabetic neuropathy). This nerve damage leads to spontaneous pain and hypersensitivity. Central sensitization leading to hypersensitivity is principally due to persistent NMDA activity.

C-fiber damage can lead to neuronal sprouting of alpha-beta fibers into lamina II of the dorsal horn. Normally, lamina II is reserved for C-fibers—it is the area of pain reception from afferent fibers. Alpha-beta fibers convey touch perception, so this extension into lamina II results in nonnoxious inputs being interpreted as painful. This is clinically evident in the severe allodynia felt by many patients with neuropathic pain.

This alteration of sensory transmission has clinical implications. Neuronal transmission of most alpha-beta fibers is through sodium channels. Sodium channel blockers such as tricyclic antidepressants can be very effective in controlling neuropathic pain in many patients. Since selective serotonin reuptake inhibitors (SSRI) antidepressants have no action on sodium channels, they would not be expected to be effective in neuropathic pain; research has confirmed their ineffectiveness. C-fibre and spinal cord transmission is directly reliant on Ca^{2+} as well. If tricyclics have been unsuccessful in controlling neuropathic pain, then a specific Ca^{2+} channel antagonist such as gabapentin may be effective. Clinical trials have confirmed that gabapentin can be as effective as tricyclic agents, with less adverse effects.[14,15]

IMPLICATIONS FOR TREATMENT

In acute severe pain, use of opioids should remain the first treatment option. Mu receptors are present cortically, in the thalamus, the spinal cord, and the DRG. The recognized adverse effects of opioids (constipation, nausea, and emesis) are due to peripheral, not central, activation.[16] Calcitonin, which increases beta-endorphins centrally, produces almost none of the adverse effects normally associated with opioids. Newer opioids without peripheral action are now entering clinical practice.[16] They will be discussed in greater detail elsewhere (Chap. 14). Opiophobia arises out of the unreasonable fear of addiction in patients who require opioids for pain control. This has chronically resulted in undertreatment of pain. Recognition that CB$_1$ receptors are the primary culprits in addictive behavior development[17] has led to development of CB$_1$ antagonists. Combining a CB$_1$ antagonist with an opioid may allow use of opioids without fear of addiction.

Anti-inflammatory nonsteroidal agents understandably have a therapeutic ceiling. Prostanoids are only one of several mediators of the inflammatory soup, so NSAIDs or COX-2 agents cannot be expected to control severe pain. It is reasonable to expect them to be effective in chronic inflammatory states where COX-2 receptors are persistently present. They should also be considered as part of the analgesic regimen plan for severe pain. They cannot be expected to be of benefit in neuropathic or maladaptive pain, for no inflammatory response has occurred.

Although directed agents such as tricyclics and gabapentin for neuropathic pain have been effective, it is unreasonable to expect that a new agent with a specific single peripheral antagonistic effect will achieve pain control. The multiple pathways involving inflammatory mediators, neuropeptides, and excitatory amino acids suggest rather that further advances in pain control will require combinations of agents based on understanding of the mechanisms of a particular pain. Use of single agents active at multiple sites (opioids and ketamine) leads to not only analgesia but often undesirable effects as well. Here again, combination therapy will allow dosage reductions, permitting pain control with minimal adverse effects.

REFERENCES

1. Woolf CJ. Pain: moving from symptom control toward mechanism-specific pharmacologic management. *Ann Intern Med.* 2004;140(6):441–451.
2. Woolf CJ. Pain: moving from symptom control toward mechanism-specific pharmacologic management. *Ann Intern Med.* 2004;140(6):441–451.
3. Silberstein SD. Neurotoxins in the neurobiology of pain. *Headache.* 2003;43(suppl 1):S2–S8.
4. Laulin JP, Maurette P, Corcuff JB, et al. The role of ketamine in preventing fentanyl-induced hyperalgesia and subsequent

acute morphine tolerance. *Anesth Analg.* 2002;94(5): 1263–1269.

5. Woolf CJ. Pain: moving from symptom control toward mechanism-specific pharmacologic management. *Ann Intern Med.* 2004;140(6):441–451.

6. Fields HL, Heinricher MM, Mason P. Neurotransmitters in nociceptive modulatory circuits. *Annu Rev Neurosci.* 1991; 14:219–245.

7. Ren K, Dubner R. Descending modulation in persistent pain: an update. *Pain.* 2002;100(1–2):1–6.

8. Sweatt JD, Weeber EJ, Levenson JM. Central neural mechanisms that interrelate sensory and affective dimensions of pain. *Mol Interven.* 2002;2:393–402.

9. Silberstein SD. Neurotoxins in the neurobiology of pain. *Headache.* 2003;43(suppl 1):S2–S8.

10. Silberstein SD. Neurotoxins in the neurobiology of pain. *Headache.* 2003;43(suppl 1):S2–S8.

11. Goutopoulos A, Makriyannis A. From cannabis to cannabinergics: new therapeutic opportunities. *Pharmacol Ther.* 2002;95(2):103–117.

12. Elphick MR, Egertova M. The neurobiology and evolution of cannabinoid signalling. *Philos Trans R Soc Lond B Biol Sci.* 2001;356(1407):381–408.

13. Walker JM, Hohmann AG, Martin WJ, et al. The neurobiology of cannabinoid analgesia. *Life Sci.* 1999;65(6–7):665–673.

14. Rowbotham M, Harden N, Stacey B, et al. Gabapentin for the treatment of postherpetic neuralgia: a randomized controlled trial. *JAMA.* 1998;280(21):1837–1842.

15. Backonja M, Beydoun A, Edwards KR, et al. Gabapentin for the symptomatic treatment of painful neuropathy in patients with diabetes mellitus: a randomized controlled trial. *JAMA.* 1998;280(21):1831–1836.

16. Bates JJ, Foss JF, Murphy DB. Are peripheral opioid antagonists the solution to opioid side effects? *Anesth Analg.* 2004;98(1):116–122.

17. Rice ASC, Farquhar-Smith WP, Bridges D, et al. Cannabinoids and pain. In: Dostrovsky JO, Carr DB, Koltzenburg M, eds. *Proceedings of the 10th World Congress on Pain: Progress in Pain Research and Management.* Seattle, WA: IASP Press; 2003:437–468.

31

Opioid-Dependent Patients in the Emergency Department

John Ward

Grant D. Innes

HIGH YIELD FACTS

- Opioid-dependent patients belong to one of two groups: those with chronic pain syndromes and those whose dependence arises from misuse.

- Aberrant or drug-seeking behavior occurs in victims of oligoanesthesia who develop such behavior in a desperate attempt to obtain pain relief as well as those who are addicted or misuse opioids.

- Complex neurochemical changes make it difficult for addicts to make rational decisions even when drug misuse is detrimental to their well-being.

- Substance abuse disorder is "a cluster of cognitive, behavioral and psychological symptoms indicating that a person is continuing to use a substance despite having clinically significant substance related problems."

- Substance dependence requires ≥3 of the following: tolerance, withdrawal, substance use in greater amounts or for longer periods than intended, desire or unsuccessful attempts to ↓ use, considerable time/effort to obtain the substance, ↓ in important activities due to drug use, continued use despite problems.

- Tolerance is the body's requirement of increasing amounts of drug to maintain the same pharmacologic effects, and can occur with many drugs.

- Physical dependence is the physiologic changes occurring with opioid exposure, which leads to withdrawal with opioid discontinuance.

- Patients with chronic pain: use opioids appropriately, opioids improve the quality of life, are aware of side effects, follow treatment plans, have saved medication from previous prescription.

- Patients with opioid abuse: opioid use is out of control, opioids impair quality of life, unconcerned about side effects, noncompliant, out of meds/lost prescription/tale of woe, commonly polydrug use, high risk of psychiatric disorder.

INTRODUCTION

Numerous studies have documented suboptimal emergency department (ED) pain management, with delayed or inadequate treatment for patients unequivocally in pain (i.e., patients with long bone fractures, burns, and multiple trauma).[1] A variety of factors have been postulated or shown to contribute to this phenomenon of oligoanalgesia. Patient characteristics such as age, ethnicity, gender, socioeconomic status, and previous analgesic usage affect treatment. Provider characteristics, particularly the reluctance to prescribe opioid analgesics, are also a major barrier to achieving pain control. Caregivers are often overly concerned about opioid use leading to addiction. Alternatively, they may wish to avoid contributing to the drug-seeking behavior of patients selling or misusing opioids. The latter issue is particularly problematic for emergency physicians. Suspicion that patients may be exaggerating a somatic complaint in order to receive a particular medication, coupled with the lack of an objective measure of pain frequently leaves physicians unsure whether they are providing appropriate care. In addition to denying the patient therapy to control pain and suffering, this uncertainty has the potential to generate frustration, anger and, ultimately, burnout on the part of the physician. With recent literature encouraging greater use of opioids for conditions such as chronic nonmalignant pain, acute severe pain, and cancer-related pain, emergency physicians will face this problem with increasing frequency.[2] Perhaps the most important cause of oligoanalgesia, treatment variability, and care provider frustration is the lack of a systematic approach to identifying, measuring, and treating pain. It is therefore surprising that few EDs have implemented systems and processes for acute pain management that could standardize care and decrease these stressors.

The purpose of this chapter is to review the management of opioid-dependent patients and provide a framework to guide physicians' decisions in the ED. This will include an overview of the biology of chronic pain and addiction syndromes, a discussion of how biology affects patient behavior, and response to therapy, and a synthesis of how this information can be applied practically in the clinical setting.

The Science of Chronic Pain versus Addiction

The opioid-dependent patients presenting to the ED generally fall into two categories: those with chronic pain syndromes and those whose dependence arises from misuse. Addiction may be seen in either group; up to 20% of patients prescribed opioids for chronic nonmalignant pain are at risk for addiction. Further, aberrant or drug-seeking behavior is not restricted to those who are addicted to or misuse opioids, as those who are victims of oligoanalgesia develop such behavior in a desperate attempt to obtain pain relief. This creates even more difficulty in identifying the patient who requires additional opioids versus those who should not receive any.

Chronic pain syndromes result from a number of anatomic, biochemical, and genetic changes to pain pathways (Fig. 31-1). At a peripheral level, repeated or prolonged exposure of nociceptors to inflammatory mediators causes sensitization. As a consequence, less intense stimuli are required to cause depolarization, with nerves continuing to send pain signals to the central nervous system (CNS) long after the inciting pain condition has resolved. Central sensitization at the level of the dorsal horn involves a process termed *windup*, in which there is a progressively increasing central response to subsequent stimuli, even those temporally distant from the original painful event. In the CNS, the degree of expression of particular forebrain receptors (e.g., *N*-methyl-D-aspartate (NMDA) receptors) appears to influence the patient's response to painful conditions. These alterations lead to hyperalgesia, a heightened response to noxious stimuli, and allodynia, where non-noxious stimuli lead to the sensation of pain. All of these critical pathophysiologic processes may be mitigated by aggressive management of the acute pain state.[3]

Genetic and biochemical changes in the CNS also contribute to addiction-related behaviors. The neuronal pathways of drug addiction reside in the mesocorticolimbic dopamine systems that originate in the ventral tegmental area of the brain (Fig. 31-2). The mesolimbic system has projections to the nucleus accumbens, the amygdala, and the hippocampus; these structures mediate the acute reinforcing effects of opioids as well as the emotional and motivational changes of the withdrawal syndrome. The mesocortical circuit projects to the prefrontal, oculofrontal, and anterior cingulate cortex; areas that mediate drug craving, the compulsion to take drugs, and the conscious experience of drug effects.[4]

All addictive drugs are both positive and negative reinforcers. Positive reinforcement is the euphoria resulting from dopamine release into the nucleus accumbens. Addictive drugs have similar effects to natural rewards like food and sex. However, the response to natural rewards exhibits habituation. Conversely, each dose of an addictive drug stimulates dopamine release, and the resulting euphoria reinforces drug-seeking behavior. The withdrawal syndrome is associated with low levels of dopamine in the nucleus accumbens, a negative reinforcement ensuring persistence of opioid use.

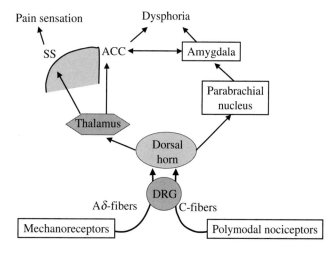

Fig. 31-1. Pain pathways. SS, somatosensory cortex; ACC, anterior cingulate cortex; DRG, dorsal root ganglion. (Reprinted with permission from Bolay H, Moskowitz MA. Mechanisms of pain modulation in chronic syndromes. *Neurology.* 2002;59(suppl 2):S2–S7.)

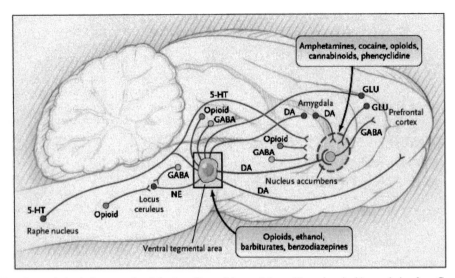

Fig. 31-2. Neural reward circuits important in reinforcing effects of drugs of abuse. (Reproduced with permission from Cami J, Farre M. Drug addiction. *N Engl J Med*. 2003;349:975–986.) As shown in the rat brain, mesocorticolimbic dopamine (DA) systems originating in the ventral tegmental area include projections from cell bodies of the ventral tegmental area to the nucleus accumbens, amygdala, and prefrontal cortex; glutamatergic (GLU) projections from the prefrontal cortex to the nucleus accumbens and the ventral tegmental area; and projections from the aminobutyric acid (GABA) neurons of the nucleus accumbens to the prefrontal cortex. Opioid interneurons modulate the GABA-inhibitory action on the ventral tegmental area and influence the firing of norepinephrine (NE) neurons in the locus ceruleus. Serotonergic (5-HT) projections from the raphe nucleus extend to the ventral tegmental area and the nucleus accumbens. The figure shows the proposed sites of action of the various drugs of abuse in these circuits.

The inability of abusers to curb their craving or to avoid relapse after prolonged periods of abstinence is difficult for nonaddicts to comprehend. Here too, specific CNS alterations that make drug cessation difficult have been documented. In this regard, the glutamate system appears to be important. With drug sensitization, there are long-lasting increases in glutamate transmission in the mesocorticolimbic dopamine system. The glutamate system is integral to learning and memory and likely leads to behavioral sensitization whereby environmental cues contribute to addiction-related behaviors and relapse.[4] Intere-stingly, initiation of drug craving and addictive behavior seems linked not to endorphin receptors but rather canna-binoid ones. Preliminary research suggests that canna-binoid antagonists combined with opioids may prevent the development of addictive traits in patients requiring long-term opioids.

Ultimately, like any other illness, addiction is associated with or caused by quantitative and qualitative biochemical changes. Unfortunately, the resultant clinical manifestations lead to behavior patterns that are misunderstood and aggravating to nonaddicts, in this case ED personnel. Although the physiologic adaptations involved in addiction do not absolve addicts of responsibility for their actions, emergency physicians should remember that addictive behavior is not merely a lifestyle choice. These real and complex neurochemical changes make it difficult for addicts to make constructive or seemingly rational decisions so that addicts demonstrate persistent misuse of drugs even when such misuse is detrimental to their health and personal and social well-being.

Chronic Pain versus Addiction: The Definition

Before deciding whether a patient's ED presentation is being driven primarily by addiction or by an underlying somatic complaint, it is important to understand what constitutes addiction. The American Psychiatric Association[5] has replaced the word addiction with the term *substance abuse disorder*, defined as "a cluster of cognitive, behavioral and physiological symptoms indicating that a person is continuing to use a substance despite having clinically significant substance related problems." For substance dependence to be diagnosed, at least three of the following must be present:

1. Symptoms of tolerance.
2. Symptoms of withdrawal.

3. Use of the substance in larger amounts or for longer periods than intended.

4. Persistent desire or unsuccessful attempts to reduce or control use.

5. Spending of considerable time in efforts to obtain the substance.

6. Reduction in important social, occupational, or recreational activities because of drug use.

7. Continued substance use despite attendant health, social, or economic problems.

Opioid Tolerance

Tolerance occurs with any prolonged use of many drugs, not just opioids. It refers to the body's requirement of increasing amounts of drug to maintain the same pharmacologic effects. Physical dependence refers to physiologic changes that occur with opioid exposure. These changes result in a withdrawal syndrome if exposure is discontinued. It is important to note that tolerance and physical dependence are distinct from the diagnosis of substance dependence disorder, and that both invariably accompany long-term opioid use.

Several types of tolerance are recognized.[6] Innate tolerance is genetically determined and is present before any exposure to the drug.[7] Pharmacokinetic tolerance involves changes in the distribution or metabolism of a drug; thus exposure to barbiturates, antiepileptic medications, and even opioids induces cytochrome P450 enzymes that enhance conversion of narcotics to their inactive metabolites.[6,7] Learned tolerance involves a reduction in the effects of a drug by voluntary adaptive changes in behavior, i.e., the improved ability to perform motor skills at previously debilitating drug levels.[8]

Two types of pharmacodynamic tolerance exist. The first relates to opioid receptors residing in the CNS, in musculoskeletal structures, in visceral and vascular smooth muscle, and at the terminals of peripheral sympathetic and sensory neurons.[9] Repeated exposure to opioids leads to down-regulation, with reduction in the number of receptors and uncoupling of receptors from cell signalling proteins. The result is fewer opioid receptors and a reduced response to receptor activation. The second form of pharmacodynamic tolerance relates to an alteration in the synthesis of cAMP, which is involved in pain generation and perception. Short-term opioid exposure decreases cAMP levels, while chronic exposure upregulates cAMP generation. Increased cAMP levels are believed to produce physical dependence and contribute to the withdrawal syndrome. Supranormal cAMP levels have been documented in the mesocorticolimbic system after discontinuation of opiates and other addictive drugs. These elevated levels decrease dopamine levels in the nucleus accumbens and contribute to the dysphoria that occurs during the early phases of abstinence.[10]

The degree of tolerance and the rate of its development vary from drug to drug and between individuals, based on the adaptations described previously. Drugs with a high intrinsic receptor activity, which require low receptor occupancy to produce their effects (e.g., sufentanil) induce tolerance much more slowly than agents with low intrinsic activity (e.g., morphine).[11]

In summary, tolerance accompanies ongoing opioid use and explains the following phenomena, which tend to create unease among physicians and nurses.[12] First, patients are likely to require and request increasing analgesic doses, particularly in the early weeks or months of treatment; second, regular opioid users often require larger than normal dose increments to achieve analgesia; third, long-term genetically-based neural adaptations mean that patients who have been opioid-free for months or years may still be relatively opioid-resistant and require higher doses for adequate pain relief.

Opioid Mechanism of Action

Opioids have the potential to act on three types of receptors: mu, kappa, and delta.[13] Most of the clinically active opioids act on mu receptors, which mediate reward and physical dependence. Mice, who have had the mu receptor genetically "knocked out" do not exhibit behavioral signs of opioid administration and do not develop withdrawal.[4,14] There are multiple mu receptor subtypes, and genetic polymorphism explains the variable efficacy and side effect profiles seen when the same drug and dose is administered to different individuals.[15] This has important ramifications for emergency physicians, who are often suspicious of patients who request specific analgesics. While some patients seek specific agents because of their euphoric effects and rapid onset, there are legitimate biologically plausible reasons for patient preferences—for example, codeine is ineffective in the 7–10% of Caucasians who cannot convert it to its active metabolite, morphine. Genetic differences may also help explain why patients who claim intolerable adverse effects to an opioid such as morphine or codeine respond well to hydromorphone even though the active metabolites are similar for these drugs (Fig. 31-3). Patients should thus not be automatically considered substance abusers when they insist on being treated with a specific opioid. The final corollary is that, because of individual variability, patients cannot be considered unresponsive to opioids until all opioids have been tried.

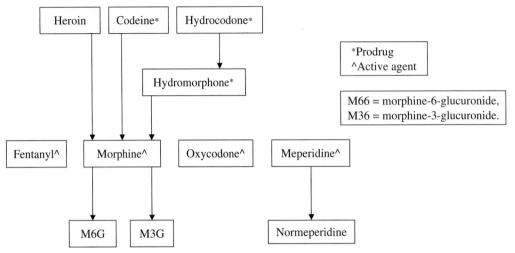

Fig. 31-3. Pure opioid agonists and key breakdown products. (Reprinted with permission from Innes GI, Zed PJ. Basic pharmacology and advances in emergency medicine. *Emerg Med Clin North Amer.* 2005;23:455.)

Chronic Pain versus Addiction: The Practice

An understanding of drug tolerance should allay many misgivings physicians have in treating opioid-dependent patients who have acute pain. This understanding is less helpful in cases when physicians believe patents are fabricating or exaggerating pain complaints in order to receive medications that will relieve addiction-related needs. Further complicating matters, there is significant overlap between chronic pain and addiction. Although most chronic pain patients eventually achieve a steady state where increases in drug requirements are uncommon (and usually reflect a change in their underlying disease process), 3–17% of these patients are also addicted.[16] No objective test exists that can identify these latter patients. Attempts have been made to identify patients at risk of addiction, for whom therapy might be altered. Techniques include the use of tools like the modified CAGE questionnaire (Table 31-1) or the Screening Instrument for Substance Abuse Potential questionnaire (Table 31-2). Once addiction is established, there are several features to help determine whether chronic pain (and the related need for analgesia) or opioid addiction is the primary reason for the ED visit (Table 31-3).[17]

It is important to assess whether patients are abusing opioids or appropriately using them to maintain quality of life. The importance of this is not primarily to deny addicts' access to these agents, but rather to develop treatment strategies that control pain while simultaneously minimizing any deleterious effects of opioid dependency. The following discussion will review the four common opioid-related scenarios that ED physicians are likely to encounter.

Opioid-Dependent Patients with Unequivocal and Uncontrolled Pain

Patients may present with uncontrolled chronic pain, the exacerbation of an underlying chronic pain syndrome, or the development of a new acute pain episode. While recognizing that multimodal analgesia (the use of nonopioid coanalgesics or therapies such as regional anesthesia) can contribute significantly to pain relief, the majority of these patients will require some adjustment of their opioid

Table 31-1. The CAGE Questionnaire[15,21]

In the past have you

felt that you wanted or needed to *cut* down on your
   drug use?

been *annoyed* or *angered* by others complaining about
   your drug use?

felt *guilty* about the consequences of your drug use?

ever used drugs to "get going" or calm down

Note: One positive response suggests the need for caution in prescribing opioids; two or more positive responses suggest increased vigilance by the physician prescribing opioids.
Source: Adapted from Refs. 15 and 21.

Table 31-2. SISAP Questionnaire

If you drink alcohol, how many drinks do you have in a typical day?
How many drinks do you have in a typical week?
Have you used marijuana or hashish in the last year?
Have you ever smoked cigarettes?
What is your age?

SISAP: Screening Instrument for Substance Abuse Potential.

Note: Increased vigilance is required by the physician prescribing opioids in men who consume more than 4 drinks a day or 16 drinks a week, women who consume more than 3 drinks a day or 12 drinks a week, patients who admit to marijuana use in the last year, and patients under 40 who smoke.

Source: Coombs RB et al. The SISAP: a new screening tool for identifying potential opioid abuse in the management of chronic non-malignant pain in general medical practice. *Pain Res Manage.* 1999;18:6–8.

regimen. This may only require increasing the dose of the medication they are receiving. Some patients develop marked tolerance within weeks of starting an initially effective medication. In such cases, *opioid rotation* will often be effective because different opioid receptor subtypes will respond to different drugs.[13] If intolerable side effects or a clear lack of efficacy suggest the need to switch to a different opioid, there are several important considerations. The addition or supplementation of short-acting opioids allows rapid titration of pain control. Because these agents have half-lives of approximately

Table 31-3. Comparison between Chronic Pain and Opioid Abuse

Chronic Pain	Opioid Abuse
Appropriate use of opioid	Opioid use out of control
Opioids improve quality of life	Opioids impair quality of life
Aware of side effects	Unconcerned about side effects
Follows treatment plan	Noncompliant with treatment plan
Has saved medication from previous prescription	Out of meds, lost prescription, a tale of woe
	Polydrug use is common
	High risk of psychiatric disorder

Source: Adapted from Ref. 17 page 217.

Table 31-4. Opioid Equianalgesic Data

Opioid	Parenteral (mg)	Oral (mg)
Morphine	10	30*
Hydromorphone	1.5	7.5
Oxycodone	–	20
Codeine	130	200
Fentanyl	0.1†	–
Methadone	–	3–5

*Oral morphine undergoes significant first pass effect. In morphine naive patients, equivalency with parenteral morphine is closer to 6:1.
†The transdermal fentanyl dose in mcg/h is approximately half the 24-hour dose of morphine (i.e., 100 mcg/h of fentanyl = 200 mg/day of morphine).

Source: Adapted from Gammaitoni et al. Clinical application of equianalgesic data. *Clin J Pain.* 2003;19:286–97.

4 hours, steady states are achieved within 24 hours, and further modifications can be instituted as necessary. If, on the other hand, the screening assessment suggests addictive or aberrant behavior, it may be appropriate to use longer acting or sustained release preparations, which have diminished euphoric effects and are associated with less intense withdrawal symptoms. In some circumstances, management will require more than dose adjustment and the ED physician may have to employ an alternative opioid. In such cases, an understanding of opioid pharmacology, and particularly knowledge of dose equivalencies is useful (Tables 31-4 to 31-6). Even prescribing longer acting forms is not without risk if there is concern of drug misuse, as some substance abusers will grind up the pills and inject through the intravenous (IV) route. Many emergency

Table 31-5. Equivalent Doses of Opioids for Acute Pain Management

Drug	Intramuscular Dose (mg)	Oral Dose (mg)
Morphine	10	60 milligrams
Meperidine	100	300
Hydromorphone	2	8
Codeine	60	180
Hydrocodone	–	20
Oxycodone	–	20
Fentanyl	0.15	

Source: Adapted from Innes GD, Zed PJ. Basic pharmacology and advances in emergency medicine. *Emerg Med Clin North Amer.* 2005;23:453.

Table 31-6. Opioids Compared to Standard Dose Morphine 10 mg IM or 20–30 mg PO

Drug	PO Dose	Parenteral Dose (IM or SC)	PR Dose	Dose Frequency
Codeine	200 mg	120 mg		q 4 h
Oxycodone				
Percocet (Acet.)	10–15 mg			q 4 h
Percodan (ASA)	(2–3 tabs)			
Hydromorphone	4 mg	2 mg	3 mg	q 4 h
– Dilaudid				
Sustained release capsule		2 × 6 mg		q 12 h
Morphine				
Solution (MOS)	20–30 mg			q 4 h
MS Contin/ MOS-SR	60–90 mg			q 12 h
Suppository*			10, 20, or 30 mg	q 6–8 h
Injectable		10 mg		q 4 h
Fentanyl				
Avoid:				
Meperidine	300 mg	75 mg		
Demerol				

*2 mg hydromorphone PO is equivalent to 10 mg morphine solution PO.

Source: Adapted from Innes GD, Zed PJ. Basic pharmacology and advances in emergency medicine. *Emerg Med Clin North Amer.* 2005;23:454.

physicians may feel more comfortable providing enough long-acting medication for a period of 24–48 hours, with the expectation that the patient will follow up with the physician who normally prescribes the opioids.

Gammaitoni et al[13] have recommended an approach to managing opioid-dependent patients with uncontrolled pain. The first step is to determine the patient's total daily dose of opioid, then convert this to total daily morphine equivalents based on equianalgesic data (Tables 31-4 to 31-6). Morphine is used because most studies have used it as the sole comparator with other potent opioids like hydromorphone or oxycodone.[18] This method allows calculation of the total daily opioid dose when patients are taking multiple medications, and it provides the basis for any medication or dosage changes.

If patients are being converted to another opioid, it is recommended that the total daily morphine equivalent dose be decreased by approximately 20–30% because of the lack of complete cross-tolerance among opioids,[15] although more aggressive dosing may be employed if pain is severe. Breakthrough dosing should be approximately 10–20% of the total daily dose of the long-acting agent. For example, a patient receiving 100 mg of long-acting morphine q 12 hour (total daily dose = 200 mg) should receive 20–40 mg q 4 hour for breakthrough pain.

Of note, methadone may be particularly effective when patients have been receiving other opioids for prolonged periods or at high doses, although it is not usually part of the emergency physicians' armamentarium.[15]

Determining equianalgesic doses is difficult in heroin addicts, given the varying purity of drugs sold on the street; however, as a rough guide, heroin is sold in *points*, and 1 point is equivalent to 0.1 g or 100 mg. Consumption can be estimated as high (>1.5 g/day), moderate (0.5–1 g/day), or low (0.5 g/day). A conservative approach to managing pain in these patients—if they had an open fracture, for example—would be to start short-acting morphine in doses of 10 mg PO q 4 hour in the low consumption group to 20 mg PO q 4 hour in the high consumption group. As noted previously, equivalent sustained release doses are sometimes preferable and easily calculated, for example, 10 mg of short-acting morphine q 4 hour is a total daily dose of 60 mg, which can be provided as 30 mg of a sustained release preparation q 12 hour.

Opioid-Dependent Patients with Acute Pathology of Questionable Validity or Severity

Patients with a history of substance abuse and those of dubious reliability often present with complaints such as back pain, dental pain, migraine headache, or renal colic. It is never easy to rate another person's pain experience and, in these conditions, the problem is often compounded by a lack of objective findings as well as the fact that the treatment offers significant potential for secondary gain. Consequently, physicians often feel they are being manipulated, which leads to anger and frustration, a compromised physician-patient relationship, and difficulty providing objective compassionate care. Attempts to avoid being "beaten" by a drug-seeking patient may lead physicians to withhold opioids from patients having real pain; however, in the absence of clear-cut indications that the patient is drug seeking, the emergency physician's fundamental responsibility is to relieve pain. The oft-quoted dictum, "pain is what the patient says it is" should guide management in most cases.

The designated medical profile (DMP) (aka frequent flyer) program is a useful ED innovation that improves care consistency and reduces physician uncertainty.[19] Patients who frequently use the ED for care that is more appropriately provided in community settings, including those who present repeatedly with pain-related complaints, may be referred to the DMP program. After ED nurses or physicians refer a patient to the program, a multidisciplinary committee, including an ED physician, nurse, social worker, and the patient's primary care provider or pain management physician, reviews the case and develops an ED care protocol defining a consistent approach to investigation, management and drug prescribing during subsequent ED visits. The DMP plan is consistent with the patient's overall care plan and is printed automatically at the triage desk each time the patient registers in the ED. Patients who do not have a primary care provider are referred to an appropriate community provider, and patients who are likely to benefit from other specialty consultation (e.g., psychiatry and chronic pain service) are referred, often during their next ED visit. Patients unwilling to participate in such a program need to be advised first that such a program can only be of benefit to their needs. If patients still refuse, they need to be informed that use of opioids may not be considered a treatment option for future visits with similar complaints.

Patients without Acute Pathology Requesting Opioids

Patients without acute pathology often present to EDs with hopes of having ED physicians prescribe drugs they cannot obtain elsewhere. Typical scenarios involve a lost or stolen prescription, running out of medication, being out of town, or being unable to access their regular physician.

Not infrequently, the inability to obtain their drug of choice has led to withdrawal, and they need something to alleviate their symptoms—preferably more opioid. There is little to guide a physician's management in this circumstance and decisions often relate more to personal philosophy than medical science. It is important that all physicians in one ED maintain the same approach for this group of patients. Varying approaches lead to patient's manipulating staff and creating confrontational situations; a standardized approach also permits rapid identification of such manipulation, allowing direct discussion with the patient.

When patients have legitimate reasons for being without medication, prescription refill is appropriate. When there is doubt about the patient's story, physicians should seek corroborating information. The patient's personal physician, if available, can clarify the patient's medication needs and usage history. Hospital records may show multiple previous visits for the same reason. Newer medical information systems are increasingly helpful, providing rapid access to hospital- and community-based data. Some states and provinces now have real-time computer-based prescription drug databases that can support or refute a patient's story. For example, the British Columbia Pharmanet system documents all drugs dispensed in the province of BC. Emergency physicians can access this database from the ED to confirm a patient's history of previous opioid requirements and assess recent utilization.

Regardless of how a physician deals with individual cases, it should be made clear to patients that their opioid management should be supervised by one physician and that the ED should be used only in exceptional circumstances. If the emergency physician does provide medication in this setting, the amount dispensed should generally be enough to allow patients time to visit their own doctor.

Patients Requesting Medication because of Withdrawal Symptoms

Patients requesting medication because of withdrawal symptoms require treatment. Physicians should be aware that the timing of onset and the severity of symptoms will depend on the opioid being used (Table 31-7), with longer acting agents having milder and more delayed presentations. In general, opioid withdrawal is rarely life threatening and is less severe than ethanol or sedative-hypnotic withdrawal. Classic findings include diaphoresis, yawning, tearing, rhinorrhea, myalgias, and piloerection. In more severe cases, abdominal cramping, diarrhea, and vomiting may occur. Altered level of consciousness, seizures, fever, or hypotension suggests the presence of an alternate explanation or concomitant illness.[20]

Table 31-7. Withdrawal Characteristics of Different Opioids

Opioid	Onset (h)	Peak Intensity	Duration
Meperidine	2–6	6–12 h	4–5 days
Fentanyl			
Morphine	6–18	36–72 h	7–10 days
Heroin			
Methadone	24–48	3–21 days	6–7 weeks

Source: Mitra S, Sinatra RS. Perioperative management of acute pain in the opioid dependent patient. *Anesthesiology.* 2004; 101:212–227.

Several types of agents are helpful in providing symptomatic relief for patients with opioid withdrawal. Clonidine (0.1–0.2 mg q 4–6 hour) acts on the autonomic nervous system, blocking sympathetic symptoms. Benzodiazepines are not cross-tolerant with opioids and reduce withdrawal-related anxiety. Antiemetics and antispasmodics can be used to treat gastrointestinal manifestations. For patients who are not recurrent ED users, it may be appropriate to offer one or two doses of opioid until they can see their regular physician. From a harm reduction perspective, it may be better to give regular, well-maintained methadone users, one or two doses of sustained release opioid than to have them leave the department in search of heroin. When addicts are discharged without symptom relief, the risk of assault or robbery is unclear but real.

Patients with Acute Pathology and a Remote History of Opioid Dependence or Abuse

Patients who were previously opioid dependent or addicted often present to the ED with acute pain problems. There are few data to guide analgesic management in this setting. However, it is prudent to involve the patient in decision making. In some cases, patients may feel that symptom severity is not sufficient to risk opioid exposure and alternative therapies can be tried. As always, a multimodal approach using physical modalities, acetaminophen, anti-inflammatories, and other adjunctive agents is appropriate, but if pain is intolerable it is hard to justify denying opioids. If opioids are employed, they should be prescribed for limited duration, and close follow-up is mandatory. Sustained release preparations may be preferable as they are associated with less risk of readdiction.[15] Opioid *contracts* have not been shown to be useful across the spectrum of ED patients, but may be of some value in this patient subset.[21]

SUMMARY

Caring for opioid-dependent patients in the ED is a difficult and uncertain experience. The misunderstanding and suspicion that often accompany these encounters are counterproductive and often result in unhappy outcomes for both physician and patient. Emergency physicians should remember that opioid addiction and dependence are physiologic processes that change the treatment needs. Because of physiologic and patient characteristics, these situations can manifest as solicitous or confrontational behavior that is annoying to ED staff, and they are often perceived as misuse of the ED. Although physicians should not enable inappropriate behaviors or use of resources, we should offer the most appropriate compassionate care possible. Addiction and dependence is the patient's problem. When we respond with anger or frustration, it becomes our problem as well.

REFERENCES

1. Rupp T, Delaney KA. Inadequate analgesia in emergency medicine. *Ann Emerg Med.* 2004;43:494–503.
2. Joranson DE, Ryan KM, Gilson AM, et al. Trends in medical use and abuse of opioid analgesics. *JAMA.* 2000;283: 1710–1714.
3. Bolay H, Moskowitz MA. Mechanisms of pain modulation in chronic syndromes. *Neurology.* 2002;59(suppl 2):S2–S7.
4. Cami J, Farre M. Drug addiction. *N Engl J Med.* 2003;349: 975–986.
5. American Psychiatric Association. *Diagnostic and Statistical Manual of Mental Disorder.* 4th ed. Text revision: DSM-IV-TR. Washington, DC: American Psychiatric Association; 2000.
6. Gurstin HB, Akil H. Opioid analgesics. In: Hardman JG, Limbird LE, eds. *Goodman and Gilman's The Pharmacological Basis of Therapeutics.* 10th ed. New York: McGraw-Hill; 2001:569–619.
7. Howard LA, Sellers EM, Tyndale RF. The role of pharmacogenetically-variable cytochrome P450 enzymes in drug abuse and dependence. *Pharmacogenomics.* 2002;3: 85–89.
8. O'Brien CP. Drug addiction and abuse. In: Hardman JG, Limbird LE, eds. *Goodman and Gilman's The Pharmacological Basis of Therapeutics.* 10th ed. New York: McGraw-Hill; 2001:641–642.
9. Austrup ML, Korean G. Analgesic agents for the post-op period. *Surg Clin North Am.* 1999;79:253–271.
10. Nestler EJ. Molecular neurobiology of addiction. *Am J Addict.* 2001;10:201–217.
11. Sosnowski M, Yalesh TL. Differential cross tolerance between intra-thecal morphine and sufentanil in the rat. *Anesthesiology.* 1990;73:1141–1147.
12. Christo PJ. Opioid effectiveness and side effects in chronic pain. *Anesthesiol Clin North Am.* 2003;21:699–713.

13. Gammaitoni AR, Fine P, Alvarez N, et al. Clinical application of equianalgesic data. *Clin J Pain.* 2003;19: 286–297.

14. DeVries TJ, Shippenberg TS. Neural systems underlying opiate addiction. *J Neurosci.* 2002;22:3321–3325.

15. Gardner-Nix J. Principles of opioid use in chronic non-cancer pain. *CMAJ.* 2003;169:38–43.

16. Fishbain DA, Rosomoff HL, Rosomoff RS. Drug abuse, dependence and addiction in chronic pain patients. *Clin J Pain.* 1992;8:77–85.

17. Mitra S, Sinatra RS. Perioperative management of acute pain in the opioid dependent patient. *Anesthesiology.* 2004;101:212–227.

18. Dunbar PJ, Chapman CR, Buckley FP, et al. Clinical analgesic equivalence for morphine and hydromorphone with prolonged PCA. *Pain.* 1996;68:265–270.

19. Grafstein E, Burton K, Innes G, et al. Evaluation of a program to address frequent emergency department users. *Acad Emerg Med.* Chan A. Personal communication. Addiction Services Team. St. Paul's Hospital, Vancouver, BC, Canada. 2004;11:455–456.

20. Chiang C, Wax PM. In: Delaney KA, Ling LJ, Frickson T, eds. *Ford: Clinical Toxicology.* Philadelphia, PA: W.B. Saunders; 2001:587–588.

21. Wilsey B, Fishman S, Rose JS, et al. Pain management in the ED. *Am J Emerg Med.* 2004;22:51–57.

22. Coombs RB, Jarry JL, Santhiapillai AC, et al. The SISAP: a new screening tool for identifying potential opioid abuse in the management of chronic non-malignant pain in general medical practice. *Pain Res Manage.* 1999;18:6–8.

Part 2: SPECIFIC PAIN SYNDROMES

32

Chest Pain

Sandra M. Schneider
James I. Syrett

HIGH YIELD FACTS

- Sixteen percent of adults complain of occasional chest pain, leading to over 5% of emergency department (ED) visits.

- Of all patients presenting to an ED with cardiac-like chest pain, 24% will have a myocardial infarction and 30% will have unstable angina.

- Although nitroglycerin rapidly relieves the pain of cardiac ischemia through improvement of blood flow, studies have found no benefit in outcomes from its use.

- Relief of pain by nitroglycerin is not specific for myocardial ischemia. There is no diagnostic value when chest pain is relieved by a trial of nitroglycerin.

- Beta-blockers do not appear to reduce the pain of cardiac ischemia.

- Most patients with cocaine-induced chest pain have normal coronary arteries; ischemia is likely due to coronary artery spasm.

- Acute chest syndrome is the leading cause of death and hospitalization among patients with sickle cell disease. It may present with chest pain, fever, and leukocytosis.

- Use of viscous lidocaine to differentiate esophageal pain from cardiac pain is not diagnostic.

Complaints of chest pain are common; when surveyed, 16% of adults complain of occasional chest pain. It leads to over 5% of emergency department (ED) visits at an annual cost to the health care system in excess of U.S. $8 billion. Most patients complaining of chest pain fear their pain is due to cardiac disease. Failure to alleviate or explain the nature of such pain may lead to ongoing anxiety and recurrent visits to the health care system.

Most cardiac pain presents as a deep aching visceral sensation. Cardiac pain is sensed through afferent nerves C8-T4. Similar innervation exists for other mediastinal structures; the great vessels (acute distention) and the esophagus (spasm or irritation) may also produce this visceral type of pain. Superficial neuropathways are shared with intercostal nerves and the pleura.

Of all patients presenting to an ED with cardiac-like chest pain (i.e., crushing, pressure, or heaviness), 24% will have myocardial infarction and 30% will have unstable angina. The other 46% of patients will have non-cardiac causes of their pain. Even when the presentation is not typical cardiac pain, differentiating that cause may be difficult. For example, while burning pain is more suggestive of esophageal pain, it occurs in 23% of patients with myocardial infarction and 21% of patients with unstable angina.

MYOCARDIAL ISCHEMIA

Since 1809, the pain of myocardial ischemia has been attributed to an imbalance in the oxygen supply and demand. An increase in left ventricular systolic pressure and wall tension (i.e., increased stretch) stimulates the nociceptors within the myocardium. Decrease in coronary artery flow can occur from a decrease in coronary artery perfusion pressure, coronary artery vasospasm, increased intramyocardial pressure and heart rate, coronary artery stenosis or thrombosis, rupture of an atheromatous plaque, increased blood viscosity, anomalous coronary artery origin, or an anomalous intramyocardial coronary artery course. Coronary atherosclerosis has been felt to be the major cause of angina, although vasospasm may cause angina in up to 10% of patients.[1] Spasm and atherosclerotic disease may coexist in the same patient.

Effort-related angina is the most common form of ischemic pain, and is due to a transient increase in oxygen demand. Carotid massage, and subsequent bradycardia, can rapidly abort angina but carries other risks, including a decrease in cerebral perfusion, and is not recommended.

Pain relief is critical in the patient with an acute myocardial infarction. A frightened, uncomfortable patient has an increased sympathetic tone, which leads to an outpouring of catecholamines. Additional coronary vasoconstriction, tachycardia, and raised systemic vascular resistance, may all increase myocardial ischemia and infarct size. Patients with prolonged pain have more severe outcomes.[2]

Nitroglycerin is extremely effective in relieving all forms of angina. Following administration of nitroglycerin, there is marked venous dilation causing a reduction in preload. This decreases left ventricular volume and results in a decrease in left ventricular wall tension. To a lesser extent, arterial vasodilation reduces afterload. Together these actions decrease myocardial oxygen demand. Nitrates are readily absorbed through the skin, oral mucosa, and intestinal mucosa. Sublingual nitroglycerin is one of the fastest acting of the common preparations, with an onset of 1–2 minutes, lasting 1 hour. Oral and transcutaneous forms are used for prophylaxis, with a slow onset of action that may last 4–24 hours. Acute reduction in preload—as seen with sublingual or intravenous nitrates—may produce transient hypotension and reflex tachycardia. This is most often seen in preload dependent patients such as the volume-depleted patient or someone with mitral stenosis.

Angiographic studies show that nitroglycerin dilates both normal and diseased coronary arteries, as well as decreasing the area of the stenosis.[3] There is an increase in the ratio of endocardial to epicardial blood flow.

Nitroglycerin rapidly relieves the pain of cardiac ischemia through improvement of blood flow. It should be given to all patients with acute onset of chest pain that appears to be of cardiac origin. While ISIS-4 and GISSI-3 studies have found no benefit in outcomes (such as 28-day survival and left ventricular function) as a result of routine use of nitroglycerin in patients with uncomplicated myocardial infarction, intravenous nitroglycerin is an effective treatment in patients with unstable angina. Infusions are begun at 5–10 mcg/min with the dose doubled every 5 minutes as tolerated until pain relief is obtained or until a change in blood pressure or pulse occurs. For prophylactic infusions and patients receiving thrombolytics, the dosage is 10–15 mcg/min.

Relief of pain by nitroglycerin is not specific for myocardial ischemia. The patient with functional origin of chest pain may express pain relief after taking nitroglycerin, but relief often takes more than a few minutes. Nitroglycerin may rapidly relieve chest pain associated with esophageal spasm, pylorospasm, biliary colic, and renal colic. One study found 90% of patients receiving nitroglycerin for chest pain obtained partial, and 72% complete relief, while demonstrating that such a response was unrelated to the cause of the pain.[4] Thus, there is no diagnostic value possible when chest pain is relieved by a trial of nitroglycerin.

Nitroglycerin in any form causes vasodilatation, and can produce postural hypotension and even syncope. This is more frequent in patients on beta-blockers, antihypertensives, phenothiazines, or in patients who have ingested alcohol. It should be used with caution in patients who have a right-sided myocardial infarction because of their dependence on preload to maintain their blood pressure. Nitroglycerin may cause hypoxemia, especially in patients with severe chronic obstructive pulmonary disease, due to an increase in venous blood admixture. Uncommon forms of angina due to severe aortic stenosis, hypertrophic subaortic stenosis, or Barlow's syndrome (mitral valve prolapse) may occasionally worsen with nitroglycerin therapy due to an increase in outflow obstruction and a decrease in preload.

The American Heart Association advises the initial use of oxygen to maintain saturation greater than 90%. Hypoxemia may result from a decrease in cardiac output and peripheral vasoconstriction brought on by the sympathetic response. Partial relief of chest pain with oxygen is reported by nearly one-third of patients. There is some evidence that the use of oxygen may limit myocardial ischemia and reduce ST elevation in patients with acute anterior wall myocardial infarctions. Patient outcomes are unchanged with oxygen use; further, opioid requirements are identical when patients are treated with oxygen or room air placebo. In uncomplicated cases, supplemental oxygen can be discontinued after the first few hours.

If pain is not completely relieved by nitroglycerin then an opiate should be administered. The ultimate goal of opiate use is complete pain relief. Morphine is the opiate most frequently used, although theoretically other opiates would be beneficial. Fentanyl may produce sympathetic blockade, so may be superior to morphine in acute ischemia but no formal studies have been done to compare fentanyl with morphine. Incremental doses of intravenous morphine (2–5 mg) are recommended. Patients should be reassessed every 10–20 minutes to assure that pain relief/comfort is obtained and there is no recurrence.

Side effects to morphine occur in 2–8% of patients. Most common is hypotension, secondary to an initial release of histamine as a reaction to the presence of morphine. Repetitive dosing will not repeat the histamine release, so recurrent hypotension and nausea are unlikely. Hypotension from morphine is most common in volume-depleted patients, patients with right ventricular infarction, or patients treated with nitrates.

Beta-blockers reduce the size of an infarct in patients who do not receive reperfusion therapy. They decrease postinfarction ischemia and nonfatal myocardial infarction in those receiving thrombolytic agents. By decreasing heart rate, arterial pressure, and left ventricular contractility, myocardial oxygen demand is decreased. They do not appear to reduce the pain of cardiac ischemia. Nearly 80% of patients suffering from acute myocardial infarction can safely be given beta-blockers although optimal doses of beta-blockers are yet unknown. Side effects include hypotension, bradycardia, atrioventricular block, left ventricular failure, and bronchospasm. Bronchospasm may be significant in patients with bronchospasm airway disease.

The use of ultra-short-acting beta-blockers may offer the potential for more patients to receive beta-blockers since their clinical effect and side effects last less than 30 minutes. Esmolol is cardioselective, 100 times more active on the cardiac beta$_1$ receptor than the vascular beta$_2$ receptors. Esmolol is given as a loading infusion of 500 mcg/kg/min, for 1 minute followed by infusion of 25 mcg/kg/min, progressively increasing the infusion by 50 mcg/kg/min every 4 minutes until a response is seen. Higher doses of esmolol are usually required in patients who have previously been on beta-blockers.

Thrombolytics restore coronary artery blood flow to infarcting myocardial tissue when given within 6 hours of the onset of chest pain, reversing the ischemic insult. Over 75% of eligible patients are treated with some form of reperfusion therapy, although the use of thrombolytic medication has become less common with the increased availability of cardiac angioplasty.

Recent evidence suggests that angioplasty may be superior to thrombolysis.[5] Reperfusion by angioplasty or stent placement is now indicated in patients with cardiogenic shock due to myocardial infarction in patients when thrombolysis has failed. When available, catheterization with angioplasty or stent placement is the preferred method of myocardial salvage.[5]

The efficacy of aspirin to improve outcome in patients with acute cardiac ischemia is well established. The ISIS-2 study showed that mortality was reduced by 2.4% in patients receiving aspirin for acute myocardial infarction and this benefit was even more pronounced when the patient was also given streptokinase.[6] Aspirin reduces platelet adhesiveness and is frequently given to patients who have suffered acute myocardial infarction prior to thrombolytic administration. Aspirin also prevents chest pain and myocardial infarction in patients with chronic stable angina. It can be given to chest pain patients at home while awaiting paramedics, in the ambulance, in the physician's office, or on entering the ED. It is inexpensive and has few adverse side effects.

COCAINE-INDUCED CHEST PAIN

In the past 10 years, cocaine-related ED visits rose by more than 33%. In 18 of 21 metropolitan areas monitored by the DAWN network, visits involving cocaine exceeded that of any other drug of abuse, including marijuana, heroin, and methamphetamine. Nearly 40% of cocaine-related visits are for chest pain. However, the incidence of cardiac arrest in ED patients with cocaine associated chest pain is only 1%. Recent cocaine use is associated with cardiac ischemia, arrhythmia, cardiomyopathy, aortic dissection, asthma, pneumomediastinum, hypersensitivity pneumo-nitis, pneumothorax, and intrapulmonary hemorrhage, all of which can produce chest pain.[7]

Most patients with cocaine-induced chest pain, including those with acute myocardial infarction, have normal coronary arteries.[8] Ischemia is likely due to coronary artery spasm. Cardiac enzymes may be elevated for a very brief period of time and may not follow a normal necrosis pattern. Nitroglycerin relieves pain in 45% of patients with cocaine-induced chest pain. Beta-blockers have been demonstrated to worsen alpha adrenergic receptor-mediated vasoconstriction, and may be harmful in cocaine-induced chest pain. Phentolamine may be of benefit in blocking alpha adrenergic vasoconstriction, but its use is still regarded as experimental. Benzodiazepines are used to treat cocaine-associated chest pain in addition to nitroglycerin. In addition, opioids and anxiolytics may be of benefit in the drug users who are experiencing withdrawal.

PERICARDITIS

The pain of pericarditis is frequently confused with that of cardiac ischemia. This is particularly true of patients with postmyocardial infarction pericarditis, which usually occurs while the memory of the acute infarction is still vivid. Other causes of pericarditis include infection, tumor, and connective tissue disease. Regardless of etiology, pain is caused by an inflammatory irritation of the nerves in the adjacent pleura. Patients often relieve their own pain by sitting upright and leaning forward.

Opioids are poor analgesics in this setting. Intravenous steroids (15 mg dexamethasone or 500 mg methylprednisolone) may provide prompt relief of pain regardless of etiology. Oral nonsteroidal anti-inflammatory drugs (NSAIDs) and even salicylates can produce a decrease in inflammation with eventual total pain relief.[9] Colchicine may be another alternative in patients unable to take NSAIDs or steroids.

VALVULAR HEART DISEASE

Patient with aortic stenosis often seek medical care for angina. Angiographic studies have shown significant coronary artery occlusion to be present in 20–60% of patients.[10] Some of these patients may have atypical angina or be asymptomatic. The cause of angina pain in the absence of atherosclerotic coronary artery disease is not clear. Coronary perfusion may be decreased in patients with aortic stenosis, or there may be decreased flow in the endomyocardium because of increased left ventricular diastolic pressure. The mismatch of oxygen supply and demand may be dependent on aortic valve area and left ventricular wall thickness. Often the angina is directly attributed to direct increased oxygen demand by the heart to maintain coronary perfusion.

Patients with acute angina and aortic stenosis can initially be treated with nitroglycerin. These patients are at high risk for death. Definitive procedures such as angiography and valve replacement should be considered early. It is common for angina to cease after valve replacement with a low resistance aortic valve.

Severe aortic regurgitation may lead to chest pain, often confused with angina. Symptomatic patients are often younger than those with aortic stenosis, and atherosclerosis is less common. Pain is due to a decrease in coronary artery blood flow from the hyperdynamic left ventricular wall. This pain responds poorly to nitroglycerin and other antianginal drugs. Surgical correction should be considered early.

Mitral stenosis causes left atrial distention, which may lead to angina-like chest pain. Surgery often corrects the situation, but in the short term, relief can be gained by rest. Pain may also occur from pulmonary hypertension.

Mitral valve prolapse is perhaps the most common valvular disease in the United States, with a prevalence of 4–7% of the population (predominantly in woman). Nearly 50% of patients with mitral valve prolapse complain of chest pain; 10–20% have pain similar to angina. The association between mitral valve prolapse and chest pain may be spurious since a similar number of patients without mitral valve prolapse complain of chest pain. Very few patients with mitral valve prolapse have coexisting coronary artery disease; subjects with mitral valve prolapse are no more likely to have chest pain than were subjects without mitral valve prolapse.

Beta-blockers have been used for the relief of chest pain due to mitral valve prolapse. There are conflicting results in the literature regarding the effectiveness of this treatment. Propranolol and other beta-blockers increase esophageal contractility both in amplitude and duration and therefore should increase esophageal pain. Beta-blockade may reduce the symptomatology of panic disorder, often coexistent in patients with mitral valve prolapse.

THORACIC AORTIC DISSECTION

Though the pressure of a large nondissecting thoracic aortic aneurysm may cause chronic chest pain, acute chest pain is more commonly associated with thoracic aortic dissection. The pain is similar to cardiac ischemia and the two conditions are often confused. Nearly 2000 new cases of thoracic aortic dissection occur each year. Untreated, 25% of patients will die within 24 hours, 50% in 1 week, 75% in 1 month, and 90% in 1 year,[11] with surgical and/or medical intervention, 60% of patients can live a normal life span.

Hypotensive therapy can reduce the shear force (dP/dT) on the aorta, and decrease the risk of further dissection. Reduction of shear force may relieve pain and stabilize the patient while the necessary imaging and consultations are obtained. Trimethaphan decreases mean systolic arterial pressure and dP/dT, and may be used in combination with reserpine and/or guanethidine. Nitroprusside (for hypotensive effect) is used in combination with beta-blockers (to decrease dP/dT).

PLEURAL CAUSES OF CHEST PAIN

The pleura itself has no nociceptive innervation, but receptors lie very close to the endothoracic fascia near the parietal pleura. Intercostal nerves supply this area. The pain of pleural irritation is usually sensed as being superficial. If the diaphragmatic pleura is involved, pain will be referred to the shoulder.

Any condition involving the pleura directly or indirectly may cause pleuritic chest pain including pulmonary embolism, pneumonia, and pneumothorax. Pain control with opioids or nitrous oxide (contraindicated in pneumothorax) should be initiated while definitive investigations and therapy such as antibiotics, anticoagulants, and so forth are initiated. Analgesia should not be withheld until a diagnosis is made.

Viral pleuritis, also known as pleurodynia, is usually of abrupt onset, but may have a typical viral prodrome. In many cases, the pain is similar to that seen with cardiac ischemia. Symptoms are generally self-limited, but often take up to 2 weeks to resolve. Nonsteroidal anti-inflammatory medications and local heat application are most commonly used. In severe or refractory cases, intercostal nerve blocks may be performed.

PULMONARY CAUSES OF CHEST PAIN

Pulmonary hypertension may cause chest pain as a result of acute dilation of the pulmonary arteries. Patients with known primary pulmonary hypertension or pulmonary hypertension secondary to valvular heart disease develop chest pain with exertion or stress. Chest pain may be seen in normal individuals when there is sudden hypoxia, such as with massive pulmonary embolism, exposure to high altitudes, or prolonged exposure to inclement conditions.

Supplemental oxygen sufficient to raise the PO_2 will decrease the pulmonary vascular resistance, causing pulmonary vasodilation and relieve the pain. Sublingual nifedipine has been shown to be effective in some patients with acute elevation of pulmonary pressure. Patients with primary pulmonary hypertension have more chronic pain, which may require the use of opioids.

ACUTE CHEST SYNDROME IN SICKLE CELL ANEMIA

Patients with sickle cell anemia and occasionally with sickle cell trait may present with chest pain, fever, and leukocytosis.[12] It is the leading cause of death and hospitalization among patients with sickle cell disease. The diagnosis of acute chest syndrome is made in the patient with sickle cell disease who has fever, cough, and arterial oxygen desaturation. Patients are likely to be adults with a history of vasoocclusive disease, thrombocytopenia, pain in the arms or legs at presentations, abnormal chest x-ray, and fever. This syndrome may be difficult to distinguish from pulmonary embolism or infarction. Postmortem examinations have shown alveolar necrosis, bone marrow emboli, and infarctions without identifiable thrombosis. Many patients will progress rapidly to acute respiratory failure requiring intubation and positive pressure ventilation. Other treatments utilized include exchange transfusion particularly in children. Some patients show improvement with early albuterol treatments.

ESOPHAGEAL CAUSES OF CHEST PAIN

Patients with esophageal causes for chest pain are frequent users of medical services, filling 1.2 prescriptions per month, making 2.2 visits to private physicians or EDs per year, and costing $40 million per year. Esophageal pain may arise from distention, spasm, or frequent contraction of the esophagus. The innervation is nearly identical to that of the heart and, therefore may produce pain indistinguishable from that seen with cardiac ischemia.

Tight, vice-like pain is described in 91% of patients with esophageal disease. Pain radiating to the left arm, shoulder, or neck is seen in 79% of such patients; exertional pain in 72% of patients. Relief with nitroglycerin is noted in 63% of patients.[13] Despite overlap, reflux esophagitis is generally responsible for heartburn, whereas esophageal spasm more likely causes dull substernal pain.

REFLUX ESOPHAGITIS

Gastroesophageal reflux disease (GERD) is the most common cause of noncardiac chest pain. Over 35% of the normal population experiences heartburn at least once a month. Nearly 25% of pregnant women experience esophageal reflux daily and an additional 27% have heartburn at least once a month. Reflux is dependent on lower esophageal sphincter tone, acid clearance, the presence of a hiatal hernia, and the efficiency of gastric emptying. Therapy is directed toward these factors.

Antacids are the drugs of choice for the acute one-time control of reflux-induced pain. Antacids neutralize any acids present in the esophagus and stomach and increase lower esophageal sphincter tone. Relief is reported in 39–95% of patients, beginning within a few minutes and lasting 1–2 hours. All liquid antacids are equally effective. Lifestyle modifications include eating small meals, avoiding food 3–6 hours before bedtime, and raising the head of the bed 15°. Foods high in fat content, alcohol, chocolate, spearmint, and peppermint decrease lower esophageal sphincter tone and should be avoided. Citrus juices, tomatoes, and caffeine have a direct irritant effect. Theophylline, prostaglandin E1 and E2, and anticholinergics should be tapered or discontinued if possible. Antianginal drugs such as calcium-channel blockers, beta-blockers, and nitroglycerin decrease lower esophageal sphincter tone and decrease contraction amplitude, thereby increasing reflux. Smoking should be prohibited. While H_2 blockers and proton pump inhibitors are effective, response may take 1 week.

When H_2 blocker therapy has failed, treatment with metoclopramide or proton pump inhibitors may be indicated. Proton pump inhibitors markedly decrease or eliminate acid production in the stomach. They are superior to H_2 blockers and seem to cure or improve pain in at least 50% of patients with doses up to 40–60 mg/day. Though effective, proton pump therapy can be expensive.

Sulcrafate binds to the ulcerative surface of the stomach and displaces pepsin, preventing diffusion of gastric acid across the barrier it creates. Although this drug is effective in patients with peptic ulcer disease, it has not been studied in patients with esophageal reflux.

ESOPHAGEAL SPASM

Much debate surrounds the actual significance of esophageal spasm. Motility and pH monitoring has shown that many episodes of chest pain occur without motor or acid reflux abnormalities. Conversely, motility abnormalities occur without causing chest pain. The chest pain itself may precipitate the motility disturbance. With this confusion, it is understandable that treatments have varied greatly and studies have failed to show any single superior treatment.

Nitrates can relieve the pain of diffuse esophageal spasm. Pain relief, when it occurs, generally does not begin until 5 minutes after medication and may last as long as 60 minutes. Long-acting nitroglycerin may provide 4 hours of relief from esophageal spasm pain. Muscle relaxants and anticholinergic medications have been effective in relieving pain in some reports. However, controlled clinical trials are lacking.

CHEST WALL SYNDROME

Tietze's syndrome, acute costochondritis, and a variety of other musculoskeletal syndromes cause chest pain often mistaken for angina by both the physician and the patient. Tietze's syndrome is classically described as point tenderness of one or more costal cartilages associated with nonsuppurative swelling. Pathologic findings have been minimal, showing only mild perichondritis. It is a very common cause of chest pain occurring in 10–69% of patients presenting with chest pain.

A wide variety of treatments are reported in the literature—nearly all of them based on anecdotal reports or with limited clinical experience. Controlled clinical trials are absent. Pain relief has been claimed with the use of short-wave diathermy, physical therapy, muscle relaxants, and oral anti-inflammatory agents. Injection of 1% lidocaine 2–11 mL into the joint space provides complete resolution of symptoms within minutes.

POSTSTERNOTOMY CHEST PAIN

Nearly 40% of patients who have had a surgical midline sternotomy have chronic pain occurring over the incision. Serious causes of chest pain include sternal or chondral infection, sternal nonunion, sternal dehiscence, fractured ribs, or costosternal separation. Patients without signs of these serious etiologies may be treated with lidocaine injection. Therapy in other patients is directed at the cause.

Patients who have undergone internal mammary artery grafting may develop numbness over the site of the donor artery, tenderness in the sternum, and allodynia (pain felt with stimuli that usually does not provoke pain). This pain is present immediately after surgery and often increases over the next several months. Local injection gives short-term pain relief, while use of a transcutaneous electrical nerve stimulation (TENS) unit very early after surgery has been reported to give long term relief of pain.

Persistent chest pain due to the sternal wires has been described in some patients related to nickel sensitivity.

When pain is localized over a sternal wire(s), removal may provide relief.

THORACIC OUTLET SYNDROME

Thoracic outlet syndrome involving the upper extremity and neck, commonly causes pain and parasthesias in the ulnar distribution. Occasionally pain is felt in the anterior chest and in some cases may be indistinguishable from cardiac ischemia. Thoracic outlet syndrome is felt to be caused by compression of the neurovascular bundle by a cervical rib, first thoracic rib, or scalene muscle. Though it generally arises spontaneously, thoracic outlet obstruction can begin after thoracic trauma. Special maneuvers may aid in the diagnosis by reproducing the pain. The Adson test is positive if a decrease or obliteration of the radial pulse occurs when the patient takes a deep breath while lifting the chin and turning the head to the affected side. This test has an accuracy (true positive rate) of 27–100% for the presence of thoracic outlet obstruction (scalene anticus syndrome)[14]; however, 50% of normal patients also have a positive test (false positive). The hyperabduction test involves raising both hands over the head. If the radial pulse decreases or disappears, thoracic outlet obstruction may be present with similar accuracy as the Adson test. If either of these tests is positive or thoracic outlet syndrome is suspected on clinical grounds, further diagnostic studies are indicated, including neurologic evaluation, sensory evoked potentials, and other neurophysiologic tests. No consistent criteria have been used to definitively diagnose thoracic outlet obstruction.

Conservative therapy of thoracic outlet obstruction is preferred. Patient education and avoidance of hyperabduction, especially while sleeping, is often successful. Physical therapy maneuvers including shoulder girdle strengthening exercises and relaxation of shortened muscles have been recommended. Refractory cases require surgery.

RIB FRACTURE

Rib fractures with or without trauma may cause severe chest pain. The fractured area irritates intercostal nerves and causes reflex intercostal muscle spasm. This spasm not only intensifies the pain but also causes splinting of that area against any movement, preventing normal respiratory exertion. Splinting (rib belts or muscle spasm) can decrease patient discomfort, but also decreases the patient's vital capacity and impairs coughing. Pooling of secretions into areas of atelectasis may lead to pneumonia. Local taping using an elastic adhesive material has largely replaced binding the entire thorax.

Oral and parenteral opioids are often necessary for patient comfort. Pain control is difficult. The most severe pain is with activity (especially abrupt activity such as coughing or sneezing). Nonsteroidal anti-inflammatory medications are also helpful, but may provide inadequate analgesia, particularly when there has been a substantial amount of soft tissue trauma.

Injection of local anesthetic allows pain-free coughing and normal respiratory movement. Intercostal nerve blocks not only give pain relief, but this relief is sufficient to avoid mechanical ventilation in some cases with multiple rib fractures. While many patients require supplemental oral analgesics such as nonsteroidal anti-inflammatory medications, the nerve bock may last for several days despite the short duration of action of the local anesthetic.

For patients with multiple rib fractures and extensive thoracic trauma, admission is usually necessary. Most of these patients have a pulmonary contusion and decrease in pulmonary function. In cases of severe chest wall trauma, early placement of an epidural catheter to provide a continuous analgesic infusion has been correlated with a decreased incidence of pulmonary complications and decreased mortality.

SPINAL DISC DISEASE

Cervical discs can rarely present as chest pain, simulating cardiac ischemia. Treatment with nonsteroidal medications, steroids, traction, and surgical removal will relieve the associated chest complaints. Thoracic disc disease is extremely rare, but over 50% of these patients have chest pain. Most patients respond to conservative measures of posture change and lifting techniques. Nonsteroidal anti-inflammatory medications and steroids are beneficial. Some patients do require surgical treatment.

MEDICATION TRIAL FOR DIAGNOSIS OF CHEST PAIN

Placebo effect in analgesia trials is positive in 20–40% of patients. Decrease in pain after receiving medication may therefore be due to this placebo effect. Many physicians have used an antacid trial to distinguish reflux symptoms from cardiac pain; however, true myocardial ischemic pain can be relieved with antacids.[15] Viscous lidocaine with or without concomitant use of antacids has been given to patients as a diagnostic test for reflux esophagitis. Though patients with reflux respond to the treatment, patients with ischemic pain may also respond. Therefore, use of viscous lidocaine to differentiate esophageal pain from cardiac pain is not diagnostic. Pain that responds to nitroglycerin may not be ischemic. Esophageal spasm responds to nitroglycerin. Reproducible chest wall tenderness may be present in 7–10% of patients with pulmonary emboli or with myocardial infarction.

CHEST PAIN IN THE PEDIATRIC POPULATION

Like their adult counterparts, chest pain is a common complaint of young children and adolescents. It accounts for 650,000 outpatient visits per year and is the third leading nontraumatic complaint following headache and abdominal pain. Musculoskeletal and posttraumatic causes account for 15–20% of patients with chest pain. Gastrointestinal (GI) disorders are common, accounting for somewhere between 7 and 16% of patients with chest pain. Primary respiratory disorders account for 10% of young people with chest pain and this is usually due to coughing and asthma, but may also be due to more serious disorders such as sickle cell anemia and cystic fibrosis.

Cardiovascular disorders are quite rare and present only in 1–6% of teenagers.[16] Serious causes such as right- or left-sided outlet obstruction may lead to sudden death. Patients who have cardiac murmurs may need to be screened for the presence of valvular disease, pulmonary hypertension, or idiopathic hypertrophic subaortic stenosis. Cardiac ischemia can be caused by congenital coronary artery abnormalities, such as anomalous left coronary artery arising from pulmonary artery or impingement of the left coronary artery between the main pulmonary artery and aorta. Polyarteritis nodosa and Kawasaki disease may lead to coronary arteritis producing ischemic coronary disease. Ischemia may also be seen in patients with coronary artery spasm, type II A (homozygous) hyperlipidemia, or cocaine use.

Idiopathic chest pain may account for up to 40% of children who present with chest pain. This syndrome seems to occur primarily in patients during rapid growth spurts and has been described more frequently in females. Pain is usually in a very specific location, often directly over the precordium. These patients are frequent users of health care and may have some psychologic component. Reassurance and symptomatic therapy is generally successful. The pain disappears in approximately 80% of patients within 3 years.

CHEST PAIN WITHOUT DEFINABLE CAUSE

Demonstrating the absence of coronary artery disease does not either relieve the chest pain or reassure the patient. Less than 40% of patients seen in an ED with atypical chest pain believe the diagnosis that was given to them. Of those who undergo a stress test with negative results, most continue to believe they have organic disease. Of patients with angiographic evidence of clean coronary arteries, 50–75% will have persistent chest pain and most will show a decrease in their social and physical activity.

Panic attack is probably the most frequent cause, occurring in approximately 40–60% of patients with normal arteriographic studies. Panic attacks may also occur in the patient with true ischemic disease. Panic attacks produce alarming physical symptoms including shortness of breath, dizziness, palpitations, choking, abdominal distress, and fear of dying, as well as atypical chest pain. Panic disorders respond to a variety of therapies including both pharmacologic and cognitive/behavioral. Tricyclic antidepressants have been shown to benefit patients with panic disorder and cardiovascular symptoms. Monoamine oxidase inhibitors are also good for relief of anxiety, but have not been specifically studied in patients with noncardiac chest pain. Beta-adrenergic antagonists can be used to control the sympathetically-mediated symptoms. Beta-blockers decrease the incidence of palpitations and diaphoresis and may decrease the effect of catecholamines on the respiratory center. In one study, nearly 50% of patients treated with a benzodiazepine responded with a decrease in panic frequency.

Hyperventilation syndrome is a common cause of chest pain, particularly in patients below the age of 40. Patients present with chest pain, palpitations, dyspnea, and occasionally parasthesias and dizziness. Such patients have increased symptoms with voluntary hyperventilation or with mental stress and may have an increased awareness of body sensations. Many people believe that hyperventilation syndrome may be a variant of panic disorder and/or depression. Patients respond to behavioral and cognitive therapy or to long-acting benzodiazepines.

SUMMARY

Relief of chest pain should be accomplished as soon as possible, not only to provide patient comfort, but because of the physiologic and psychologic consequences of the pain. In the patient with cardiac chest pain, persistent discomfort leads to elevated catecholamines and an increase in myocardial oxygen demand. Unrelieved pain from musculoskeletal pain may lead to splinting and dysfunction of the respiratory tract, possibly atelectasis or pneumonia. Persistent pain in the patient without an obvious organic cause may increase anxiety, increasing intercostal muscle tension, increasing chest pain, and lead to a pattern of psychologic and physiologic dysfunction.

Selection of appropriate medication for each entity requires knowledge of the analgesic qualities of the drug and the hemodynamic changes and side effects that may be expected. Nitroglycerin and opioids cause hemodynamic changes that may actually improve myocardial oxygen supply/demand ratio. Other agents may provide similar pain relief, but without the changes in preload or afterload; their role in ischemic pain is therefore limited.

Relief of pain cannot be used as a diagnostic trial; there is tremendous overlap in conditions that can be relieved by opioids, nitroglycerin, antacids, and even calcium channel blockers. Diagnostic trials with these medications are not reliable. A careful history combined with physical findings remains the best diagnostic tool.

REFERENCES

1. Ishii K, Miwa K, Makita T, et al. Diagnosis of coronary vasospasm by detection of postischemic regional left ventricular delayed relaxation using echocardiographic evaluation of color kinesis. *Clin Cardiol.* 2003;26:477–482.
2. Sametz W, Metzler H, Gries M, et al. Perioperative catecholamine changes in cardiac risk patients. *Eur J Clin Invest.* 1999;29:582–587.
3. Brown G, Bolson E, Peterson RB, et al. The mechanisms of nitroglycerin action: stenosis vasodilation as a major component of drug response. *Circulation.* 1981;64:1089–1097.
4. Shry EA, Dacus J, Van De Graaff E, et al. Usefulness of the response to sublingual nitroglycerin as a predictor of ischemic chest pain in the emergency department. *Am J Cardiol.* 2002;90(11):1264–1266.
5. Cucherat M, Bonnefoy E, Tremeau G. Primary angioplasty versus intravenous thrombolysis for acute myocardial infarction. *Cochrane Database Syst Rev.* 2003(3):CD001560.
6. ISIS-2 (Second International Study of Infarct Survival) Collaborative Group). Randomised Trial of intravenous streptokinase, oral aspirin, both, or neither among 17 187 cases of suspected acute myocardial infarction: ISIS-2. *Lancet.* 1988;332(8607):349–360.
7. Weber JE, Chudnofsky CR, Boczar M, et al. Cocaine-associated chest pain: how common is myocardial infarction? *Acad Emerg Med.* 2000;7:873–877.
8. Kontos MC, Jesse RL, Tatum JL, et al. Coronary angiographic findings in patients with cocaine-associated chest pain. *J Emerg Med.* 2003;24:9–13.
9. Goyle KK, Walling AD. Diagnosing pericarditis. *Am Fam Physician.* 2002;66(9):1695–1702.
10. Rapp AH, Hillis LD, Lange RA, et al. Prevalence or coronary artery disease in patients with aortic stenosis with and without angina pectoris. *Am J Cardiol.* 2001;87(10):1216–1227.
11. Suzuki T, Mehta RH, Ince H, et al. International registry of aortic dissection. Clinical profiles and outcomes of acute type B aortic dissection in the current era: lesions from the International Registry of Aortic Dissection (IRAD). *Circulation.* 2003;108(suppl 1):11318–11223.

12. Vichinsky EP, Newmayr LD, Earles AN, et al. Causes and outcomes of acute chest syndrome in sickle cell disease. *N Engl J Med.* 2000;342:1855–1865.

13. Rothstein RD, Ouyang A. Chest pain of esophageal origin. *Gastroenterol Clin North Am.* 1989;18:257–273.

14. Murphy TO, Clinton AP, Kanar EA, et al. Subclavian approach to first rib resection. *Am J Surg.* 1980;139:634–636.

15. Schwartz GR. Xylocaine viscous as an aid in the differential diagnosis of chest pain. *J Am Coll Emerg Physician.* 1976;5: 981–983.

16. Milov DE, Kantor RJ. Chest pain in teenagers: when is it significant? *Post Grad Med.* 1990;88:145–154.

33

Sickle Cell Disease-Related Pain

James Ducharme

HIGH YIELD FACTS

- Vasoocclusive crises (VOC) do not occur to the same degree in all patients with sickle cell disease (SCD): 8% of adult sickle cell patients account for over 70% of all emergency inpatient days.

- The demographics of those most often seeking treatment for VOC resemble those for problem drug users, resulting in mistaken labeling of patients as drug seekers.

- Fifty-three percent of emergency physicians believe that greater than 20% of SCD patients are addicted, while 22% think more than 50% are addicted; actual addiction rates are 1–2%.

- Sicklers have dysfunctional vasodilation in VOC as a result of depletion of nitric oxide (NO) levels, allowing uninhibited vasoconstriction.

- In VOC, opioid analgesia must be provided rapidly and consistently. *In addition to* ongoing medication administration, *as needed (prn) orders* for breakthrough pain are recommended.

- Meperidine should be avoided in the management of VOC.

- Oral morphine protocols can be as effective as parenteral protocols.

- Hydroxyurea appears to be an effective treatment modality for preventing VOC.

INTRODUCTION

Approximately 70,000–100,000 Americans suffer from sickle cell disease (SCD).[1] Vasoocclusive crises (VOC) are the most common cause for hospitalization. Although patients on an average experience 0.8 pain episodes each year, this misrepresents the actual clinical experience of patients. Up to 40% do not report a VOC during a 5-year period, while 5% of patients suffer approximately one-third of all episodes.[2] More revealing is that 8% of adult sickle cell patients account for over 70% of all emergency inpatient days.

The minority of patients represent the majority of visits, which risks having them identified as "frequent flyers" or "drug seekers." It is therefore important to define why a subgroup of patients is at higher risk for these painful ischemic episodes. The greatest incidence of VOC occurs in males, age 15–30. Patients with poor coping strategies or those with adverse social situations are more affected by their pain.[3] Adolescent males have increased hemoglobin levels, leading to increased likelihood of sickling. Young males are more exposed to exertion, stress, cold, and alcohol, all of which can lead to intracellular dehydration and greater sickling. The result is that the demographics of those most often seeking treatment for VOC resemble those for problem drug users.[3].

Women are less likely to suffer VOC, thought to be due to estrogen-related factors. This decreased risk of VOC and its complications result in women surviving on average 6 years longer than males with SCD.

PATHOPHYSIOLOGY

Although the basic principles of VOC have been recognized for almost a century, we are just now defining this complex process. Erythrocyte dehydration leads to sludging in small capillaries. This decrease in flow, or decrease in ambient oxygen, allows greater deoxygenation of hemoglobin S; rigid polymerization occurs, leading to sickling of erythrocytes. Concurrently, leukocytes release cytokines, creating increased endothelial adhesion. Erythrocytes bind to this "sticky" endothelium, further narrowing the vascular lumen thereby creating a cycle of sickling, hypoperfusion, and ischemic injury.

It has been recently recognized that sicklers have impaired vasodilation in VOC, allowing uninhibited vasoconstriction. Nitric oxide (NO) is most responsible for vasodilation. It is rapidly neutralized in the presence of stroma-free hemoglobin. Nitrous oxide neutralization occurs up to 1000 times faster in the presence of free hemoglobin than with erythrocyte-contained hemoglobin.[4] This increased neutralization can result in the elimination of NO-mediated vasoregulation.

L-Arginine is the substrate precursor of NO. As a VOC commences, both L-arginine and NO levels are rapidly depleted, probably due to even higher rates of hemolysis during the VOC. Of note, men have fourfold greater circulatory levels of free hemoglobin, partially explaining their increased frequency of VOC compared to women.[4] It would appear there is a potential to decrease the severity and duration of VOC if L-arginine and NO levels could be maintained. Once a VOC is established, a painful episode will last 5–14 days, as the ischemic/inflammatory process is completed.

BARRIERS TO PAIN MANAGEMENT

The report of pain by any patient should be considered valid. Unfortunately, the most common complaint by SCD patients is that staff unjustly suspect or accuse them of drug dependency.[5] In one survey, 53% of emergency physicians believed that greater than 20% of SCD patients were addicted, while 22% thought more than 50% were addicted.[6] Undertreatment of pain often leads to "pseudo-addiction," a state where patients have to resort to exaggerated or manipulative pain behaviors to obtain relief.[7] Their behaviors often reinforce staff perceptions of substance abuse.

As Todd et al. have indicated, ethnic minorities are less likely to receive analgesia in the emergency department (ED).[8] Hospital staff rate pain at lower levels when there is no objective medical evidence of injury, as is the case with VOC. Valid home coping strategies such as distraction by watching television or talking with others are often interpreted by staff as indicative of drug-seeking behavior.[5]

Substance dependence is a relatively rare condition in those with SCD. Rates of 1–2% are usually quoted, in stark contrast to the numbers cited previously by surveyed physicians. In a study by Elander et al., reasons for this disparity were identified.[9] When pain-related symptoms were included, 31% met DSM-IV criteria for dependence, whereas only 2% met diagnostic criteria when only non-pain-related symptoms were assessed. Almost all pain-related symptoms were due to pseudo-addiction: 100% of sicklers feel they have to justify their pain in order to have staff recognize the severity of their pain. The need for sympathy and understanding, rather than disbelief and confrontation cannot be over emphasized.[10]

MANAGEMENT OF AN ACUTE VASCOOCCLUSIVE CRISIS

An integrated approach is required. In addition to a standardized analgesic regimen, efforts should be made to identify a precipitating factor. Hydration, compassion, and understanding from all staff along with appropriate discharge analgesics need to be considered.

Standardized pain regimens, individualized to each patient, are the crux of pain management. A sickle cell day hospital succeeded not only in decreasing admissions by a factor of 5 over that seen in the ED, but also was able to decrease admission duration by 1.5 days.[11] The principles used in this study can readily be applied to the ED setting. Analgesia must be provided rapidly and consistently. *In addition to* ongoing medication, administration, *as needed (prn) orders* for breakthrough pain are recommended.

Opioids

Intramuscular (IM) injections of meperidine should not be considered a valid analgesic regimen. Rapid titration to relief is not possible. Serum levels of meperidine after IM injections are only approximately half those seen in non-sicklers.[12] Due to ongoing renal disease, patients with SCD are at higher risk of seizures from normeperidine accumulation. Sterile abscesses and muscular degeneration are other complications associated with the IM approach.

Morphine clearance can vary by as much as a factor of 10 between individual patients during steady-state infusions.[13] Factors that increase morphine clearance include younger age and more severe symptoms. It is not possible to develop a simple "one-dose-fits-all" morphine protocol. Several have suggested the maintenance of a treatment book, indicating morphine requirements for each individual. This would allow rapid initiation of appropriate doses, providing more rapid control of the painful episode.

One way to individualize opioid dosing is with the use of patient-controlled analgesia (PCA) after initial morphine dosing. Patients are able to titrate to their desired end point on the time interval they choose, giving them the impression of being in control of their pain management. PCA initiated in the ED also avoids the "pain window" often seen between last dose in the ED and first dose on the ward. On the negative side, the patient may feel loss of contact with nursing staff. In addition, many older children and adolescents have been shown to inadequately treat their pain with PCA.[14]

Patients do not have to routinely receive intravenous morphine. Oral morphine protocols for VOC have been published for the past 20 years.[15,16] As with every regimented protocol of pain management, these studies have demonstrated decreases in ED length of stay, number of ED visits within a given year, and in hospitalization rates. See Table 33-1 for examples of published parenteral and oral morphine dosing regimens.

Although the risk of addiction is low with opioid use in VOC, morphine use may pose another more immediate risk. In 2004, Kopecky et al. suggested (in a posthoc analysis)

Table 33-1. Morphine Dosing Regimens for VOC

Authors	Age Group	Route	Dosing Regimen
Melzer-Lange et al.[14]	<18 years	PCA	2 mg IV bolus, up to four times 0.025–0.05 mg/kg demand dose, lockout of 10 minutes
Cole et al.[23]	Children	IV	0.15 mg/kg bolus 0.07—0.1 mg/kg/h
Jacobson et al.[24]	Children	IV and oral	0.15 mg/kg IV bolus 1.9 mg/kg sustained release tablet q 12 h Rescue oral dose
Conti et al.[15]	Adults	Oral	60 mg elixir first dose 20 mg q 30 minutes until relief 800 mg ibuprofen as adjunct
Friedman et al.[16]	Adults	Oral	60 mg elixir first dose 15 mg q 20 minutes until relief q 2 h dosing of cumulative secondary doses
Brookoff and Polomano[25]	Adult	IV	5 mg IV bolus Titrated infusion (2–12 mg/h), adjusted q 2 h Rescue dose available

an association of increased risk of acute chest syndrome with higher serum morphine and morphine-6-glucuronide levels.[17] This risk was even higher in those receiving oral morphine. No causality or mechanism of action was suggested.

Anti-Inflammatory Medications

Due to increased cytokine activity, several regimens have suggested the routine additions of ibuprofen to the opioid protocol. Intravenous ketorolac does not appear to provide adequate analgesia as a sole agent for severe VOC pain,[18] nor does it appear to provide any opioid-sparing effect when used in conjunction with meperidine.[19] Its role seems to be limited at best to cases of mild-to-moderate pain.

Other Interventions

In some cases of VOC, hemolysis may produce even more than the usual decrease of 1 g of hemoglobin. Patients with ongoing pain and a hemoglobin ≤5 g or a drop of 2 g from baseline may require transfusions. Investigation for infection: chest x-ray, urinalysis, and so forth should occur in patients with fever. Oxygen has been recommended as a baseline treatment modality for decades, despite no evidence of benefit in the management of VOC.

Its use can be limited to patients with decreased oxygen saturation levels or those with low hemoglobin levels.

PREVENTION OF VOC

Hydroxyurea appears to be an effective treatment modality for preventing VOC.[20] It stimulates fetal hemoglobin levels to as high as 20% of all hemoglobin, thereby inhibiting sickling. It also appears to act as a substrate for providing L-arginine, increasing NO levels.

Future Possibilities in the Management of VOC

As discussed in the pathophysiology section, increasing levels of L-arginine and thereby NO levels should diminish vascular occlusion and decrease ischemic injury and pain. Preliminary studies of inhaled NO in pediatric patients with VOC suggest some potential, with decreases in hospitalization and some decreases in morphine usage.[21] Similar modest results have been found using a nonionic surfactant.[22] This agent, Poloxamer 188, has anti-thrombotic properties that might improve microvascular flow. Neither treatment modality is yet ready for general clinical practice.

CONCLUSION

Rapid standardized opioid protocols are the key to VOC treatment. Once pain is controlled, hydration and identification of precipitants should occur. New understandings of VOC pathophysiology may soon allow directed management.

REFERENCES

1. Morgan MT. Don't blame the patients. *West J Med.* 1999;171 (5–6):313–314.
2. Yaster M, Kost-Byerly S, Maxwell LG. The management of pain in sickle cell disease. *Pediatr Clin North Am.* 2000;47 (3):699–710.
3. Fuggle P, Shand PA, Gill LJ, et al. Pain, quality of life, and coping in sickle cell disease. *Arch Dis Child.* 1996;75(3): 199–203.
4. Reiter CD, Gladwin MT. An emerging role for nitric oxide in sickle cell disease vascular homeostasis and therapy. *Curr Opin Hematol.* 2003;10(2):99–107.
5. Sutton M, Atweh GF, Cashman TD, et al. Resolving conflicts: misconceptions and myths in the care of the patient with sickle cell disease. *Mt Sinai J Med.* 1999;66(4):282–285.
6. Shapiro BS, Benjamin LJ, Payne R, et al. Sickle cell-related pain: perceptions of medical practitioners. *J Pain Symptom Manage.* 1997;14(3):168–174.
7. Weissman DE, Haddox JD. Opioid pseudoaddiction—an iatrogenic syndrome. *Pain.* 1989;36(3):363–366.
8. Todd KH. Pain assessment and ethnicity. *Annals of Emergency Medicine.* 1996;27(4):421–423.
9. Elander J, Lusher J, Bevan D, et al. Pain management and symptoms of substance dependence among patients with sickle cell disease. *Soc Sci Med.* 2003;57(9):1683–1696.
10. Pollack CV Jr, Sanders DY, Severance HW Jr. Emergency department analgesia without narcotics for adults with acute sickle cell pain crisis: case reports and review of crisis management. *J Emerg Med.* 1991;9(6):445–452.
11. Benjamin LJ, Swinson GI, Nagel RL. Sickle cell anemia day hospital: an approach for the management of uncomplicated painful crises. *Blood.* 2000;95(4):1130–1136.
12. Abbuhl S, Jacobson S, Murphy JG, et al. Serum concentrations of meperidine in patients with sickle cell crisis. *Ann Emerg Med.* 1986;15(4):433–438.
13. Dampier CD, Setty BN, Logan J, et al. Intravenous morphine pharmacokinetics in pediatric patients with sickle cell disease. *J Pediatr.* 1995;126(3):461–467.
14. Melzer-Lange MD, Walsh-Kelly CM, Lea G, et al. Patient-controlled analgesia for sickle cell pain crisis in a pediatric emergency department. *Pediatr Emerg Care.* 2004;20(1): 2–4.
15. Conti C, Tso E, Browne B. Oral morphine protocol for sickle cell crisis pain. *Md Med J.* 1996;45(1):33–35.
16. Friedman EW, Webber AB, Osborn HH, et al. Oral analgesia for treatment of painful crisis in sickle cell anemia. *Ann Emerg Med.* 1986;15(7):787–791.
17. Kopecky EA, Jacobson S, Joshi P, et al. Systemic exposure to morphine and the risk of acute chest syndrome in sickle cell disease. *Clin Pharmacol Ther.* 2004;75(3): 140–146.
18. Beiter JL Jr, Simon HK, Chambliss CR, et al. Intravenous ketorolac in the emergency department management of sickle cell pain and predictors of its effectiveness. *Arch Pediatr Adolesc Med.* 2001;155(4):496–500.
19. Wright SW, Norris RL, Mitchell TR. Ketorolac for sickle cell vaso-occlusive crisis pain in the emergency department: lack of a narcotic-sparing effect. *Ann Emerg Med.* 1992;21(8): 925–928.
20. Charache S, Terrin ML, Moore RD, et al. Effect of hydroxyurea on the frequency of painful crises in sickle cell anemia. Investigators of the Multicenter Study of Hydroxyurea in Sickle Cell Anemia. *N Engl J Med.* 1995;332(20): 1317–1322.
21. Weiner DL, Hibberd PL, Betit P, et al. Preliminary assessment of inhaled nitric oxide for acute vaso-occlusive crisis in pediatric patients with sickle cell disease. *JAMA.* 2003;289 (9):1136–1142.
22. Orringer EP, Casella JF, Ataga KI, et al. Purified poloxamer 188 for treatment of acute vaso-occlusive crisis of sickle cell disease: a randomized controlled trial. *JAMA.* 2001;286 (17):2099–2106.
23. Cole TB, Sprinkle RH, Smith SJ, et al. Intravenous narcotic therapy for children with severe sickle cell pain crisis. *Am J Dis Child.* 1986;140(12):1255–1259.
24. Jacobson SJ, Kopecky EA, Joshi P, et al. Randomised trial of oral morphine for painful episodes of sickle-cell disease in children. *Lancet.* 1997;350(9088):1358–1361.
25. Brookoff D, Polomano R. Treating sickle cell pain like cancer pain. *Ann Intern Med.* 1992;116(5):364–368.

34

Ischemic Pain

James Ducharme

HIGH YIELD FACTS

- Acidotic tissue stimulates pain fibers through dedicated acid-sensing channels.
- Ischemic tissue produces "pain out of proportion" to findings as part of a mechanism of self-preservation.
- High rates of pain fiber depolarization produce high local levels of vasodilators in an effort to maintain tissue oxygenation.
- The five *P*s associated with compartment syndromes are rarely present prior to irreversible tissue damage.
- Pain in cases of suspected compartment syndromes should not be completely removed: increasing pain or increasing analgesic requirements may be the only early symptoms prior to ischemic damage.
- Abnormal lab results (for example, elevated white blood cell (WBC) and serum lactate) are found with ischemic bowel only after tissue damage is present—disproportionate pain alone should raise suspicion.
- Painful peripheral diabetic neuropathy cannot be controlled with opioids. It requires directed therapy as with tricyclics or gabapentin.

INTRODUCTION

Pain related to hypoxic tissue injury is often described as being so painful as to be "out of proportion with physical findings." Despite this well-known adage, there are published cases of compartment syndromes—well identified as a cause of ischemic pain—being painless.[1] Certain visceral forms of ischemic injury as in coronary artery disease may produce *pressure* or *heaviness* rather than pain. This chapter will be focusing on ischemic pain related to compartment syndrome, peripheral vascular disease, and ischemic bowel, with some discussion on the microvascular ischemic pain as seen in diabetes.

Chest pain and vasoocclusive crisis associated with sickle cell disease will be discussed in Chapters 32 and 33. The final section of this chapter will deal with medication options for control of ischemic pain.

PATHOPHYSIOLOGY

Ischemia occurs as a result of oxygen deprivation leading to an increasingly acidotic tissue environment. This hypoxic insult may directly lead to nerve depolarization and painful sensation, as seen in diabetes. With worsening arteriolosclerosis, there is gradual obliteration of the *vaso nervosum*. Patients initially have decreased proprioception, for the largest delta fibers are first impacted by decreased circulation. As the microvascular disease progresses, alpha-delta and C-fibers suffer from ischemia.

Indirect nerve stimulation occurs in an acidotic extracellular milieu as a result of an anaerobic metabolism. Such acidosis develops not only from vascular occlusion, but also inflammation, infection, crush injuries, hematoma, edema, and even blisters. The excitatory effect of hydrogen protons on sensory neurons are potentiated by proinflammatory mediators.[2] The inflammatory group of bradykinin, serotonin, prostaglandins, and histamine—seen with tissue injury or inflammation—sensitizes nociceptors to the effect of hydrogen ions. Further, only nociceptors are sensitive to low pH, so the first symptom of tissue hypoxia will be pain. Specific channels on nociceptive fibers—acid-sensing ion channels (ASIC)—are stimulated and create a higher rate of depolarization of neurons than seen with any other single stimulus.

The presence of persistent inflammation can induce the production of ASIC channels to a level as much as 15 times greater than seen at baseline. This increased induction can be aborted by corticosteroids. With more numerous ASIC channels, sensing neurons are further sensitized to low pH levels, producing a hyperalgesic state. A patient with Crohn's disease, for example, will suffer much more intense abdominal pain with bowel spasms or obstruction than a similar patient without Crohn's disease.

Why have we developed such a reaction to tissue ischemia? Why is pain from ischemia so much more intense? Certainly, exercise or increased activity will worsen tissue acidosis causing further injury. The pain, therefore, is a strong signal to avoid activity. It appears that heightened nociceptor response to low tissue pH may also be a protective mechanism. When afferent C-fibers are stimulated by ischemia/acidosis, these sensory neurons automatically locally release neuropeptides. Patients with vasoocclusive crisis in sickle cell disease often succumb to prolonged pain episodes due to depletion of L-arginine and nitric oxide.[3]

Infusion of L-arginine can potentially decrease the severity and duration of a vasoocclusive crisis. In conditions such as ischemic bowel, the release of nitric oxide, calcitonin gene-related peptide, and vanilloids from nociceptive neurons seems to induce local vasodilation, increasing perfusion.[4] In animal studies, preapplication of capsaicin—which depletes substance P and other neuropeptides, preventing vasodilation—results in more extensive tissue injury on an experimental ischemia bowel model. The heightened response to ischemia—severe pain—appears therefore to be related to an autoprotective mechanism.

CLINICAL CONDITIONS

Compartment Syndrome

Compartment syndrome is a clinical condition characterized by elevated pressure within a confined fascial space, causing circulatory compromise, ischemia, and ultimately tissue necrosis.[5] Although the eponym of the five Ps (pain, pallor, paresthesia, paralysis, and pulselessness) has been classically used, some of these may present only after irreversible tissue damage has occurred. In addition, certain compartments have no major artery within the fascial limits, so a peripheral pulse may never diminish. In a review of pediatric cases, Bae et al., found pain present in 88%, pallor in 30%, paresthesia in 61%, paralysis in 36%, and pulselessness in only 18%.[5] Many of the cases were discovered because of increased demand for analgesia or by the increased usage of patient-controlled analgesia (PCA) pumps.

It appears, therefore, that subjective symptoms may be all that are present prior to tissue damage. Physicians must be attentive to such complaints when clinical scenarios that can lead to a compartment syndrome are present (Table 34-1). Use of analgesia is encouraged in conjunction with measurement of intracompartmental pressures in patients at risk.

Trauma patients or victims of overdoses may have diminished mental status, preventing pain recognition. Overuse of analgesics or sedation of patients postoperatively may also prevent recognition of the only consistent symptoms associated with compartment syndrome—pain.[6] Increased analgesic requirements should alert the caretaker to the possibility of a compartment syndrome. Similarly, in patients with altered mental status, the clinician should have a low threshold for measuring the pressures of compartments at risk.

Ischemic Bowel

Although normally only considered in patients with acute vascular occlusion, ischemia is probably the major source

Table 34-1. Conditions Associated with Compartment Syndromes

Fractures
    Supracondylar humeral or femoral
    Femoral shaft
    Tibia
Prolonged tissue pressure
    Unconscious patient
    IV drug users
Vascular reconstruction or recannulation
Hereditary bleeding disorders
Infection
    Myositis
    Necrotizing fasciitis
Intravenous fluid infiltration
Full thickness circumferential burns
Crush injuries
Exertion

of pain in small bowel obstruction due to adhesions or volvulus. Prolonged bowel spasm, as with any sustained muscular contraction, can result in severe pain. In the latter condition, sustained contraction depletes adenosine triphosphate (ATP) and initiates an anaerobic state leading to a lowering of tissue pH. With volvulus or obstruction from twisting of bowel around adhesions, vascular flow is compromised, leading to tissue hypoxia and acidosis.

Ischemia must be present for a certain time interval before tissue injury (and a secondary inflammatory response) can occur. Until inflammation initiates the release of interleukins into the circulation, there will not be a rise in neutrophil count. Until tissue hypoxia leads to cellular damage and leakage of lactate and hydrogen protons, there can be no increase in serum lactate or drop in serum pH. Biochemical or hematologic abnormalities become abnormal therefore only well after the onset of ischemia. The clinician must be alert to the possibility of ischemia prior to abnormal lab results, relying on the patient describing severe pain while still having a relatively benign physical exam. The clinician should be cautious in completely alleviating pain, for this may eliminate the only early warning sign of ischemic bowel.

Peripheral Vascular Disease

Ischemic limb pain can arise from both macro and microangiopathic abnormalities. Claudication is pain arising from muscle becoming ischemic as a result of insufficient perfusion by major vessels during physical activity. Exertional compartment syndrome can mimic claudication: muscle edema naturally occurs with physical activity. In some people fascial compartments may be too small, restricting the natural muscle engorgement. Further activity results in increased compartmental pressure, thereby decreasing local circulation, leading to ischemic pain.

As peripheral vascular disease progresses, flow diminishes to the point where there is inadequate perfusion to maintain an aerobic state even at rest. Patients complain of severe burning pain, somewhat alleviated when the affected limb is lowered. Ischemic limb pain is very difficult to control; oral opioids are rarely sufficient, even with high doses. Persistent ischemic pain rapidly induces changes in the central pain system so that amputation of a limb that has produced pain even for a few days may leave the patient with severe phantom limb pain for years. It appears that epidural control of ischemic limb pain—using bupivacaine and fentanyl—for a period of 72 hours prior to amputation can decrease considerably the duration and severity of phantom limb pain.[7]

Microangiopathic ischemia, as seen in diabetes, can lead to severe pain as a result of damage to peripheral nerves. Standard analgesics are usually inadequate; diabetic neuropathic pain is best treated as with other painful neuropathies using a tricyclic antidepressant or gabapentin.[8] Selective serotonin reuptake inhibitors (SSRI) antidepressants having no action on sodium or calcium channels are ineffective for neuropathic pain.

EFFECTIVE ANALGESIC FOR PAIN OF ISCHEMIC ORIGIN

As with any severe pain, combination therapy is recommended. Nonsteroidal anti-inflammatory drugs (NSAIDs) can be effective as part of the management of ischemic pain. Only four NSAIDs—ibuprofen, flurbiprofen, ASA, and diclofenac—inhibit ASIC channels independently of cyclooxygenase inhibition.[2] Since pain from ischemia can arise prior to inflammation, probably only one of these four should be considered.

Opioids should be the mainstay for management of acute ischemic pain, be it crush injury, circumferential burn, or vascular occlusion. Rapid intravenous titration can usually effectively control pain. Caution should be used in lowering, not eliminating, pain in patients suspected of ischemic bowel or compartment syndrome, for progression of pain may be the sentinel symptom indicating need for urgent surgery. In patients with severe pain, addition of a ketamine infusion (starting at 0.1 mg/kg/h) after an initial bolus (0.1 mg/kg) may provide

additive analgesic effect.[9] Combination therapy allows lower dosing of all agents minimizing the risk of adverse effects. Another *N*-methyl-D-aspartate (NMDA) antagonist, dextramethorphan, has not been found to provide analgesia in an ischemic pain model.[10]

Other analgesic options that have been studied include topical nitrates, acupuncture, and spinal cord stimulation. Locally applied nitrate patches were found to be effective in one small study for ischemic pain at rest.[11] Acupuncture was found to provide no benefit for experimentally induced ischemic pain.[12] Spinal cord stimulation appears to be a valid treatment option for pain associated with inoperable peripheral vascular disease, although its use to date has been primarily in Europe.[13]

CONCLUSION

Ischemia may produce severe pain requiring aggressive pain management. Pain control should be managed in conjunction with consideration for need of urgent surgery. Care must be taken to not remove pain entirely in those patients at risk for ischemic bowel or compartment syndrome for progressive pain may be the only symptom prior to irreversible tissue injury.

REFERENCES

1. O'Sullivan MJ, Rice J, McGuinness AJ. Compartment syndrome without pain! *Ir Med J.* 2002;95(1):22.
2. Voilley N. Acid-sensing ion channels (ASICs): new targets for the analgesic effects of non-steroid anti-inflammatory drugs (NSAIDs). *Curr Drug Targets Inflamm Allergy.* 2004;3(1):71–79.
3. Morris CR, Kuypers FA, Larkin S, et al. Patterns of arginine and nitric oxide in patients with sickle cell disease with vaso-occlusive crisis and acute chest syndrome. *J Pediatr Hematol Oncol.* 2000;22(6):515–520.
4. Pawlik WW, Thor P, Sendur R, et al. Myoelectric bowel activity in ischemia/reperfusion damage. Role of sensory neurons. *J Physiol Pharmacol.* 1998;49(4):543–551.
5. Bae DS, Kadiyala RK, Waters PM. Acute compartment syndrome in children: contemporary diagnosis, treatment, and outcome. *J Pediatr Orthop.* 2001;21(5):680–688.
6. Thonse R, Ashford RU, Williams TI, et al. Differences in attitudes to analgesia in post-operative limb surgery put patients at risk of compartment syndrome. *Injury.* 2004;35(3):290–295.
7. Jahangiri M, Jayatunga AP, Bradley JW, et al. Prevention of phantom pain after major lower limb amputation by epidural infusion of diamorphine, clonidine and bupivacaine. *Ann R Coll Surg Engl.* 1994;1994 Sep;76(5):324–326.
8. Rowbotham M, Harden N, Stacey B, et al. Gabapentin for the treatment of postherpetic neuralgia: a randomized controlled trial. *JAMA.* 1998;280(21):1837–1842.

9. Persson J, Hasselstrom J, Wiklund B, et al. The analgesic effect of racemic ketamine in patients with chronic ischemic pain due to lower extremity arteriosclerosis obliterans. *Acta Anaesthesiol Scand*. 1998;42(7):750–758.

10. Plesan A, Sollevi A, Segerdahl M. The *N*-methyl-D-aspartate-receptor antagonist dextromethorphan lacks analgesic effect in a human experimental ischemic pain model. *Acta Anaesthesiol Scand*. 2000;44(8):924–928.

11. Fletcher S, Wright M, Wilkinson A, et al. Locally applied transdermal nitrate patches for the treatment of ischaemic rest pain. *Int J Clin Pract*. 1997;51(5):324–325.

12. Barlas P, Lowe AS, Walsh DM, et al. Effect of acupuncture upon experimentally induced ischemic pain: a sham-controlled single-blind study. *Clin J Pain*. 2000;16(3):255–264.

13. Erdek MA, Staats PS. Spinal cord stimulation for angina pectoris and peripheral vascular disease. *Anesthesiol Clin North Am*. 2003;21(4):797–804.

35

Visceral Pain

Marc Leder
Ann M. Dietrich

HIGH YIELD FACTS

- Difficulty in distinguishing pain as being visceral in origin may arise because visceral pain is often referred to somatic areas with resultant somatic symptoms.
- Distension, ischemia, and inflammation are the most likely to induce visceral pain.
- Specific somatic sensation can be expected in the dermatomes representing the involved thoracic or lumbar nerves.
- Each year emergency departments (EDs) in the United States evaluate close to 5 million adult and pediatric patients with the chief complaint of abdominal pain.
- The medical practice of withholding analgesics from patients with abdominal pain was not based on evidence, but rather on medical care in the 1920s.
- No study evaluating the use of opioids for acute abdominal pain has demonstrated negative outcomes.
- National associations including the American College of Emergency Physicians (ACEP) endorse the use of opioid analgesia for patients with abdominal pain.

INTRODUCTION

Visceral pain produces its own unique symptoms, distinct from those of somatic pain. It is typically perceived as a deep, vague, poorly discriminated, diffuse pain with a dull, heavy, or oppressive quality. It is commonly associated with autonomic symptoms (pallor, sweating) and emotional reactions (anxiety, sense of impending doom). Difficulty in distinguishing pain as being visceral in origin may arise because visceral pain is often referred to somatic areas with resultant somatic symptoms. In fact, cutaneous hyperalgesia may be present secondary to a visceral pain origin. With several viscera converging to the same spinal segment, an overlap in patterns of referred sensations may further confuse interpretation of the patient's pain.

Initiation of Visceral Pain Stimuli

Visceral pain stimuli differ from those required to evoke pain in somatic structures. Crushing, cutting, and burning do not appear to elicit pain in viscera as they would in somatic tissues. Instead, distension, ischemia, and inflammation are the most likely to induce visceral pain.[1] Several studies have examined the methods of pain production that result from distension. Such pain appears related to the pressure within the distending lumen rather than the actual volume of the lumen.[2] Lipkin and Sleisinger reported that increasing intensity of the distending stimulus shortened the latency from the onset of the stimulus to patient reporting of pain.[3] Lewis et al. reported that distension of the gut was most painful when greater lengths of continuous segments were affected.[4] Inflammation induces visceral pain directly; it also creates a visceral allodynia by sensitizing visceral tissues to nonpainful stimuli. Experimentally induced ischemia has been demonstrated to produce significantly increased rates of afferent nociceptor depolarization. Such afferent activity may be a form of tissue survival mechanism, for heightened nociceptor activity stimulates release of calcitonin gene-related peptide (CGRP) and nitric oxide by efferent fibers in an effort to induce vasodilation. Unfortunately, the severity of the pain does not necessarily reflect the severity of the disease process.

Visceral Nociceptors

Current research suggests that there are two classes of viscerosensory receptors (afferent receptors-nociceptors): *high-threshold* and *low-threshold* receptors.[5] High-threshold receptors respond to mechanical stimuli within the noxious range and exclusively innervate organs from which pain is the only conscious sensation (ureter, kidneys, lung, heart). They have little presence in organs that provide both innocuous and noxious sensation. The low-threshold receptors encode the stimulus intensity in the magnitude of their discharge, ranging from innocuous stimuli to stimuli in the noxious range.[6] Evidence also exists to suggest that the viscera contain spinal nociceptive afferent fibers that are normally silent and are sensitized by inflammation.[7] It appears that local agents such as prostaglandins, kinins, and hydrogen ions increase the sensitivity of certain nociceptors such that continuous low-frequency firing can be detected. As with somatic windup, the peripheral receptive fields enlarge with persistent inflammation; mildly painful stimuli may therefore be exquisitely painful when acting on inflamed tissues.

Spinal Cord and Pain Modification

The viscera, in contrast to somatic tissue, are innervated by two sets of primary afferent fibers that project to distinct areas of the neuroaxis. Visceral afferent fibers travel through both sympathetic and parasympathetic efferent nerves, reaching the spinal cord (cell bodies in the dorsal root ganglia) and the brain stem (cell bodies in nodose ganglion).

NOCICEPTOR CONVERGENCE

Second-order neurons that receive the input are mostly located in laminae I and V of the dorsal horn as well as the ventral horn of the spinal cord. Viscerosomatic convergence is normal so that visceral sensations can be mediated only through the common somatosensory pathways. Viscerovisceral convergence also occurs onto the same second-order neurons.

Referral of Visceral Pain

A fundamental feature of visceral pain is pain referral.[8] If a visceral pain process either recurs or becomes prolonged and intense, the sensation is not felt in a common site, irrespective of the viscus of origin. Instead it tends to be perceived in superficial somatic structures. Referral sites vary based on the viscera and may be distant from the primary site. During this process, the pain tends to become sharper, better defined, more localized, and more like somatic pain. The initial autonomic response tends to dissipate as the pain becomes more somatic in nature.

Evidence exists that suggests that altered central mechanisms may play an important part in visceral sensations. Several animal studies have demonstrated that convergent, cutaneous receptive fields expand in size after repetitive distention of a viscus, supporting a central mechanism. Two types of referred pain have been recognized: referred pain without hyperalgesia and referred pain with hyperalgesia.[5] It has been theorized that referred pain with hyperalgesia consists of both peripheral and central nervous system components and may be initiated and maintained by either system, although the mechanisms are incompletely understood. The central nervous system is believed to be induced by abnormal visceral input that create a point of heightened sensitivity in the spinal cord thereby facilitating subsequent messages from somatic structures.[9]

COMMON ABDOMINAL VISCERAL PAIN SYNDROMES

Abdominal Pain

Although abdominal pain is usually secondary to injury or inflammation to viscera in the abdominal cavity, the common somatic and visceral nerve supply shared by the thorax and abdomen should make thoracic etiologies a consideration for patients with abdominal pain. Specific somatic sensation can be expected in the dermatomes representing the indicated thoracic or lumbar nerves.

Gastrointestinal Tract

Patients with gastrointestinal tract pain are believed to have nociception via sympathetic fibers to the celiac plexus and spinal cord through splanchnic nerves T5–T9.

Liver or Spleen

Inflammation of the liver or spleen may result in pain that radiates to the diaphragmatic pleura. The pain may radiate to the left shoulder as a result of distention of the descending colon with secondary irritation of the diaphragm. Afferent sympathetics from the liver capsule are believed to transmit the pain. Nociception is initiated via sympathetic fibers and splanchnic nerves to the spinal cord at the T6–T10 level.

Biliary System

Inflammatory disease of the biliary system is localized to the right upper quadrant secondary to stimulation of afferent nerve fibers of the parietal peritoneum.

Pancreas

Nociception is carried from the pancreas to thoracic splanchnic nerves T5–T9 via the celiac plexus and ganglion to the spinal cord.

Genitourinary Pain

The kidney is innervated by sympathetic, parasympathetic, and sensory contributions. Preganglionic sympathetic fibers from T10 to L1 transmit afferent information via the white rami and paravertebral ganglia and synapse in celiac and aorticorenal ganglia. Postganglionic fibers travel to the renal plexus.

Pelvic Pain

Many types of pelvic pain are cyclic and difficult to diagnose. Since the lower gastrointestinal tract shares sensory innervation with the pelvic viscera, disease processes such as irritable bowel syndrome should be in the differential for this type of pain. Urologic etiologies may also result in pelvic pain and should be considered.

THE PROVISION OF ANALGESIA TO PATIENTS WITH ACUTE UNDIFFERENTIATED ABDOMINAL PAIN

Oligoanalgesia—the provision of inadequate pain control to patients by physicians—has been attributed to multiple practical and attitudinal barriers.[10] Each year emergency departments (EDs) in the United States evaluate close to 5 million adult and pediatric patients with the chief complaint of abdominal pain.[11] The decision to provide analgesia for these patients can be particularly challenging. During the diagnostic workup, while management and therapeutic decisions are being made, patient and/or parental expectations for the provision of adequate pain control may conflict with the practitioner's belief that providing pain relief in these circumstances may hinder a timely diagnosis and increase patient morbidity and mortality.[12]

The first edition of Cope's textbook the *Early Diagnosis of the Acute Abdomen* stated that providing analgesia to the patient with acute abdominal pain would mask signs and symptoms, delay diagnosis, and lead to increased morbidity and mortality.[13] Such a position was perhaps defendable at the time due to concerns over limitations of diagnostic tools, operative risk, and variable purification techniques for producing opioids. The latter difficulty made physicians, at times, unsure of the dose of morphine they were actually giving to patients. As a result, the standard medical practice became the withholding of analgesics from these patients until a definitive diagnosis and management plan had been established.[14] Since emergency medicine did not exist, the burden of evaluation fell to the surgeon. There has never been evidence or a study published that supports Cope's initial position. Rather, the recent literature in this field concludes that the early use of analgesia in these patients probably facilitates diagnostic evaluation. Diagnostic accuracy may actually be improved by relieving patient pain and thereby providing a more comfortable patient to interview and examine.[15–18]

Despite these recent articles it appears that the timely treatment of acute abdominal pain in the ED setting is not practiced consistently. A survey in 1998 by Wolfe et al. concluded that 80% of emergency medicine physician respondents would withhold narcotic analgesia pending assessment by a surgeon.[14] In similar surveys of pediatric emergency medicine physicians and pediatric surgeons there was considerable reluctance to provide analgesia for children with acute abdominal pain by both groups of physicians.[12,19] A myriad of explanations for the reluctance to provide analgesia in these groups of patients include the concern for surgical misdiagnosis once these patients receive analgesia, a "masking" of physical examination findings and thus a delay in diagnosis.[20] Currently there are no evidence-based studies to support these concerns.[21]

The contemporary emphasis on minimizing patient pain in the acute care setting has become a priority focus of multiple regulatory agencies including the U.S. Department of Health and Human Services Agency for Healthcare Research and Quality, and the Joint Commission for the Accreditation of Healthcare Organizations (JCAHO).[10] These agencies have provided standards for the evaluation of pain and have recommended punitive financial consequences for health care institutions that do not meet them.[22,23]

Recognizing the disparity between the recommendations of currently available studies on the treatment of abdominal pain and what is being practiced clinically, attitudinal changes toward providing analgesia to the patient with acute abdominal pain are reflected in multiple texts[24] and in published guidelines advocated by organizations such as the American College of Emergency Physicians (ACEP).[11] This paradigm shift recognizes that laboratory and imaging modalities (computed tomography [CT]/ultrasound) that are increasingly used by health care providers to make a definitive diagnosis for patients with abdominal pain as well as the ability to titrate narcotic analgesics were unavailable when initial recommendations advocating withholding of analgesia for the patient with abdominal pain were propagated.[25]

The latest edition of Cope's *Early Diagnosis of the Acute Abdomen* reflects this by acknowledging that "the judicious use of analgesics in the setting of acute abdominal pain is appropriate."[26] The ACEP clinical policy: Critical Issues for the Initial Evaluation and Management of Patients Presenting with a Chief Complaint of Nontraumatic Acute Abdominal Pain states that the administration of narcotics to these patients is a safe and humane option that does not obscure the physical examination findings nor increase morbidity and mortality.[11]

Physicians who continue to withhold analgesia from patients with abdominal pain often do so based on anecdotal case reports with alleged bad outcomes or argue that the literature supporting the provision of early analgesia has methodologic limitations. They conclude the evidence accrued to date is not definitive.[27] One manuscript found that a study addressing this issue would need close to 1500 patients to make statistically significant outcome conclusions about safety.[28] Given that the total number of subjects studied in all the relevant literature reviewed to make guideline recommendations fall significantly below this number, one can argue that we lack a definitive statement.[21] It should be recognized that no study establishing negative outcomes of any sort has been published. Humane treatment of suffering should therefore be the only argument required to treat abdominal pain.

Communication between the emergency physician and the surgical consultant will vary depending on the practice setting. University hospitals may have multiple layers of house staff evaluation before a final decision is made on patient management by a surgical attending. In community hospitals there may be more direct communication with surgical staff but individual patient evaluation and decision

making in the ED may be delayed if the surgeon is in the operating room or involved in other clinical matters.[20] To address individual emergency physician or surgeon concerns about the timely provision of analgesia to these patients, both departments should work cooperatively to develop institutional practice guidelines and departmental standards which would lead to more consistent practice patterns.[29] Issues to be addressed could include medication type, dosing, end point, and administration timing. As a review of the cumulative studies thus far on the subject was unable to identify even one patient with a poor outcome secondary to analgesia provision, the impetus to develop these protocols is great.[29]

Analgesics should normally be given after the initial history and physical examination is completed in the patient presenting to the ED with undifferentiated abdominal pain. It will arise, however, that the physician should not delay analgesia even that long, rather intravenous opioids may be initiated for patients in severe pain simultaneously with the

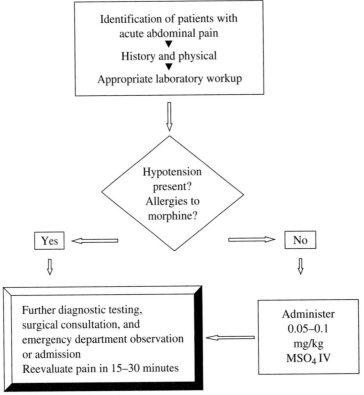

Fig. 35-1. Algorithm for treatment of acute abdominal pain. MSO_4 = morphine sulfate; IV = intravenous. (Reprinted with permission from McHale PM, LoVecchio F. Narcotic analgesia in the acute abdomen—a review of prospective trials. *Eur J Emerg Med.* 2001;8:131–136.)

initial assessment. To withhold opioid analgesia from someone in agony while waiting for a physician to complete his or her assessment is to encourage exactly the same mindset we have criticized in surgeons. McHale and LoVecchio have proposed one such algorithm for the approach toward the treatment of acute abdominal pain that should be applicable to patients 5 years and older[30] (see Fig. 35-1).

Disease entities causing abdominal pain in children younger than 5 years of age are different. The use of analgesics for undifferentiated abdominal pain has not been adequately studied for this approach to be recommended in this group.[14] Although, most physicians are uncomfortable assessing acute abdominal pain in small children, it is difficult to condone allowing an infant to continue to suffer. For these and all patients, early communication with surgical consultants is encouraged, as is interdepartmental cooperation.

Future directions in studying analgesia for abdominal pain should include multicenter randomized clinical trials with adequate power to address issues of optimal drug, dose, and timing of administration, for e.g., morphine versus fentanyl versus nonsteroidal medications; patient outcomes and diagnostic accuracy; and adverse events and applicability to the younger pediatric patient. Pending further research the judicious provision of analgesia appears safe, reasonable, and in the best interests of patients in pain and has become accepted by many as the standard of care.

REFERENCES

1. Procacci P, Maresca M, Cersosimo R. Visceral pain: pathophysiology and clinical aspects. In: Costa M, ed. *Sensory Nerve and Neuropeptides in Gastroenterology*. New York: Plenum Press; 1991.
2. Goligher JC, Hughes ESR. Sensibility of the rectum and colon: its role in the mechanism of anal continence. *Lancet*. 1951;1–2:543–548.
3. Lipkin M, Sleisinger MH. Studies of visceral pain: measurements of stimulus intensity and duration associated with the onset of pain in esophagus, ileum and colon. *J Clin Invest*. 1957;37:28–34.
4. Lewis T. *Pain*. London: MacMillan; 1942.
5. Vecchiet L, Giamberardino MA, Dragani L. Pain from renal/ureteral calculosis: evaluation of sensory thresholds in the lumbar area. Pain. 1989;36:289–295.
6. Sengupta JN, Gebhart GF. Gastrointestinal afferent fibers and sensation. In: Johnson LR, ed. *Physiology of the Gastrointestinal Tract*. 3rd ed.. New York: Raven; 1994:483–519.
7. McMahon SB, Koltzenburg M. Silent afferents and visceral pain. In: *Pharmacologic Approaches to the Treatment of Chronic Pain: New Concepts and Critical Issues. Progress in Pain Research and Management*. Vol I. Seattle, WA: IASP press; 1994:11–30.
8. Bonica JJ. General considerations of acute pain. In: Bonica JJ, ed. *The Management of Pain*. Philadelphia, PA: Lea & Febiger; 1990:159–179.
9. Cervero F. Pathophysiology of referred pain and hyperalgesia from viscera. In: Vecchiet L, Albe-Fessard D, Lindblom U, eds. *New Trends in Referred Pain and Hyperalgesia, Pain Research and Clinical Management*. Amsterdam, The Netherlands: Elsevier science; 1993:35–46.
10. Rupp T, Delaney K. Inadequate analgesia in emergency medicine. *Ann Emerg Med*. 2004;43(4):494–503.
11. Clinical policy: critical issues for initial evaluation and management of patients presenting with a chief complaint of nontraumatic acute abdominal pain. *Ann Emerg Med*. 2000;36(4):406–415.
12. Green R, Kabani A, et al. Analgesic use in children with acute abdominal pain. *Pediatr Emerg Care*. 2004;20(11):725–729.
13. Cope Z. *Early Diagnosis of the Acute Abdomen*. 15th ed. New York: Oxford University Press; 1979.
14. Wolfe JM, Lein DY, Lenkoski K, et al. Analgesic administration to patients with an acute abdomen: a survey of emergency medicine physicians. *Am J Emerg Med*. 2000;18:250–253.
15. Zoltie N, Cust MP. Analgesia in the acute abdomen. *Ann R Coll Surg Engl*. 1986;68:209–210.
16. Attard AR, Corlett MJ, Kidner NJ, et al. Safety of early pain relief for acute abdominal pain. *Br Med J*. 1992;305:554–556.
17. Pace S, Burke TF. Intravenous morphine for early pain relief in patients with acute abdominal pain. *Acad Emerg Med*. 1996;3:1086–1092.
18. LoVecchio F, Oster N, Sturmann K, et al. The use of analgesics in patients with acute abdominal pain. *Emerg Med*. 1997;15:775–779.
19. Kim M, Galustyan S, Sato T, et al. Analgesia for children with acute abdominal pain: a survey of pediatric emergency physicians and pediatric surgeons. *Pediatrics*. 2003;112(5):1122–1126.
20. Thomas SH, Silen W. Effect on diagnostic efficiency if analgesia for undifferentiated abdominal pain. *Br J Surg*. 2003;90:5–9.
21. Brewsters GS, Herbert ME, Hoffman JR. Medical myth: analgesia should not be given to patients with an acute abdomen because it obscures the diagnosis. *West J Med*. 2000;172(3):209–210.
22. Joint Commission for the Accreditation of Healthcare Organizations. Background on the development of the Joint Commission standards on pain management. Available at *http://www.jcaho.org/news+room/health+care+issues/pain.htm*. Accessed September 1, 2003.
23. Hill C. Joint Commission focuses on pain management [Joint commission for the accreditation of healthcare organizations web site]. Available at *http://www.jcaho.org/news+room/health+care+issues/pain.htm*. Accessed September 1, 2003.
24. Rosen P. *Emergency Medicine: Concepts and clinical Practices*. 3rd ed. St. Louis, MO: CV Mosby; 1992:P1513.

25. Thomas Sh, Silen W, Cheema F, et al. Effects of morphine analgesia on diagnostic accuracy in emergency department patients with abdominal pain: a prospective, randomized trial. *J Am Coll Surg*. 2003;196(1):18–31.

26. Silen W. Cope's early diagnosis at the acute abdomen. 20th ed. New York: Oxford University Press; 2000.

27. Nissman SA, Kaplan LJ, Mann BD. Critically reappraising the literature-driven practice of analgesia administration for acute abdominal pain in the emergency room prior to surgical evaluation. *Am J Surg*. 2003;185(1):1291–1296.

28. Lee JS, Stiell IG, Wells GA, et al. Adverse outcomes and opioid analgesic administration in acute abdominal pain. *Acad Emerg Med*. 2000;7:980–987.

29. McHale PM, LoVecchio F. Narcotic analgesia in the acute abdomen—a review of prospective trials. *Eur J Emerg Med*. 2001;8(2):131–136.

30. Kim MK, Strait RT, Sato TT, et al. A randomized clinical trial of analgesia in children with acute abdominal pain. *Acad Emerg Med*. 2002;9(4):281–287.

36

Renal (Ureteral) Colic

William H. Cordell

HIGH YIELD FACTS

- Increase in the intraluminal pressure from ureteral obstruction stretches nerve endings in the mucosa and produces severe pain.
- Opioids are a mainstay of renal colic analgesia.
- Intravenous (IV) ketorolac (an NSAID) is highly efficacious in many patients with renal colic.
- Opioids and NSAIDs may be combined ("balanced analgesia" or "multimodal analgesia") during ED, hospital or out-patient treatment.
- Prostaglandins have been shown to directly increase the phasic and tonic contractile activity of isolated human ureteric smooth muscle.
- Analgesics should *not* be withheld from hemodynamically stable patients with suspected ureteral colic until the diagnosis is confirmed.
- Consider the possibility of a leaking or dissecting aortic abdominal aneurysm (AAA) in age groups at risk.
- Ensure there is no associated urinary infection.
- Intravenous (IV) ketorolac is effective, but not for all patients.
- *Balanced analgesia* or *multimodal analgesia* is the ideal approach to renal colic.

INTRODUCTION

The excruciating flank or abdominal pain caused by acute ureteral obstruction has been likened in severity to childbirth, the "gold standard" of pain. This chapter will emphasize the nature and pathophysiology of this severe pain, review analgesics used to treat the pain of renal colic, and propose a clinical approach for evaluating and treating patients with acute symptoms suggestive of ureteral obstruction.

Throughout this chapter, for simplicity sake, the term renal colic will be applied to the pain and symptom complex produced by acute ureteral obstruction. Readers should note that other terms for this condition appear in the medical literature. These include acute ureteric obstruction, renoureteral colic, ureteral colic, and ureteric colic.

Patients with acute ureteral obstruction typically present with sudden onset of severe pain in the flank, abdomen, and/or groin and genitalia, depending on the location of the stone in the ureter. The pain associated with acute ureteral obstruction is typically acute, severe, incapacitating, and unilateral. It frequently occurs in the middle of the night or early morning while the patient is sedentary. As the stone descends in the ureter, the pain may localize in the abdominal area overlying the stone and radiate to the gonad[1] and often is associated with a great desire to void. The pain typically waxes and wanes, but rarely completely disappears. Nausea and vomiting are common.

PATHOPHYSIOLOGY

Urinary tract stones are the most common cause of ureteral obstruction. The lifetime risk of developing an acute attack of flank pain is estimated at 1–10%.[2] Stones in the renal calyces are often asymptomatic or produce painless hematuria. Those in the renal pelvis are too large to enter the ureter though they may intermittently obstruct the pelvi-ureteric junction. It is stones in the ureter that produce ureteral colic. ("It is little stones, like little dogs, that are likely to produce the most noise.")[3]

In addition to uroliths, any intraluminal or extraluminal etiology that obstructs the ureter may produce the ureteral colic symptom complex. Noncalculous conditions that can produce ureteral colic include the passage of sloughed renal tissue, blood clots, inspissated pus, oxalate crystals, and uratic debris, and lower ureteral strictures caused by bilharzial (schistosomal) infections.[4] Pain may occasionally be produced by sudden kinking of the ureteropelvic junction (UPJ) when there is an unduly mobile kidney (Dietl's crisis).

How do tiny uroliths, a few millimeters in diameter, produce one of humankind's most agonizing pains? The resulting increase in the intraluminal pressure from ureteral obstruction stretches nerve endings in the mucosa and produces the colicky pain.[5] If the stone becomes lodged, the ureteral muscles go into spasm. A prolonged isotonic contraction leads to increased production of lactic acid, which irritates both slow-type A- and fast-type C-fibers. Afferent impulses are generated that travel to the spinal cord at the

T11–L1 levels.[5] The pain can thus be perceived in any organ sharing the urinary tract innervation.

Small, circular stones more effectively block urinary flow than large, irregularly shaped stones, explaining why small stones can produce such severe pain. Uroliths are most likely to cause obstruction at one of the five regions of narrowing in the urinary system—the renal calyx, the UPJ, where the ureter crosses over the iliac vessels at the pelvic brim, in the posterior pelvis in females, and the ureterovesical junction (UVJ). The ureteral wall also becomes edematous and swollen at the stone site, further worsening the obstruction.

Obstruction causes an increase in urinary tract pressures above the stone as well as an increase in tension in the urinary tract walls. The increase in renal pelvic wall tension is probably responsible for the excruciating pain of renal colic.[6] Since the renal pelvis has a considerably larger radius than the ureter, the tension there is greatest according to Laplace's law (mural tension is dependent on both the pressure and radius of the cylinder lumen). Irrespective of the site of the stone, severe pain will be located in the region of the flank which corresponds to that of the renal pelvis. Increased pressure in the renal pelvis secondary to the ureteral obstruction induces synthesis and secretion of renal prostaglandins. Prostaglandins, primarily E_2, in turn produce a diuresis via vasodilatation of the afferent arteriole (increased renal blood circulation), further increasing pressure in the renal pelvis. Prostaglandins have also been shown to directly increase the phasic and tonic contractile activity of isolated human ureteric smooth muscle.[7]

Emergency Department Approach to Patients with Suspected Renal Colic

The administration of potent analgesics is integrated into a process aimed at providing comfort and controlling pain, confirming the diagnosis and/or excluding life-threatening conditions (especially ruptured abdominal aortic aneurysm and urosepsis), and making a proper disposition (Table 36-1).

Prompt and adequate pain relief is the aim in treating acute renal colic. Analgesics should *not* be withheld from hemodynamically stable patients with suspected ureteral colic until the diagnosis is confirmed, a process which can take hours. Once vital signs have been obtained and the focused history and physical are expeditiously undertaken, analgesics should be administered. At the same time, it cannot be overemphasized that pain control is more than administering pharmacologic analgesic agents. Pain management includes the important "art of medicine" humanistic steps of reassuring patients, placing them in a quiet, warm environment, and addressing their fears and needs.

The physician and nurse should assure the patient that pain relief will be rapidly provided while the cause for the pain is being evaluated.

History and Physical Examination

Patients with renal colic may writhe in bed or pace the floor in an attempt to find relief. This behavior is in contrast to patients with an acute abdominal inflammatory process who prefer to lie still because of the increased pain associated with body movement. The remainder of the physical examination may be remarkably benign. Since ileus often accompanies renal colic, bowel sounds may be diminished. Peritoneal signs are absent.[1] Though there may be tenderness on deep palpation over the location of the calculus,[8] peritoneal signs usually signify an inflammatory process. An examination of the testes should be performed since torsion and other scrotal disease may mimic ureteral colic. Rectal and pelvic examinations should be performed if the diagnosis of renal colic remains in doubt.

Consider the Possibility of a Leaking or Dissecting Aortic Abdominal Aneurysm

Though the symptom complex of renal colic is often highly suggestive of urolith passage through the ureters, the pain may also be a symptom of other disease states including several life-threatening conditions. Physicians should be aware of conditions that mimic renal colic, in particular a leaking or dissecting aortic abdominal aneurysm (AAA). This condition should be suspected in any elderly person presenting with ureteral colic. An AAA may present with symptoms identical to renal colic or other genitourinary conditions,[9] and misdiagnosis may delay surgery and increase morbidity.[10] Morgan et al. noted that the spread of a retroperitoneal hematoma into the paranephric space could put extraluminal pressure on the ureter and produce renal colic.[11] They recommended that the diagnosis of leaking aortic aneurysm be entertained in any patient over 55 presenting with a first episode of renal colic. When a leaking AAA is suspected, surgical consultation should be immediately obtained. For equivocal cases, diagnostic imaging such as abdominal ultrasonography or computerized tomography should be obtained.

Is there a Urinary Tract Infection in the Presence of Obstruction?

A urine specimen should be evaluated by dipstick with or without microscopy to determine the presence of infection and hematuria. Pyuria is uncommon and fever and

Table 36-1. A Patient Care Process for Suspected Renal Colic

Triage and initial evaluation

Triage: Rapidly triage patients with suspected renal colic for pain control and diagnostic evaluation.

Reassurance: Reassure patients that their pain will be rapidly treated and that the cause of their severe discomfort will be sought.

Vital signs: Check vital signs and assess pain intensity.

Focused history and physical examination

IV access and fluid management

IV access such as saline lock should be established to allow administration of analgesics, antiemetics, and fluids if the patient is dehydrated.

The administration of forced IV fluids to "flush out stones" is controversial.

Instruct the patient to remain NPO (until other causes of abdominal pain are considered and in case the patient becomes or is nauseous).

Differential diagnosis and special considerations

Renal infarction, renal artery thrombosis/embolism, renal parenchymal tumors, papillary necrosis, pyelonephritis, hemorrhage (blood clot), ureteral strictures, testicular torsion, intra-abdominal or retroperitoneal disease, ruptured ectopic pregnancy, ruptured ovarian cyst, adnexal torsion, endometriosis, musculoskeletal.

Consider the possibility of a leaking or dissecting aortic abdominal aneurysm: In older patients, a leaking aortic abdominal aneurysm (which can mimic renal colic by retroperitoneal compression of the ureter from the expanding hematoma).

Is there a urinary tract infection in the presence of obstruction? Urinary tract infection + acute ureteral obstruction = medical/urologic emergency.

Diagnostic testing

Imaging: Helical CT, IVP, or abdominal ultrasound (depending on availability; order for first episode or when the diagnosis is uncertain).

Urinalysis: Strain the urine, urine pregnancy test, check evidence of urinary tract infection.

Analgesia

For patients in moderate-to-severe pain, administer an NSAID and/or titrate an opioid. One example of an analgesic treatment regimen:

Ketorolac 30 mg IV or 60 mg SC or IM (if IV access unavailable) if there are no contraindications to NSAIDs.

Morphine titration (in nonfrail adult): 5–10 mg IV loading dose → 3–5 mg IV increments every 5 minutes with monitoring of pain intensity and vital signs.

Hospitalization vs. discharge from the emergency department (ED)

Hospitalization: Patients with intractable pain or vomiting or evidence of infection should be hospitalized.

Arrange follow-up care: The majority of patients will be successfully evaluated and treated in the ED and released to follow-up. If this is the patient's first urinary stone, consult the patient's primary care physician and/or urologist for follow-up and possible metabolic evaluation and stone (if passed) analysis.

Follow-up instructions: Instruct patients to return immediately to the ED for recrudescence of the pain, fever, or development of new symptoms. Instruct the patient to strain the urine and save any stones in a dry container.

Analgesia: Prescribe an NSAID and/or an opioid. Consider instructing patients to carry some of the medications with them in the future to serve as an "emergency pain kit."

CT: computed tomography; IVP: intravenous pyelogram; NSAIDs: nonsteroidal anti-inflammatory drugs.

Note: These steps should not be construed as applicable to all patients, appropriate in all medical care settings, or a complete care guide. Nor are they intended to imply a standard of care. Individualized patients require individualized, tailored care as well as clinician judgment which cannot be distilled into a single set of recommendations. Many of the actions may occur simultaneously or in a different order based on the needs of the patients and practice pattern of the physician. For example, during the initial evaluation, an intravenous (IV) can be inserted by another member of the emergency medical team and preparations for symptom management and diagnostic testing can be initiated.

bacteriuria typically do not occur unless there is an infection behind an obstructing renal stone. Urinary tract infection plus obstruction is a medical emergency. An obstructing stone, by impeding the normal flow of urine, predisposes to urinary infection and urosepsis. Under these circumstances, severe renal parenchymal damage can rapidly occur. Antibiotic therapy active against gram negative bacteria should be immediately administered. In addition, immediate urologic consultation should be obtained since relief of the obstruction of urine outflow by percutaneous nephrostomy or another drainage procedure may be urgently required.

The Controversy of Intravenous Fluids

The administration of IV fluids to patients with renal colic is controversial. Large volumes of IV fluids are often administered to produce a fluid diuresis that mechanically "flushes out" the stone. Such a rationale has not been consistently borne out in animal and human studies. In experimental models, Holmlund was unable to demonstrate that high pressure above a stone could be used to make an arrested stone pass.[6] A clinical study by Grenabo et al., in which plasma antidiuretic hormone (ADH) levels were measured as an indicator of the state of hydration, suggested the therapeutic effect of indomethacin was most notable in patients whose fluid balance tended toward deficit.[12] Edna and Hesselberg, however, compared IV fluid administration (3 L over 6 hours) to fluid restriction in renal colic patients who received pethidine intramuscular (IM) and found no significant difference in pain relief between the two groups measured at 6 hours.[13] Nor did their results suggest an increased likelihood that stones would be spontaneously passed with forced IV fluid therapy. Fluid therapy might also diminish the effect of other therapies, particularly indomethacin. Sjodin and Holmlund demonstrated in an anesthetized pig model that rapid infusion of saline or x-ray contrast medium counteracted the fall in renal pelvic pressure induced by indomethacin.[14] Edna et al., however, compared the effect of fluid load and fluid restriction on pain in patients with acute renal colic treated with indomethacin 50 mg IV and found no difference in pain after 1, 3, and 6 hours of observation.[15] In summary, there are different views concerning the consequences of forced fluids versus fluid restriction during the acute episode and treatment phase of renal colic. However, for the prevention of new stones, there seems to be general agreement that patients should be instructed to increase their PO fluid intake.

Indications for Hospitalization

The majority of patients with acute ureteral obstruction from stones will spontaneously pass the stones. Patients should be hospitalized for intractable pain or vomiting or evidence of infection. Relative indications for admission include high-grade obstruction, urinary extravasation on intravenous pyelogram (IVP), solitary kidney, intrinsic renal disease, and stone size greater than 5 mm.

ANALGESIA FOR RENAL COLIC

A surprising number and variety of analgesics to treat renal colic have been studied. In this chapter, these have been categorized as opioids, nonsteroidal anti-inflammatory drugs (NSAIDs), antispasmodics, and combination drugs.

Opioids

Opioids, particularly morphine, remain a cornerstone of analgesic therapy until the stone spontaneously passes or is removed or pulverized by various surgical techniques. Opioids are efficacious, safe when properly administered, relatively inexpensive, and possess a long "track record." Opioids used and studied in the treatment of renal colic include morphine, meperidine (pethidine), butorphanol, buprenorphine, and ciramadol. *Butorphanol tartrate* is a totally synthetic agonist-antagonist that exhibits less spasmogenic activity in smooth muscle than other opioids, a property that may be advantageous in the treatment of renal colic. *Buprenorphine*, a synthetic opioid closely related in structure to morphine, is a potent analgesic with longer duration of action than meperidine or morphine. *Ciramadol* is a partial agonist opioid analgesic pain control which has been discontinued by the manufacturers because of a high incidence of adverse effects and therefore is not available.

Administration of Opioids

Opioids are typically administered parenterally for severe pain with the IV route typically preferred to the IM route. IV administration of opioids permits *titration*, the technique of administering a loading dose of medication followed by increments at time intervals until either the desired effect is achieved or clinically significant side effects occur. Such an approach allows a more "individualized" dosing of opioids, affords better monitoring, and avoids the attendant problems and erratic drug absorption associated with the IM route. In general, the patient should be titrated to the point of comfort and not necessarily total pain ablation. In the uncommon event hypotension or respiratory depression occur, further incremental doses may be withheld and naloxone and/or IV fluids administered. The total dose of opioid required to treat renal colic may be considerably higher than doses considered customary or "usual." Nevertheless, it is prudent to set "stop-and-think points" every

10–15 mg of morphine for reassessing the patient and rethinking the situation. The axiom that pain refractory to opioid therapy may be of vascular origin (arterial dissection or rupture) should be considered. Though PCA (patient-controlled analgesia) pumps allow patients to self-titrate opioids and are frequently used postsurgery and in hospitalized patients, they are, in general, infrequently used in emergency departments (EDs). Barriers to their use include equipment cost and maintenance, lack of familiarity, and pharmacy charges for filling the opioid syringes.

Adverse events associated with opioid therapy include drowsiness, hallucinations, confusion, nausea, vomiting, decreased intestinal motility and constipation, orthostatic hypotension, and risk of dependence. Morphine produces spasmogenic effects on the urinary tract, causing contraction of the smooth muscles of the ureter and bladder. On balance, however, opioids remain an efficacious, relatively safe, inexpensive treatment option in severe pain states. Concern about infrequent adverse reactions or abuse potential should not lead to the misguided and unfortunate withholding of opioids from patients in severe pain.

Nonsteroidal Anti-Inflammatory Drugs (NSAIDs)

NSAIDs are an important advance in the treatment of renal colic. Prostaglandins play an integral role in inflammation and inflammatory pain throughout the body. The effects of prostaglandins on the urinary tract include increased renal blood flow, increased diuresis, increased ureteral smooth muscle activity, and local ureteral inflammation. NSAIDs inhibit the enzyme cyclooxygenase (COX), which is the ratelimiting step in producing prostaglandins from arachidonic acid. There are both constitutive (COX-1) and inducible isoforms (COX-2) of the COX enzyme.

Treatment of pain due to ureteral stones is therefore directed at reducing the pressure above the stone first by improving flow past the stone and second by reducing urine production. In particular, NSAIDs have been shown to increase the afferent arteriolar resistance, reduce glomerular capillary pressure, and thus block the diuresis and increase in pelvic pressure usually associated with acute obstruction. Anti-inflammatory agents appear to reduce the inflammatory reaction in the ureteral wall so that stones are more rapidly passed[16] and have been demonstrated to directly reduce or abolish the smooth muscle activity of ureteral and renal pelvis smooth muscle.[17]

Several systematic reviews[18–20] have assessed NSAIDs in renal colic. The systematic review by Holdgate and Pollock concluded that patients with acute renal colic who received NSAIDs achieved greater reductions in pain scores were less likely to require further analgesia in the short

term than those receiving opioids. Opioids, particularly pethidine (meperidine), were associated with a higher rate of vomiting. The presently available NSAIDs are predominantly COX-1 inhibitors (flurbiprofen, ketoprofen) or nonselective COX inhibitors (indomethacin, diclofenac), which are often associated with gastrointestinal (GI) side effects.[21] NSAIDs studied and used to treat renal colic include indomethacin, ketorolac, diclofenac, ketoprofen, aspirin, naproxen, and pirprofen. The availability and formulations of various NSAIDs approved for clinical use varies considerably from country-to-country.

Indomethacin

Indomethacin was introduced for clinical trial in 1962 for the treatment of arthritic disorders. The "indomethacin era" of ureteral colic treatment was ushered in by research conducted primarily in Sweden. In 1974, Holmlund had published a study of the NSAID Tanderil in the treatment of ureteral stone disease.[22] In 1978, Holmlund and Sjodin published a randomized, double-blind, crossover study comparing indomethacin 50 mg IV to placebo IV in relieving renal colic.[23] Pain relief following indomethacin IV injection was rapid. Other trials have confirmed the efficacy of parenteral indomethacin in relieving ureteral colic.[14,24] Although IV indomethacin is not approved for analgesia by the Food and Drug Administration (FDA) in the United States, formulations for rectal administration are widely available. Cordell et al.[25] compared indomethacin 100 mg rectal suppositories to IV titrated morphine (5 mg followed by two 2.5 mg increments) and demonstrated both regimens reduced pain associated with acute ureteral obstruction. The suppository form of indomethacin provides reliable absorption in patients who are vomiting and unable to take oral medications. In addition, the suppository form can be prescribed as an out-patient treatment should pain return. The disadvantages of indomethacin suppositories include slower onset of pain relief compared to morphine or IV indomethacin, objection by many patients to suppositories, inadvertent expelling of the suppository, and lack of availability or inability to compound the suppository in many pharmacies.

Ketorolac Tromethamine (Toradol)

In 1989, ketorolac became the first NSAID in the United States to be approved for parenteral use as an analgesic. The efficacy of parenteral ketorolac—alone or in combination with other agents—has been confirmed by numerous studies.[26–31] *Balanced analgesia* or *multimodal analgesia* is the combination of pharmacologic agents whose goal is to achieve sufficient analgesia through additive or synergistic effects between different analgesics with concomitant reduction of adverse events as a result of lower doses of analgesics and differences in side effects profile.[32] Cordell et al. compared ketorolac 60 mg IV, meperidine 50 mg IV, and a combination of both (balanced analgesia) in patients with renal colic.[28] By 30 minutes, 75% of the ketorolac group, 74% of the combination group, and 23% of the meperidine group had a 50% reduction in pain scores. (Clinicians should note that while this study was being completed in 1995, the manufacturers' prescribing recommendations or ketorolac were changed to an IV dose of 30 mg and IM dose of 60 mg for single-dose injections and 30 mg for both IV and IM administration of multiple doses with a maximum daily dose not to exceed 120 mg.)

Diclofenac Sodium (Voltaren)

Many studies,[4,29,33–36] some including large numbers of subjects, have demonstrated the efficacy of diclofenac sodium in renal colic. A study by Cohen et al. concluded that diclofenac and ketorolac are equally effective.[29]

COX-2 Inhibitors

The newer selective COX-2 inhibitors include celecoxib (Celebrex), rofecoxib (Vioxx), and valdecoxib (Bextra). In an in vitro ureteral model, the selective COX-2 inhibitor (NS-398) reduced ureteral contractility as effectively as indomethacin[21]; however, the clinical use of COX-2 inhibitors in renal colic has not yet been reported. Because of the concern regarding the increased risk of significant heart disease and GI bleeding, warnings have been issued for the COX-2 inhibitors and the drugs; rofecoxib and valdecoxib have been withdrawn from the market.

Administration of NSAIDs

Because they have a ceiling effect, NSAIDs are not amenable to titration. NSAIDs are contraindicated or should be used with caution in patients with a history of hypersensitivity to the agent, active GI bleeding, active peptic ulcer disease, allergic diseases (chronic urticaria or nasal polyps), and chronic renal insufficiency. (Clinicians should consult prescribing instructions relevant to their practice locale for individual NSAIDs.)

Antispasmodics

Because ureteral spasm is one of the factors in producing the pain of ureteral obstruction as well a cause of stone retention,[37] spasmolytics have long been employed in the treatment of renal colic. Anticholinergic agents have been used alone or in combination with other agents to treat renal colic by relaxing the smooth muscle within the wall of the ureter.[38] Hyoscyamine sulfate (Levsin) is an orally active anticholinergic agent that inhibits the action of acetylcholine at postganglionic receptors of smooth muscle. Jones and Dula compared hyoscyamine sulfate sublingual to ketorolac tromethamine IV in ED patients with renal colic.[30] Although both reduced pain, the rate of pain relief was faster in those receiving ketorolac tromethamine compared to hyoscyamine. Jones et al. later studied sublingual hyoscyamine in combination with IV ketorolac.[31] Side effects of antimuscarinic agents include decreased salivary secretions, blurred vision, and ileus.

Other spasmolytic agents including ceruletide, glucagon, metoclopramide, nifedipine, and tamsulosin have been studied, though with often conflicting results regarding efficacy in renal colic.

Ceruletide is a decapeptide structurally and is pharmacologically similar to cholecystokinin that produces relaxation of the cystic duct and sphincter of Oddi. Though it has been shown to be effective in alleviating biliary colic, one study[39] concluded that ceruletide was significantly inferior to pentazocine in treating renal colic.

Glucagon is a polypeptide hormone consisting of 29 amino acids produced by the pancreas. Because glucagon is a smooth muscle relaxant, it has been used to treat meat impactions of the lower esophagus and in GI radiologic studies to relax the duodenum, ampulla of Vater, and colon. Glucagon has been studied in renal colic,[40–43] though some of these studies concluded glucagon did not relieve renal colic or promote stone passage.

Metoclopramide, a cholinergic agonist with central dopamine antagonism, is widely used to treat nausea, migraine, and gastroparesis. One study which compared metoclopramide 20 mg IV to Spasmofen IV to treat renal colic concluded both drugs had equal pain-reducing capacity without serious side effects.[44] The authors did not know if the pain-reducing property of metoclopramide was due to any of its known pharmacologic effects and speculated metoclopramide could have been effective to some extent by relieving nausea, a symptom frequently seen in patients with renal colic.

Nifedipine is a calcium channel blocker that has been studied alone[45,46] or in combination with a corticosteroid[37] to treat renal colic and facilitate stone expulsion. One study, however, concluded nifedipine did not differ from placebo in providing relief from renal colic.

Tamsulosin, a selective alpha-1A adrenergic receptor antagonist commonly used to treat lower urinary tract symptoms (LUTS), has been studied in the medical management of juxtavesical ureteral stones.[47] The authors concluded that tamsulosin decreased stone expulsion time and the need for hospitalization and endoscopic procedures and provided control of colic pain.

Avafortan, Baralgin, Ketogan, and *Spasmofen* are the trade names of four fixed dose *spasmoanalgesics* that combine one or more spasmolytics with opioids or NSAIDs. They are mentioned since they are used outside the United States to treat renal colic.

Other Treatments

Desmopressin nasal spray, subcutaneous paravertebral block, trigger point injections, acupuncture, and local active warming have also been studied or described in the treatment of renal colic. These treatments, though intriguing avenues to be further explored, lack the breadth of research and clinical experience of opioids, NSAIDs, and spasmolytic agents.

SUMMARY

The care process for patients with suspected ureteral colic emphasizes rapid triage and evaluation, search for mimicking conditions and complications, individualized analgesia, and careful monitoring. While a surprising number of agents and combination drugs have been studied, opioids and NSAIDs remain the cornerstone of analgesia in patients suffering from renal colic.

REFERENCES

1. Teichman JM. Clinical practice. Acute renal colic from ureteral calculus. *N Engl J Med.* 2004;350:684–693.
2. Shokeir AA. Renal colic: pathophysiology, diagnosis and treatment. *Eur Urol.* 2001;39(3):241–249.
3. Boyd W. *A Textbook of Pathology.* 7th ed. London: Klimpton; 1961.
4. Khalifa MS, Sharkawi MA. Treatment of pain owing to acute ureteral obstruction with prostaglandin-synthetase inhibitor: a prospective randomized study. *J Urol.* 1986;136:393–395.
5. Shokeir AA. Renal colic: new concepts related to pathophysiology, diagnosis and treatment. *Curr Opin Urol.* 2002;12 (4):263–269.
6. Holmlund D. The pathophysiology of ureteral colic. *Scand J Urol Nephrol Suppl.* 1983;75:25–27.
7. Cole RS, Fry CH, Shuttleworth KE. The action of the prostaglandins on isolated human ureteric smooth muscle. *Br J Urol.* 1988:61:19–26.
8. Abber JC, McAninch JW. Renal colic: emergency evaluation and management. *Am J Emerg Med.* 1985;3:56–63.
9. Northwall WH. Ureteral colic and aortic aneurysm. *Nebr Med J.* 1976:61:427–430.
10. Johar JS, Cordell WH, Nelson DR. Misdiagnosis of abdominal aortic aneurysm as renal colic in an ED [abstract]. *Ann Emerg Med.* 1997;30:383.
11. Moran CG, Edwards AT, Griffith GH. Ruptured abdominal aortic aneurysm presenting with ureteric colic. *Br Med J* (Clin Res Ed). 1987:294:1279.
12. Grenabo L, Holmlund D. The significance of fluid restriction in indomethacin treatment of pain from ureteral stone. *Scand J Urol Nephrol Suppl.* 1983:75:39–40.
13. Edna TH, Hesselberg F, Loe B. Indomethacin in the treatment of ureteral colic: is fluid restriction necessary? *J Urol.* 1986: 136:390–392.
14. Sjodin JG, Holmlund D. Indomethacin by intravenous infusion in ureteral colic. A multicentre study. *Scand J Urol Nephrol.* 1982:16:221–225.
15. Edna TH, Hesselberg F. Acute ureteral colic and fluid intake. *Scand J Urol Nephrol.* 1983:17:175–178.
16. Holmlund D. Ureteral stones. An experimental and clinical study of the mechanism of the passage and arrest of ureteral stones. *Scand J Urol Nephrol.* 1968;(suppl 1):80.
17. Lundstam S, Wahlander L, Kral JG. Treatment of ureteral colic by prostaglandin synthetase inhibition with diclofenac sodium. *Curr Ther Res Clin Exp.* 1980;28:355–358.
18. Labrecque M, Dostaler LP, Rousselle R, et al. Efficacy of nonsteroidal anti-inflammatory drugs in the treatment of acute renal colic. A meta-analysis [see comments]. *Arch Intern Med.* 1994;154(12):1381–1387.
19. Holdgate A, Pollock T. Systematic review of the relative efficacy of non-steroidal anti-inflammatory drugs and opioids in the treatment of acute renal colic. *BMJ.* 2004;328 (7453):1401.
20. Holdgate A, Pollock T. Nonsteroidal anti-inflammatory drugs (NSAIDs) versus opioids for acute renal colic. *Cochrane Database Syst Rev.* 2004(1):CD004137.
21. Nakada SY, Jerde TJ, Bjorling DE, et al. Selective cyclooxygenase-2 inhibitors reduce ureteral contraction in vitro: a better alternative for renal colic? *J Urol.* 2000;163: 607–612.
22. Holmlund D. Tanderil in the treatment of ureteral stone disease. *Helvetica Chiruryca Acta.* 1974:41:333.
23. Holmlund D, Sjodin JG. Treatment of ureteral colic with intravenous indomethacin. *J Urol.* 1978:120:676–677.
24. Lehtonen T, Kellokumpu I, Permi J, et al. Intravenous indomethacin in the treatment of ureteric colic. A clinical multicentre study with pethidine and metamizol as the control preparations. *Ann Clin Res.* 1983;15(5–6):197–199.
25. Cordell WH, Larson TA, Lingeman JE, et al. Indomethacin suppositories versus intravenously titrated morphine for the treatment of ureteral colic. *Ann Emerg Med.* 1994;23(2): 262–269.
26. Oosterlinck W, Philp NH, Charig C, et al. A double-blind single dose comparison of intramuscular ketorolac tromethamine and pethidine in the treatment of renal colic. *J Clin Pharmacol.* 1990:30:336–341.
27. Larsen LS, Miller A, Allegra JR. The use of intravenous ketorolac for the treatment of renal colic in the emergency department. *Amer J Emerg Med.* 1993:11:197–199.
28. Cordell WH, Wright SW, Wolfson AB, et al. Comparison of intravenous ketorolac, meperidine, and both (balanced

analgesia) for renal colic.[see comment]. *Ann Emerg Med.* 1996;28(2):151–158.

29. Cohen E, Hafner R, Rotenberg Z, et al. Comparison of ketorolac and diclofenac in the treatment of renal colic. *Eur J Clin Pharmacol.* 1998;54(6):455–458.

30. Jones JB, Dula DJ. The efficacy of sublingual hyoscyamine sulfate and intravenous ketorolac tromethamine in the relief of ureteral colic. *Am J Emerg Med.* 1998;16(6):557–559.

31. Jones JB, Giles BK, Brizendine EJ, et al. Sublingual hyoscyamine sulfate in combination with ketorolac tromethamine for ureteral colic: a randomized, double-blind, controlled trial. *Ann Emerg Med.* 2001;37(2):141–146.

32. Kehlet H, Dahl JB. The value of "multimodal" or "balanced analgesia" in postoperative pain treatment. *Anesth Analg.* 1993;77:1048–1056.

33. Sanahuja J, Corbera G, Garau J, et al. Intramuscular diclofenac sodium versus intravenous baralgin in the treatment of renal colic. *DICP.* 1990;24:361–364.

34. Lundstam SO, Leissner KH, Wahlander LA, et al. Prostaglandin-synthetase inhibition with diclofenac sodium in treatment of renal colic: comparison with use of a narcotic analgesic. *Lancet.* 1982;1:1096–1097.

35. Thompson J, Pike J, Chumas P, et al. Rectal diclofenac compared with pethidine injection in acute renal colic. *Br Med J.* 1989;299:1140–1141.

36. Marthak KV, Gokarn AM, Rao AV, et al. A multi-centre comparative study of diclofenac sodium and a dipyrone/spasmolytic combination, and a single-centre comparative study of diclofenac sodium and pethidine in renal colic patients in India. *Curr Med Res Opin.* 1991;12(6):366–373.

37. Porpiglia F, Destefanis P, Fiori C, et al. Effectiveness of nifedipine and deflazacort in the management of distal ureter stones. *Urology.* 2000;56:579–582.

38. Risholm L. Conventional methods of treating pain from ureteral stone. *Scand J Urol Nephrol Suppl.* 1983:75:29–30.

39. Lishner M, Lang R, Jutrin I, et al. Analgesic effect of ceruletide compared with pentazocine in biliary and renal colic: a prospective, controlled, double-blind study. *Drug Intell Clin Pharm.* 1985:19:433–436.

40. Bahn Zobbe V, Rygaard H, Rasmussen D, et al. Glucagon in acute ureteral colic. A randomized trial. *Eur Urol.* 1986;12:28–31.

41. Webb DR, Nunn IN, McOmish D, et al. Glucagon and ureteric calculi. *Med J Aust.* 1986;144(3):124.

42. Kahnoski RJ, Lingeman JE, Woods JR, et al. Efficacy of glucagon in the relief of ureteral colic following treatment by extracorporeal shock wave lithotripsy: a randomized double-blind trial. *J Urol.* 1987:1124–1125.

43. Minkov N, Shumleva V, Pironkov A, et al. A new method for the management of ureteral colic after extracorporeal shock wave lithotripsy. *Int Urol Nephrol.* 1988;20(3):251–255.

44. Hedenbro JL, Olsson AM. Metoclopramide and ureteric colic. *Acta Chir Scand.* 1988;154:439–440.

45. Caravati EM, Runge JW, Bossart PJ, et al. Nifedipine for the relief of renal colic: a double-blind, placebo-controlled clinical trial [see comment]. *Ann Emerg Med.* 1989;18:352–354.

46. Porpiglia F, Ghignone G, Fiori C, et al. Nifedipine versus tamsulosin for the management of lower ureteral stones. *J Urol.* 2004;172:568–571.

47. Dellabella M, Milanese G, Muzzonigro G. Efficacy of tamsulosin in the medical management of juxtavesical ureteral stones. *J Urol.* 2003;170:2202–2205.

37

Complex Regional Pain Syndrome
Reflex Sympathetic Dystrophy and Causalgia

Sharon E. Mace

HIGH YIELD FACTS

- Characterized by spontaneous pain in an extremity that does not follow a dermatone.
- Onset varies but is usually within a month after initiating event.
- Precipitating event is commonly due to minor trauma, surgery, or illness. In 10–52% of patients no initiating event is identified.
- Vasomotor, sudomotor, integument abnormalities, muscle atrophy, and osteoporosis can occur.
- May be due to an abnormally prolonged and exaggerated response of the sympathetic nervous system to an injury.
- Treatment includes rehabilitation, psychologic support, and pain management.
- Specific therapy includes physiotherapy, psychologic support, medications, neuromodulation, and sympathectomy (by drugs, local/regional blocks, surgery).

DEFINITION AND TERMINOLOGY

Complex regional pain syndrome (CRPS) is the terminology for the conditions formerly referred to as reflex sympathetic dystrophy (RSD) (CRPS I) and causalgia (CRPS II), although there is a wide array of other terms by which CRPS has been referred to in the past (Table 37-1).[1,2] Some of the terms are descriptive, detailing clinical signs and symptoms that are characteristic of the disorder. *Algodystrophy* or *algoneurodystrophy* are from algo for the Greek word for pain and dystrophy meaning degeneration.

Causalgia is pain secondary to nerve injury and is characterized by a burning sensation (from the Greek *kausis* for burning). Other nomenclature refers to the proximate cause of CRPS, specifically trauma, including *posttraumatic painful osteoporosis, posttraumatic vasomotor syndrome*, or *posttraumatic sympathetic dystrophy*. Still other terms refer to findings that occur in patients with acute or chronic disease. For example, with acute CRPS; *transient osteoporosis* or *acute bone atrophy* can occur. With long standing CRPS, atrophy may result, thus, the name *Sudeck's atrophy*. Although the exact etiology and pathophysiology of CRPS are unknown, the causative factors appear to center around dysfunction of the sympathetic division of the autonomic nervous system.[3,4] This is reflected in the terms posttraumatic sympathetic dystrophy, *reflex neurovascular dystrophy*, and RSD (Table 37-1).

OVERVIEW OF CRPS

Incidence

The incidence of CPRS is unclear, ranging from 1 to 2% with fractures to 2 to 5% with peripheral nerve injuries, and 5% with the shoulder-hand syndrome after myocardial infarction.[5,6] Other studies have reported much higher levels: 28% in one prospective study and 17–35% in a report of patients with Colles' fractures.[7,8]

The variable clinical presentations, the occurrence of spontaneous resolution in some patients, the previous lack of uniform terminology and diagnostic criteria, the changeable clinical course with some signs/symptoms appearing/disappearing in an unpredictable fashion, and the often inconsistent response to treatment; all make CRPS a difficult entity to diagnose.

Diagnostic Criteria

In order to create consistent diagnostic criteria and terminology, the International Association for the Study of Pain (IASP) developed a new classification: CRPS.[1,2] The criteria for CRPS are spontaneous pain or allodynia/ hyperesthesia not limited to the territory of a single peripheral nerve accompanied by (at some point in time) specific vasomotor/ sudomotor/integument findings (e.g., edema, skin blood flow abnormality, or abnormal sudomotor activity) in the region of the pain following the precipitating event, and the exclusion of other conditions that could account for the pain and dysfunction. CRPS I and CRPS II develop after a precipitating event. With CRPS II, a peripheral nerve injury is the initiating event (Table 37-2).[1,2]

Table 37-1. Terminology Previously Used for Complex Regional Pain Syndrome

Descriptive Terms (painful involvement of an extremity)
Algodystrophy
Algoneurodystrophy
Causalgia
Shoulder-hand syndrome

Terms Reflecting Characteristic Findings
Bony changes
   Acute bone atrophy
   Migratory osteolysis
   Transient osteoporosis
   Posttraumatic painful osteoporosis
Neuromuscular/vasomotor involvement
   Sudeck's atrophy
   Posttraumatic vasomotor syndrome
   Traumatic angiospasm
   Traumatic vasospasm
   Postinfarction sclerodactyly

Sympathetic Nervous System Involvement
Reflex sympathetic dystrophy
Posttraumatic sympathetic dystrophy
Sympathetically maintained pain (SMP)
Reflex neurovascular dystrophy

CLINICAL CHARACTERISTICS

CRPS is characterized by severe pain precipitated by an injury. It usually occurs in an extremity and is often accompanied by muscular atrophy and bony changes (e.g., osteopenia). Dysfunction of the sympathetic nervous system is theorized to play a role in the pathophysiology (Table 37-3).[3,4,9]

Table 37-2. Diagnostic Criteria for Complex Regional Pain Syndrome

Spontaneous pain or allodynia/hyperalgesia
   Not limited to a single peripheral nerve territory
   Disproportionate to the inciting event
Evidence (past or present) of edema, skin blood flow
   abnormality, or abnormal sudomotor activity in the
   region of the pain since the inciting event
CRPS diagnosis excluded by conditions that can
   account for the pain and dysfunction
CRPS I and CRPS II occur after an initiating event with
   CRPS II the precipitating event is a peripheral nerve
   injury

Table 37-3. Clinical Characteristics of Complex Regional Pain Syndrome

History
Pain
   Spontaneous
   Can also be evoked
   Mild ache to excruciating pain
   Usually severe
   Greater than expected based on precipitating incident
   Constant with acute exacerbations
   Burning, throbbing, aching
   Most commonly in an extremity
   Does not follow a dermatone or the territory of
      a peripheral nerve
   Circumferential, regional
   Onset, usually within 1 month after initial traumatic
      event
Precipitating event
   Diverse types of injury
   From peripheral locations to central structures/organs
   Commonly orthopedic injuries
   May be iatrogenic (major or minor surgery, pressure
      of cuff on an extremity creating a bloodless field)
   Original triggering event may be very minor,
      forgotten, resolved
   In 52% of pediatric and 10% of adults,
      no precipitating event identified

Physical Examination
Hyperesthesia*
   Hyperalgesia
   Dysesthesia
   Allodynia
Edema: variable, transient
Sudomotor: ↑ sweating
Vasomotor
   Temperature perception: ↑ or ↓ or both in
      involved limb
   Skin color changes: redness, blueness, mottling
Integument
   Skin: shiny, glossy appearance, thinning,
      or flaky thickened
   Hair: alopecia or coarse hair
   Nails: thickening
Changes secondary to immobilization
   Muscle atrophy
   Joint stiffness, contractures
   Osteopenia

*May be triggered by movement (passive or active), touch, pressure, temperature.

The diagnosis of CRPS is a clinical one, there being no diagnostic test developed for the disorder.[10] The hallmark of CRPS is neuropathic pain, often described as burning or searing, but it may be a throbbing or aching sensation. Although the pain may be a mild ache, it is usually severe and seemingly disproportionate to the original inciting cause.[10] It is constant with episodes of exacerbations and is usually distal in location but also has been described in the face and neck.[10,11] The distribution of the pain is important in the differential diagnosis and aids in ruling out other disorders, for it does not follow a dermatone or the territory of a single nerve[12] as seen with peripheral nerve injuries. It is regional, extending beyond the distribution of a single peripheral nerve or dermatome even when a peripheral nerve injury is the precipitating incident. It is typically circumferential.

The onset of pain of CRPS may be hours, weeks, or even months after the initial inciting traumatic event, although typically it is within the first few weeks.[13,14] In one large prospective study of adult patients, symptom onset began within 1 day in 75% of the patients while beginning more than 1 year after the precipitating traumatic event in 0.8% (7/829).[5] In a pediatric study, the duration from the initial noxious event to symptom onset ranged from 9 days to 1 year.[15]

The average time from the initial injury to diagnosis varied from 1 week to 24 months[5,15,16] Most of the patients had been seen previously by another physician or physicians suggesting that the disorder is underrecognized, especially in pediatric patients. The initial events that can trigger the onset of CRPS are varied and extensive (Table 37-4). Various injuries, thrombosis, surgery, or even a heart attack (*shoulder-hand syndrome*) can precipitate CRPS.[5,14] In adults, the precipitating events are trauma (65%), following surgery (19%), an inflammatory process (2%), other suspected causes (4%) (such as injections, intravenous infusion, cerebrovascular accident), with no identified precipitant in 10%.[5] In children, minor trauma is a common precipitant. Indeed, the initial precipitating trauma may have been extremely minor, easily forgotten, and long since resolved when the pain and other symptoms of CRPS begin.[5,15]

Both CPRS I and CPRS II have similar clinical features. The main distinguishing feature between CPRS I and CPRS II is the type of precipitating event. By definition, CRPS II or causalgia occurs after a peripheral nerve injury.[1,2] The pain with CRPS is a spontaneous pain characterized by an oversensitivity or overreaction to stimuli. CRPS patients typically have hyperesthesia, with hyperalgesia, dysesthesia, and allodynia.[2] Hyperesthesia is an excessive sensibility to stimuli including pain, touch, or other sensory stimuli and

Table 37-4. Precipitating Factors of Complex Regional Pain Syndrome

Orthopedic injuries
Soft tissue, contusions, sprains, strains, fasciitis
Bone/joints: arthritis, bursitis, fractures, dislocations

Nervous system
Peripheral: peripheral nerve injuries/disease, postherpetic neuralgia
Brachial plexus injuries/disease
Spinal cord injuries/disease
Central nervous system (CNS): head trauma, CNS disease

Visceral
Thoracic: disease/trauma, myocardial infarction (especially shoulder-hand syndrome)
Abdomen: disease/trauma

Dermatologic
Burns
Lacerations, abrasions

Vascular
Deep vein thrombosis

Iatrogenic
Surgery/procedures: major or minor surgery (even outpatient procedures such as arthroscopy), use of a tourniquet during surgery
Dental procedures: especially with facial/neck CRPS

Idiopathic
In some CRPS patients, no precipitating incident is identified (up to 10% of adults, 52% of children)

special senses. Hyperalgesia is defined as an extreme sensitivity to painful stimuli. Dysesthesia is the condition in which ordinary stimuli produce a disagreeable sensation. Allodynia is the perception of pain from a stimulus that is normally not considered noxious or painful. Allodynia may be precipitated by touch, pressure, temperature, or movement of the limb/joint in the affected area.

The sensory changes may be so severe that any movement (active or passive) of the affected limb or any contact (even merely touching the involved region) can produce extreme pain. The patient attempts to shield or protect the affected limb, leading to loss of function.[17] Prolonged immobilization leads to joint stiffness/contractures, osteopenia, and muscle atrophy.[18] Tremor or dystonia occurs infrequently (<5% of patients).[12] Swelling is present at some time during the course of the disease, although it is often not present when the patient is being examined. Characteristics of the edema have not been well defined.

Findings of autonomic dysfunction may be vasomotor or sudomotor. Vasomotor signs include redness, blueness, and mottling or blotchiness of the extremity; temperature changes in the extremity with a perceived temperature increase, decrease, or both in the involved extremity.[14] Any one or multiple vasomotor signs in any permutation may be present in a given patient during the course of their disease. Sudomotor changes usually involvs increased sweating. Alterations in the integument that have been reported include thinning of the skin with a shiny appearance or a flaky thickened skin, alopecia or coarse hair, and thickened nails (Table 37-3).[14]

The severe pain combined with loss of function can create psychologic dysfunction ranging from anxiety to fear and depression.[19,20]

DIAGNOSTIC TESTING FOR CRPS

Unfortunately, there is no one diagnostic test for CRPS; however, some radiologic and laboratory tests can support the diagnosis of CRPS and are used to rule out other disorders. Plain radiographs of the affected limb may reveal bone resorption, a patchy demineralization, or osteopenia.[20] Soft tissue swelling may or may not be present on the roentgenogram.[1] The longer the disease has been present, the more likely spotty or diffuse osteopenia will be present[5]; however, normal radiographs do not rule out the disease, especially early in the course of the disease.

Three-phase bone scans of the affected extremity typically demonstrate increased patchy uptake of the radiotracer on the delayed images, increased perfusion on the radionuclide angiogram, and increased tissue uptake on the blood pool phase.[21] Sensitivity of the three-phase bone scans varies widely.[22] Skin thickening and contrast enhancement have been reported in 88.6% (31/35) of CRPS patients on magnetic resonance imaging (MRI).[23] Synovial effusion may be seen on MRI in CRPS I.

Various tests of sensory function have also been used in the detection of allodynia and hyperalgesia that may occur with CRPS.[24] Simple objects: a cotton swab (broken to obtain a sharp end or with the handle-end sharpened); metal objects at room temperature cooled in a refrigerator or by vapocoolants, or warmed in the physician's hand or by a water bath, and a tuning fork have been used to test for allodynia (heat, cold, mechanical), hyperalgesia (heat, mechanical), and for temporal summation to mechanical stimulation.[24]

Bedside testing for allodynia includes static mechanical allodynia—touching the skin with manual light pressure, dynamic mechanical allodynia—stroking the skin with a cotton swab (cotton end) or gauge or a brush; cold allodynia-touching the skin with a coolant or a metal or nonmetal refrigerated object, and comparing with an object warmed to room temperature.[24] Ice water, alcohol, acetone, or fluorometholone have been used as coolants. Heat hyperalgesia is tested using skin contact with an object immersed in a water bath at 45–47°C. Mechanical hyperalgesia is tested by manual pinprick to a safety pin or the sharp end of a broken cotton swab. More detailed testing for various types of allodynia and hyperalgesia can be performed in a specialty clinic.

In the past, a positive response with a decrease in pain to sympathetic block or surgical sympathectomy had been used as diagnostic criteria for CRPS.[18,25] While this viewpoint has been discarded, sympathetic blockade and sympathectomy may still be used as treatment in some cases.

PATHOPHYSIOLOGY OF COMPLEX REGIONAL PAIN SYNDROMES

The etiology of CRPS is thought to be an abnormally prolonged exaggerated response of the sympathetic nervous system to injury.[26] A normal response to a traumatic injury involves the sympathetic reflex arc.[27] Efferent sympathetic impulses from the spinal cord are transmitted via the ventral roots to the white communicating ramus into the sympathetic chain to synapse in the sympathetic ganglion[3]. Failure of the sympathetic reflex arc to turn off causes the persistent and increasing functioning of the sympathetic reflex. The (now) hyperdynamic sympathetic nervous system leads to greater vasoconstriction and worsening tissue ischemia further increasing pain.[3] A vicious cycle ensues.

Sympathetically maintained pain (SMP) is maintained by efferent sympathetic activity or by circulating catecholamines.[17] Pain that is relieved by a specific sympatholytic procedure, whether a sympathetic nerve block or a sympatholytic pharmacologic agent, is considered SMP. Sympathetically independent pain (SIP) is not maintained by and is independent of the sympathetic nervous system. SMP is believed to be involved in CRPS I and CRPS II, although SIP may also be part of CRPS.[17] Recent research has expanded on the theorized participation of the sympathetic nervous system reflex arc in the etiology of CRPS.[28] In addition to an abnormal linkage of peripheral sensory afferents with the efferent sympathetic nervous system, there is also involvement of inflammatory processes in the peripheral tissues plus the development of secondary changes in the central nervous system.[14]

When peripheral nerves suffer severe damage, as occurs when a nerve is transected, multiple changes can occur. The somatosensory fibers develop an increased sensitivity to catecholamines.[29] This effect is dependent on α-receptor activity. The nerve growth factor released by stimulation of the sympathetic trunk and circulating catecholamines stimulate the growth of the damaged sensory nerve fibers, and also stimulates inflammation, which activates complement.[30–33] Sympathetic stimulation releases norepinephrine, which leads to the release of prostaglandin, a mediator of inflammation.[34]

Peripheral nerve damage results in an increased firing of neurons, especially the wide dynamic range neurons (WDRN) in the dorsal root ganglion. Sympathetic stimulation, at least initially, results in an even greater discharge of dorsal root ganglions.

Several human studies do indicate an effect of the sympathetic nervous system on pain after peripheral nerve damage, a situation that occurs with CRPS II or causalgia.[35] For example, administration of norepinephrine causes severe pain in the involved limb in patients with causalgia and those with an amputation stump neuroma.[36,37] Direct simulation of the sympathetic chain worsens the pain with causalgia.[38] The pain mechanisms involved in CRPS may be similar to other types of neuralgias or neuropathic pain including phantom limb pain and herpetic neuralgia. A study documented allodynia and worsening pain when norepinephrine or epinephrine was administered to patients with postherpetic neuralgia.[39]

The sympathetic nervous system may also play a role in the development of pain in patients without nerve damage (a situation similar to CRPS I). Again, both peripheral and central components are implicated. In one study, administration of norepinephrine to an area of skin inflammation produced hyperalgesia.[40] In some situations, chemical sympathectomy with phentolamine decreased the pain caused by local inflammation.[41]

There is some evidence that the sensitization of somatosensory afferents can result from a direct effect of the neurotransmitters, e.g., norepinephrine, or may be mediated by inflammatory substances, such as, prostaglandins.[34,40] Free radical damage has also been proposed as a factor contributing to CRPS.[42] There is also some suggestion that alterations in the central nervous system may occur from extended nociceptive input.[43]

Nociceptors (pain receptors) are the terminal ends of sensory nerves (A-delta and C-fibers.).[44] The receptors of the peripheral sensory nerve are located within a given dermatone. Nociceptors are responsible for transduction of noxious stimuli into specific electrical activity at sensory nerve endings. The A-delta fiber mechanoreceptors respond as nociceptors to severe mechanical stimulation but are otherwise silent.[45] Polymodal nociceptors (PMN) are C-fibers that have a nociceptive response to severe mechanical, thermal, or chemical stimuli.[45] Stimulation of a nociceptor may cause the release of various mediators of inflammation ranging from prostaglandin, substance P, thromboxanes, platelet-activating factor, and serotonin to the leukotrienes and bradykinins. These inflammatory mediators can result in the conduction of nociceptive stimuli and/or sensitization of receptors.

Nerve damage releases nerve growth factor, which creates nerve sprouts.[30] These nerve sprouts are extremely sensitive, creating an ongoing barrage of stimuli or sensory input into the dorsal horn. The result is allodynia. α_2-Adrenoreceptors, which respond to circulating norepinephrine, are located on these nerve sprouts. A condition known as *central hypersensitivity* or *windup*, is when there is a maximal activity of the nociceptors (pain receptors). This central hypersensitivity may be a component of CRPS.

Multiple hypotheses have been proposed to account for the hyperalgesia occurring in CRPS patients. These mechanisms include increased nociceptor sensitivity, with lower levels of threshold stimulation, alterations in the dorsal horn neurons, neuroanatomical restructuring, and central hypersensitivity or windup.[27,28,46] There are several ways in which this heightened nociceptor response can be mediated. An increased affinity of the receptor or a greater density of receptors could occur. Intracellular mechanisms might involve a greater influx of intracellular calcium. Localized inflammation leading to the release of chemical mediators such as histamine or serotonin could cause indirect stimulation of nociceptors.

Activation of WDRN in the dorsal horn by C-nociceptors could lower the pain threshold of C-fibers by a feedback loop. Sympathetic (noradrenergic) perivascular axons extend into the dorsal root ganglion enveloping sensory neurons following nerve injury. This is an additional possible linkage between the sympathetic nervous system and the peripheral nerves.

CRPS IN PEDIATRIC PATIENTS

As with adults, CRPS in children is underrecognized and frequently diagnosed late (up to 24 months in one study).[5,15,16] There are some differences between CRPS in children and adults (Table 37-5). CRPS occurs more in the upper extremities in adults, while the lower extremities are more frequently involved in children.[15,16,47–49] The precipitating event may be associated with an injury, illness, psychologic distress, or a combination of these events. No inciting event can be identified in 52% of pediatric patients

Table 37-5. Comparison of Pediatric and Adult Patients with CRPS

	Peak Age (Years)*	Female: Male	Average Time to Diagnosis (Months)	Most Commonly Involved Extremity	Treatment	Prognosis
Pediatric	9–13 (diagnosed as young as 3 years)	Females >> males	12 9 days to 24 months (range)	Lower extremity	Active physiotherapy, drugs, sympathetic blocks, neuromodulation. Generally conservative therapy	Better than adults
Adult	Middle age (can occur in elderly)	Females >> males	11	Upper extremity	Active physio-therapy, drugs, sympathetic blocks, neuro-modulation	More patients progress to atrophy, osteoporosis

*Can occur at any age.

with CRPS.[15] CRPS in children usually responds to conservative therapy including physiotherapy, psychologic support, and pharmacologic agents for pain.[15,16,47–50]

There is a strong female gender predilection for CRPS (up to 84% in one series). Although CRPS has been diagnosed in a patient as young as 3 years old, the peak incidence is from 9 to 13 years.[15,16,47–49] Often pediatric patients with CRPS are participants in team sports and other athletic activities. Such activities may predispose them to musculoskeletal injuries; however, it has been theorized that their pain allows them to get out of activities and avoid parental expectations.[51] Some experts believe that psychologic factors may have a greater role in children.

There is no standardized universally accepted CRPS management algorithm for children or adults, although the various treatments offered are similar.[12] Although some children with CRPS will need long-term care, the prognosis is better in pediatric patients than adults.[15,16,] Fewer children have osteoporosis or atrophy, fewer children require interventions, and they usually respond to physical therapy and cognitive-behavioral treatment.[45–50]

PSYCHOLOGIC FEATURES OF CRPS

There is no direct relationship between CRPS and a pre-existing psychologic disorder.[19] Because CRPS patients often have chronic ongoing pain and disuse secondary to fear of pain, supportive psychotherapy can be an important part of management and helps patients cope with the anxiety and depression related to their disease.[14,19]

DIFFERENTAL DIAGNOSIS

There is a wide range of diseases that can be mistaken for CRPS. Thrombosis or infection should be ruled out when considering the diagnosis.[3,4,17] Many acute and chronic musculoskeletal disorders present with pain and sometimes with swelling. Acute musculoskeletal disorders from contusions, to sprains and strains and even fractures are in the differential. Chronic musculoskeletal pathology to be considered include bursitis, tendonitis, tennis elbow, overuse syndrome, repetitive strain injury, and cumulative trauma disorder.

Neurologic disorders, especially those presenting with severe pain, weakness, paresthesias, or limited range of motion can be confused with CRPS. Peripheral neuropathies, various neuralgias, and generalized neurologic disorders from multiple sclerosis to the various dystrophies (especially if paresthesias, neuralgias, atrophy, or contractures are present) can also be considered.

Vasomotor changes with cold pale or blue fingers/extremities can occur with Raynaud's syndrome and rheumatologic disorders (such as systemic lupus erythematosus); and vascular diseases (thrombosis, Buerger's disease) as well as with CRPS. When the presentation involves a hot red painful extremity, it is critical to rule out an infection

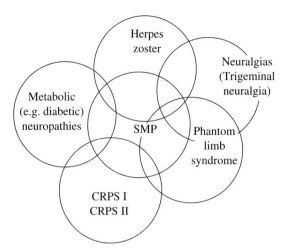

Fig. 37-1. Neuropathic pain disorders with sympathetically maintained pain (SMP).

Table 37-6. Treatment of Complex Regional Pain Syndrome

Appropriate therapy for initial injury*
    Eliminate or limit any ongoing injury/illness/injury
        that may stimulate nociceptors
    Active physiotherapy
        Avoids the adverse effects of disuse
        Increases circulation and bone mineralization
Therapies for pain
    Regional anesthesia: sympathetic blockade
        Stellate ganglion (C6 or C7)
        Lumbar sympathetic blockade (L3)
        Brachial plexus
        Lumbar plexus
        Central neural block
        Peripheral nerve block
    Neuromodulation
        Spinal cord stimulation
        Peripheral nerve stimulation
    Pharmacologic agents for epidural administration
        Clonidine: α_2-adrenergic agonist
    Oral drugs
        α-Receptor agonist: phenoxybenzamine
        Calcium channel blocker: nifedipine
        Anticonvulsants (for neuropathic pain):
            gabapentin, phenytoin
    Tricyclic antidepressants
    Calcitonin
    Corticosteroids
    Nonsteroidal anti-inflammatory drugs:
        ↓ prostaglandin

*Early diagnosis and treatment give best outcome.

(e.g., cellulitis, septic joint, and osteomyelitis) as well as undiagnosed trauma (such as a fracture).

Other disorders with similar presenting complaints are: the numerous pain disorders (from fibromyalgia to the neuropathic pain disorders) and even psychiatric illnesses, malingering and factitious disease.

There are numerous pain disorders that may have a component of SMP. These include phantom limb syndrome, metabolic neuropathies, neuralgias, and herpes zoster. Whether all these pain disorders have a common underlying pathophysiology as have been suggested, remains to be confirmed (Fig. 37-1).

TREATMENT

Early diagnosis and treatment ensure the best outcome with CRPS.[14,17,18,52] Principles of therapy focus on appropriate therapy for the initial injury, removing or limiting any ongoing illness/injury/infection that could stimulate nociceptors (Table 37-6). Active physiotherapy is critical in order to maintain and hopefully, regain function of the affected extremity.[18,52] Active physiotherapy enhances circulation and bone mineralization and avoids the adverse effects of disuse. Since specific guidelines for physical therapy do not exist, rehabilitation programs must be individualized in order to reestablish normal function without reinjuring the affected extremity.[4,52]

There is no universal consensus on subsequent therapy. Randomized controlled clinical trials with large numbers of patients regarding CRPS therapy are few.[4,18] Many treatments focus on eliminating or minimizing sympathetic

efferent activity to the affected limb. This can be accomplished by sympathectomy, either by pharmacologic agents, by sympathetic blockade (local or regional) or infrequently surgical sympathectomy.[3,18]

Sympathetic ganglion blocks have been recommended by some clinicians who feel that this treatment improves the long-term outcome.[53-55] Regional anesthetic techniques are used for symptom relief when pharmacotherapy has not been successful and to document that the pain is sympathetically maintained. Such sympathetic nervous system blocks disrupt vasomotor, sudomotor, and visceromotor efferent fibers; visceral and somatic afferents, and nociceptor fibers. A cervicothoracic sympathetic block (sometimes, inappropriately called a stellate ganglion block) done paratracheally at a C6 level or at the C7 level, achieves upper extremity sympatholysis.[55] A successful sympathetic block is indicated by Horner's syndrome (ptosis, miosis, enopthalmos).[52] Lumbar sympathetic block at L3 under fluoroscopy attains sympatholysis in the lower extremity.[55,56] A finger pulp temperature rise to 35°, loss of sympathetic response by the cold pressor test (placing the extremity in ice cold water) or by laser Doppler flowmetry document successful sympatholysis.

Attainment of symptomatic relief with regional anesthesia sympatholysis suggests prolonged sympathetic block by neurolysis with phenol or radio frequency may be beneficial. Successful sympathetic blockage indicates a trial of an α-adrenoreceptor blocker (e.g., terazosin) is likely to achieve symptomatic relief.[52] Other options to sympatholysis include regional anesthesia blocks: brachial plexus, lumbar plexus, a central neural, or a mixed conduction peripheral nerve block.

Continuous conduction analgesia for 1–2 weeks can be attained by insertion of a catheter in the brachial or lumbosacral plexus.[57] Tunneling of an epidural catheter allows long-term (e.g., months) provision of local anesthesia and other medications. However, technical problems can occur ranging from infection and breakage to displacement, which occurs more commonly at the skin entrance than in the deeper tissues. Catheter removal with treatment of any infection is mandatory when such technical complications occur. Intrathecal programmable pumps may be useful in patients with refractory CRPS.

Neuromodulation or neurostimulation is the alteration of the central or peripheral nervous system via spinal cord or peripheral nerve stimulation, respectfully.[52] It is now preferred over surgical sympathectomy. The posterior columns, the descending inhibitory pathways, and the dorsal root fibers are all involved in the effect of spinal cord stimulation on nociception. Alterations of the preganglionic autonomic nervous system may lead to better circulation in the stimulated area. Good results have been reported with neuromodulation in CRPS with spinal cord stimulators for CRPS I and peripheral nerve stimulators for CRPS II.[52,58–60] The exact mechanism of action of spinal cord stimulators is unknown but may act by interference of transmission of impulses from the nociceptors.[60]

Oral drugs have shown variable success in CRPS patients. Some of these pharmacologic agents include α-receptor antagonists (phenoxybenzamine), calcium channel blockers (nifedipine), anticonvulsant drugs (gabapentin, phenytoin), tricyclic antidepressants, calcitonin, corticosteroids, nonsteroidal anti-inflammatory drugs (NSAIDs), and opioids.[17,18,52] Other drugs that have been employed to treat CRPS include capsaicin, and especially in pediatric patients, ketamine, which is an *N*-methyl-D-aspartate (NMDA) blocker.[49]

For intravenous regional blocks, the following drugs have been used: guanethidine (blocks norepinephrine reuptake), bretylium (decreases norepinephrine release), and NSAIDs (e.g., ketorolac) (decreases prostaglandin release, ameliorates thromboxane-induced vasoconstriction).[17,18,52]

It should be remembered that the goal of all these various therapies is to maintain and return limb function by allowing active physiotherapy. Treatment involves a three-pronged approach: rehabilitation, pain management, and psychologic support.[61] For pain management, pharmacologic agents or TENS should be tried first before more invasive measures are used.[14,16]

When should the emergency physician intervene?

For most patients with CRPS, the emergency physician can best serve the patient by discussion and explanation of the problem as well as referral to physiotherapy and a pain specialist when indicated. Opioids are of little if any value in pain management, as with most neuralgic type pain. Their use is discouraged. Initiation of novel analgesics without a detailed past treatment history is unjustified; rather referral to someone who can initiate such treatment and follow the patient is the better option. Emergency physicians do need to recognize indications for admission. Severe pain flare-ups will not respond well to increased doses of oral agents. At these times admission for pain control may be required. One therapeutic option is a lidocaine infusion of 1–2 mg/min after a 1.5 mg/kg bolus. Other options for aggressive pain control include low-dose ketamine infusions (0.1 mg/kg bolus with a 0.1 mg/kg/h infusion) due to its specific NMDA antagonistic effect.

SUMMARY

CRPS is characterized by spontaneous pain, allodynia, hyperesthesia that extends beyond the territory of a single peripheral nerve, and vasomotor/sudomotor/integument abnormalities. In some patients, an initialing event including minor trauma (such as a sprain), surgery, or an illness can precipitate CRPS. In other patients (10–52%), no precipitating incident can be identified. CRPS is underdiagnosed and/or diagnosed late. CRPS occurs in both children and adults. Conservative therapy including physical therapy, psychologic support, and medications for relief may be effective, especially in pediatric patients. Other more invasive therapies include local or regional sympathetic blockade, neuromodulation, and even surgical sympathectomy.

REFERENCES

1. Stanton-Hicks M, Janig W, Hassenbusch S, et al. Reflex sympathetic dystrophy: changing concepts and taxonomy. *Pain.* 1995;63:127–133.
2. Merskey H, Bogduk N, eds. *Classification of Chronic Pain: Descriptions of Chronic Pain Syndrome and Definitions of Pain Terms Syndromes, and Definitions of Pain Terms.* 2nd ed. Seattle, WA: IASP; 1994:40–43.
3. Manning DC, Loar CM, Raj PP, et al. Neuropathic pain. In: Raj PP, ed. *Pain Medicine: A Comprehensive Review.* 2nd ed. St. Louis, MO: Mosby; 2003:77–94.
4. Wilson PR. Reflex sympathetic dystrophy. In: Low PA, ed. *Clinical Autonomic Disorders Evaluation and Management.* 2nd ed. Philadelphia, PA: Lippincott-Raven; 1997:537–544.
5. Veldman P, Reyman HM, Arntz IE, et al. Signs and symptoms of reflex sympathetic dystrophy: prospective study of 829 patients. *Lancet.* 1993;342:1012–1016.
6. Rosen PS, Graham W. The shoulder-hand syndrome: historical review with observations on 73 patients. *Can Med Assoc J.* 1957;77:86–91.
7. Blickerstaff DR, Kanis JA. Algodystrophy: an under-recognized complication of minor trauma. *Br J Rheumatol.* 1994;33:240–248.
8. Atkins RM, Duckworth T, Kavis JA. Features of algodystrophy after Colles fracture. *J Bone Joint Surg.* 1990;72:105–110.
9. Low PA, Wilson PR, Sandroni P, et al. Clinical characteristics of patients with reflex sympathetic dystrophy (sympathetically maintained pain) in the USA. In: Janig W, Stanton-Hicks M, eds. *Reflex Sympathetic Dystrophy: A Reappraisal. Progress in Pain Research and Management.* Vol 6. Seattle, WA: IASP; 1996:49–66.
10. Boas RA. Complex regional pain syndromes: symptoms, signs, and differential diagnosis. In: Janig W, Stanton-Hicks M, eds. *Reflex Sympathetic Dystrophy: A Reappraisal. Progress in Pain Research and Management.* Vol 6. Seattle, WA: IASP; 1996:79–92.
11. Waldman SD. Reflex sympathetic dystrophy of the face. In: *Atlas of Common Pain Syndromes.* Philadelphia, PA: W.B. Saunders; 2002:39–41.
12. Wilson PR, Low PA, Bedder MD, et al. Diagnostic algorithm for complex regional pain syndromes. In: Janig W, Stanton-Hicks M, eds. *Reflex Sympathetic Dystrophy: A Reappraisal. Progress in Pain Research and Management.* Vol 6. Seattle, WA: IASP; 1996:93–106.
13. Maillard SM, Davies K, Khubchandani R, et al. Reflex sympathetic dystrophy: a multidisciplinary approach. *Arthritis Rheum.* 2004;51(2):284–290.
14. Hendler NH. Complex regional pain syndrome, types I and II. In: Weiner RS, ed. *Pain Management—A Practical Guide for Clinicians.* Boca Raton, FL: CRC Press; 2002:213–233.
15. Bernstein BH, Singsen BH, Kent JT, et al. Reflex neurovascular dystrophy in children. *J Pediatr.* 1978;93(2):211–215.
16. Wilder RT. Reflex sympathetic dystrophy in children and adolescents. In: Janig W, Stanton-Hicks M, eds. *Reflex Sympathetic Dystrophy: A Reappraisal. Progress in Pain Research and Management.* Vol 6. Seattle, WA: IASP; 1996:67–78.
17. Walker SM, Cousins MJ. Complex regional pain syndromes: including "reflex sympathetic dystrophy" and "causalgia". *Anaesth Intens Care.* 1997;25:113–125.
18. Scadding JW. Complex regional pain syndrome. In: Melzack R, Wall PD, eds. *Handbook of Pain Management.* Edinburgh: Churchill Livingstone; 2003:275–288.
19. Covington EC. Psychological issues in reflex sympathetic dystrophy. In: Janig W, Stanton-Hicks M, eds. *Reflex Sympathetic Dystrophy: A Reappraisal. Progress in Pain Research and Management.* Vol 6. Seattle, WA: IASP; 1996:191–216.
20. Genant HK, Kozin F, Beckman C, et al. The reflex sympathetic dystrophy syndrome. A comprehensive analysis using fine detail radiography, photon absorptiometry, and bone and joint scintigraphy. *Radiology.* 1975;117:21–32.
21. Holder LE, Cole LA, Myerson MS. Reflex sympathetic dystrophy in the foot: clinical and scintigraphic criteria. *Radiology.* 1992;184:531–535.
22. McGill J, Wilson C, Wright WC, et al. Diagnosis: reflex sympathetic dystrophy. *Orthopedics.* 2004;27(3):334–336.
23. Schweitzer ME, Mandel S, Schwartz RJ, et al. Reflex sympathetic dystrophy revisited: MR imaging findings before and after infusion of contrast material. *Radiology.* 1995;195:211–214.
24. Gracely RH, Price DD, Roberts WJ, et al. Quantitative sensory testing in patients with complex regional pain syndrome (CRPS) I and II. In: Janig W, Stanton-Hicks M, eds. *Reflex Sympathetic Dystrophy: A Reappraisal. Progress in Pain Research and Management.* Vol 6. Seattle, WA: IASP; 1996:151–172.
25. Stanton–Hicks M, Raj PP, Racj CB. Use of regional anesthetics for diagnosis of reflex sympathetic dystrophy and sympathetically maintained pain: a critical evaluation. In: Janig W, Stanton-Hicks M, eds. *Reflex Sympathetic Dystrophy: A Reappraisal. Progress in Pain Research and Management.* Vol 6. Seattle, WA: IASP; 1996:217–237.
26. Bonica JJ. Causalgia and other reflex sympathetic dystrophies. *Postgrad Med.* 1973;53:143–148.
27. Janig W. The puzzle of "reflex sympathetic dystrophy," mechanisms, hypotheses, open questions. In: Janig W, Stanton-Hicks M, eds. *Reflex Sympathetic Dystrophy: A Reappraisal. Progress in Pain Research and Management.* Vol 6. Seattle, WA: IASP; 1996:1–24.
28. Bennett GJ, Roberts WJ. Animal models and their contribution to our understanding of complex regional pain syndromes I and II. In: Janig W, Stanton-Hicks M, eds. *Reflex Sympathetic Dystrophy: A Reappraisal. Progress in Pain Research and Management.* Vol 6. Seattle, WA: IASP; 1996:107–122.
29. Bennett CJ. The role of the sympathetic nervous system in painful peripheral neuropathy. *Pain.* 1991;45:221–223.
30. Levi-Montalcini R, Shaper SD, Toso RD, et al. Nerve growth factor: from neuroscience to neurokine. *Trends Neurosci.* 1996;19:514–520.

31. Webster CF, Schwartzman RJ, Jacoby RA, et al. Reflex sympathetic dystrophy: occurrence of inflammatory skin lesions in patients with stages II and III disease. *Arch Dermatol*. 1991;127:1541–1544.

32. Knobler R. The pathogenesis of reflex sympathetic dystrophy: immune and viral mechanisms. *Am J Pain Manage*. 1996;6(3):83–85.

33. Schwartzman RJ, McKellan TL. Reflex sympathetic dystrophy: a review. *Arch Neurol*. 1987;44:555–561.

34. Levine JD, Taiwo YO, Collins SD, et al. Noradrenaline hyperalgesia is mediated through interaction with sympathetic postganglionic neurone terminals rather than acti-vation of primary afferent nociceptors. *Nature*. 1986;323: 158–160.

35. Roberts MA. Hypothesis on the physiological basis for causalgia and related pain. *Pain*. 1986;24:297–311.

36. Wallin BG, Torebjork HE, Hallin RG. Preliminary observations on the pathophysiology of hyperalgesia in the causalgic pain syndrome. In: Zolterman Y, ed. *Sensory Functions of the Skin in Primates*. Oxford: Pergamon Press; 1976:489–499.

37. Chabal C, Jacobson L, Russell LC, et al. Pain response to perineuronal injection of normal saline epinephrine, and lidocaine in humans. *Pain*. 1992;49:9–12.

38. Walker AE, Nielsen F. Electrical stimulation of the upper thoracic portion of the sympathetic chain in man. *Arch Neurol Psychiatr*. 1948;59:559–560.

39. Choi B, Rowbotham MC. Effects of adrenergic receptor activation on post-herpetic neuralgia pain and sensory disturbances. *Pain*. 1997;69:55–63.

40. Drummond PD. Noradrenaline increases hyperalgesia to heat in skin sensitized by capsaicin. *Pain*. 1995;60:311–315.

41. Kinman E, Nygards EB, Hausson P. Peripheral alpha adrenoreceptors are involved in the development of capsaicin induced ongoing and stimulus evoked pain in humans. *Pain*. 1997;69:79–85.

42. vander Laan L, ter Laak HJ, Gabreels Festen A, et al. Complex regional pain syndrome type I (RSD). Pathology of skeletal muscle and peripheral nerve. *Neurology*. 1998;51:20–25.

43. Doubell TP, Mannion RJ, Woolf CJ. The dorsal horn: state–dependent sensory processing, plasticity and the generation of pain. In: Wall PD, Melzack R, eds. *Textbook of Pain*. 4th ed. Edinburgh: Churchill-Livingston; 1999:165–182.

44. Paris PM, Stewart R. Pain management. In: Rosen P, Barkin R, Danzl DF, et al, eds. *Emergency Medicine Concepts and Clinical Practice*. 4th ed. Vol 1. St. Louis, MO: Mosby; 1998: 276–300.

45. Willis WD Jr. The somatosensory system. In: Berne RM, Levy MN, Koeppen BM, et al, eds. *Physiology*. St. Louis, MO: Mosby; 2004:100–117.

46. Koltzenburg M. Afferent mechanisms mediating pain and hyperalgesias in neuralgia. In: Janig W, Stanton-Hicks M, eds. *Reflex Sympathetic Dystrophy: A Reappraisal. Progress in Pain Research and Management*. Vol. 6. Seattle, WA: IASP, 1996:123–150.

47. Wilder RT, Berde CB, Woloham M, et al. Reflex sympathetic dystrophy in children. *J Bone Joint Surg*. 1992;6:910–919.

48. Fermaglich DR. Reflex sympathetic dystrophy in children. *Pediatrics*. 1977;60(6):881–883.

49. Olsson GL. Neuropathic pain in children. In: McGrath PJ, Finley GA, eds. Chronic and recurrent pain in children and adolescents. *Progress in Pain Research and Management*. Vol 13. Seattle, WA: IASP; 1999:75–98.

50. Lee BH, Scharff L, Sethna N, et al. Physical therapy and cognitive–behavioral treatment for complex regional pain syndromes. *J Pediatr*. 2002;141(1):135–140.

51. Sherry DD, Weisman R. Psychological aspects of reflex neurovascular dystrophy. *Pediatrics*. 1988;81:572–578.

52. Stanton-Hicks M. Complex regional pain syndrome. In: Warfield CA, Bajwa ZH, eds. *Principles and Practice of Pain Medicine*. New York: McGraw-Hill; 2004:405–416.

53. Wang JK, Johnson KA, Ilstrup DM. Sympathetic blocks for reflex sympathetic dystrophy. *Pain*. 1985;23:13–17.

54. Korin F. Reflex sympathetic dystrophy: a review. *Clin Exp Rheumatol*. 1992;10:401–409.

55. Rowlingson JC, Murphy TM. Chronic Pain. In: Miller RD, Cucchiara RF, Miller ED Jr, et al, eds. *Anesthesia*. 5th ed, Vol 1. Philadelphia, PA: Churchill Livingstone; 2000: 2351–2376.

56. Hatangdi DS, Boas RA. Lumbar sympathectomy: a single needle technique. *Br J Anesth*. 1985;57:285–289.

57. Raj PP. Continuous epidural infusion and patient–controlled epidural analgesia in the management of pain. In: Waldman S, Winnie A, eds. *Interventional Pain Management*. Philadelphia, PA: W.B. Saunders; 1996:333–338.

58. Kessler MA, DeVet HCW, Barendse CAM, et al. The effect of spinal cord stimulation in patients with chronic reflex sympathetic dystrophy: two years' follow-up of the randomized controlled trial. *Ann Neurol*. 2004;55:13–18.

59. Grabow TS, Tella PK, Raja SN. Spinal cord stimulation for complex regional pain syndrome: an evidence-based medicine review of the literature. *Clin J Pain*. 2003;19: 371–373.

60. Goldstein DS. Spinal cord stimulation for chronic reflex sympathetic dystrophy. *Ann Neurol*. 2004;55(1):5–6.

61. Stanton-Hicks M, Baron R, Boas R, et al. Complex regional pain syndromes: guidelines for therapy. *Pain*. 1998;12: 155–166. icksHH;45:221–223.

38

Headache

Anne-Maree Kelly

HIGH YIELD FACTS

- The pathophysiologic basis of headache is traction or inflammation of the extracranial structures, the basal dura or the large intracranial arteries and veins, or dilatation/distension of cranial vascular structures.
- A normal physical examination does not rule out serious pathology.
- Nonsteroidal anti-inflammatory drugs (NSAIDs) are the most effective treatment for episodic tension headache.
- As most patients with migraine have already tried oral medications, parenterally administered agents are usually indicated.
- Based on current evidence, the most effective agents for treating migraine are triptans and phenothiazines. Meperidine is not indicated because it is less effective than other agents and is associated with a high rebound headache rate.
- Carbamazepine is the agent of choice for treatment of trigeminal neuralgia.

INTRODUCTION

A chief complaint of headache accounts for approximately 1% of visits to emergency departments (EDs).[1,2] The vast majority of headaches are benign, self-limiting, and managed by patients in the community. Patients coming to the ED with headache represent a small proportion of all headache patients. For those who do present, emergency physicians face the challenge of distinguishing potentially life-threatening causes from the more benign while simultaneously managing the headache pain. The latter forms the basis for this chapter.

PATHOPHYSIOLOGY

In order to treat headache effectively, it is important to understand its pathophysiologic basis. Headache is often due to a combination of physical and psychologic causative factors.

There are a limited number of structures in the head capable of producing pain. The brain parenchyma, the subarachnoid, pia mater, and most of the dura mater are incapable of producing painful stimuli. Structures that can produce pain are the main arteries at the base of the skull, the great venous sinuses and their branches, the basal dura and dural arteries and extracranial structures (including skin and mucosa, blood vessels, nerves, muscles, and fascial planes).

There are four main pathologic processes implicated in the production of headache: tension, traction, inflammation, and vascular processes.

Tension, thought to be a major factor in so-called tension headache, refers to contraction of muscles of the head and/or neck. Traction is caused by the stretching of intracranial structures as the result of mass effect, as with a tumor, abscess or hematoma. Pain caused by this mechanism is characteristically constant, but may vary in severity. Inflammation may involve the dura at the base of the skull or the nerves or soft tissues of the head and neck. This mechanism is responsible for the initial pain of meningitis and subarachnoid hemorrhage (SAH) as well as for sinusitis, mastoiditis, and probably neuralgias. Vascular mechanism includes dilatation or distension of vascular structures, and usually results in pain that is throbbing in nature. Much of migraine pain and the headache associated with severe hypertension are due to vascular mechanisms. These mechanisms are not mutually exclusive, so more than one mechanism may be involved for any given cause of headache, either simultaneously or sequentially.

ASSESSMENT

History is the most important component in the assessment of a patient complaining of headache. Key information includes the timing of the headache (in terms of both overall duration and speed of onset), the site and quality of the pain, the presence of associated features such as nausea and vomiting, photophobia and alteration in mental state, relieving factors, medical and occupational history, and drug use. Identification of underlying pathology may be critical in headache evaluation. Patients with HIV disease may pose a particular diagnostic challenge as they are at risk for opportunistic intracranial infections, tumors, and progressive multifocal leukoencephalopathy. The risk is increased if the headache is accompanied by altered mental status, seizure, focal neurology, or a low CD4 count.[3–5]

Pain intensity is important from the viewpoint of management but is an unreliable indicator of the severity of underlying pathology. This being said, sudden, severe headache and chronic, unremitting, or progressive headache are considered ominous features.

Physical assessment will be influenced by the history but should include vital signs, assessment of conscious state, careful neurologic examination, and examination for associated features such as neck stiffness, rash, and local tenderness over the temporal artery. It is important to note that while physical findings are uncommon, the presence of neurologic findings makes a serious cause more likely.

Headache Patterns

Some headaches have *classic* clinical presentations: these are listed in Table 38-1.[6] There will be a spectrum of presenting symptoms so absence of these classic features does not rule out a particular diagnosis. If symptoms persist without reasonable explanation, further investigation should be undertaken.

INVESTIGATION

For the vast majority of headaches no investigation is required. If SAH is suspected, the initial investigation of choice is noncontrast CT scan.[7] Initial sensitivity may be between 90 and 100%,[8–11] but this decreases with time, with

Table 38-1. Classical Clinical Complexes and Causes of Headache

Subarachnoid Hemorrhage
Sudden onset
Severe occipital headache, like a "blow"
Worst headache ever

Meningitis
Acute, generalized headache
Fever, nausea, and vomiting
Neck stiffness
Altered level of consciousness
Rash (meningococcemia)

Migraine
Preceeded by aura
Throbbing, unilateral
Nausea
Past/family history

Tumor
Persistent, deep-seated headache
Increasing duration/intensity
Worse in the morning
Aching in character

Temporal Arteritis
Unilateral with superimposed stabbing
Claudication on chewing

Associated malaise, myalgia
Tender artery with reduced pulsation

Neuralgia
Paroxysmal, fleeting pain
Distribution of nerve
Trigger maneuvers cause pain
Hyperalgesia of the nerve distribution

Glaucoma
Unilateral, aching, related to the eye
Nausea and vomiting
Raised intraocular pressure

Sinusitis
Throbbing, constant, frontal
Worse with cough, leaning forward
Recent URTI
Pain on percussion of sinuses

Dental Pain
Aching, facial region
Worse at night
Tooth sensitive to heat, pressure

URTI: Upper respiratory tract infection.
Source: Modified from Kelly AM. Headache. In: Cameron P, Jelinek G, Kelly AM, Murray L, Brown AFT, Heyworth J, eds. *Textbook of Adult Emergency Medicine.* 2nd ed. Edinburgh: Churchill Livingstone; 2004.

only 80% of scans positive at 3 days and 50% positive at 1 week.[12] If the CT is normal, current practice is to perform a lumbar puncture to measure red blood cell count and xanthochromia. The sensitivity of lumbar puncture for the diagnosis of SAH is unclear as is the cell count that should be regarded as positive. If CT or LP is positive, angiography (conventional 4-vessel or CT) is performed to determine the presence and location of aneurysms and plan further management by neurosurgeons. Magnetic resonance imaging (MRI) with FLAIR (fluid attenuated inversion recovery) is reliable in demonstrating early SAH and is superior to CT in detecting extravasated blood in the days after the initial bleed. Availability and logistical considerations make MRI impractical for use in the initial diagnostic workup of all patients with potential SAH but it may have a role in patients who present 1–2 weeks postsymptom onset.[13]

For suspected bacterial meningitis, it should be remembered that outcome is related to time-to-antibiotics, not time-to-investigations. Antibiotics should not be withheld awaiting tests if clinical suspicion of bacterial meningitis is high. The investigation of choice is lumbar puncture, unless contraindicated. Although some clinicians prefer to have a CT scan before performing a lumbar puncture in case of a mass effect, the risk of serious adverse events is extremely low. Risk factors for mass effect in patients with suspected meningitis are: age greater than 60 years, an immunocompromised state, altered mental status, history of central nervous system (CNS) disease, focal neurology, and seizure. In one study, if these were absent, only 1% of patients demonstrated any mass effect and all of these underwent lumbar puncture without adverse consequence.[14] Other investigations that may be useful, particularly when lumbar puncture is not possible are blood cultures, antigenic studies of blood or urine, polymerase chain reaction (PCR) analysis of blood, skin lesion aspiration for gram stain and culture, and throat swab culture.[15]

There should be a low threshold for CT in patients with HIV disease, particularly if they have altered mental status, seizure, focal neurologic findings, or a low CD4 count. If tumor is suspected, the investigations of choice are MRI or a contrast CT scan. An elevated erythrocyte sedimentation rate (ESR) may be supporting evidence for a diagnosis of temporal arteritis. With respect to sinusitis, facial x-rays are of very limited value.

TREATING HEADACHE

Given the range of causes of headache, no single approach to pain management is possible. Initiate specific treatment for the underlying cause when faced with severe hypertension,

temporal arteritis, glaucoma, or infection, while providing analgesia as an adjunct. With little published evidence in these cases, clinicians must take a symptom-based approach rather than a mechanism-based one. Options include simple analgesics such as acetaminophen, nonsteroidal anti-inflammatory agents, tramadol, and oral or parenteral opiates. As with all pain management, regular pain quantification from patients should be obtained and doctors should be prepared to move to more potent agents if pain is not controlled.

TENSION-TYPE HEADACHE

Tension-type headache (TTH) is very common with up to 78% of the population suffering from it at some time.[16] The annual prevalence is of the order of 11%.[17] TTH can be further divided into episodic and chronic subtypes, based on the frequency of symptoms. Episodic TTH may last between 30 minutes and 7 days and is present less than 180 days/year whereas chronic TTH has episodes on more than 180 days/year. In both cases, pain is usually bilateral, "pressing" or "tight" in quality, mild-to-moderate in intensity, does not prohibit routine activity, and is not associated with vomiting.

The pathologic basis of tension headaches remains unclear. Current theories suggest that myofascial nociception is the main factor in episodic TTH.[18] In chronic TTH it is suggested that nociceptive input to the CNS may be increased as a result of activation/sensitization of peripheral sensory afferent nerves and that central sensitization may be a key factor in headache generation.[18,19]

Epidemiologically, a family history of headaches is common and there is an association with an injury in childhood or adolescence. The most common precipitants are stress and alteration in sleep patterns.

Treatment of Episodic TTH

The number of high quality, comparative studies evaluating treatment of episodic TTH is small. Aspirin,[20] nonsteroidal anti-inflammatory agents such as ibuprofen,[21–24] ketoprofen,[21,22,25,26] naproxen,[22,27] diclofenac,[28] and acetaminophen[23,25,27] (paracetamol) have all been shown to be efficacious in the treatment of tension headaches with success rates between 50 and 70%. Of these, ibuprofen 400 mg or ketoprofen 25–50 mg appear to be the most effective, followed by aspirin 600–1000 mg and acetaminophen 1000 mg.

Two small studies have investigated the effectiveness of chlorpromazine 0.1 mg/kg intravenously (IV)[29] and dipyrone (metamizole) 1 g IV.[30] Sixty-three percent of patients treated with dipyrone and 70% of those treated with chlorpromazine were reported to be pain-free at 1 hour. Metamizole administered orally has also been compared to aspirin 1 g and found to have similar effectiveness.[31] Dipyrone is an NSAID. Drug induced neutropenia and agranulocytosis has been associated with dipyrone. It is not approved for use in the United States.

Treatment of Chronic TTH

Tricyclic antidepressants such as amitriptyline are the agents of choice for prevention of chronic TTH.[32] Recent evidence suggests that nitric oxide synthase inhibitors,[33] *N*-methyl-D-aspartate (NMDA) receptor antagonists,[34] magnesium,[35] and botulinum toxin type A[36] might also be useful. Psychologic and behavioral management[37] and physiotherapy[38] may also have a role in selected cases.

MIGRAINE

Most migraine headaches are successfully managed by patients and their family doctors, but a small number fail to respond to treatment at home. As oral medications have already been tried in the vast majority of cases,[39,40] parenterally administered agents are usually indicated for ED treatment.

Migraine is a clinical diagnosis and, in the ED setting, a diagnosis of exclusion. Pain management should be initiated while other causes of severe headache, such as subarachnoid hemorrhage and meningitis, are ruled out. The response of the headache to antimigraine therapy should not be used to assume that the cause was migraine. There have been several published case reports where headaches associated with SAH and meningitis have responded to these agents.

Pathophysiology

The pathophysiology of migraine is complex and still being clarified. Formerly thought to be vascular in etiology, there is increasing evidence that the primary stimulus is neural, setting off a cascade of events in susceptible individuals. This susceptibility has, at least in part, a genetic basis.

The nature of the initiating central dysfunction is not clear. It may involve the phenomenon of *cortical spreading depression,*[41] a short-lasting depolarization wave that moves across the cerebral cortex. A brief phase of excitation is followed by prolonged depression of nerve cells. At the same time, there is failure of brain ion homeostasis and an efflux of excitatory amino acids from nerve cells. Migraine seems to result from the activation of the trigeminovascular system by local dilatation of intracranial, extracerebral blood vessels.[41] Consequent release of vasoactive sensory

neuropeptides increases the pain response. Nociceptive information is transmitted via activated trigeminal nerves to the trigeminal sensory nuclei in the brain stem and then onto higher centers. There is growing evidence that these central neurons can become sensitized as a migraine attack progresses resulting in variations in response to treatment.[42]

Definition and Clinical Features

Migraine is defined as an idiopathic recurring headache disorder with attacks that last 4–72 hours. Typical migraine is unilateral, pulsating in quality (at some point during the headache), moderate or severe in intensity, and aggravated by routine physical activity. It is often accompanied by nausea, photophobia, and phonophobia.

In some patients, migraine is preceded by an "aura" of neurologic symptoms localizable to the cerebral cortex or brain stem. Examples include visual disturbance, paraesthesia, diplopia, or limb weakness. These develop gradually over 5–20 minutes and last less than 60 minutes. Headache, nausea, and/or photophobia usually follow after an interval of less than an hour. Several variant forms of migraine have been defined, including ophthalmoplegic, abdominal, and retinal migraine, but all are uncommon.

Treatment

A wide variety of pharmacologic agents and combinations of agents have been tried for the treatment of migraine, with varying results. Interpreting the evidence is challenging as the majority of the studies have small sample sizes, compare different agents or combinations of agents, and the outcome measure tested varies widely. It is further compounded by the variety of settings for studies (e.g., home, neurology clinics, and general practice) making generalization to ED patients difficult. The data presented here are based on studies in EDs unless otherwise stated.

Available evidence suggests that the most effective agents are the triptans (sumatriptan and related agents) and phenothiazines (chlorpromazine and prochlorperazine). Metoclopramide and ketorolac are also commonly used. The pooled clinical success rates and number needed to treat from published studies are shown in Table 38-2.

Meperidine (Pethidine) is commonly used in some countries.[55] There are no placebo-controlled studies demonstrating its effectiveness in the treatment of migraine. One small clinical trial[40] investigated the effectiveness of meperidine without adjuvant antiemetic or phenothiazine, reporting a clinical success rate of 56%. The potential for development of dependence should not be a factor when considering use of opioids as a therapeutic option for acute episodic headache in the ED. Rather, its low success rate

Table 38-2. Pooled Effectiveness Data from Emergency Department Studies of the Treatment of Migraine

Agent	No. of Studies	Total Patients	Clinical Success Rate (%)	NNT: Clinical Success*	References
Chlorpromazine	6	189	85	1.7	37, 43–47
Sumatriptan	1	88	75	2	48
Prochlorperazine	3	70	76	2	49–51
Metoclopramide	4	121	59	2.9	47, 50–52
Ketorolac	4	75	57	3.11	39, 40, 53, 54

*Calculated as $\dfrac{1}{\% \text{ success of active agent}-\% \text{ success placebo (assumes placebo success of 25\%)}}$.

combined with a high headache recurrence rate suggest it should be reserved for use when other agents have failed or are contraindicated. Opioids should rarely be used for pain control in chronic headache, as shown in a study of 1900 patients, where 5% were narcotic abusers.[56] In addition, daily use of opioids can give rise to analgesic rebound headache.

Triptans

Triptans are specific and selective serotonin (subtype 1B/1D) agonists that have no effect on other serotonin receptor subtypes. The antimigraine effect of sumatriptan was initially thought to be due to its effect on the 5HT subtype 1D receptors in cranial blood vessels. More recent evidence suggests that it may act presynaptically to block synaptic transmission between axon terminals of peripheral trigeminovascular neurons and cell bodies of their central counterparts.[41]

Triptans can be administered intranasally, orally, or by subcutaneous injection. The recommended dose of the exemplar, sumatriptan, is 6 mg subcutaneously, 20 mg intranasally, or 50–100 mg orally. Clinical response begins within 10–15 minutes of subcutaneous injection and within 30 minutes of oral administration. Adverse effects include drowsiness, weakness, dizziness, flushing, rash, pruritus, elevation of blood pressure, chest pain, or chest tightness. Triptans are contraindicated in patients with a history of ischemic heart disease, uncontrolled hypertension, or the concomitant use of ergot preparations. There are a significant number of nonresponders (up to 25%),[48] which may be related to sensitization of central neurons.[42]

In addition, headache recurrence at 24 hours may be as high as 50% in undifferentiated *migraineurs* treated with sumatriptan. This may limit its role for such patients in the ED, where follow-up is uncertain.

A range of triptan agents are now available (including rizatriptan, zolmitripan, and eletriptan). Efficacy seems to be similar[57] but some (e.g., naratriptan) report less reduction in coronary blood flow.

Phenothiazines

The mechanism by which phenothiazines act in migraine is uncertain. It is possibly the result of a combination of actions: anti-5HT effect, antidopamine effect in the chemoreceptor trigger zone, vascular effects via its α-adrenergic receptor blocking action, and modulation of serotonin receptors.

Prochlorperazine is usually administered at a dose of 5–10 mg intravenously, with the 5-mg dose demonstrating almost equal benefit while having less adverse events. Dosing regimens of chlorpromazine include 25 mg in 1 L normal saline over 30–60 minutes repeated if necessary or bolus doses of 12.5 mg intravenously, repeated every 20 minutes as needed to a maximum dose of 37.5 mg accompanied by intravenous saline to avert postural hypotension. Both agents may cause sedation, akathesia, or uncommonly a dystonic reaction. Akathesia and dystonia may be prevented with concomitant use of 1 mg IV benztropine. Postural hypotension is not uncommon with the use of chlorpromazine.

Other Agents

Other agents that have been tried in the management of migraine are metoclopramide, ergot alkaloids (e.g., dihydroergotamine), lidocaine, magnesium and dipyrone, haloperidol, and valproate. Most of these studies have small sample sizes making interpretation of the findings challenging.

The data on dihydroergotamine are difficult to interpret because it is often used in combination with metoclopramide, making it uncertain which medication was responsible for the documented pain relief. It has been shown to be less effective than chlorpromazine[44] and sumatriptan[58] in acute treatment, and to have a high rate (<55%) of adverse effects.[44] Intravenous lidocaine has not been shown to be superior to placebo.[59]

Civamide, a vanilloid receptor agonist and neuronal calcium channel blocker which inhibits the neuronal release of excitatory neurotransmitters, showed moderate efficacy.[60] Civamide (Zucapsaicin) has undergone some clinical trials in the United States but is not currently scheduled for release in the United States. Intravenous valproate sodium showed pro-mising results in a small case series,[61] but was not shown to illicit significant improvement in a randomized trial.[49] The efficacy of intravenous magnesium sulphate (1 or 2 mg) remains unclear. It was shown to be effective in one small placebo-controlled trial.[62] Another study found the combination of magnesium with metoclopramide was less effective than metoclopramide and placebo.[63] Intramuscular droperidol 2.5 mg has been shown to be moderately effective, but with a 13% rate of akasthisia.[64]

TRIGEMINAL NEURALGIA

Introduction

Trigeminal neuralgia is a debilitating condition. Patients describe lancinating pain like "lightening" or a "'hot poker" that is severe and follows the distribution of the trigeminal nerve. Individual episodes of pain last seconds but may recur repeatedly within a short period. They can be triggered by minor stimuli such as light touch, eating or drinking, shaving, or passing gusts of wind. Bouts last weeks to months, between which there may be long periods of remission. There is often associated mild impairment of temperature and light touch sensation in the distribution of the affected nerve, although this is not usually clinically significant.[65]

The incidence of trigeminal neuralgia is 4–5 per 100,000 and onset[66] is usually in middle or older age.[67] MRI has been reported to be 94% sensitive and 100% specific for identifying a vascular cause.[68]

Pathophysiology

Evidence suggests that the pathologic basis of trigeminal neuralgia is demyelination of sensory fibers of the trigeminal nerve in the proximal (CNS) portion of the nerve root or rarely in the brain stem.[67] In 80–90% of cases, this is due to compression of the nerve root by an overlying artery or vein.[67] Uncommonly, compression can be caused by a space-occupying lesion. Two percent of cases are associated with multiple sclerosis.[66] Microscopic examination in cases due to vascular compression shows focal demyelination in the area of compression with close apposition of neurons and loss of intervening glial processes.[67] This is thought to result in spontaneous generation of nerve impulses and ephaptic conduction to adjacent fibres.[67]

Treatment

The mainstay of therapy for trigeminal neuralgia is carbamazepine. Patients should unfortunately not expect to obtain relief in the ED from medication given acutely. Opioids are ineffective at controlling this severe neuralgic pain. The usual starting dose of carbamazepine is 200–400 mg/day in divided doses increased by 200 mg/day until relief up to a maximum of 1200 mg/day. The average dose required is 800 mg/day. The number needed to treat or have one patient with 50% pain relief has been estimated at between 1.7 and 2.3.[69,70] Single trials suggest that baclofen alone (NNT 1.4) and the addition of lamotrigine or carbamazepine or phenytoin (NNT 2.1) are also effective.[69] Case series suggest that in acute crises of trigeminal neuralgia, intravenous infusions of lidocaine,[69] phenytoin,[69] or fosphenytoin[71] may be helpful. Patients with new onset symptoms should be referred for further evaluation and to ensure pain relief from medication initiated in the ED.

REFERENCES

1. Morgenstern LB, Huber JC, Luna-Gonzales H, et al. Headache in the emergency department. *Headache*. 2001;41:537–541.
2. Locker T, Mason S, Rigby A. Headache management—are we doing enough? An observational study of patients presenting with headache to the emergency department. *Emerg Med J*. 2004;21:327–332.
3. Gifford AL, Hecht FM. Evaluating HIV-infected patients with headache: who needs computed tomography *Headache*. 2001;41:441–448.
4. Graham CB III, Wippold FJ III. Headache in the HIV patient: a review with special attention to the role of imaging. *Cephalalgia*. 2001;21:169–174.
5. Tso EL, Todd WC, Groleau GA, et al. Cranial computed tomography in the emergency department evaluation of HIV-infected patients with neurologic complaints. *Ann Emerg Med*. 1993;22:1169–1176.
6. Kelly AM. Headache. In Cameron P, Jelinek G, Kelly AM, Murray L, Brown AFT, Heyworth J, eds. *Textbook of Adult Emergency Medicine*. 2nd ed. Edinburgh: Churchill Livingstone; 2004.
7. Rosengarten P. Subarachnoid haemorrhage. In: Cameron P, Jelinek G, Kelly AM, Murray L, Brown AFT, Heyworth J, eds. *Textbook of Adult Emergency Medicine*. 2nd ed. Edinburgh: Churchill Livingstone; 2004.
8. Morgenstern LB, Luna-Gonzales H, Huber JC Jr, et al. Worst headache and subarachnoid hemorrhage: prospective,

modern computed tomography and spinal fluid analysis. *Ann Emerg Med.* 1998;32:297–304.

9. Sidman R, Connolly E, Lemke T. Subarachnoid hemorrhage diagnosis: lumbar puncture is still needed when the computed tomography scan is normal. *Acad Emerg Med.* 1996;3: 827–831.

10. van der Wee N, Rinkel GJ, Hassan D, et al. Detection of sub-arachnoid haemorrhage on early CT: is lumbar puncture still needed after a negative scan? *J Neurol Neurosurg Psychiatry.* 1995;58:357–359.

11. Perry JJ, Stiell IG, Wells GA, et al. The sensitivity of computed tomography for the diagnosis of subarachnoid haemorrhage in ED patients with acute headache. *Acad Emerg Med.* 2004;11:435–436.

12. Schievink WI. Intracranial aneurysms. *N Eng J Med.* 1997; 336:28–40.

13. van Gijn J, Rinkel GJE. Subarachnoid haemorrhage: diagnosis, causes and management. *Brain.* 2001;124:249–278.

14. Hasbun R, Abrahams J, Jekel J, et al. Computed tomography of the head before lumbar puncture in adults with suspected meningitis. *N Engl J Med.* 2001;345:1727–1733.

15. Singer A. Meningitis. In: Cameron P, Jelinek G, Kelly AM, Murray L, Brown AFT, Heyworth J, eds. *Textbook of Adult Emergency Medicine.* 2nd ed. Edinburgh: Churchill Living-stone; 2004.

16. Jensen R. Diagnosis, epidemiology and impact of tension-type headache. *Curr Pain Headache Rep.* 2003;7:455–459.

17. Waldie KE, Poulton R. The burden of illness associated with headache disorders among young adults in a representative cohort. *Headache.* 2002;42:612–619.

18. Vanderheede M, Schoenen J. Central mechanisms in tension-type headaches. *Curr Pain Headache Rep.* 2002;6: 392–400.

19. Bendtsen L. Central and peripheral sensitisation in tension-type headache. *Curr Pain Headache Rep.* 2003;7:460–465.

20. Steiner TJ, Lange R, Voelker M. Aspirin in episodic tension-type headache: placebo-controlled dose-ranging com-parison with paracetamol. *Cephalgia.* 2003;23:59–66.

21. van Gerven JM, Shoemaker RC, Jacobs LD, et al. Self-medication of a single headache episode with ketoprofen, ibuprofen or placebo, home monitored with an electronic patient diary. *Br J Clin Pharmacol.* 1996;42:475–481.

22. Lange R, Lentz R. Comparison of ketoprofen, ibuprofen and naproxen sodium in the treatment of tension-type headache. Drugs *Exp Clin Res.* 1995;21:89–96.

23. Schachtel BP, Furey SA, Thoden WR. Nonprescription ibuprofen and acetaminophen in the treatment of tension-type headache. *J Clin Pharmacol.* 1996;36:1120–1125.

24. Packman B, Packman E, Doyle G, et al. Solubilized ibuprofen: evaluation of onset, relief and safety of novel formulation in the treatment of episodic tension-type headache. *Headache.* 2000;40:561–567.

25. Steiner TJ, Lange R. Ketoprofen (25 mg) in the symptomatic treatment of episodic tension-type headache: double-blind, placebo-controlled comparison with acetaminophen (1000 mg). *Cephalalgia.* 1998;18:38–43.

26. Mehlisch DR, Weaver M, Fladung B. Ketoprofen, aceta-minophen and placebo in the treatment of tension headache. *Headache.* 1998;38:579–589.

27. Prior MJ, Cooper KM, May LG, et al. Efficacy and safety of acetaminophen and naproxen in the treatment of tension-type headache. A randomised, double-blind, placebo-controlled trail. *Cephalgia.* 2002;22:740–748.

28. Kubitzek F, Ziegler G, Gold MS, et al. Low dose diclofenac potassium in the treatment of episodic tension-type headache. *Eur J Pain.* 2003;7:155–162.

29. Bigal ME, Bordini CA, Speciali JG. Intravenous chlor-promazine in the acute treatment of episodic tension-type headache: a randomised, placebo-controlled, double-blind study. *Arq Neuropsiquiatr.* 2002;60:537–541.

30. Bigal ME, Bordini CA, Speciali JG. Intravenous dipyrone in the acute treatment of episodic tension-type headache: a randomised, placebo-controlled, double-blind study. *Braz J Med Biol Res.* 2002;35:1139–1145.

31. Martinez-Martin P, Raffaelli E Jr, Titus F, et al. Efficacy and safety of metamizol vs, acetylsalicylic acid in patients with moderate episodic tension-type headache: a randomised, double-blind, placebo and active-controlled, multicentre study. *Cephalalgia.* 2001;21:604–610.

32. Ashina S, Ashina M. Current and potential future drug therapies for tension-type headache. *Curr Pain Headache Rep* 2003;7:466–474.

33. Ashina M. Nitric oxide synthase inhibitors for the treatment of chronic tension headache. *Exp Opin Pharmacother.* 2002;3:395–399.

34. Zhao C, Stillman MJ. New developments in the pharma-cotherapy of tension-type headaches. *Expert Opin Pharma-cother.* 2003;4:2229–2237.

35. Altura BM, Altura BT. Tension headaches and muscle tension: is there a role for magnesium? *Med Hypotheses.* 2001;57:705–713.

36. Relja M, Telarovic S. Botulinum toxin in tension-type headache. *J Neurol* 2004;251(suppl 1):I12–I14.

37. Nash JM. Psychologic and behavioural management of tension-type headache: treatment procedures. *Curr Pain Headache Rep.* 2003;7:475–481.

38. Torelli P, Jensen R, Olesen J. Physiotherapy for tension-type headache: a controlled study. *Cephalalgia.* 2004;24:29–36.

39. Shrestha M, Singh R, Moreden J, et al. Ketoroloc vs chlor-promazine in the treatment of acute migraine without aura: A prospective, randomised, double-blind trial. *Arch Int Med.* 1996;156:1725–1728.

40. Larkin GL, Prescott JE. A randomized, double-blind, com-parative study of the efficacy of ketorolac tromethamine versus meperidine in the treatment of severe migraine. *Ann Emerg Med.* 1992;21:919–924.

41. Hargreaves RJ, Shepheard SL. Pathophysiology of migraine—new insights. *Can J Neurol Sci.* 1999;26:S12–S19.

42. Burstein R, Cutrer MF, Yarnitsky D. The development of cutaneous allodynia during a migraine attack clinical evidence for the sequential recruitment of spinal and supraspinal noci-ceptive neurons in migraine. *Brain.* 2000;123:1803–1809.

43. Bigal ME, Bordini CA, Speciali JG. Intravenous chlorpromazine in the emergency department treatment of migraines: a randomized controlled trial. *J Emerg Med.* 2002; 23:141–148.

44. Bell R, Montoya D, Shuaib A, et al. A comparative trial of three agents in the treatment of migraine headache. *Ann Emerg Med.* 1990;19:1079–1082.

45. Lane PL, McLellan BA, Baggoley CJ. Comparative efficacy of chlorpromazine and meperidine with dimenhydrinate in migraine headache. *Ann Emerg Med.* 1989;18:360–365.

46. Kelly AM, Ardagh M, Curry C, et al. Intravenous chlorpromazine versus intramuscular sumatriptan for acute migraine. *J Accid Emerg Med.* 1997;14:209–211.

47. Cameron JD, Lane PL, Speechley M. Intravenous chlorpromazine vs intravenous metoclopramide in acute migraine headache. *Acad Emerg Med.* 1995;2:597–602.

48. Akpunonu BE, Mutgi AB, Federman DJ, et al. 1995 Subcutaneous sumatriptan for the treatment of acute migraine in patients admitted to the emergency department. *Ann Emerg Med.* 25:464–469.

49. Tanen DA, Miller S, French T, et al. Intravenous valproate versus prochloperazine for the emergency department treatment of acute migraine headache—a prospective, randomised, double-blind trial. *Ann Emerg Med.* 2003;41:847–853.

50. Coppola M, Yeally DM, Leibold RA. Randomized, placebo-controlled evaluation of prochlorperazine versus metoclopramide for emergency department treatment of migraine headache. *Ann Emerg Med.* 1995;26:541–546.

51. Jones J, Sklar D, Dougherty J, et al. Randomized double-blind trial of intravenous prochlorperazine for the treatment of acute headache. *JAMA.* 1989;261:1174–1176.

52. Tek DS, McClellan DS, Olshaker JS, et al. A prospective, double-blind study of metoclopramide hydrochloride for the control of migraine in the emergency department. *Ann Emerg Med.* 1990;19:1083–1087.

53. Duarte C, Dunnaway F, Turner L, et al. Ketoroloc versus meperidine and hydroxyzine in the treatment of acute migraine headache: A randomized, prospective, double-blind trial. *Ann Emerg Med.* 1992;21:1116–1121.

54. Davis CP, Williams C, Barrett K, et al. Ketoroloc versus meperidine plus promethazine treatment of migraine headache: evaluation by patients. *Am J Emerg Med.* 1995:13:146–150.

55. Vinson DR. Treatment patterns of isolated benign headaches in US emergency departments. *Ann Emerg Med.* 2002;39: 215–222.

56. Granella F, Farina S, Malferrari G, et al. Drug abuse in chronic headache: a Clinico-epidemiological study. *Cephalalgia.* 1987:7:15–19.

57. McCrory DC, Gray RN. Oral sumatriptan for acute migraine. *Cochrane Database Syst Rev.* 2003;(3):CD002915.

58. Winner P, Ricalde O, Le Force B, et al. A double-blind study of subcutaneous dihydroergotamine vs subcutaneous sumatriptan in the treatment of acute migraine. *Arch Neurol.* 1996;53:180–184.

59. Reutens DC, Fatovich DM, Stewart-Wynee EG, et al. Is intravenous lidocaine clinically effective in acute migraine? *Cephalalgia.* 1991;11:245–247.

60. Diamond S, Freitag F, Phillips SB, et al. Intranasal civamide for the acute treatment of migraine headache. *Cephalalgia.* 2000;20:597–602.

61. Mathew NT, Kailasam J, Maedors L, et al. Intravenous valproate sodium (depacon) aborts migraine rapidly: a preliminary report. *Headache.* 2000;40:720–723.

62. Demirkaya S, Vural O, Dora B, et al. Efficacy of intravenous magnesium sulphate in the treatment of acute migraine attacks. *Headache.* 2001;41:171–177.

63. Corbo J, Esses D, Bijur PE, e al. Randomised clinical trial of intravenous magnesium sulphate as an adjunctive medication in the emergency department treatment of migraine. *Ann Emerg Med.* 2001;38:621–627.

64. Richman PB, Allegra J, Eskin B, et al. A randomised clinical trial to assess the efficacy of intramuscular droperidol for the treatment of acute migraine headache. *Am J Emerg Med.* 2002;20:39–42.

65. Bowsher D, Miles JB, Haggett CE, et al. Trigeminal neuralgia: a quantitative sensory perception threshold study in patients who had not undergone previous invasive procedures. *J Neurosurg.* 1997;86:190–192.

66. Merrison AFA, Fuller G. Treatment options for trigeminal neuralgia. *BMJ.* 2003;327:1360–1361.

67. Love S, Coakham HB. Trigeminal neuralgia. *Brain.* 2001: 12:2347–2360.

68. Balansard ChF, Meller R, Bruzzo M, et al. Trigeminal neuralgia—results of microsurgical and endoscopy assisted vascular decompression. *Ann Otolaryngol Chir Cervicofac.* 2003;120:330–337.

69. Sindrup SH, Jensen TS. Pharmacotherapy of trigeminal neuralgia. *Clin J Pain.* 2002;18:22–27.

70. Wiffen P, Collins S, McQuay H, et al. Anticonvulsant drugs for acute and chronic pain. *Cochrane Database Syst Rev.* 2000;(3):CD001133.

71. Cheshire WP. Fosphenytoin: an intravenous option for the management of acute trigeminal neuralgia crisis. *J Pain Symptom Manage.* 2001;21:506–510.

39

Myofascial Pain

James Ducharme

HIGH YIELD FACTS

- Short-acting opioids use should be minimal in managing patients with chronic pain or patients already receiving opioids as they risk increasing tolerance and even increasing the severity of chronic pain.
- Opioids with high intrinsic activity may be preferred if an opioid-tolerant patient arrives with new pain.
- Patients with fibromyalgia (FM) often consult because of new or worsening pain with a goal of being reassured, not to receive additional medication.
- In the emergency department (ED), a decision to initiate a "new" medication without complete assessment of not only the chronic illness but also the medication history can rarely be expected to benefit the patient with myofascial pain.
- Lack of specific criteria has lead to ongoing debate over the validity of myofascial pain syndrome (MPS) as a medical condition, ensuring a varying evaluation and management style.
- FM is a condition where facilitation of downward modulation results in nonpainful stimulus producing a painful sensation.
- Treatment of FM responds best to a multidisciplinary approach, including psychotherapy, antidepressant medication, and a moderate exercise program—pain medication offers little to the treatment plan.

INTRODUCTION

Muscular pain and injury can occur after exposure to an episode or episodes of biomechanical overloading. Myofascial pain is felt to account for 85% of muscular injury and 85–90% of patients treated in pain clinics.[1] One study found myofascial pain to be present in 37% of men and 65% of women aged 30–60 years.[2]

Direct injury leads to macrotrauma whereas microtrauma usually occurs after repetitive overloading. In the latter, pain usually occurs hours after exertion, maximizing 1–3 days after onset. Acute pain from muscular injury lasts less than 6 weeks and normally responds well to short-term rest, thermal therapy (ice for first 48 hours, followed by heat), compression, or splinting. Gradual reconditioning and return to full activity are the final steps. Failure in any of these recuperative steps can lead to chronic myofascial symptoms. Chronic pain is defined as pain lasting longer than 12 weeks. It is this group of painful conditions that will be discussed in greater depth in this chapter.

NEUROBIOLOGY

Chronic muscle pain may be caused by contractures, spasms, or dystonia. Contractures refer to a local muscle end plate injury resulting in excessive acetylcholine release. This focal contracture is felt to produce local ischemia which not only lowers tissue pH but also leads to the release of an inflammatory soup comprised of bradykinin, prostanoids, and interleukins that sensitize and activate nociceptors. Reflex spasm is induced by nociceptive input, again leading to ischemia, but on a much larger scale. In dystonic conditions, true contraction lowers pH and releases adenosine triphosphate (ATP), both of which lead to a hyperalgesic state. While myofascial pain is believed to develop after trauma, overuse or prolonged spasm, fibromyalgia (FM) is a systemic disease process, possibly caused by dysfunction of the limbic system or neuroendocrine axis.[3] Myofascial pain will often respond to structured medical management whereas FM will require a multidisciplinary approach.

OPIOIDS USE IN OPIOID-TOLERANT PATIENTS

Systemic opioids are unlikely to be effective for managing acute pain in patients chronically treated with opioids.[4] They risk being equally ineffective in other conditions with centrally mediated hyperalgesia such as neuropathic or persistent nociceptive pain. Individuals maintained on methadone will have especially high tolerance for mu opioids. Recurrent short-acting dosing of opioids will increase tolerance and hyperalgesia in patients on chronic therapy. In addition, prolonged intense painful stimulation (as with oligoanalgesia) will also decrease responsiveness to opioids.[4] Constant, even balancing of pain control is thus critical in avoiding tolerance and escalating doses of opioids in patients with chronic pain.

Opioids have different intrinsic activity levels. For example, sufentanil may provide adequate relief occupying only 10% of opioid receptors whereas meperidine would require 70% occupancy to attain the same degree of analgesia.[4] Sufentanil would be able to control further increases in pain with minimal dosing changes whereas meperidine would have to be increased by proportionally much larger amounts to achieve similar control. It may well arise that increasing doses may be unable to control pain adequately if all receptors for that medication are occupied. In morphine-tolerant animals, large increases of meperidine were required to demonstrate incremental improvement in pain control, while buprenorphine was ineffective.[5] In the emergency department (ED), agents such as fentanyl or sufentanil, as an infusion or with patient-controlled analgesia (PCA) pump, would appear to be the agents of choice for new acute pain in morphine-tolerant patients. Use of meperidine cannot be condoned in this setting due to its low intrinsic activity. Furthermore, use of short-acting opioids—as a quick solution to treat pain or as a way to discharge the patient—risks worsening tolerance and augmenting opioid-induced hyperalgesia.

EMERGENCY DEPARTMENT APPROACH TO CHRONIC NONMALIGNANT PAIN

When encountering a patient with chronic pain, it is important to establish the specific purpose of the visit to the ED. Despite a triage complaint of "pain," such patients rarely present specifically because of the pain. It is therefore necessary to establish the more specific problem. Some patients have poor coping mechanisms and catastrophize when faced with changes in their pain—they identify pain changes with the worst possible clinical situations. Others, especially those with myofascial pain, are unsure not only of their diagnosis, but of the etiology of their pain. They are more likely to believe they have a serious unidentified physiologic disturbance and be more dissatisfied with their management.[6] Such fear and frustration leads to frequent consultation of new health care specialists in an effort to identify and treat their problem. Patients with a better understanding of their pain process, such as those with FM, often consult because of new or worsening pain with a goal of being reassured, not to receive additional medication. They wish to verify that this "different" pain does not represent a more serious illness such as a myocardial infarction. Once reassurance is received, such patients are usually willing to return home.

It should be infrequent that patients with chronic myofascial pain receive a new pain medication prescription in the ED. Similarly, offering opioids either in the ED or as a short-term discharge prescription should be discouraged. Most patients with chronic pain will have attempted several treatment modalities in the effort to control their pain. A decision to initiate a new medication without complete assessment of not only their chronic illness but also their medication history can rarely be expected to benefit these patients. It may also place the patient at risk for adverse effects that had been present when the primary care physician had previously attempted a similar medication and had abandoned it for those reasons.

Acute treatment options are therefore limited. It is more important to identify and respond to the true reason for the ED visit. When faced with a new type of pain, it is reasonable to perform investigations, as with any patient. In patients with myofascial pain who are castastrophizing or frustrated from lack of results, it is more important to educate the patient. Establish the limitations of what the ED can or cannot do. Reinforce the need for patients to take control of their treatment and rehabilitation. Explain the need for ongoing, not episodic, care for treatment planning and medication usages. Make use of referrals to multidisciplinary pain clinics when indicated.

MYOFASCIAL PAIN SYNDROME

Chronic myofascial pain syndrome (MPS) is one of the most common findings in patients presenting to pain clinics.[3] The condition is associated with regional pain and is revealed by deep palpation of hyperirritable spots called trigger points. Trigger points appear as nodular masses within taut bands of skeletal muscle. Similar nodules may also be present in asymptomatic people. Injection of local anesthetic into a trigger will relieve the pain of MPS. Although this generalized description of regional location and trigger points combined with a normal neurologic examination has been accepted by pain physicians, there are still no consensus-generated criteria. The IASP chronic pain taxonomy provides no specific criteria for the diagnosis of MPS. Lack of specific criteria has lead to ongoing debate over the validity of MPS as a syndrome. In addition, lack of criteria guarantees research of different subject groups, with inability to compare results. Inconsistency has ensured a varying evaluation and management style as well.

Further adding to the confusion over MPS is that the pathogenesis of myofascial pain and trigger points remain unproven.[7] To date myofascial dysfunction with trigger points appears to be a spinal segmental reflex disorder.[8]

Treatment of MPS

When musculoskeletal pain persists for greater than 6 weeks, responsibility for rehabilitation and recovery should be transferred to the patient.[1] Patients should have been educated in self-care. The goal of treatment in MPS should be the restoration of function. Massage and physical therapy along with lifestyle changes to reduce psychosocial stressors should be the basis of initial and ongoing treatment.

Nonsteroidal agents can be effective in dealing with pain flare-ups. Addition of muscle relaxants, such as cyclobenzaprine, is not felt to provide any benefit.[9] As for any acute muscular pain or injury, splinting may be of use either for temporary relief, complete rest, or to allow activity in a controlled fashion. Needling of trigger points may also be an effective intervention for controlling the pain of MPS. While there have been numerous studies evaluating the injection of local anesthetics, steroids, or even saline, a systematic review failed to identify additional benefit from these therapies over dry needling.[10] Dry needling, where no substance is injected, appeared to be as effective, but even here the authors concluded that there was insufficient data to demonstrate that needling had any efficacy beyond placebo.

Other measures that have been studied include repetitive magnetic stimulation[11] and the injection of botulinum toxin (BT).[12] BT_A is Food and Drug Administration (FDA) approved for strabismus, blepharospasm, and hemifacial spasm while BT_B is approved for cervical dystonia. Recent literature suggests that when other treatment modalities for MPS have failed, local injection of BT may produce considerable pain relief. Here again, the proposed mechanism of action remains theoretical, for pain relief often occurs days before any expected effect on muscle relaxation by BT. There are as of yet insufficient high quality trials to confirm or refute the efficacy of BT in MPS.

FIBROMYALGIA

Although the American College of Rheumatology established classification criteria for FM in 1990,[13] many physicians remain skeptical about its existence. Disbelief of medical pathology guarantees misunderstanding of patient complaints and inadequate treatment plans. The original criteria included widespread pain for at least 3 months, along with abnormal pain sensitivity in 11 or more of 18 specific anatomical sites. These vague clinical criteria have been criticized, with authors even stating "the construct of FM does not survive critical analysis."[14] The failure of 15-year-old criteria does not distract from the clinical problems suffered by patients with FM, but does further increase skepticism.

FM, chronic fatigue syndrome (CFS), and major depressive disorders (MDD) share many behavioral changes and symptoms.[15] In addition many patients with FM and CFS experience similar comorbidity such as irritable bowel syndrome. The presence of allodynia and lower pain thresholds to mechanical stimulation are what distinguish FM from CFS. Objective testing has confirmed the existence of FM. Studies using functional magnetic resonance imaging[16] and single photon emission computed tomography,[17] have both demonstrated abnormal brain stimulation and blood flow in patients with FM compared to controls, MDD, or CFS. Their cerebrospinal fluid has consistently elevated levels of substance P.[18,19] Sleep electroencephalogram (EEG) studies have demonstrated sleep disturbances similar to other patients with chronic pain.[20] This nonrecuperative sleep further exacerbates the systemic malaise of patients with FM.

Quality of life in patients with FM is considerably worse in comparison to women with MPS or with no body pain.[21] It has also been found to be extremely low when compared to other patients with chronic illness such as rheumatoid arthritis, osteoarthritis, diabetes, or chronic lung disease. FM impacts therefore not just on physical health, but on mental health as well, demonstrating characteristics of severe depre-ssion and poor social functioning.

Treatment of Fibromyalgia

Treatment of FM responds best to a multidisciplinary approach, including psychotherapy, antidepressant medication, and a moderate exercise program.[3] Almost all patients with FM suffer from muscular deconditioning, with many having considerable lessening of their pain within weeks of starting even a mild regular exercise program. Sedative-hypnotics do not improve sleep or increase the amount of recuperative sleep. Management in the ED is therefore very limited. Investigation of new painful conditions should be undertaken as with any patient, recognizing the old adage that previous pathology does not preclude new pathology. Once any potentially serious problems have been ruled out, understanding and support are the best that can be offered. Physicians should ensure that these patients understand the limited role of the ED in their management, all the while ensuring that the patient does have appropriate continuity of care. If the patient does not appear to have a multidisciplinary approach established, such recommendations can be made to the patient and the primary care physician.

Emergency physicians can offer little in the form of pain control to patients with FM. Since the basis of their pain appears to be from altered perception of stimulus, not from inflammation or injury, analgesics offer little benefit. Some benefit may be found from non-steroidal analgesics; most patients will either already be taking one or will have tried them in the past. It appears that the pain is what is classified as *functional*, where there is increased facilitation of downward modulation—normal sensation signals from the periphery are interpreted as being painful. This is conveyed mainly by pathways involving serotonin and norepinephrine, for which as of now we have no effective treatment. Medications that increase inhibition of downward modulation—opioids or GABA-mimetics—do not appear to provide much pain control without further adversely affecting quality of life. Tricyclic antidepressant use for pain control is strongly supported by research whereas selective serotonin reuptake inhibitors (SSRI) antidepressants have at best mixed results, and do not appear to be as analgesic as tricyclic agents.

SUMMARY

Both MPS and FM are myofascial pain disorders that are still inadequately defined and not universally recognized as specific illnesses. Ongoing care is the cornerstone of treatment. Understanding, support, and education from us are essential to their care, given the limited role of the ED in their management. Ensure that new onset or type of pain is not attributed to the chronic pain disorder *before* being evaluated. Use or prescription of short-acting opioids offers little if any benefit, while risking negative behavioral changes and increasing the risk of tolerance in patients on chronic opioids for pain control.

REFERENCES

1. Wheeler AH, Aaron GW. Muscle pain due to injury. *Curr Pain Headache Rep*. 2001;5(5):441–446.
2. Drewes AM, Nielsen KD, Taagholt SJ, et al. Sleep intensity in fibromyalgia: focus on the microstructure of the sleep process. *Br J Rheumatol*. 1995;34(7):629–635.
3. Raj PP. Botulinum toxin therapy in pain management. *Anesthesiol Clin North America*. 2003;21(4):715–731.
4. Abram SE. Acute pain management in the chronic pain sufferer. In: Dostrovsky JO, Carr DB, Koltzenburg M, eds. *Proceedings of the 10th World Congress on Pain: Progress in Pain Research and Management*. Seattle, WA: IASP Press; 2002:739–749.
5. Paronis CA, Holtzman SG. Development of tolerance to the analgesic activity of mu agonists after continuous infusion of morphine, meperidine or fentanyl in rats. *J Pharmacol Exp Ther*. 1992;262(1):1–9.
6. Roth RS, Horowitz K, Bachman JE. Chronic myofascial pain: knowledge of diagnosis and satisfaction with treatment. *Arch Phys Med Rehabil*. 1998;79(8):966–970.
7. Wheeler AH. Myofascial pain disorders: theory to therapy. *Drugs*. 2004;64(1):45–62.
8. Rivner MH. The neurophysiology of myofascial pain syndrome. *Curr Pain Headache Rep*. 2001;5(5):432–440.
9. Turturro MA, Frater CR, D'Amico FJ. Cyclobenzaprine with ibuprofen versus ibuprofen alone in acute myofascial strain: a randomized, double-blind clinical trial. *Ann Emerg Med*. 2003;41(6):818–826.
10. Cummings TM, White AR. Needling therapies in the management of myofascial trigger point pain: a systematic review. *Arch Phys Med Rehabil*. 2001;82(7):986–992.
11. Smania N, Corato E, Fiaschi A, et al. Therapeutic effects of peripheral repetitive magnetic stimulation on myofascial pain syndrome. *Clin Neurophysiol*. 2003;114(2):350–358.
12. Mense S. Neurobiological basis for the use of botulinum toxin in pain therapy. *J Neurol*. 2004;251(suppl 1):I1–II7.
13. Wolfe F, Smythe HA, Yunus MB, et al. The American College of Rheumatology 1990 Criteria for the Classification of Fibromyalgia. Report of the Multicenter Criteria Committee. *Arthritis Rheum*. 1990;33(2):160–172.
14. Bradley LA, Cohen ML, Fors EA. A biopsychosocial appro-ach to fibromyalgia and chronic fatigue syndrome. In: Dostrovsky JO, Carr DB, Koltzenburg M, eds. *Proceedings of the 10th World Congress on Pain, Progress in Pain Research and Management*. Seattle, WA: IASP Press; 2002:865–877.
15. Aaron LA, Burke MM, Buchwald D. Overlapping conditions among patients with chronic fatigue syndrome, fibromyalgia, and temporomandibular disorder. *Arch Intern Med*. 2000; 160(2):221–227.
16. Gracely RH, Petzke F, Wolf JM, et al. Functional magnetic resonance imaging evidence of augmented pain processing in fibromyalgia. *Arthritis Rheum*. 2002;46(5):1333–1343.
17. Mountz JM, Bradley LA, Alarcon GS. Abnormal functional activity of the central nervous system in fibromyalgia syndrome. *Am J Med Sci*. 1998;315(6):385–396.
18. Russell IJ. The promise of substance P inhibitors in fibromyalgia. *Rheum Dis Clin North Am*. 2002;28(2): 329–342.
19. Herpfer I, Lieb K. Substance P and substance P receptor antagonists in the pathogenesis and treatment of affective disorders. *World J Biol Psychiatry*. 2003;4(2):56–63.
20. Mahowald ML, Mahowald MW. Nighttime sleep and daytime functioning (sleepiness and fatigue) in less well-defined chronic rheumatic diseases with particular reference to the 'alpha-delta NREM sleep anomaly.' 2000;1(3):195–207.
21. Tuzun EH, Albayrak G, Eker L, et al. A comparison study of quality of life in women with fibromyalgia and myofascial pain syndrome. *Disabil Rehabil*. 2004;26(4):198–202.

40

Prehospital Pain Management and Sedation

Salvatore Silvestri
George A. Ralls
L. Connor Nickels
Blake O'Brien

HIGH YIELD FACTS

- Appropriate prehospital pain control does not interfere with a patient's ability to provide consent.

- Careful titration of prehospital pain medications and/or sedatives is safe and effective.

- Prehospital pain protocols include assessment, reliable tools, indications/contraindications, monitoring, documentation, information transfer, QI, and medical oversight.

- Both nonpharmacologic and pharmacologic interventions are part of prehospital pain management.

- Indications for prehospital sedative agent use include procedures, treatment of specific medical conditions, and managing violent patients.

INTRODUCTION

The field of emergency medical services (EMSs) has evolved over the years to include patient care that reflects advances in emergency medicine. Literature on the management of acute pain has reported that emergency health care providers (prehospital and hospital) underestimate pain and underprescribe analgesics thus contributing to *oligoanalgesia* but this is changing. Stewart emphasized these principles in prehospital care in 1988[1] and efforts to improve prehospital pain management have continued to progress.

STUDIES OF PREHOSPITAL PAIN MANAGEMENT

Several studies have shown that failure to acknowledge pain and administer analgesics in the prehospital setting results in further analgesic delays once the patient has arrived in the emergency department (ED).[2-4] In a study of 123 patients with lower extremity or hip fractures, transported by EMS, McEachin et al. found that only 22 (18.3%) received prehospital analgesics.[2] Almost all (91.7%) of the patients ultimately received analgesics in the ED. Patients who received prehospital analgesics were younger and more likely to have lower extremity injuries other than hip fractures. Gender did not seem to play a role and the age discrimination was of unclear etiology. In this study, the mean time to analgesic administration was 28.4 (±36) minutes for those patients who received prehospital analgesics and 145.9 (±74) minutes for those patients who did not receive prehospital analgesics ($P < 0.001$).[2] In a retrospective study by Vassiliadis, of 128 patients, with an admission diagnosis of femoral neck fracture, patients were given a higher ED triage category if they had been given prehospital analgesics.[3] Although the triage category did not affect the time interval between arrival and assessment by the physician, those patients who received prehospital analgesics were given further ED analgesics 2 hours and 3 minutes earlier on average than patients who had not received prehospital analgesics ($P = 0.002$).[3]

Other studies have focused on the tendency of EMS providers to underassess and underestimate pain. In a study by Luger et al., the assessment of pain intensity by an EMS team (physician, emergency medical technician, and EMS driver) was compared to the patient's self-assessment.[4] The EMS providers were graded as having correctly assessed the patient's pain intensity if they had categorized the pain (mild, moderate, or severe) in agreement with the patient's self-assessment. The study results showed that there was a general underestimation of pain at all levels of training. Physician level providers and emergency medical technicians underestimated severe pain in 60% of the cases, whereas EMS drivers underestimated severe pain in 68% of the cases.[4]

McLean et al. studied the feasibility of prehospital pain assessment using verbal and numeric rating scales.[5] Results showed that the use of protocol-driven rating scales required little paramedic training and successful assessment was achieved.[5]

Richard-Hibon et al. conducted a trial to evaluate methods for improving prehospital pain management.[6] This was a two-part study held in France over an 8-month period. In part one, pain management was analyzed before any modifications were made, and the choice of medication and decision to treat was left to the EMS provider's discretion. After part one, the EMS providers underwent a 2-week training session to improve their pain management skills. The program subsequently modified protocols that encouraged the use of opioids. In part two of the study, EMS providers administered small boluses of morphine, taking into account the patient's pain intensity, respiratory rate, hemodynamic status, and level of consciousness. Patients were continuously monitored and naloxone was available if needed. The results comparing the two parts showed that more patients expressed adequate pain relief in part two (67%, $n = 105$) versus part one (49%, $n = 108$).[6]

An article by Jones et al. explored paramedics' perceptions of pain evaluation and factors which influence pain management decision making.[7] The study design involved detailed interviews with six urban EMS system paramedics. Results of these interviews are summarized in Table 40-1.[7]

CONFOUNDING ISSUES IN PREHOSPITAL PAIN MANAGEMENT

Some long-standing medical opinions and beliefs have influenced the approach to prehospital pain management and raised confounding issues.[8] One such issue involves the competency of patients to provide informed consent for procedures or release of medical information after the administration of analgesics in the field. When addressing this issue, one should consider the following: there are four requirements that must be met to consider informed consent valid:

1. Patients must have the capacity to understand the information and treatment options.

2. They must be able to clearly communicate their choice.

Table 40-1. Paramedics' Perspective of Factors Influencing Prehospital Pain Management

Theme Identified	Influential Factors
Patient's experience of pain	Age Cultural background
Evaluation of pain	Patient's behavior 　Facial expressions, guarding painful areas, withdrawal from examination Physical signs 　Deformity, swelling, loss of function
Decision making	Patient-focused factors 　Patients' perspective of pain Non-patient-focused factors 　Time to hospital arrival, road conditions, possible hospital delayed off-load
Alternative methods	Psychologic, communicative, acupuncture, TENS units, if proven to be effective

TENS: transcutaneous electrical nerve stimulation.
Source: Richard-Hibon A, Chollet C, Saada S. A Quality control program for acute pain management in out-of-hospital critical care medicine. *Ann Emerg Med.* 1999;34:738–744.

3. They must not be coerced into making a decision.

4. The information must be presented in a way that patients can comprehend the choices and consequences of those choices.[8]

Based on these criteria, the appropriate use of pain control measures, including the judicious use of narcotic agents, should not interfere with a patient's ability to communicate their wishes when providing consent. Furthermore, it has been speculated that withholding analgesics from a patient in acute pain for the sake of obtaining consent can be interpreted as a form of coercion.[8] Another commonly encountered concern affecting the approach to prehospital pain control is that of narcotic-induced respiratory arrest.[8] Respiratory depression is a known side effect of narcotics, however, careful titration of medications to decrease pain has been shown to be safe and effective.

Yet another issue surrounding the application of prehospital pain control is the use of analgesics in the setting of abdominal pain prior to a physician/surgeon evaluation. In the opinion of some practitioners, the reduction in pain may mask key physical examination findings, thus making

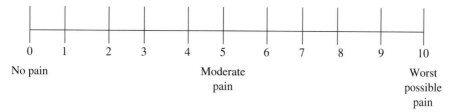

Fig. 40-1. 0–10 Numeric pain intensity scale.

diagnosis more difficult. Although the treatment of abdominal pain in the field may never be considered standard treatment, a hospital-based study in 1996 suggested that the concern for masking physical examination findings may be overstated. In this double-blinded study, Pace et al. randomized two groups of patients with abdominal pain to receive either morphine or normal saline. The patients were examined by emergency physicians and surgeons before and after the medications were given. Not only did the presence of peritoneal signs not change, but the accuracy of the diagnosis did not differ between the emergency physicians and the surgeons or between the two groups of patients. Also of note in this study, morphine was titrated to make the patients more comfortable, not necessarily to eradicate their pain.[9]

The variety of opinions that shape the approach to prehospital pain management emphasizes the value of establishing evidence-based treatment protocols, whenever evidence for a particular intervention exists. The paucity of large randomized control trials on this topic has sustained a rather inconsistent approach to dealing with pain control in the field.

PREHOSPITAL PAIN MANAGEMENT PROTOCOLS

Pain is a subjective symptom, which can be dealt with objectively. Protocol-driven assessment and treatment of pain may help eliminate the subjectivity of an individual provider's evaluation of the need for pain control. The National Association of EMS Physicians (NAEMSP) has stated that prehospital pain relief for patients in

distress must be a priority.[10] They have recommended the following items as part of prehospital pain management protocols:

1. Mandatory assessment of both the presence and severity of pain.
2. Use of reliable tools for the assessment of pain.
3. Indications and contraindications for prehospital pain management.
4. Nonpharmacologic interventions for pain management.
5. Pharmacologic interventions for pain management.
6. Mandatory patient monitoring and documentation before and after analgesic administration.
7. Transferal of relevant patient care information to receiving medical personnel.
8. Quality improvement and close medical oversight to ensure appropriate use of prehospital pain management.[10]

Mandatory assessment of pain enables the provider to recognize the presence and intensity of pain that may otherwise be unrecognized. Choosing an appropriate assessment tool is crucial in the development of an effective prehospital pain management strategy. An ideal pain assessment tool measures the presence and severity of pain, as well as any change experienced throughout prehospital treatment and transport. Some examples include the numeric rating scale (Fig. 40-1),[11] the verbal rating scale (Fig. 40-2),[11] and the Wong-Baker faces pain rating scale (Fig. 40-3).[12,13] Table 40-2 is a standard protocol for prehospital adult pain management and Table 40-3 is a standard protocol for prehospital pediatric pain management.[14]

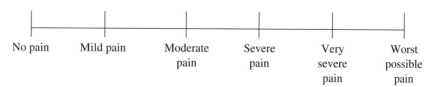

Fig. 40-2. Simple descriptive pain intensity scale.

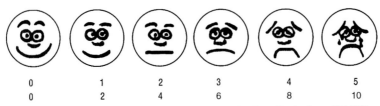

Fig. 40-3. Wong-Baker FACES pain rating scale. (Reproduced with permission from Hockenberry MJ, Wilson D, Winkelstein ML: *Wong's Essentials of Pediatric Nursing*, ed. 7, St. Louis, MI; 2005, p.1259).

Table 40-2. Prehospital Adult Pain Management Protocol

Basic Life Support
Secure airway
Supplemental 100% oxygen
Record and monitor vital signs
Assess baseline pain level (0–10 scale) (0 = no pain, 10 = worst pain)
Provide therapeutic communication whenever applicable
Administer nothing by mouth

Advanced Life Support
Advanced airway/ventilatory management as needed
Perform cardiac monitoring and evaluate 12-lead ECG
Record and monitor O_2 saturation
Record and monitor microstream capnography
IV 0.9% NaCl KVO or IV lock
    If BP <90 mmHg systolic, administer boluses of 0.9% NaCl at 250 mL until systolic BP >90 mmHg
    Contraindicated if evidence of congestive heart failure (e.g., rales)
Analgesic indications
    Isolated extremity injury
    Burn without airway, breathing, or circulatory compromise
    Sickle crisis with pain that is typical for that patient's sickle cell disease
    Acute chest pain (see Chap. 32)
    History and assessment consistent with renal colic (see Chap. 36)
Agents for pain control
    Morphine sulfate 2 mg slow IVP every 2 minutes until pain relief achieved (maximum 6 mg)
    Contraindicated if systolic BP <90
    Nalbuphine HCl (Nubain) 2.5 mg every 2 minutes slow IV
    If patient is allergic to morphine sulfate or SBP <90 mmHg
    Maximum 5 mg if patient <50 kg, 10 mg if patient >50 kg
    May induce acute withdrawal symptoms in patients who take narcotic medication chronically (i.e.,
        methadone, oxycodone, and fentanyl), therefore nalbuphine is contraindicated in this setting
    Nitrous oxide (use nitrous oxide procedural protocol)
After drug administration
    Reassess the patient's pain
    Note adequacy of ventilation and perfusion
    Monitor oxygen saturation and end-tidal CO_2 continuously
Reassess the patient frequently

Medical Control
Contact medical control for additional orders or questions

ECG: electrocardiogram; KVO: keep vein open; IV: intravenous; IVP: intravenous push; SBP: systolic blood pressure.
Source: Orange County EMS System Protocols. Orange County, FL; 2004.

Table 40-3. Prehospital Pediatric Pain Management Protocol

Basic Life Support

Establish responsiveness

Assess airway, breathing, circulation, and perfusion

If trauma suspected, stabilize spine

Supplemental 100% oxygen if any respiratory signs or symptoms present

Record and monitor vital signs

Advanced Life Support

Advanced airway/ventilatory management as needed

When condition warrants

Perform cardiac monitoring

Record and monitor O_2 saturation

Record and monitor microstream capnography

IV 0.9% NaCl KVO or IV lock

   If signs of shock administer boluses of 0.9% NaCl at 20 mL/kg until signs of shock resolve or 60 mL/kg total

Analgesic indications

   Isolated extremity injury

   Burn without airway, breathing, or circulatory compromise

   Typical sickle cell crisis for patient

Agents for pain control

   Morphine sulfate 0.1 mg/kg IV or SC (maximum single dose 2 mg; maximum total dose 6 mg)

   Nitrous oxide (if available)

After drug administration

   Reassess the patient's pain

   Note adequacy of ventilation and perfusion

   Monitor oxygen saturation and end-tidal CO_2 continuously

Reassess frequently

Medical Control

Contact Medical Control for questions concerning pain control in children not meeting above criteria

---

KVO: keep vein open; IV: intravenous; SC: subcutaneous.

Note: Contact Medical Control for questions concerning pain control in children not meeting above criteria.

Source: Orange County EMS System Protocols. Orange County, FL; 2004.

NONPHARMACOLOGIC INTERVENTIONS

Nonpharmacologic techniques can be used to achieve pain relief. Examples include biofeedback, distraction, parental attention for children, and immobilization, elevation and/or cold therapy for injured extremities. Generally, these techniques can be categorized into psychologic, verbal, and physical interventions.

The use of psychologic interventions can be significantly limited by age (pediatric and elderly), level of consciousness, and language barriers. With pediatric patients, especially infants, having their parents present can soothe them in ways that would otherwise be unachievable. Furthermore, support from friends or family during painful episodes can be therapeutic to patients of all ages.

Pain can also be influenced by verbal interventions. This can be termed the *therapeutic communication technique* and can be performed by health care providers or family members. It involves careful use of appropriate wording, music, or other forms of distraction, drawing attention away from the painful stimulus.

Lastly, physical interventions can prove beneficial in the relief of pain. For example, if a patient with an extremity fracture is placed in proper immobilization, he or she may experience significant reduction in pain. Elevation and application of cold packs to extremity injuries are also effective physical interventions.

Nonpharmacologic interventions can greatly contribute to pain relief, when used properly. They are especially useful when used in conjunction with pharmacologic interventions.[10,15]

PHARMACOLOGIC INTERVENTIONS

Pharmacologic interventions have been available for years. However, few clinical studies have focused on prehospital use of analgesics. While the most well-known and frequently used prehospital medications are opioids, there are other classes of drugs used in the field, such as nonsteroidal anti-inflammatory drugs (NSAIDs), opioid receptor agonist-antagonists, and inhalational agents such as nitrous oxide. A detailed description of these agents is contained elsewhere in this textbook; However, some of the evidence to support the prehospital use of these agents will be discussed further.

NARCOTIC ANALGESICS

Opiates have been the standard in analgesia for centuries. The physiologic effects of opioids are mediated principally through mu and kappa receptors in the central nervous system (CNS) and periphery. Common classifications divide the opioids into agonist, partial agonist, or agonist-antagonist agents and natural, semisynthetic, or synthetic. Opioids decrease the perception of pain rather than eliminate or reduce the painful stimulus. Inducing slight euphoria, opioid agonists reduce the sensitivity to exogenous stimuli. Peak effects generally are reached in 10 minutes with the intravenous (IV) route, 10–15 minutes after nasal insufflation (e.g., butorphanol and heroin),

30–45 minutes with the intramuscular (IM) route, 90 minutes with the PO route, and 8 hours after dermal application (i.e., fentanyl).

Morphine Sulfate

Morphine is considered, by many, a benchmark agent against which other analgesics are measured. Prehospital use of morphine has centered on management of acute ischemic chest pain (i.e., refractory to nitrates) and isolated extremity trauma. These subsets of patients are usually normovolemic and narcotic-induced hypotension is less likely. Bruns et al.[16] reported a prospective study evaluating the safety of morphine use in patients with presumed ischemic chest pain and/or pulmonary edema in the prehospital setting. They reported that overall appropriateness of paramedic therapy was 88% ($n = 89$) and noted a 6% complication rate.[16] A 2002 study by Fullerton-Gleason et al. demonstrated efficacy of a prehospital protocol for morphine use in isolated extremity fractures.[17] In this study, paramedics administered a mean dose of 6.7 mg to a sample of 963 patients and no adverse events were reported.[17] Richard-Hibon showed dramatic improvement in post-transport pain scores in patients treated with morphine. This study included 108 patients and there were no cases of respiratory failure or hemodynamic compromise after a mean dose of 7.2 mg of morphine.[6]

Yaster discussed management of pediatric pain with opioid analgesia.[18] He noted that 0.1 mg/kg morphine IV or IM produced adequate analgesia without loss of consciousness. However, infants less than 2 months of age are highly sensitive to respiratory depression, and any narcotic in this age group must be limited to the intensive care setting.[18]

The lack of an authoritative reference on the use of morphine in the prehospital setting makes it difficult to establish rigid dosing protocols. With the availability of blood pressure, oxygen saturation, and end-tidal CO_2 monitoring, IV morphine titration for prehospital analgesia can be safe and effective. Adverse effects such as hypotension and respiratory depression can be controlled with fluid boluses and naloxone, respectively. The ready availability of a pure antagonist (naloxone) makes this method of analgesia relatively safe. While no standard dosing regimen has been cited in any prehospital studies, in adults an IV starting dose of 2 mg with titration to pain (or maximum dosing limit) is generally accepted as safe.

Fentanyl

While fentanyl has not been prospectively studied in the prehospital setting, several critical care air transport teams have used it. A frequently cited study by Devellis showed effective analgesia in 98 patients receiving fentanyl for isolated extremity fractures, with 20.4% not requiring additional analgesia in the ED.[19] This study did not report any significant side effects.

In 1998, a retrospective cohort study by Devellis showed that fentanyl was safely tolerated by 131 pediatric patients with a mean age of 6.2 years.[20] Each patient was given 0.33–0.5 mg/kg of fentanyl and there were no reported episodes of hypotension, chest wall rigidity, or respiratory depression.[20] In a 2002 Australian study of intranasal fentanyl use, effective analgesia was achieved in children aged 3–12 years.[21] In a recently published study by Kotwal et al.,[22] field use of oral transmucosal fentanyl citrate was evaluated in 22 soldiers during Operation Iraqi Freedom. In this study, hemodynamically stable soldiers with isolated, uncomplicated orthopedic injuries or extremity wounds self-administered oral doses (1600 mcg) of transmucosal fentanyl citrate via a lozenge on a stick. Results demonstrated the median verbal (0–10) numeric rating scale was 7.0 at time 0, 1.0 at 15 minutes, and 0.5 at 5 hours post oral fentanyl administration. The differences in pain scores at time 0 and 15 minutes were statistically significant, and not significantly different between 15 minutes and 5 hours. The authors concluded this demonstrated the sustained action of the oral fentanyl preparation.[22]

Fentanyl is a promising drug for prehospital pain management. Its potency, shorter duration of action, and lower incidence of hemodynamic effects and respiratory depression make it a particularly useful drug to consider in the multiple-system trauma patient. However, further prospective prehospital trials are still needed to assess the safety and efficacy of fentanyl in the EMS setting.

Alfentanil

Alfentanil is a short-acting synthetic opioid similar to fentanyl. It has been extensively used in the prehospital care setting in Finland. A comparison study by Silfvast explored alfentanil and morphine in the prehospital treatment of acute chest pain.[23] Alfentanil 0.5 mg showed a more rapid onset and better efficacy of ana-lgesia than morphine without respiratory or hemodynamic compromise. The main side effect was dizziness, likely related to rapid penetration of the blood-brain barrier.[23]

Meperidine

Meperidine is a synthetic narcotic with a potency about one-tenth that of morphine. This drug is associated with increased histamine release and CNS excitation with the potential of increased agitation progressing to tonic clonic seizures. The drug's metabolite, normeperidine, is a highly active proconvulsant. Meperidine inhibits serotonin reuptake in the CNS and has been linked to serotonin syndrome especially when used in conjunction with tricyclic antidepressants (TCAs), selective serotonin reuptake inhibitors (SSRIs), and monoamine oxidase inhibitors (MAOIs). A critical review of meperidine by the Duke University Department of Pharmacy explored these side effects and cited that its poor efficacy, toxicity, and multiple drug interactions supported a movement to replace meperidine with more efficacious and less toxic opioid analgesics.[24] Many EMS systems have removed this drug from their list of authorized pharmaceuticals. Meperidine, however, remains in use in emergency medicine, and is present in some EMS systems.

NONNARCOTIC ANALGESICS

Nalbuphine

Nalbuphine is a mixed opioid receptor agonist/antagonist. Its advantages include less respiratory and cardiovascular side effects. Also, it is not a controlled substance, and therefore, not regulated. These attributes have made this drug very popular in many prehospital analgesic protocols. An early study by Stene demonstrated efficacious treatment of 46 patients with a variety of medical, orthopedic, and surgical complaints, with no side effects.[25] Chambers et al. studied nalbuphine in the prehospital setting. They were able to show a clinically significant visual analog scale (VAS) score reduction in patients who received the drug. This study was done in the absence of a placebo.[26] More recently the use of the drug has come under scrutiny. Houlihan reported a 10-patient case review showing increased analgesic requirements in the ED in those who had received prehospital nalbuphine.[27] Robinson and Burrows questioned the efficacy of nalbuphine while examining patients who had received prehospital nalbuphine. The study showed no difference in pain levels on presentation to the ED and a less dramatic decline in pain scores within the ED when compared to a control group who did not receive prehospital nalbuphine.[28] EMS systems that utilize nalbuphine should also educate their paramedics that use of this class of drug, i.e., partial agonist-antagonists, may precipitate an acute narcotic withdrawal syndrome in patients who chronically use narcotic agents.

Tramadol

Tramadol is a centrally acting analgesic with a weak affinity for mu opioid receptors. Ward studied the efficacy of tramadol versus nitrous oxide in the treatment of analgesia in the prehospital setting.[29] This poorly controlled trial of questionable clinical significance found tramadol to be more efficacious.[29] Vergnion et al., studied prehospital 50-mg tramadol as an alternative to 5-mg morphine IV.[30] This double-blinded trial concluded that analgesia and side effects where not significantly different and recommended this as an acceptable alternative analgesic.[30] Tramadol may be supported for use in the prehospital setting since it is an unregulated drug with comparable efficacy. However, IV tramadol is not currently available in the United States.

Ketorolac

NSAIDs affect peripheral pain transmission by inhibiting prostaglandins. Ketorolac, the only available injectable NSAID, has analgesic, anti-inflammatory, and antipyretic effects without CNS or respiratory depression. While ketorolac has proven effective in the hospital setting, its use in the prehospital setting is not well studied. It is currently used in some EMS systems, as single therapy or in combination with centrally acting analgesics.

Nitrous Oxide

Nitrous oxide is a gas rapidly absorbed when inhaled and produces central analgesia and sedation. In the United States it is delivered in a mixture of 50% nitrous oxide and 50% oxygen called Nitronox. The Food and Drug Administration (FDA)-approved delivery system has a safety mechanism such that pure nitrous oxide is not inhaled, but this mode of delivery requires two cylinders and is bulky. Entonox, a single cylinder system, is used in Europe. This self-administered analgesic has been utilized by EMS systems since the early 1980s. A 1983 study of over 1200 patients by Stewart et al., demonstrated the efficacy and safety of nitrous oxide in the prehospital setting.[31] Johnson et al. studied prehospital self-administered nitrous oxide analgesia in 200 patients.[32] Both studies reported only mild or minimal side effects: dizziness, nausea, and drowsiness being the most common.[31,32] Kaplan et al. suggested nitrous oxide use during transcutaneous pacing.[33] Nitrous oxide is extensively used in the prehospital setting, with a low incidence of reported adverse outcomes related to the drug.

Methoxyflurane/Enflurane

This inhalational agent is administered through a mask at concentration of 25–35%. It has been utilized in the international prehospital community for years. The inability to supply supplemental oxygen in combination with this agent, and the slow onset and recovery time in comparison to nitrous oxide have made this agent less popular in the United States. No large randomized controlled trials exist to clearly support the use of this inhalational agent in the prehospital setting.

PREHOSPITAL SEDATION

General Comments

Prehospital sedation is not a well-defined topic in EMS. The majority of information supporting sedation in the field is extrapolated from literature on procedural sedation and analgesia in the ED. Sedation may be required to perform a procedure such as transcutaneous pacing, or to treat a condition such as seizures or excited delirium. The American College of Emergency Physicians (ACEP) developed their own clinical policy on the topic of procedural sedation in 1998, with a recent update released in 2005.[34] ACEP defines procedural sedation as "a technique of administering sedatives or dissociative agents with or without analgesics to induce a state that allows the patient to tolerate unpleasant procedures while maintaining cardiorespiratory function."[34] They further explain its application by stating, "Procedural sedation and analgesia requires personnel who have an understanding and experience with the drugs used; the ability to monitor the patient's condition and recognize changes in clinical status; and the skills necessary to manage a compromised airway and to perform CPR."[34] Although procedural sedation represents one indication for the prehospital use of sedative agents, these guidelines can be applied to all situations where a sedative or analgesic agent is used by EMS personnel.

The concept of psychologic, verbal, and pharmaceutical interventions discussed earlier in the chapter applies to prehospital sedation as well. This is especially applicable to violent or combative patients, where the initial therapeutic intervention may be verbal de-escalation.

Indications

Indications for prehospital sedative agent use include the performance of procedures, the treatment of specific medical conditions, or for management of violent or combative patients exhibiting excited delirium (see Table 40-4).

Procedural Sedation

Procedural sedation is much more limited in the prehospital setting as compared to the ED. Caution must be used when defining indications for prehospital procedural sedation due to the limited ability to monitor, recognize, and deal with the potential complications that may arise. Common indications for procedural sedation include symptomatic bradycardia

Table 40-4. Common Indications for Prehospital Sedative Agent Use

Procedural sedation
Transcutaneous pacing
Synchronized cardioversion
Sedative-facilitated intubation
Rapid sequence intubation

Agitated, combative states*
Cocaine/sympathomimetic toxicity
Drug overdose
Postictal states
Acute brain injury
Acute psychotic states
CNS infection
Postresuscitation combativeness
Ethanol (or other drug) withdrawal

*End point of sedative agent use is patient control for adequate monitoring and safe transport.

requiring transcutaneous pacing, tachydysrhythmias requiring synchronized cardioversion, sedative-facilitated intubation and rapid sequence intubation (RSI). In the right setting, a sedative drug that allows for the performance of life or limb-saving procedures by relieving pain, anxiety, or awareness can assist in more rapid stabilization and transport of patients to the hospital. The drugs used in procedural sedation may vary from system to system.

Table 40-5. Agitation Scale

Score	Agitation Category	Criteria
5	Extremely combative	Continuous, vigorous fighting against restraints
4	Moderately combative	Occasional vigorous efforts against restraints, still agitated
3	Minimally combative	Minimal efforts against restraints, occasional verbal hostility
2	Resting	No efforts against restraints, awake, may be cooperative
1	Somnolent	Sleeping or sleepy

Source: Hick JL, Mahoney BD, Lappe M. Prehospital sedation with intramuscular droperidol: a one-year pilot. *Prehosp Emerg Care* 2001;5:391–394.

Agitated, Combative Patient Management

Management of the agitated, combative patient is a difficult and dangerous situation for prehospital providers (Table 40-5). Establishing an organized, stepwise approach to these patients, which includes a plan for the use of physical and chemical restraints, represents an important EMS system risk management strategy (see Fig. 40-4). Protocols for the restraint of agitated patients must address medical conditions which may present as combativeness,

such as hypoglycemia, head injury, or hypoxia. They must also provide for both the safety of EMS providers, as well as the patient. The NAEMSP released a position paper on patient restraint in the prehospital setting.[35]

The safe restraint of violent, combative patients may require the use of verbal, physical, and chemical interventions. Verbal interventions include verbal de-escalation techniques, whereas physical restraint may employ manpower from law enforcement, or the use of straps or belts to protect the patient from harming themselves or others.

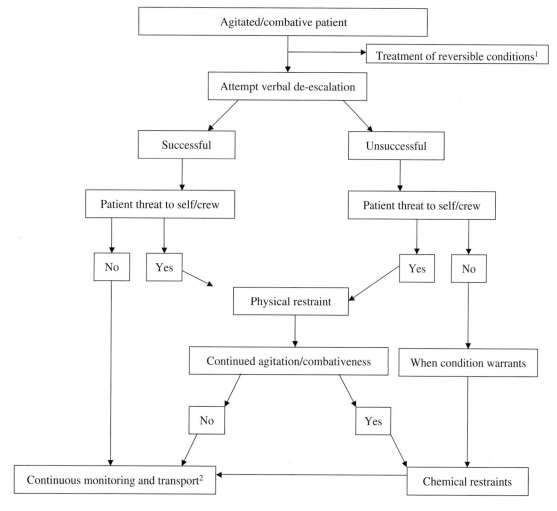

[1]Treatment examples: oxygen, glucose, or naloxone as needed.

[2]Cardiac, oxygen saturation, and end-tidal CO_2 monitoring.

Fig. 40-4. Agitated/combative patient management algorithm.

Chemical restraint is the term used to describe the use of sedative agents to assist in the care and transport of agitated, violent, or combative patients. The goal of chemical restraint is to suppress the continued and excessive struggling against physical restraints. Preferably, the patients' behavior would be subdued without significantly altering their overall level of consciousness.

It is possible to encounter a scenario when sedatives are indicated for behavioral issues when physical restraints are not needed. This may be the case for children or elderly patients who are not physically endangering caregivers, but whose behavioral state may interfere with their care and transport. When designing a treatment algorithm, consideration should be given to conditions when this is appropriate.

Contraindications

Contraindications to sedative agent use are similar to contraindications for pain relief. They include obvious reasons such as allergies, hemodynamic instability, and preexisting medical conditions contraindicating use. Because of these contraindications, continuous assessment and monitoring must be heavily emphasized.

PHARMACOLOGIC INTERVENTIONS FOR PREHOSPITAL SEDATION

The two most commonly employed types of sedative agents in the prehospital setting are butyrophenones and benzodiazepines.

Benzodiazepines preferentially act on the limbic system of the brain where they potentiate inhibitory neurotransmission in those systems where γ-aminobutyric acid (GABA) is a neurotransmitter. Lorazepam and midazolam are the two most commonly used benzodiazepines for prehospital sedative use.[36]

Butyrophenones, also known as the major tranquilizers, basically act by blocking dopamine D2 receptors. The true mechanism of action is quite complex and poorly understood. Of the butyrophenones, haloperidol and droperidol are the most commonly employed in the EMS setting. High-potency butyrophenones, such as haloperidol, are less sedating than other drugs in this category. Extrapyramidal symptoms and orthostasis are the most common adverse effects associated with use of this class of drugs.[36]

Midazolam

Midazolam is a benzodiazepine with sedative and amnestic properties. It can be administered IM with reliable absorp-

tion. Most respiratory suppression occurs with rapid IV administration. Midazolam is employed in many EMS systems for the management of seizures, behavioral emergencies, and the facilitation of intubation.

Midazolam has been shown to be effective in the prehospital treatment of seizures. Gilbert et al. found that midazolam IM was superior to diazepam and had the lowest mortality rate of all prehospital seizure medications.[37]

In a recent study by Nobay, the role of midazolam was evaluated in violent, agitated patients.[38] This prospective, randomized, double-blind study compared midazolam (5 mg), haloperidol (5 mg), and lorazepam (2 mg) in the chemical restraint of violent and agitated patients.[38] Results showed that midazolam had the shortest time to sedation (18.3 min) and arousal (81.9 min) when compared to haloperidol and lorazepam ($P < 0.05$ for both comparisons).[38] Although midazolam had a shorter time to sedation than haloperidol and lorazepam individually, it was not evaluated against the combination of haloperidol and lorazepam.

The use of midazolam to facilitate prehospital endotracheal intubation has been reported in the literature.[39–41] In the prehospital setting, Davis et al. has described dose-dependent hypotension associated with the use of midazolam to perform RSI in severe brain-injured patients.[42] A detailed discussion of the role of midazolam in the prehospital performance of RSI is beyond the scope of this chapter.

Midazolam remains a commonly used drug in the prehospital setting. EMS systems must decide on the indications, the authorized dosage, and the accepted route(s) of administration for the use of midazolam.

Lorazepam

Lorazepam is a benzodiazepine with anxiolytic, CNS depressant, and sedative properties. The onset and duration of action is longer with lorazepam than midazolam. In addition, lorazepam has been the accepted first line treatment of choice for seizing patients in the ED setting for many years. Lorazepam can be given sublingually, orally, intramuscularly, or intravenously. Lorazepam is contraindicated in patients with a known allergy to benzyl alcohol, propylene glycol, or polyethylene glycol. Recommended dosages vary based on route and indication, whether treating an acute problem versus a chronic disorder.

The evidence supporting the use of lorazepam for the management of acutely agitated, combative patients favors combination drug therapy over single agent use. Battaglia et al. studied 98 patients needing rapid tranquilization in a double-blind, prospective trial that showed that a combination of lorazepam (2 mg) and haloperidol (5 mg) was superior to either drug alone ($P < 0.05$).[43] In another randomized controlled trial, Bieniek et al. evaluated lorazepam (2 mg) compared to the combination of lorazepam (2 mg) and haloperidol (5 mg) in managing 20 acutely agitated patients. A significantly higher percentage of patients who received the combination therapy had improved overt aggression scale (OAS) scores at 1 hour ($P < 0.05$).[44] One other randomized controlled trial, by Garza-Tevino et al., evaluated lorazepam (4 mg) versus haloperidol (5 mg) versus lorazepam (4 mg) and haloperidol (5 mg). The combination therapy arm of the study demonstrated significantly better tranquilization at 30 minutes compared to the other two arms ($P < 0.05$).[45]

Although these studies demonstrate the superiority of the combination of lorazepam and haloperidol, none of them evaluated the time interval to sedation or arousal as in the Nobay study discussed previously. In the prehospital management of acutely agitated, combative patients, the time-to-sedation interval may likely be the most important characteristic of the treatment option chosen. Results of a randomized controlled trial comparing the time-to-sedation intervals of midazolam to the combination of lorazepam and haloperidol would be a valuable addition to the scientific literature.

Ketamine

Ketamine is a dissociative anesthetic that induces a cataleptic state with effective sedation and analgesia. Green et al. reported a study of 1021 children who received IM ketamine in the ED setting, and concluded that there was no significant ketamine dose relationship with airway complications, emesis, or recovery agitation.[46] In addition, a British study examined the use of ketamine in the prehospital setting and found it to be a safe and effective option in extrication and fracture splinting.[47]

Droperidol

Droperidol is a butyrophenone with major tranquilizing effects similar to haloperidol. It is commonly used as an adjunct medication for anesthesia. It has pharmacologic actions similar to those of phenothiazines with antiemetic properties. Side effects include hypotension, decreased pulmonary arterial pressure, and tardive dyskinesia (40%). Life-threatening arrhythmias may occur in patients receiving this medication. Droperidol received a black box warning because of the drug's ability to prolong the QT interval, which led to a dramatic decrease in its use. In a randomized controlled trial in the ED setting, Thomas

compared IM and IV droperidol (5 mg) to IM and IV haloperidol (5 mg). IM Droperidol decreased combativeness significantly more than IM haloperidol at 10, 15, and 30 minutes ($P < 0.05$ for all comparisons).[48] There was no significant difference between the two groups treated via the IV route. In another ED setting study, Richards et al. demonstrated IV droperidol to be superior to IV lorazepam by producing better sedation and requiring fewer repeat dosages than lorazepam.[49] Although these studies were performed in the ED setting, the comparative analysis can be extrapolated to the prehospital setting.

Droperidol has been experimentally evaluated in the prehospital setting. In a randomized controlled trial of IV droperidol (5 mg) versus normal saline, Rosen et al. revealed significantly less agitation in combatativs patients 5 and 10 minutes after receiving droperidol. In addition, patients in the normal saline-treated group required more sedation after arrival at the ED.[50] In another prehospital setting evaluating droperidol, Hick published a study of 53 patients with an average agitation score of 4.7 (scale range: 1[least] to 5[most]) and concluded that 5 mg IM droperidol contributed to adequate sedation in this population.[51]

While this drug has demonstrated efficacy in the prehospital sedation of agitated patients, its use may still be limited unless a pretreatment QT interval can be obtained.

Haloperidol

Haloperidol is a high-potency antipsychotic that acts centrally by blocking dopamine. The usual dosage IM is 5–10 mg. This drug has low anticholinergic side effects with a high frequency of extrapyramidal side effects. It has been used for many years in the chemical restraint of acutely agitated patients. Although literature on the use of this drug in the prehospital setting is lacking, evidence from well-designed clinical trials, in the hospital setting, has demonstrated its efficacy.[35,38,43–45,48]

It provides excellent sedation when combined with a benzodiazepine, especially lorazepam as described previously. Its advantages and disadvantages are reviewed in Table 40-6, and a sample prehospital protocol demonstrating the role for haloperidol use is depicted in Table 40-7.

Etomidate

Etomidate is a hypnotic analgesic with minimal cardiovascular side effects. Evidence supporting prehospital use has been mostly limited to its role in sedative-facilitated intubation[52–54] and its role in RSI.[55–56] It has been extensively studied in ED procedural sedation. At doses of 0.2 mg/kg

Table 40-6. Advantages and Disadvantages of the Prehospital Use of Haloperidol

Advantages	Disadvantages
IM or IV use	Extrapyramidal side effects
Rapid onset of action	Cautious use in patients on narcotics or MAOIs
Can be combined with a benzodiazepine	
Minimal respiratory effects	
Achieves effective tranquilization	

effective sedation is achieved with minimal side effects.[57] Extrapolation of this data into the prehospital use for sedation in cardioversion, extrication, and pacing are promising.

SUMMARY

Overall, the area of prehospital pain management and sedation remains poorly studied. Furthermore, emergency care providers at all levels underestimate and undertreat pain, although this may be changing. Pain management by prehospital providers may be improved by providing EMS personnel with expanded education on the subject, and the use of protocols which include an objective pain management scale. The pharmaceutical choices for pain management and sedation will vary depending on the needs of the individual EMS environment. Prehospital pain

Table 40-7. Prehospital Behavioral Emergencies Protocol

Basic Life Support

Secure airway

Administer supplemental oxygen

Record and monitor vital signs

Apply physical restraints if needed to ensure patient/crew safety. Adhere to EMS Procedural Protocol on Physical Restraint of Agitated Patients when this process is deemed necessary

Advanced Life Support

Advanced airway/ventilatory management as needed

Begin cardiac monitoring, record and evaluate ECG strip

Record and monitor O_2 saturation continuously

IV 0.9% NaCl KVO or IV lock if condition warrants

    If BP <90 mmHg systolic, administer boluses of 0.9% NaCl at 250 mL until systolic BP >90 mmHg

    Contraindicated if evidence of congestive heart failure (e.g., rales)

Blood glucose check

Continuous microstream capnography, if patient restrained

For patients with severe agitation resulting in interference with patient care or patient/crew safety, or for patients who continue to struggle against physical restraints

    If cocaine/sympathomimetic toxicity strongly suspected, refer to the cocaine/sympathomimetic toxicity protocol

    Haloperidol (Haldol) 5 mg IV or IM if <60 kg and 10 mg if >60 kg.

    Not to be administered to patients on MAO inhibitors or with allergy

    Administer IM if unable to administer IV

Medical Control Options:

Call Medical Control if further sedation needed

Repeat Haloperidol (Haldol) 5 mg IV or IM or,

Diazepam (Valium) 5 to 10 mg IV or,

Lorazepam (Ativan) 1 to 2 mg IV (can be combined in same syringe with haloperidol) or,

    Midazolam (Versed) 3 – 5 mg IV or IM

ECG: electrocardiogram; KVO: keep vein open.

Note: Select MAO inhibitors: phenelzine(Nardil) and tranylcypromine (Parnate).

management and sedation can be done safely. When performing pain control or sedation EMS providers should maintain a constant level of monitoring, and be prepared to deal with adverse events.

REFERENCES

1. Stewart RD. Pain Control in pre-hospital care. In: Paris PM, Stewart RD, eds. *Pain Management in Emergency Medicine*. Norwalk, CT: Appleton-Lange; 1988:313–321.
2. McEachin DD, McDermott JT, Swor R. Few emergency medical services patients with lower-extremity fractures receive pre-hospital analgesia. *Prehosp Emerg Care*. 2002; 6:406–410.
3. Vassiliadis J, Hitos K, Hill CT. Factors influencing pre-hospital and emergency department analgesia administration to patients with femoral neck fractures. *Emerg Med* (Fremantle). 2002;14:261–266.
4. Luger TJ, Lederer W, Gassner M, et al. Acute Pain is under-assessed in out-of-hospital emergencies. *Acad Emerg Med*. 2003;10:627–632.
5. McLean SA, Domeier RM, DeVore HK, et al. Feasibility of pain measurement in the pre-hospital setting. *Acad Emerg Med*. 2003;10:474–475.
6. Richard-Hibon A, Chollet C, Saada S. A Quality control program for acute pain management in out-of-hospital critical care medicine. *Ann Emerg Med*. 1999;34:738–744.
7. Jones GE, Machen I. Pre-hospital pain management: the paramedics' perspective. *Accid Emerg Nurs*. 2003;11: 166–172.
8. Myers J. Myths of pre-hospital analgesia. *JEMS*. 2003:72–73.
9. Pace S, Burke TF. Intravenous morphine for early pain relief in patients with acute abdominal pain. *Acad Emerg Med*. 1996;3:108–192.
10. Alonso-Serra HM, Wesley K. Position paper: pre-hospital pain management. *Prehosp Emerg Care*. 2003;7:482–488.
11. Acute Pain Management Guideline Panel. *Acute Pain Management: Operative Medical Procedures and Trauma. Clinical Practice Guideline No. 1—AHCPR Publication No. 92–0032*. Rockville, MD: Agency for Health Care Policy and Research; Feb 1992.
12. Wong, DL. *Whaley and Wong's Nursing Care of Infants and Children*. 5th ed. St Louis, MO: Mosby; 1999.
13. Yaster, M. *Pediatric Pain Management and Sedation Handbook*. St Louis, MO: Mosby-Yearbook; 1997.
14. Orange County EMS System Protocols. Orange County, FL; 2004.
15. Bledsoe B, Myers J. Pain and comfort: the pathophysiology of pain and prehospital treatment options. *JEMS*. 2003;28:50–67.
16. Bruns BM, Dieckmann R, Shagoury C, et al. Safety of pre-hospital therapy with morphine sulfate. *Am J Emerg Med*. 1992;10:53–57.
17. Fullerton-Gleason L, Crandall C, Sklar DP. Prehospital administration of morphine for isolated extremity injuries: a change in protocol reduces time to medication. *Prehosp Emerg Care*. 2002;6:411–416.
18. Yaster M, Deshpande JK. Management of pediatric pain with opioid analgesics. *J Pediatr*. 1988;113:421–427.
19. Devellis P, Thomas SH, Wedel SK, et al. Prehospital and emergency department analgesia for air-transported patients with fractures. *Prehosp Emerg Care*. 1998;2:293–296.
20. Devellis P, Thomas SH, Wedel SK, et al. Prehospital fentanyl analgesia in air-transported pediatric trauma patients. *Ped Emerg Care*. 1998;14:321–323.
21. Borland ML, Jacobs I, Geelhoed G. Intranasal fentanyl reduces acute pain in children in the emergency department: a safety and efficacy study. *Emerg Med*. 2002;14:275–280.
22. Kotwal RS, O'Connor KC, Johnson TR, et al. A novel pain management strategy for combat casualty care. *Ann Emerg Med*. 2004;44:121–127.
23. Silfvast T, Saarnivaara L. Comparison of alfentanil and morphine in the prehospital treatment of patients with acute ischaemic-type chest pain. *Eur J Emerg Med*. 2001;8:275–278.
24. Golembiewski J. Safety concerns with meperidine. *J Perianesth Nurs*. 2002;17:123–125.
25. Stene JK, Stofberg L, MacDonald G, et al. Nalbuphine analgesia in the prehospital setting. *Am J Emerg Med*. 1988; 6:634–639.
26. Chambers JA, Guly HR. Prehospital intravenous nalbuphine administered by paramedics. *Resuscitation*. 1994;27:153–158.
27. Houlihan KP, Mitchell RG, Flapan AD, et al. Excessive morphine requirements after pre-hospital nalbuphine analgesia. *J Accid Emerg Med*. 1999;16:29–31.
28. Robinson N, Burrows N. Excessive morphine requirements after pre-hospital nalbuphine analgesia. *J Accid Emerg Med*. 1999;16:392.
29. Ward ME, Radburn J, Morant S. Evaluation of intravenous tramadol for use in the prehospital situation by ambulance paramedics. *Prehospital Disaster Med*. 1997;12:158–162.
30. Vergnion M, Degesves S, Garcet L, et al. Tramadol, an alternative to morphine for treating posttraumatic pain in the prehospital situation. *Anesth Analg*. 2001;92:1543–1546.
31. Stewart RD. Nitrous oxide sedation/analgesia in emergency medicine. *Ann Emerg Med*. 1985;14:139–148.
32. Johnson JC, Atherton GL. Effectiveness of nitrous oxide in a rule EMS system. *J Emerg Med*. 1991;9:45–53.
33. Kaplan RM, Heller MB, McPherson J, et al. An evaluation of nitrous oxide analgesia during transcutaneous pacing. *Prehospital Disaster Med*. 1990;5:145–149.
34. American College of Emergency Physicians. Clinical policy for procedural sedation and analgesia in the emergency department. *Ann Emerg Med*. 1998;31:663–677.
35. Kupas DF, Wydro GC. Position paper: National Association of EMS Physicians. Patient restraint in emergency medical services systems. *Prehosp Emerg Care Online*. 2002;6:1–6.
36. Bosse GM. Benzodiazepines. In: *Emergency Medicine: A Comprehensive Study Guide*. 4th ed. New York: McGraw-Hill; 1996: 759–761.
37. Gilbert DL, Gartside PS, Glauser TA. Efficacy and mortality in treatment of refractory generalized convulsive status epilepticus in children: a meta-analysis. *J Child Neurol*. 1999;14;602–609.

38. Nobay F, Simon BC, Levitt MA, et al. A prospective, double-blind, randomized trial of midazolam versus haloperidol versus lorazepam in the chemical restraint of violent and severely agitated patients. *Acad Emerg Med.* 2004;11:744–749.

39. Wang HE, O'Connor RE, Megargel RE, et al. The utilization of midazolam as a pharmacological adjunct to endotracheal intubation by paramedics. *Prehosp Emerg Care.* 2000;4:14–18.

40. Dickinson ET, Cohen JE, Mechem CC. The effectiveness of midazolam as a single pharmacologic agent to facilitate endotracheal intubation by paramedics. *Prehosp Emerg Care.* 1999; 3:191–193.

41. Swanson ER, Fosnocht DE, Jensen JC. Comparison of etomidate and midazolam for prehospital rapid-sequence intubation. *Prehosp Emerg Care.* 2004;8:273–279.

42. Davis DP, Kimbro TA, Vilke GM. The use of midazolam for prehospital rapid-sequence intubation may be associated with a dose-related increase in hypotension. *Prehosp Emerg Care.* 2001;5:163–168.

43. Battaglia J, Moss S, Rush J, et al. Haloperidol, lorazepam, or both for psychotic agitation? A multicenter, prospective, double-blind, emergency department study. *Am J Emerg Med.* 1997;15:335–340.

44. Bieniek SA, Ownby RL, Penalver A, et al. A double-blind study of lorazepam versus the combination of haloperidol and lorazepam in managing agitation. *Pharmacotherapy.* 1998;18:57–62.

45. Garza-Trevino ES, Hollister LE, Overall JE, et al. Efficacy of combinations of intramuscular antipsychotics and sedative-hypnotics for control of psychotic agitation. *Am J Psychiatry.* 1989;146:1598–1601.

46. Green SM, Kuppermann N, Rothrock SG, et al. Predictors of adverse events with intramuscular ketamine sedation in children. *Ann Emerg Med.* 2000;35:35–42.

47. Porter K. Ketamine in prehospital care. *Emerg Med J.* 2004; 21:351–354.

48. Thomas H, Schwartz E, Petrilli R. Droperidol versus haloperidol for the chemical restraint of agitated and combative patients. *Ann Emerg Med.* 1992;21:407–413.

49. Richards JR, Deriet RW, Duncan DR. Chemical restraint for the agitated patient in the emergency department: lorazepam versus droperidol. *J Emerg Med.* 1998;16:5 67–573.

50. Rosen CL, Ratliff AF, Wolfe RE, et al. The efficacy of intravenous droperidol in the prehospital setting. *J Emerg Med.* 1997;15:13–17.

51. Hick JL, Mahoney BD, Lappe M. Prehospital sedation with intramuscular droperidol: a one-year pilot. *Prehosp Emerg Care.* 2001;5:391–394.

52. Reed DB, Snyder AG, Hogue TD. Regional EMS experience with etomidate for facilitated intubation. *Prehosp Emerg Care.* 2002;6:50–53.

53. Bozeman WP, Young S. Etomidate as a sole agent for endotracheal intubation in the prehospital air medical setting. *Air Med J.* 2002;21:32–35, discussion 35–37.

54. Kociszewski C, Thomas SH, Harrison T, et al. Etomidate versus succinylcholine for intubation in an air medical setting. *Am J Emerg Med.* 2000;18:757–763.

55. Deitch S, Davis DP, Schatterman J, et al. The use of etomidate for prehospital rapid-sequence intubation. *Prehosp Emerg Care.* 2003;7:380–383.

56. Swanson ER, Fosnocht DE, Neff RJ. The use of etomidate for rapid-sequence intubation in the air medical setting. *Prehosp Emerg Care.* 2001;5:142–146.

57. Vinson DR, Bradbury DR. Etomidate for procedural sedation in emergency medicine. *Ann Emerg Med.* 2002;39: 592–598.

41

Management of Pain and Sedation in Neonates

Ghazala Q. Sharieff

HIGH YIELD FACTS

- Newborns have the neuroendocrine mechanisms to feel pain.
- Newborns who undergo multiple painful procedures have increased distress levels during future painful procedures.
- Breast-feeding or administration of a sucrose solution during painful procedures reduces newborn pain scores.
- Due to slower renal clearance of morphine, use 25% of the recommended dose in newborns and titrate as necessary.

Neonates often undergo painful procedures such as lumbar puncture, intravenous (IV) catheter placement, intubation, circumcision, and heel sticks for blood draws without analgesia. Although there is an increasing awareness that neonates do experience pain, many clinicians still limit their use of analgesics in this patient population.[1] While medical personnel often base administration of pain medications to neonates on their own perceptions, newborns have been proven to have the neuroendocrine mechanisms that permit the transmission of pain.[2,3] Studies have shown that neonates, between 28 and 32 weeks' gestational age, who were exposed to multiple painful stimuli had increased distress during future painful procedures when compared with neonates who did not experience these earlier painful stimuli.[4,5]

Pain scales for preterm and term neonates have been developed and use physiologic indicators (such as heart rate, respiratory rate, oxygen saturation, plasma cortisol or catecholamine levels, palmar sweating, and blood pressure) and behavioral changes (such as crying, body position, and facial expression). The Premature Infant Pain Profile (PIPP) uses physiologic indicators and facial expressions (such as the nasolabial furrow, tightly closing the eyes, and the brow bulge) to evaluate pain.[6] The Neonatal Infant Pain Scale (NIPS) uses crying, arm and leg movement, state of arousal, and crying and facial expressions. The CRIES scale specifically addresses Crying, Requirement for oxygen supplementation (for SaO_2 >95%), Increases in heart rate and blood pressure, facial Expression, and Sleeplessness.[7] Other signs of pain include pallor, flushing, diaphoresis, dilated pupils, hyperglycemia, alterations in sleep and wakeful states, fussiness or listlessness, limb withdrawal, arching, or thrashing movements.

NONSTEROIDAL ANTI-INFLAMMATORY DRUGS

Acetaminophen (Paracetamol) can be safely given to preterm and term infants. The usual dosage is 10–15 mg/kg orally and is 20–30 mg/kg rectally. The maximum daily dosage should not exceed 60 mg/kg/day for neonates over 32 weeks' gestational age and 40 mg/kg/day for preterm neonates 28–32 weeks' gestational age.[8,9] If multiple doses are necessary in 28–32-week-old newborns, a time interval of more than 8 hours in between doses is necessary to avoid increasing serum concentrations.[10] While there are several studies investigating the use of ibuprofen for use in neonates for ductal closure,[11,12] there are no studies to date regarding the efficacy or safety of ketorolac or ibuprofen for neonatal pain management.

TOPICAL AND INFILTRATIVE MEDICATIONS

Eutectic mixture of local anesthetic (EMLA), a eutectic formulation of lidocaine and prilocaine is effective in decreasing the pain of procedures such as circumcision, IV catheter insertion, and lumbar puncture.[13–15] EMLA may cause redness and blistering of the penis, so a small area should be tested for hypersensitivity prior to the full application. EMLA has not been shown to be effective for pain reduction from heel sticks.[16,17] EMLA is not recommended for use in newborns less than 36 weeks of age or in preterm infants less than 2 weeks of age due to the potential for systemic drug absorption. EMLA is also contraindicated in patients with G6PD (glucose-6-phosphate dehydrogenase) deficiency or congenital or idiopathic methemoglobinemia. Patients who are taking phenobarbital, phenytoin, sulfonamides, and acetaminophen and use EMLA are at risk for developing methemoglobinemia.[18] The onset of action is 1 hour with duration of action of 1–2 hours after cream removal. Due to concern about systemic absorption, repeat application is not recommended particularly in neonates.

Infiltrative medications are also effective in newborns; however, high doses of local anesthetics may result in seizures and cardiac instability, particularly when using the amide medications, lidocaine and bupivacaine, due to decreased metabolic clearance rates in children. The recommended dose of these agents is therefore lower in neonates. The maximal dose of lidocaine is 4 mg/kg without epinephrine and 5 mg/kg of lidocaine with epinephrine. The maximal dose of bupivacaine is 2 mg/kg regardless of the use of epinephrine.[19] Dorsal penile nerve blocks and penile ring blocks have been shown to be useful in decreasing the pain of circumcision and can be used in conjunction with topical EMLA.[20]

SEDATIVES

Several sedatives have been used successfully in neonates (Table 41-1 lists dosages). Diazepam is not routinely recommended in neonates due to its long half-life and long-acting metabolites. Midazolam is approved for use in neonates, although hypotension, paradoxical agitation, and abnormal movements have been reported. Lorazepam is also used for sedation in newborns but as with all benzodiazepines has been associated with respiratory depression, hypotension, and seizures.[21]

Chloral hydrate has been used in neonates; however, its metabolites may be detrimental. Trichloroethanol may induce hyperbilirubinemia due to interference with the glucuronidation process. Other metabolites of chloral hydrate are trichloracetic acid and trichloroethanol, which have long half-lives and may cause dysrhythmias and renal failure particularly in preterm newborns.[22] If a sedative is to be used in addition to narcotic analgesics, lower doses of both agents should be considered in order to decrease the risk of respiratory depression. Ketamine a dissociative sedative agent is not generally recommended

for sedation in infants less than 3 months of age due to laryngeal hyperexcitability, smaller airway size, and resultant difficulty maintaining a patent airway.[23]

Etomidate is an ultra-short-acting sedative hypnotic with onset of action less than 1 minute and duration of 3–5 minutes; it has minimal cardiorespiratory effects. Standard dose is 0.1–0.3 mg/kg IV. Although etomidate has been used for intubations in infants, there are no studies to date addressing its safety and efficacy for sedation in neonates.[24,25]

Propofol is also an ultra-short-acting sedative hypnotic with no analgesic or amnestic properties. It has an onset of action within one circulation time following IV infusion and an effective duration of action of less than 5–10 minutes. Standard initial dose is 0.5–3 mg/kg, followed by either repeated boluses or a constant infusion at 125–300 µg/kg/min. It can cause pain at the site of infusion, has potent respiratory depressant effects, and can produce significant hypotension. Specific studies regarding the routine use of propofol in neonates in the emergency department setting are lacking; however, a recent study of newborns sedated with propofol in the critical care setting found that increased peripheral distribution volume and reduced metabolic clearance particularly after surgery prolonged elimination time.[26]

OPIOIDS

While many opioids do not have formal Food and Drug Association approval for use in children, their use is widespread and effective in children. Adverse effects are related to the dose, combination agents, and the rate at which the medication is given. Chest wall rigidity may occur with rapid IV administration and/or high doses of fentanyl.

Table 41-1. Commonly Used Medications for Analgesia and Sedation in Neonates*

Agent	Dose	Adverse Effects
Morphine	Start with 0.025 mg/kg IV, SC, IM Maximum first dose: 0.1 mg/kg	Long half-life in neonates
Fentanyl	0.05–1 mcg/kg	Chest wall rigidity, hypotension
Midazolam	0.05 mg/kg IV, 0.1–0.2 mg/kg SC, IM, 0.3–0.5 mg/kg PO, PR	Hypotension, abnormal movements
Lorazepam	0.05–0.1 mg/kg IV	Hypotension, respiratory depression, seizures
Chloral hydrate	25–100 mg/kg PO or PR	Hyperbiliruminemia, cardiac dysrhythmias, and renal failure

IM, intramuscular; PO, oral; PR, rectal; SC, subcutaneous.
*Dosages may vary. Withe drugs such as Morphine, we recommend starting at the lower dose in neonates and titrating to the desired effect. SC is preferred over IM.

Although morphine has been used in neonates, renal clearance is slower resulting in the accumulation of active metabolites. The average half-life of morphine in preterm infants is 9 hours versus 6.5 hours in term neonates. The half-life in older children is only 2 hours. The accumulation of metabolites may cause respiratory depression and seizures. Therefore, in infants less than 6 months of age, initial per kilogram dosing should begin with 25% of the recommended dose for older children[27] Meperidine should be avoided in neonates as accumulation of its metabolite normeperidine can lead to seizures. Fentanyl may be used with starting doses of 0.5–1 µg/kg. Neonates who receive opioids should be placed on continuous cardiac monitoring and pulse oximetry and personnel trained in advanced airway management should be immediately available.

NONPHARMACOLOGIC INTERVENTIONS

Several studies have shown that suckling and breast-feeding is analgesic in neonates.[28,29] A prospective, randomized trial of neonates undergoing heel lances for blood tests revealed that infants who were held and breast-fed by their mothers during the procedure had a reduction in crying and grimacing of 91% and 84%, respectively, when compared to infants who were swaddled in their bassinet.[30]

Another method under investigation is the use of kangaroo care (KC)—maternal skin-to-skin contact.[31] KC was recently shown to significantly lower the PIPP scores in preterm neonates (32–36 weeks' gestational age) undergoing heel lancing procedures. Patients are held in KC for 30 minutes prior to the procedure and remain in this position throughout the heel lancing.[32]

The use of a 12–50% oral sucrose solution has also been shown to control pain effectively in neonates.[33,34] Typically, the newborn is given up to 2 mL of the sucrose solution approximately 2 minutes prior to a painful procedure via a dropper, syringe, or pacifier. Smaller volumes of less than 1 mL should be used in preterm infants.

The effectiveness of oral glucose was recently demonstrated in a study of 201 newborns undergoing venipuncture for clinical reasons. Ninety-one newborns received EMLA on the skin and oral sterile water placebo and 102 newborns received a 1 cc dose of 30% glucose orally placed by syringe into the mouth and placebo on the skin. Staff members or family members were encouraged to pacify the infants with a pacifier or their own fingers. Symptoms associated with pain at venipuncture were measured using the PIPP scales, which have also been validated for full-term infants. Heart rate and crying time were recorded. There was no difference in background variables between the two groups. PIPP scores were lower in the glucose group than the EMLA group and duration of crying in the first 3 minutes was also lower in the glucose group (median 1 second) versus a median of 18 seconds in the EMLA group. Only 19.3% of the glucose group was scored as having pain (defined as a PIPP score of greater than 6) versus 41.7% in the EMLA group. Changes in heart rate and time to successful venipuncture were equivalent in both groups.[35]

Furthermore, combining sucrose, oral tactile stimulation, and parental holding has been associated with reduced crying in infants receiving multiple immunization injections or undergoing painful procedures.[36,37] Table 41-2 lists possible combination therapies for neonatal pain management.[38]

Table 41-2. Pain Control Combination Therapies for Common Neonatal Procedures

Procedure	Suggested Therapy
Heel lance	Consider venipuncture Sucrose pacifier Kangaroo care/swaddling
Percutaneous venous catheter placement/ venipuncture	Sucrose pacifier Kangaroo care/swaddling EMLA
Lumbar puncture	Sucrose pacifier EMLA Subcutaneous lidocaine infiltration
Subcutaneous or intramuscular injection	Use IV medication if possible Sucrose pacifier Kangaroo care/swaddling EMLA
Circumcision	Sucrose pacifier EMLA Dorsal penile nerve block, caudal nerve block Acetaminophen for postoperative analgesia
Umbilical catheter insertion	Sucrose pacifier Swaddling
Nasogastric or orogastric tube placement	Sucrose pacifier Kangaroo care/swaddling Topical lidocaine
Catheterization for urinalysis	Sucrose pacifier Swaddling Topical lidocaine

REFERENCES

1. Simons S, van Dijk M, Anand K, et al. Do we still hurt newborn babies? A prospective study of procedural pain and analgesia in neonates. *Arch Pediatr Adolesc Med*. 2003;157:1058–1064.
2. Klimach VJ, Cooke RW. Maturation of the neonatal somato-sensory evoked response in preterm infants. *Dev Med Child Neurol*. 1988;30:208–214.
3. Warnock F, Sandrin D. Comprehensive description of newborn distress behavior in response to acute pain (newborn mail circumcision. *Pain*. 2004;107:242–255.
4. Bushila D, Zmora E, Bolotin A. Pain sensitivity in prematurely born adolescents. *Arch Pediatr Adolesc Med*. 2003;157:1079–1082.
5. Taddio A, Katz JK, Ilersich AL, et al. Effect of neonatal circumcision on pain response during subsequent routine vaccination. *Lancet*. 1997;349:599–603.
6. Stevens B, Johnston C, Petryshen P, et al. Premature infant pain profile: development and initial validation. *Clin J Pain*. 1996;12:13–22.
7. Krechel SW, Bildner J. CRIES: A new neonatal postoperative pain measurement score: initial testing of validity and reliability. *Pediatr Anaesth*. 1995;5:53–61.
8. Anderson BJ, van Lingen RA, Hansen TG, et al. Acetaminophen developmental pharmacokinetics in premature neonates and infants: a pooled population analysis. *Anesthesiology*. 2002;96:1336–1345.
9. van Linger RA, Deinum HT, Quak CM, et al. Multiple-dose pharmacokinetics of rectally administered acetaminophen in term infants. *Clin Pharmacol Ther*. 1999;66:509–515.
10. van Lingen RA, Deinum JT, Quak JM, et al. Pharmacokinetics and metabolism of rectally administered paracetamol in preterm neonates. *Arch Dis Child Fetal Neonatal Ed*. 1999; 80:F59–F63.
11. Heyman E, Morag I, Batash D, et al. Closure of patent ductus arteriosus with oral ibuprofen suspension in premature newborns: a pilot study. *Pediatrics*. 2003;112(5):e354.
12. Lago P, Bettiol T, Salvadori S, et al. Safety and efficacy of ibuprofen versus indomethacin in preterm infants treated for patent ductus arteriosus: a randomized controlled trial. *Eur J Pediatr*. 2002;161(4):202–207.
13. Taddio A, Stevens B, Craig K, et al. Efficacy and safety of lidocaine-prilocaine cream for pain during circumcision. *N Engl J Med*. 1997;336:1197–1201.
14. Kaur G, Gupta P, Kumar A. A randomized trial of eutectic mixture of local anesthetics during lumbar puncture in newborns. *Arch Pediatr Adolesc Med*. 2003;157:1065–1070.
15. Taddio A, Ohlsson A, Einarson TR, et al. A systematic review of lidocaine-prilocaine (EMLA) cream in the treatment of acute pain in neonates. *Pediatrics*. 1998;101:(2)e1.
16. Stevens B, Johnston C, Taddio A, et al. Management of pain from heel lance with lidocaine-prilocaine (EMLA) cream: is it safe and efficacious in preterm infants? *J Dev Behav Pediatr*. 1999;20:216–222.
17. Larsson BA, Jylli L, Lagercrantz H, et al. Does a local anesthetic cream (EMLA) alleviate pain from heel-lancing in neonates. *Acta Anaesthesiol Scand*. 1995;23:1028–1031.
18. American Academy of Pediatrics, Committee on Drugs. Alternate routes of drug administration: advantages and disadvantages. *Pediatrics*. 1997;100:143–152.
19. Larsson BA, Lonnqvist PA, Olsson GL. Plasma concentrations of bupivacaine in neonates after continuous epidural infusion. *Anesth Analg*. 1997;84:501–505.
20. Holliday MA, Pinckert TL, Kieman SC, et al. Dorsal penile nerve block vs topical placebo for circumcision in low-birth-weight neonates. *Arch Pediatr Adolesc Med*. 1999; 153:476–480.
21. Ng E, Klinger G, Shah V, et al. Safety of benzodiazepines in newborns. *Ann Pharmacother*. 2002;36:1150–1155.
22. American Academy of Pediatrics. Prevention and management of pain and stress in the neonate. *Pediatrics*. 2000;105:454–461.
23. Proudfoot J. Pediatric procedural sedation and analgesia (PSA): keeping it simple and safe. *Pediatr Emerg Med Rep*. 2002;7:13–23.
24. Guldner G, Schultz J, Sexton P, et al. Etomidate for rapid-sequence intubation in young children: hemodynamic effects and adverse events. *Acad Emerg Med*. 2003;10:134–139.
25. Sokolove PE, Price DD, Okada P. The safety of etomidate for emergency rapid sequence intubation of pediatric patients. *Pediatr Emerg Care*. 2000;16:18–21.
26. Rigby-Jones AE, Nolan JA, Priston MJ, et al. Pharmacokinetics of propofol infusions in critically ill neonates, infants and children in an intensive care unit. *Anesthesiology*. 2002;97:1393–1400.
27. Berde C, Sethna N. Analgesics for the treatment of pain in children. *N Engl J Med*. 2003;347:1094–1103.
28. Gray L, Miller LW, Philipp BL, et al. Breastfeeding is analgesic in healthy newborns. *Pediatrics*. 2002;109:590–593.
29. Campbell C. Analgesic effects of sweet solutions and pacifiers in term neonates. Suckling at the breast is better than sweet solutions and pacifiers. *BMJ*. 2000;320(7240):1002.
30. Carbajal R, Veerapen S, Couderc S, et al. Analgesic effect of breast-feeding in term neonates: randomized controlled trial. *BMJ*. 2003;326:13.
31. Gray L, Watt L, Blass EM. Skin-to-skin contact is analgesic in healthy newborns. *Pediatrics*. 2000;105:e14.
32. Johnston C, Stevens B, Pinelli J, et al. Kangaroo care is effective in diminishing pain response in preterm neonates. *Arch Pediatr Adolesc Med*. 2003;157:1084–1088.
33. Stevens B, Taddio A, Ohlsson A, et al. The efficacy of sucrose for relieving procedural pain in neonates: a systematic review and meta-analysis. *Acta Paediatr*. 1997;86:837–842.
34. Stevens B, Ohlsson A. Sucrose for analgesia in newborn infants undergoing painful procedures (Cochrane Review). In: *The Cochrane Library, Issue 4, 1999*. Oxford: Updated Software.

35. Gradin M, Erikson M, Holmqvist G, et al. Pain reduction at venipuncture in newborns: oral glucose compared with local anesthetic cream. *Pediatrics*. 2002;110: 1053–1057.

36. Reis E, Roth E, Sypham J, et al. Effective pain reduction for multiple immunization injections in young infants. *Arch Pediatr Adolesc Med*. 2003;157:1115–1120.

37. Johnston CC, Stremler RL, Stevens BJ, et al. Effectiveness of oral sucrose and simulated rocking on pain response in preterm neonates. *Pain*. 1997;72:193–199.

38. Anand KJS, the International Evidence-Based Group for Neonatal Pain. Consensus statement for the prevention and management of pain in the newborn. *Arch Pediatr Adolesc Med*. 2001;155:174–180.

42

Procedural Sedation and Analgesia in Children with Special Health Care Needs

Alfred D. Sacchetti
Thomas F. Turco

HIGH YIELD FACTS

- Children with special health care needs (CSHCN) frequently need emergency department (ED) procedural sedation and analgesia but present unique challenges.

- No one procedural sedative agent is ideal for every patient in every clinical situation.

- It is critical to establish a child's baseline abnormalities before administering any medications.

- Increases in P_{CO_2} can cause pulmonary vasoconstriction and pulmonary hypertension with changes in pulmonary-aortic shunts.

- In children with central nervous system (CNS) lesions or shunts, increases in P_{CO_2} can cause cerebral vasodilation and increases in intracranial pressure.

- Macroglossia, micrognathia, cervical spine limitations, and hydrocephalus can cause airway problems.

- Head positioning and continuous anterior jaw displacement may limit upper airway obstruction. The laryngeal mask airway should be available along with other airway equipment.

- Underlying medical conditions need to be considered in choosing a sedative and/or analgesic agent.

INTRODUCTION

As a result of tremendous successes in the treatment of childhood illnesses, children with special health care needs (CSHCN) are living longer, healthier, and more normal lives.[1] Like any child, these unique children occasionally require emergency department (ED) care. Some of these ED visits will be for common problems such as minor trauma or febrile illnesses while others will be related to underlying medical conditions. The real challenge for emergency physicians occurs when either of these presentations requires some form of procedural sedation.[2]

PATIENT ASSESSMENT

Preprocedure patient assessment does not change because of a child's underlying medical condition. A focused history and related physical examination define their ED care and the parameters of their procedural sedation. As with any ED patient, the treatment of these children may include simple analgesia, anxiolysis, or sedation for a painless or painful procedure. The same definitions of minimal, moderate, and deep sedation apply equally to CSHCN and those without chronic conditions. Additional information on last meal, medications, prior sedation experiences, and allergies are collected in the same manner as with any other ED patient. Obviously the existence of a prior medical condition necessitates a more extensive history and physical examination prior to delivery of any procedural sedation or analgesia (PSA).[3]

PSA-specific historical questions should attempt to identify as specifically as possible the child's special health care needs. The parents of some patients are extremely knowledgeable concerning the condition of their child while others may have difficulty communicating their child's special needs.[4,5] To address this problem the American College of Emergency Physicians and the American Academy of Pediatrics in conjunction with other agencies have created an Emergency Information Form (EIF) for CSHCN.[6–8] These forms contain all the information required by a health care provider to treat a patient under any emergency situation and can function as a surrogate consultant until a patient's physician is contacted. Other parents may carry a letter describing their child's condition or use some form of medical identification jewelry with a database access to provide information to unfamiliar health care providers. It is certainly worth inquiring as to the existence of an EIF or other related tool when approaching these children.[2]

The physical examination of these children should look specifically for baseline abnormalities. It is important to establish a child's unique physical findings prior to administration of central nervous system (CNS) altering medications. Particular note should be made of preexisting gait abnormalities, coordination problems, and variances between ages and developmental stages or cognitive level to avoid confusion with assessment during the postprocedure period.

The child's presenting problem and underlying special health care needs determine the remainder of the PSA decisions. Modifications in the route of administration are generally not required for CSHCN. Older children with neurodevelopmental problems may present difficulties in obtaining vascular access for parenteral drug administration necessitating use of an intramuscular or preferably subcutaneous route. In these children it is important that an adequate dose of a reliable medication be administered on the first injection because a second approach to these children is likely to be strongly resisted. Similarly, children with chronic medical conditions may suffer loss of peripheral veins secondary to overuse during prior admissions or procedures limiting intravenous (IV) drug administrations.

MONITORING

Standard monitoring approaches to PSA are generally appropriate for CSHCN.[9–11] A more intensive schedule for blood pressure sampling or a slightly longer duration of postprocedure observation may be required in some patients, although this is rarely warranted. The exact value of end-tidal capnometry is unclear in procedural sedation in any patients.[10] Transient elevations in carbon dioxide levels are common during sedative procedures with multiple medications, but appear to have no deleterious effects in American Society of Anesthesiologists (ASA) class I patients.[12–14] The clinical impact of sedation-induced hypercapnia has not been well studied in other ASA classes. Elevated alveolar carbon dioxide tensions can produce pulmonary vasoconstriction and pulmonary hypertension.[15] In children with susceptible cardiac lesions such changes can lead to changes in pulmonary-aortic shunts. Increases in serum CO_2 tensions also produce cerebral vasodilation and elevated intracranial pressures in children with CNS lesions or shunts. Both of these problems are theoretical with little data demonstrating clinically significant adverse effects from transient elevations in carbon dioxide levels.[2,7,12] At this time the role of continuous capnometry in CSHCN is no more defined than that for children without medical problems.

CSHCN can also present unique anatomic challenges for treating clinicians. Macroglossia, micrognathia, cervical spine limitations, and even hydrocephalus can create potential airway problems during moderate or deep sedation. Since most airway obstructions result from skeletal muscle relaxation, the use of agents such as ketamine, etomidate, or fentanyl can help minimize this problem. Meticulous head positioning, as well as

conservative airway maneuvers such as continuous anterior jaw displacement may limit upper airway obstruction. The laryngeal mask airway has proven effective in the operating room management of these patients and should be readily available along with other airway adjuncts and intubation equipment.[16–18]

Selection of Procedural Sedation and Analgesia Agents

The selection of a specific PSA agent for a given child is a function of patient characteristics, clinical presentation, physician preference, and facility capabilities. Although all the pharmacologic characteristics of a medication must be considered, it is frequently the interrelation between the child's underlying condition and a specific drug action that determines it use. Cardiovascular effects may be most important for a child with a cardiac lesion while metabolic pathways are more relevant for a child with liver failure. Table 42-1 describes the pharmacologic actions of commonly used PSA agents.

Selection of a safe agent may be difficult in a child with complex medical problems. Use of an agent that is within the class of drugs a child is already receiving may eliminate concerns regarding drug interactions.[2] For example, if a child is receiving phenobarbital for a seizure disorder, then another barbiturate such as pentobarbital may be used for magnetic resonance imaging (MRI) sedation. Short-acting titratable agents also permit the greatest flexibility when treating unfamiliar patients. The ability to titrate a medication allows administration of small doses while monitoring clinical effects. Similarly, selection of drugs with brief durations of action may limit the severity of any adverse effects that do occur.[19,20]

Neurodevelopmental and Behavioral Conditions

For children with neurologic, developmental, or behavioral problems, recognition of the need for analgesia can be a major problem. Both exaggerated and subdued responses to uncomfortable or painful stimuli may mask true analgesic requirements in this population. Failure to even consider analgesic needs can occur in a child with an abnormal baseline mental status.[19,21] Extrapolation from experiences with similar procedures in other children or even adults can help guide the use of analgesics or local anesthetics when direct evaluation of a patient's pain perception is confusing. In higher functioning nonverbal children a pictorial pain scale may be considered. Most of these children tolerate opioid analgesics well and the

Table 42-1. Characteristics of Analgesic and Sedative Agents

Medication	Ventilations/ Airway Reflexes	Peripheral Vascular Resistance	Intracranial Pressure	Comments
Opioids				
Meperidine	↓	↓	↑*	
Morphine	↓	↓	↑*	10% hepatobiliary excretion
Hydromorphone	↓	↓	↑*	
Fentanyl	↓↓	SL↓	±	Hepatobiliary excretion
Remifentanil	↓↓↓	SL↓	?	Metabolized by nonspecific esterases
Sedative hypnotics				
Chloral hydrate	↓	—	?	
Diazepam	↓	↓	↓	
Lorazepam	↓	↓	↓	
Midazolam	↓↓	↓↓	↓	
Pentobarbital	↓	↓	↓↓	
Thiopental	↓↓↓	↓↓↓	↓↓	
Methohexital	↓↓↓	↓↓↓	↓↓	May lower seizure threshold
Propofol	↓↓↓	↓↓↓	↓↓	
Other agents				
Etomidate	↓	↓	±	
Ketamine	—	SL↑	↑↑	
Nitrous oxide	—	—	—	
Diphenhydramine	—	—	?	
Droperidol	—	↓	?	

↓ Decreases; ↑ increases; ?: insufficient data; ±: studies indicating effects in both directions; -: no effect; ≤: no effect or slight decrease; ≥: no effect or slight increase.

*Rise in intracranial pressure (ICP) may occur as a secondary effect from hypoventilation.

treating clinician can feel comfortable using these medications liberally for acute painful conditions.[21]

For painless diagnostic procedures any of the sedative hypnotics may be considered.[22–24] Disinhibition following normal or low doses of Midazolam has been well described in developmentally normal children and should be anticipated in this population as well. The barbiturates have been used extensively in children in this group for seizure management with predictable reliable actions and have similar profiles for sedation for painless diagnostic studies.[25,26] One caution with this group of drugs involves methohexital, which unlike any of the other barbiturates can lower rather than raise a child's seizure threshold.[27] CAT scan sedation failures in children receiving pentobarbital have been reported in those greater than 12 years of age when a non-weight-based ceiling was placed on the drug dose. Propofol, with its easily titratable dosing has proven effective in children undergoing extended MRI and computed tomography (CT) studies.[24,25]

As noted, theoretical elevations in intracranial pressure can result from hypoventilation and the increased arterial carbon dioxide tension that can result from most sedative agents. Conversely both propofol and the barbiturates directly lower cerebral metabolism and intracerebral pressure producing a protective effect in these patients. These offsetting actions may explain the lack of clinically significant adverse effects with these drugs. If elevated ICP is a serious concern, a protocol employing pentobarbital (2–6 mg/kg) with or without fentanyl (1–3 μg/kg) successfully sedated children for MRI with no detectable hypercapnia.[28] Droperidol has proven effective in the control of acute agitation in older adolescents and psychiatric patients and may be considered in violent or particularly difficult patients.[2] It has been used as part of both procedural sedation and general anesthesia in younger pediatric patients as well.[29]

Cooperation for painful procedures may be accomplished through any of the sedative opioid combinations. All of the drugs in these categories are well tolerated by neurodevelopmental and behavioral patients. Ketamine, a drug commonly used for painful procedures in children, may produce vivid dreaming and should be used with caution in this population. If this drug must be used, it should probably be combined with midazolam to limit recall of ketamine-induced dreams.[2] It should be noted that midazolam will not limit the development of emergence reactions in any children. Etomidate is another drug used for painful procedures and may be considered in these patients. It remains controversial as to whether this drug is truly epileptogenic, however, if possible an alternative should be considered in children with seizure disorders.[27]

Cardiovascular Lesions

Cardiovascular lesions represent a spectrum of diseases in children. From the minimally symptomatic ASA II child with a coronary artery aneurysm to an ASA IV child with a severe cardiomyopathy, these children present a significant physiologic challenge.

Children with cardiac lesions may be particularly sensitive to changes in either their systemic or pulmonary vascular resistance. The preload and after load effects of many sedative and opioid agents can produce dramatic hemodynamic effects in these patients. These actions can be particularly severe in those patients with open communications between the pulmonary and systemic.[15,30-32] Decreases in the vascular resistance of either of these circulations can produce a devastating shift of blood from the higher pressure bed to the lower pressure bed. Medications which decrease peripheral vascular resistance, as many of the sedative and narcotic analgesics do, may produce a right to left shunt with an increase in systemic blood flow at the expense of pulmonary blood flow.[30,31] This is the exact pattern produced in the classic hypercyanotic or Tet spell seen in children with surgical shunts and tetralogy of Fallot. Similar physiologic effects can be produced if pulmonary hypertension develops as a result of drug-induced respiratory depression with hypoxia or hypercarbia.[15]

In other patients, a chronic state of hypoxia-induced pulmonary hypertension is produced following placement of a central surgical shunt. In these patients reversal of their baseline hypoxia with supplemental oxygen can induce a left to right shunt creating systemic hypoperfusion and shock.[33] In such patients a determination of their baseline pulse oximetry will identify a target value to be maintained during the procedural sedation. In most instances this will generally be in the range of 85–90%. As counterintuitive as it seems, supplemental oxygen may need to be withheld in these patients to reverse systemic hypoperfusion or shock that develops following overaggressive oxygen therapy with procedural sedation.[33]

Children with univentricular heart syndromes have a single ventricle which pumps blood to the aorta with a completely passive blood flow to the pulmonary circulation. These patients are preload dependent and rely on vena caval pressure for any blood flow to the pulmonary circulation. Medications that produce peripheral venous dilation will decrease this pressure and drop any return to the heart leading to an overall loss of systemic cardiac output. Similarly, patients with cardiomyopathies may also be very preload dependent requiring higher filling pressures to maintain ventricular wall tension and their cardiac output.[2,32]

For simple analgesia, most of these patients can tolerate standard doses of morphine or other opioid agents. Similarly, in well-hydrated patients, reasonable doses of benzodiazepines or barbiturates for anxiolysis will also be well tolerated. Selection of a cardiovascular neutral agent is preferred whenever possible for PSA in patients with cardiovascular pathology. Most of the literature in this area is based on observations performed during cardiac catheterizations or other interventional procedures.[30-37] Ketamine has been extensively studied in children with cardiac lesions and is well tolerated even in very young infants with complex anatomic lesions.[37] Fentanyl and remifentanil both exhibit flat cardiovascular curves and have been used successfully in this population of patients.[36] Propofol has both respiratory depressant and peripheral vascular actions and has the potential to produce right to left shunts in children with open circulations. Observational studies in children undergoing transesophageal echocardiography and cardiac catheterization demonstrated mixed results on propofol's impact on pulmonary-systemic shunts. In some studies, reductions in systemic pressures increased pulmonary to systemic shunts,[31,32] while in other studies no circulatory effects could be demonstrated.[30] In children undergoing electrophysiologic procedures, propofol produced no significant hemodynamic effects but did slow AV nodal conduction and prevented induction of certain atrial arrhythmias.[33,34,38] Propofol's physiologic effects are most likely the result of direct peripheral vascular actions with no demonstrable effects on cardiac contractility, pulmonary vascular resistance, or heart rate.[32]

Different cardiac catheterization sedation regimens employing propofol-fentanyl, midazolam-fentanyl, or ketamine, all produced statistically significant elevations in end-tidal capnometry raising the possibility of exacerbation of pulmonary hypertension.[15] Again the clinical significance of this hypercapnia remains uncertain.

Respiratory Problems

Because of the large number of asthmatic children, this group accounts for the largest percentage of CSHCN. More than any of the other conditions discussed, respiratory problems can be extremely labile in their clinical presence. Children with severe reactive airway disease may change from being completely asymptomatic to severely bronchospastic within minutes after exposure to a specific antigen. Some PSA agents may be particularly antigenic and may place such children at risk.[2]

During assessment of the patients, parents should be questioned as to baseline pulse oximetry even though preprocedure readings will be obtained in the ED. Anxiety, hyperventilation, or the nature of the presenting complaint can effect a child's oxygen saturation and mislead the clinician into assigning too high or too low of a target value during the PSA.

As has been discussed many procedural agents produce respiratory depression. Decreases in minute ventilation in children with lung pathology and poor alveolar gas exchange may lead to more rapid oxygen desaturation than in those with healthy lungs. Continuous capnometry in these patients will detect hypoventilation before the development of clinical hypoxia.[12–14]

Standard doses of opioids or sedatives are well tolerated by these children for simple analgesia and anxiolysis. With attentive monitoring both the barbiturates and benzodiazepines can be used for procedural sedation in this population.[39–42] Ketamine is frequently advocated for rapid sequence intubation in children with asthma and has much to recommend it for procedural sedation in this population as well.[43] Ketamine has little to no respiratory depression and its sympathomimetic actions can produce bronchodilation. Conversely, ketamine does increase respiratory secretions, which may present a problem in children with cystic fibrosis or similar conditions. The addition of atropine or glycopyrolate with ketamine may help limit this problem.[19,44–46] Etomidate also has less respiratory depression than other agents and may be considered in these children.[47]

Propofol's pharmacokinetics makes it very attractive for painless procedures although some preparations utilize eggs to form the drug's emulsion while others have high concentrations of sulfites and can trigger bronchospasm in asthmatics.[2,44] Midazolam has been used effectively for sedation for pediatric dental patients with no evidence of hypoxia.[39]

Endocrine/Metabolic Problems

Children with endocrine or metabolic disorders present a unique problem for clinicians administering procedural sedation agents. Unlike other CSHCNs, there are few generalizations that can be made about this group of patients and each specific condition responds differently to PSA approaches.

Endocrine patients in general tolerate sedatives and opioid analgesics without difficulty. Diabetic children placed on long-term propofol infusions may require adjustments in their management due to this drug's high caloric content.[2] Etomidate has been shown to produce a clinically insignificant suppression of adrenal function for 6–8 hours in healthy patients. Although never proven to be a problem, an alternative drug should probably be considered in children with an abnormal adrenal-pituitary axis.[48–51]

Children with inborn errors of metabolism must be managed on an individual basis. With so many different conditions now described, no pattern of safety or efficacy can be applied to any of the standard PSA agents. Individual case reports describe the success or failure of different agents in individual children and may be used as a rough guide for children with similar problems. A number of such articles report success with propofol in a wide variety of patients with metabolic disorders.[52–55] Specific problems have also been described with individual PSA agents. Barbiturates induce hepatic enzymes such as 5-aminolevulinic acid synthase, which can lead to exacerbations of intermittent porphyria. Droperidol produces a dose-dependent increase in serum prolactin levels while lorazepam clearance is reduced in children with Gilbert syndrome.[2] Aside from propofol, the safety of opioid analgesics, benzodiazepines and ketamine, have all been reported for various metabolic conditions. When time permits it is probably safest in these patients to examine an online medical database or literature search engine for use of a particular PSA agent in a specific condition.

Hepatic/Renal Problems

Children with liver or kidney abnormalities generally respond well to procedural sedation and analgesic agents. The major problem with PSA in this class of patients is their ability to either metabolize or eliminate the specific drugs. With the exception of remifentanil which is metabolized by nonspecific esterases in the muscle and intestines and nitrous oxide which is excreted unchanged through the lungs, virtually every other PSA agent is metabolized by the liver.[56] In children with liver problems the duration of action of these drugs can be significantly prolonged. Clinically this effect does not impact the initial administration of a sedative or analgesic but could markedly modify the duration of action and subsequent dosing and titration of these agents. When managing children with liver problems it is probably prudent to begin with the smallest effective dose and titrate slowly any additional medication to avoid overtly prolonged actions.

Similarly children with kidney dysfunction or those on renal dialysis will have difficulty excreting administered medications or their metabolites. Aside from fentanyl which does have significant hepatic excretion and nitrous oxide which is excreted entirely by the lungs, all other PSA agents or their metabolites are excreted in the urine. The same approaches used in patients with liver problems apply to those with kidney failure. Minimal effective doses of PSA agents are used initially and titrated cautiously to produce a desired action.

Hematologic/Oncologic Problems

Children with hematologic or oncologic problems frequently undergo procedures requiring sedation and/or analgesia and the use of almost all of the commonly used PSA agents have been very well described in this population.[57–61] Differences in the efficacy of some agents have been noted in studies of children undergoing lumbar punctures or bone marrow biopsies, but none of the drugs listed in Table 42-1 have been regarded as contraindicated in these children. Acetaminophen and aspirin have been reported to produce hemolysis in children with G6PD deficiency.[2]

More of a concern with these patients is the potential for oligoanalgesia in children with chronic painful conditions such as sickle cell anemia. Many of these children develop a tolerance of opioid analgesics and may require doses in excess of the typical mg/kg amounts commonly referenced. In managing acute painful conditions such as

Table 42-2. Procedural Analgesia, Anxiolysis, and Sedation Options

Special Health Care Need	Analgesia	Anxiolysis	Procedural Sedation	
			Painless	**Painful**
Neuro/developmental	Morphine, fentanyl, hydromorphone	Lorazepam, Droperidol, Pentobarbital	Pentobarbital, Propofol, Methohexital	Propofol/fentanyl, Ketamine*, Etomidate
Cardiovascular	Fentanyl, hydromorphone, morphine	Lorazepam, Diazepam, Morphine	Fentanyl, Ketamine, Midazolam	Fentanyl, Ketamine, Etomidate
Respiratory	Hydromorphone, morphine, fentanyl	Lorazepam, Diazepam, Morphine	Ketamine, Propofol, Etomidate	Ketamine, Etomidate, fentanyl
Hepatic/renal	Morphine, remifentanil, fentanyl	Lorazepam, Diazepam, Morphine	Midazolam, Propofol, Nitrous Oxide	Ketamine, Etomidate, Remifentanil
Endocrine/metabolic	Morphine, hydromorphone, nitrous oxide	Lorazepam, Pentobarbital†, Diazepam	Propofol, Methohexital, Midazolam	Propofol/fentanyl, Ketamine, Remifentanil
Heme/oncologic	Hydromorphone, morphine, fentanyl	Lorazepam, Diazepam, Morphine	Propofol, Methohexital, Etomidate	Propofol/fentanyl Ketamine Etomidate

*Consider adding midazolam for psychiatric patients.
†Caution with porphyria.

fractures or burns, the amount of analgesic administered should be based on the child's clinical response and not be limited by weight-based dosing regimens.[2]

One other precaution in the treatment of these patients is the use of pulse oximetry in patients with severe anemias. Supplemental oxygen should be used liberally in these patients to maintain oxygen saturation between 97 and 100%. A child with a serum hemoglobin of 7 g/dL and 100% oxygen saturation will have a tissue oxygen delivery similar to that of a child with a hemoglobin of 14 g/dL and a 70% oxygen saturation.

Scenario-Specific Medications

No single PSA agent is ideal for any patient or any scenario. For CSHCN this is even more accurate. For most clinical encounters any number of agents can be used safely and effectively. Table 42-2 lists some options that might be considered for use in different ED situations. It is also very clear that because of the unique needs of these patients, treating clinicians will require access to a complete formulary of PSA agents to provide the safest care for these children.

SUMMARY

CSHCN will continue to become more frequent visitors to all EDs. The effective application of analgesia and procedural sedation in these children will now be an ongoing emergency medicine expectation.

REFERENCES

1. The Future of Pediatric Education II (FOPE): organizing pediatric education to meet the needs of infants, children, adolescents, and young adults in the 21st century. *Pediatrics.* 2000;105(suppl):161–212.
2. Sacchetti A, Turco T, Carraccio C, et al. Procedural sedation for children with special health care needs. *Pediatr Emerg Care.* 2003;19:231–239.
3. Sacchetti AD. Procedural sedation and analgesia. In: Gausche-Hill M, Fuchs S, Yamamaoto L, eds. *APLS The Pediatric Emergency Medicine Resource.* 4th ed. Sudbury, MA: Jones and Bartlett; 2004.
4. Sacchetti A, Sacchetti C, Carraccio C, et al. The potential for errors in children with special health care needs. *Acad Emerg Med.* 2000;7:1330–1333.
5. Carraccio CL, Dettmer KS, duPont ML, et al. Family member knowledge of children's medical problems: the need for universal application of an emergency data set. *Pediatrics.* 1998;102:367–370.
6. Sacchetti AD, Gerardi M, Barkin R, et al. Emergency data set for children with special needs. *Ann Emerg Med.* 1996;28: 324–327.
7. American College of Emergency Physicians. Emergency information form for children with special health care needs. *Ann Emerg Med.* 1999;34:577–582.
8. Committee on Pediatric Emergency Medicine, American Academy of Pediatrics. Emergency preparedness for children with special health care needs. *Pediatrics.* 1999;104:e53.
9. American Academy of Pediatrics. Guidelines for monitoring and management of pediatric patients during and after sedation for diagnostic and therapeutic procedures. *Pediatrics.* 1992;89:1110–1115.
10. American Academy of Pediatrics. Guidelines for monitoring and management of pediatric patients during and after sedation for diagnostic and therapeutic procedures: addendum. *Pediatrics.* 2002;110:836–838.
11. American College of Emergency Physicians. Clinical policy for procedural sedation and analgesia in the emergency department. *Ann Emerg Med.* 1998;31:663–677.
12. McQuillen KK, Steele DW. Capnography during sedation/ analgesia in a pediatric emergency department. *Pediatr Emerg Care* 2000;16:401–404.
13. Friesen RH, Alswang M. End-tidal P_{CO_2} monitoring via nasal cannula in pediatric patients: accuracy and sources of error. *J Clin Monit.* 1996;12:155–159.
14. Hart LS, Berns SD, Houck CS, et al. The value of end-tidal CO_2 monitoring when comparing three methods of conscious sedation for children undergoing painful procedures in the emergency department. *Pediatr Emerg Care.* 1997;13:189–193.
15. Friesen RH, Alswang M. Changes in carbon dioxide tension and oxygen saturation during deep sedation for paediatric cardiac catheterization. *Paediatr Anaesth.* 1996;6:15–20.
16. Ezri T, Szmuk P, Warters RD, et al. Difficult airway management practice patterns among anesthesiologists practicing in the United States: have we made any progress? *J Clin Anesth.* 2003;156:418–422.
17. Bogetz MS. Using the laryngeal mask airway to manage the difficult airway. *Anesthesiol Clin North Am.* 2002;204: 863–870.
18. Infosino A. Pediatric upper airway and congenital anomalies. *Anesthesiol Clin North Am.* 2002;20:747–766.
19. Sacchetti AD, Schafermeyer R, Gerardi M, et al. Pediatric analgesia and sedation. *Ann Emerg Med.* 1994;23:237–250.
20. Dial S, Silver P, Bock K, et al. Pediatric sedation for procedures titrated to a desired degree of immobility results in unpredictable depth of sedation. *Pediatr Emerg Care.* 2001;17: 414–420.
21. Gakal B, Scott CS, MacNab AJ. Comparison of morphine requirements for sedation in Down's syndrome and non-Down's patients following paediatric cardiac surgery. *Paediatr Anaesth.* 1998;8:229–233.
22. D'Agostino J, Terndrup TE. Chloral hydrate versus midazolam for sedation of children for neuroimaging: a randomized clinical trial. *Pediatr Emerg Care.* 2000;16:1–4.
23. Moro-Sutherland D, Algern JT, Penelope TL, et al. Comparison of intravenous midazolam with pentobarbital for sedation for head computed tomography imaging. *Acad Emerg Med.* 2000;7:1370–1375.

24. Havel CJ, Strati RT, Hennes HA. Clinical trial of propofol vs midazolam for procedural sedation in a pediatric emergency department. *Acad Emerg Med.* 1999;6:989–997.

25. Bloomfield ED, Masaryk TJ, Caplin A, et al. Intravenous sedation for MR imaging of the brain and spine in children: pentobarbital vs propofol. *Radiology.* 1993;186:93–97.

26. Beekman RP, Hoorntje TM, Beek FJ, et al. Sedation for children undergoing magnetic resonance imaging: efficacy and safety of rectal thiopental. *Eur J Pediatr.* 1996;155: 820–822.

27. Modica PA, Tempelhoff R, White PF. Related articles, pro- and anticonvulsant effects of anesthetics (Part II). *Anesth Analg.* 1990;70:433–444.

28. Connor L, Burrows PE, Zurakowski D, et al. Effects of IV pentobarbital with and without fentanyl on end-tidal carbo dioxide levels during deep sedation of pediatric patients undergoing MRI. *Am J Roentgenol.* 2003;181:1691–1694.

29. Milnes AR, Maupome G, Cannon J. Intravenous sedation in pediatric dentistry using midazolam, nalbuphine and dro-peridol. *Pediatr Dent.* 2000;22:113–119.

30. Gozal D, Rein AJ, Nir A, et al. Propofol does not modify the hemodynamic status of children with intracardiac shunts undergoing cardiac catheterization. *Pediatr Cardiol.* 2001; 22:488–490.

31. Wodey E, Chonow L, Beneurx S, et al. Haemodynamic effects of propofol vs thiopental in infants: an echocardio-graphic study. *Br J Anaesth.* 1999;82:516–520.

32. Williams GD, Jones TK, Hanson KA, et al. The hemo-dynamic effects of propofol in children with congenital heart disease. *Anesth Analg.* 1999;89:1411–4416.

33. Sacchetti A, Wernovsky G, Paston C, et al. Hypoventilation and hypoxia in reversal of cardiogenic shock in an infant with congenital heart disease. *Emerg Med J.* in press.

34. Wu MH, Lin JL, Lai LP, et al. Radiofrequency catheter ablation of tachycardia in children with and without con-genital heart disease: indications and limitations. *Int J Cardiol.* 2000;72:221–227.

35. Lai LP, Lin JL, Wu MH, et al. Usefulness of intravenous propofol anesthesia for radiofrequency catheter ablation in patients with tachyarrhythmias pacing. *Clin Electrophysiol.* 1999;22:1358–1364.

36. Donmez A, Kizilkan A, Berksun H, et al. One center's experience with remifentanil infusions for pediatric cardiac catheterization. *J Cardiothorac Vasc Anesth.* 2001;15:736–739.

37. Pees C, Haas NA, Ewert P, et al. Comparison of analgesic/ sedative effect of racemic ketamine and S(+)-ketamine during cardiac catheterization in newborns and children. *Pediatr Cardiol.* 2003;24:424–429.

38. Erb TO, Kanter RJ, Hall JM, et al. Comparison of electro-physiologic effects of propofol and isoflurane-base anes-thetics in children undergoing radiofrequency catheter ablation for supraventricular tachycardia. *Anesthesiology.* 2002;96:1386–1394.

39. Kil N, Zhu JF, VanWagnen C, et al. The effects of midazolam on pediatric patients with asthma. *Pediatr Dent.* 2003;25:137–142.

40. Newman DH, Azer MM, Pitetti RD, et al. When is a patient safe for discharge after procedural sedation? The timing of adverse effect events in 1367 pediatric procedural sedations. *Ann Emerg Med.* 2003;42:627–635.

41. Egelhoff JC, Ball WS Jr, Koch BL, et al. Safety and efficacy of sedation in children using a structured sedation program. *Am J Roentgenol.* 1997;168:1259–1262.

42. Greenberg SB, Adams RC, Aspinall CL. Initial experience with intravenous pentobarbital sedation for children under-going MRI at a tertiary care pediatric hospital: the learning curve. *Pediatr Radiol.* 2000;30:689–691.

43. Godambe SA, Elliot V, Matheny D, et al. Comparison of propofol/fentanyl versus ketamine/midazolam for brief orthopedic procedural sedation in a pediatric emergency department. *Pediatrics.* 2003;112:116–123.

44. Green SM, Kuppermann N, Rothrock SG, et al. Predictors of adverse events with intramuscular ketamine sedation in children. *Ann Emerg Med.* 2000;35:35–42.

45. Havel CJ Jr, Strait RT, Hennes H. A clinical trial of propofol vs midazolam for procedural sedation in a pediatric emergency department. *Acad Emerg Med.* 1999;6:989–997.

46. Kim G, Green SM, Denmark K, et al. Ventilatory response during dissociative sedation in children—a pilot study. *Acad Emerg Med.* 2003;10:140–145.

47. Vinson DR, Bradbury DR. Etomidate for procedural seda-tion in emergency medicine. *Ann Emerg Med.* 2002;30: 592–598.

48. Absalom A, Pledger D, Kong A. Adrenocortical function in critically ill patients 24 hours after a single dose of etomidate. *Anaesthesia.* 1999;54:861–867.

49. Allolio B, Dorr H, Stuttmann R, et al. Effect of a single bolus of etomidate upon eight major corticosteroid hor-mones and plasma ACTH. *Clin Endocrinol* (Oxf). 1985;22:281–286.

50. Dickinson R, Singer A, Wesley C. Etomidate for pediatric sedation prior to fracture reduction. *Acad Emerg Med.* 2001;8:74–77.

51. Schenarts CL, Burton JH, Riker RR. Adrenocortical dys-function following etomidate induction in emergency depart-ment patients. *Acad Emerg Med.* 2001;8(1):1–7.

52. Bennun M, Goldstein B, Finkelstein Y, et al. Continuous propofol anaesthesia for patients with myotonic dystrophy. *Br J Anaesth.* 2000;85:407–409.

53. Sarantopoulos CD, Brantanow NC, Stowe DF, et al. Une-ventful propofol anesthesia in patients with coexisting here-ditary coproporphyria and hereditary angioneurotic edema. *Anesthesiology.* 2000;92:607–609.

54. Pazvanska EE, Hinkov OD, Stojnovska LV. Uneventful pro-pofol anaesthesia in patients with acute intermittent porphyria. *Eur J Anaesthesiol.* 1999;16:485–492.

55. Williams KS, Hankerson JG, Ernst M, et al. Use of propofol anesthesia during outpatient radiographic imaging studies in patients with Lesch-Nyhan syndrome. *J Clin Anesth.* 1997;9:61–65.

56. Schwinn DA, Shafer ST. Basic principles of pharmacology related to anesthesia. In: Miller RD, ed. *Anesthesia.* 5th ed. Philadelphia, PA: Churchill Livingstone; 2000:15–44.

57. Neirotti MT. Intravenous methohexital for brief sedation of pediatric oncology outpatients: physiologic and behavioral responses. *Pediatrics.* 1997;99(5):E8.

58. Guenther E, Pribble CG, Junkins EP, et al. Propofol sedation by emergency physicians for elective pediatric outpatient procedures. *Ann Emerg Med.* 2003;42:783–791.

59. Hertzog JH, Dalton HJ, Anderson BD, et al. Prospective evaluation of propofol anesthesia in the pediatric intensive care unit for elective oncology procedures in ambulatory and hospitalized children. *Pediatrics.* 2000;106: 742–747.

60. Jayabose S, Levendoglu-Tugal O, Giamelli J, et al. Intravenous anesthesia with propofol for painful procedures in children with cancer. *J Pediatr Hematol Oncol.* 2001;23: 290–293.

61. Keidan I, Berkenstadt H, Sidi A, et al. Propofol/remifentanil versus propofol alone for bone marrow aspiration in paediatric haemato-oncological patients. *Paediatr Anaesth.* 2001;11:297–301.

43

Pain Management and Procedural Sedation for Pediatric Patients

Sharon E. Mace

HIGH YIELD FACTS

- Individuals of all ages, even newborns, experience pain.
- Infants have similar or greater physiologic/hormonal responses to pain than older children and adults.
- Failure to treat pain can have negative short-term and long-term effects on the individual.
- Evidence indicates that pediatric patients receive less analgesia (oligoanalgesia) than adults.
- Early experiences with pain may affect later responses and behaviors.
- Inadequate analgesia for initial procedures decreases analgesic effectiveness for later procedures.
- Pharmacologic differences exist between infants, older children, and adults that affect a drug's activity/effectiveness.
- Nonpharmacologic techniques are safe, effective, based on age/development, may not work in all patients, do not necessarily eliminate drug therapy.
- Choice of drugs for procedural sedation and analgesia (PSA) depends on the patient (age, developmental level, comorbidity, allergies, medications, special needs), the procedure (painful vs. painless, the specific procedure, the duration of procedure), and institution/emergency department (ED) factors.

DEVELOPMENTAL ASPECTS OF PAIN

The fetus, by late gestation, has all the requisite anatomic, hormonal, and neurophysiologic elements to perceive pain and respond to stress.[1–4] Cutaneous sensory nerve terminals (nociceptors) appear by 7 weeks of gestation and exist throughout the body by 20 weeks' gestation.[5] The entire quota of cortical neurons in the central nervous system is present by 20 weeks' gestation. Synapses between the sensory nerve fibers and the interneurons located in the dorsal horn of the spinal cord are also formed by 20 weeks gestation.[4] Myelination of the pain transmission pathways between the spine and brain is completed by 22–30 weeks' gestation, to the thalamus by 30 weeks gestation, and to the cortex by 37 weeks gestation.[6,7] The cortical descending inhibitory pathways develop postterm.[7]

Both excitatory and inhibitory neurotransmitters and neuromodulators exist in the fetus with a preponderance toward the excitatory neurotransmitters.[3] Receptors for the excitatory neurotransmitters are widespread in the neonate with postnatal regression to the adult model.[3]

Differences between neonates and infants with children and adults exist. Neonates are considered *hypersensitive* to noxious stimuli.[3,7,8] This is evidenced by the following:

- A lower threshold for reflex withdrawal to mild stimuli in neonates than adults.[3]
- Painful stimuli cause a more protracted discharge from spinal cord neurons in neonatal animals compared to adults.[7–9]
- There is a greater overlap of cutaneous nociceptor fields in neonates.[7]
- The spinal dorsal horn neurons receive input from a wider body surface area in newborns.[7–9]
- Inhibitory pain pathways only become fully functional later during development.[7–8]

The net result is that infants exhibit similar or even more intense physiologic and hormonal responses to pain than older children and adults.[2] The neonate has a nonspecific and more poorly organized response to sensory stimuli that occurs at a lower threshold than the older child or adult.[3] The infant has similar physiologic and behavioral responses to both painful and nonpainful stimuli confounding the ability to adequately assess pain intensity in infants.[3]

OVERVIEW OF PEDIATRIC PAIN ASSESSMENT AND MANAGEMENT

There is evidence indicating that children and infants receive less analgesia than adults for equivalent surgical procedures and types of pain, especially in the youngest patients.[10–16] This may be at least partly related to ill-conceived assumptions about pain in children and infants.[17,18] Such myths and misperceptions have lead to inadequate pain management in pediatric patients and have been disproved by much research in recent years.[17,18] The idea that children and infants are unable to experience pain because of an immature nervous system and that there are no untoward effects of untreated pain has been disproved and should be abandoned.[18]

In Eland's study of postoperative pain management in the mid-1970s, 25 children ages 4–8 years status post major surgery including amputations, nephrectomies, and cardiac surgery for atrial septal defect were compared with 18 adult postoperative patients.[10] Only 48% (12/25) of the pediatric patients received any pain medications during their entire hospital stay. Furthermore, the pediatric patients received a total of 24 doses of analgesics, while the adults were given 671 doses of analgesics, which consisted of 372 doses of narcotics and 299 doses of nonnarcotic pain medications.[10]

In a 1988 survey of British pediatric anesthesiologists, 13% stated that neonates (from birth to 1 month of age) did not feel pain and another 2% replied they did not know. In this same survey, even though they were aware that infants (age 1–12 months) did feel pain, over 10% of the pediatric anesthesiologists failed to provide them with adequate postoperative analgesia following major surgery for a variety of reasons.[11] One reason given for this oligoanesthesia or lack of anesthesia was a concern over *potential side effects or toxicity* with the use of potent analgesics in infants/younger children.[11] The risks of using "strong" pain relievers was thought to be greater than the benefits so that "milder" safer drugs were chosen to treat pediatric pain.[11]

Later studies again documented undertreatment of pediatric pain.[12–19] One reason given for this oligoanesthesia is a lack of knowledge of and/or a disbelief in the recommended safe dose of pain medications in the pediatric patient. Barriers to effective pediatric pain management include the following:

- Lack of knowledge.
- A failure to assess/reassess for pain.
- Difficulty or misunderstanding of how to conceptualize and measure the subjective pain experience in a child.
- Fears of possible addiction.
- Concern over medication side effects/complications including respiratory depression.
- The perception that pain management in infants/children consumes too much time and effort.
- The misbelief that pain may be useful ("pain builds character").[12,13,19]

Additional barriers to the assessment of pain and the appropriate management of pain in pediatric patients include age and developmental issues. Pain assessment in infants and young children is difficult. Self-report is thought to be the best way to assess pain but is not possible in infants and young children. The inability to communicate or verbalize their pain complicates pain assessment in children. Failure to understand the magnitude of *numbers* or abstract concepts such as pain makes it difficult to quantify pain in young children. Behavioral observations and physiologic parameters are nonspecific and can be affected by many variables including infection, illness, injury and fear, as well as pain. Notwithstanding these confounding issues, reliable pain scales in infants and very young children have been constructed based on such behavioral and physiologic variables.

ED reports/surveys from 1987 to 2000 have repeatedly identified oligoanesthesia and the use of less desirable medications and techniques for sedation and analgesia of infants and children.[20–27] In one study, no child with an extremity fracture was discharged from the ED with an analgesic prescription.[23]

More recent surveys indicate that this trend of oligoanesthesia is changing. Health care professionals have a greater awareness of both the assessment and management of pain in infants and children.[28–31] There is now the widespread use of procedural sedation and analgesia (PSA) for children with appropriate pharmacologic agents in EDs.[28–31]

In spite of these barriers and confounding factors, pain assessment and adequate pain management in pediatric patients can and should be a goal of all practitioners who care for infants and children. There have been numerous policy statements, clinical reports, and other documents from many professional organizations delineating the key principles of pain assessment and management in infants, children, and adolescents.[2,19,32–34]

EFFECTS OF INADEQUATE PAIN MANAGEMENT AT A YOUNG AGE

There is evidence that failure to adequately treat pain in pediatric patients has both short-term and long-term consequences.[3,7,19] Animal and human studies indicate that early painful experiences affect later physiologic responses and behaviors.[3,7,19]

Persistent anatomical changes in the receptive fields of dorsal horn neurons occurred in young rats that endured skin wounds.[35,36] Increased innervation and decreased pain thresholds were present for months following the injury.[35,36] Another murine study demonstrated greater responses to both painful and nonpainful stimuli in young rats that underwent repeated needlepricks over several days than the control rats that had no needlepricks.[37] When examined histologically, the young rats that endured the painful needlepricks had changes in brain tissue histology suggesting increased plasticity of the neonatal brain, which increased their vulnerability to stress disorders and anxiety as adults.[37] This study found a lower pain threshold in young rats subjected to early repeated painful stimuli. When adult rats were exposed to repeated noxious stimuli, they demonstrated greater stress responses than the control rats.[37]

Studies in humans indicate that there may be short-term and long-term effects of painful stimuli in the newborn period. The response to a painful stimuli (heel stick) was evaluated in newborns.[38] The newborn's experience (increased incidence of invasive procedures) affected their pain response. Behavioral immaturity was associated with a greater frequency of invasive procedures.[38] Studies in male newborns who were circumcised at ≤2 days of age had higher pain scores and longer episodes of crying than uncircumcised male infants.[39] Older male infants who were circumcised without anesthesia as newborns were compared with uncircumcised male infants when they received an immunization.[39] The previously circumcised infants had greater distress during the immunization than the uncircumcised infants.[39]

Evidence indicates that experiences in the Neonatal Intensive Care Unit (NICU) also affect the pain response. NICU graduates who had blood sampling via heel stick as newborns demonstrated greater sensitivity in their heels and a broader receptive area of sensitivity than the location of the initial heel stick.[7] Such research suggests that early pain experiences can modify or sensitize the developing sensory nervous system. Additional factors that modify behavioral and physiologic responses to pain in heel stick studies include younger (postconceptional) age and recently having undergone a painful event.[40]

When NICU graduates were compared with full-term normal newborn nursery graduates at 18 months of age, the NICU graduates were less sensitive or reactive to painful stimuli but had more somatic complaints.[41] Another report that compared preterm infants with full-term infants at 4 months of age found no significant difference in behavioral responses after a finger prick, but did find differences in the cardiac autonomic responses and in the behavioral recovery.[42] Pain complaints in 3–4-year-olds were associated with length of stay in the NICU.[43] The longer the NICU stay, the greater number of invasive procedures (and painful experiences) endured, and a greater sensitivity to pain in the 3–4-year-olds.[43] In another study, 8–10-year-old children were queried about a series of pictures of children in potentially painful situations. The low-birth rate NICU graduates assigned significantly higher pain scores for medical pain intensity than for psychosocial pain, in marked contrast to infants with birth weights >2500 g.[44]

Neonates exposed to multiple painful stimuli have greater distress during later painful procedures than neonates who did not endure these earlier painful stimuli.[45,46] Similar findings occurred in older children (<8 years old) undergoing painful procedures associated with cancer therapy. Inadequate analgesia for initial procedures decreased the effectiveness of analgesia in later procedures.[47]

The impact of pain and the benefits of pain therapy in infants in the short term have been documented. Inadequate anesthesia in neonates undergoing surgery results in a tremendous release of stress hormones.[7] This surge of stress hormones leads to hemodynamic instability, marked variability in intracranial pressure, catabolism, and immunosuppression. Studies of newborns requiring ventilatory support who received opioids documented improved hemodynamic stability.[7,48] In the No Pain Trial, neonates in the NICU had better outcomes when their management included limiting their painful experiences.[48]

In summary, although much of this information is preliminary and more research is needed, when infants and children have painful experiences there are both short-term and long-term consequences. Furthermore, appropriate pain management in such infants appears to have many beneficial effects. Early pain experiences responses affect later pain behaviors and physiologic response.

DEVELOPMENTAL PHARMACOLOGY

These are many age-related physiologic parameters that can affect the metabolism and action or effectiveness of drugs used for analgesia and procedural sedation.

The compartments of the body (water, muscle, fat) vary with age.[49] Total body water is greatest in infants (preterm infants > term infants > child > adult) and decreases from over 80% in preterm infants to about 60% in adults.[49] This high total body water creates a larger volume of distribution for water-soluble drugs in infants and younger children.[50] The net result is that a larger initial mg/kg dose of drug is needed to attain a similar blood drug level (e.g., succinylcholine and most antibiotics).[51] The larger volume of distribution also delays excretion of the drug, producing an increased dosing interval in neonates.[50]

On the other hand, infants have comparatively less fat and muscle compared to children and adults.[49] This produces a smaller reservoir for drugs that depend on redistribution into these tissues for termination of drug effects. The consequence is that drugs dependent on redistribution into these tissues for their termination of action may have a longer clinical effect (e.g., thiopental and fentanyl).[51]

The distribution of the cardiac output differs in older children than infants. A larger percent of cardiac output goes to the liver and kidneys in children >2 years of age compared to infants. Young children (ages 2–6 years), have a higher mass per kilogram of body weight of liver and kidneys compared to adults and infants.[52] These are factors at least partly responsible for the shorter drug half-life in children over 2 years of age. As an example, pediatric cancer patients are given PO morphine sustained release every 8 hours instead of every 12 hours as in adults. During adolescence, the drug half-life lengthens approaching that of adults, while infants have a longer drug half-life (Fig. 43-1).

Drug clearance, both hepatic and renal, is generally decreased in newborns, especially in the premature infant.[53] (Fig. 43-1) Overall hepatic drug metabolism depends on several factors: metabolic activity of the specific hepatic microsomal enzyme system (cytochrome P-450), the size of the liver, and the free drug available.[52] The amount of free drug available is determined by the plasma protein binding which is affected by the concentration of albumin and α_1-acid glycoprotein.[50] The limited metabolic clearance of some medications in infants, because of the immature cytochrome P-450 and glucuronyl transferases, leads to an increased dosing interval in infants (e.g., morphine and benzodiazepines).[50]

Infants, especially neonates, have fewer plasma proteins (such as albumin and α_1-acid glycoprotein) that bind drugs.[50] Neonates because of their lower plasma protein concentrations have a greater fraction of free or unbound drug when drugs with high protein binding are used, which may result in increased drug effect or even drug toxicity.

The decreased glomerular filtration rate seen in neonates, and to a lesser degree in infants, may limit the renal excretion of a parent drug and its renally excreted

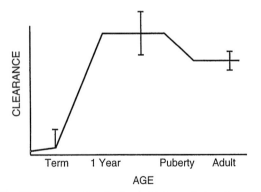

Fig. 43-1. Representative developmental changes in drug clearance. (Reprinted with permission from Nies AS. Principles of therapeutics. In: Hardman JG, Limbird LE, eds. *Goodman & Gilman's The Pharmacological Basis of Therapeutics*. 10th ed. New York: McGraw-Hill; 2001:52.)

metabolites leading to accumulation.[50] This issue may be addressed by increasing the dosing interval and/or lowering the infusion rate.[50]

Infants and children have a reduced pulmonary reserve relative to adults due to the following:

- Smaller airway caliber leading to greater work of breathing related to increased airways resistance.
- Higher ratio of oxygen consumption to functional residual capacity (FRC) so they desaturate more quickly even if preoxygenated.
- Decreased amount of laryngeal and tracheal cartilage (leading to decreased rigidity of the larynx and trachea).
- FRC close to alveolar closing volume.
- Lesser number of diaphragmatic type 2 muscle fibers leading to faster diaphragmatic fatigue.
- Decreased control of the extrinsic respiratory muscles.
- Diminished ventilatory responses to hypercarbia and hypoxia.

Infants, particularly neonates, have high metabolic rates and oxygen consumption. Coupled with a limited pulmonary reserve this makes them even more vulnerable to medications that produce hypoventilation and apnea.[50]

PAIN THERAPY FOR PEDIATRIC PATIENTS

Both nonpharmacologic and pharmacologic modalities are employed in pediatric pain management.

Nonpharmacologic Approaches to Pain Therapy

Nonpharmacologic interventions are valuable tools in the management of pediatric pain serving as adjuncts to the pharmacologic agents, or as stand-alone therapies. However, the use of nonpharmacologic therapy may not be sufficient for some patients, necessitating the addition of analgesic agents. Nonpharmacologic modalities must be tailored to the patient's age and developmental level, and are typically employed to relieve fear and anxiety in addition to pain. Nonpharmacologic methods are safe and have been documented to be effective. Cognitive behavioral therapy is valuable in dealing with acute pain, may assist the child in dealing with new challenges and situations, and provides a sense of accomplishment in mastering the symptoms of an acute situation (Table 43-1).

Addressing the immediate environment in which the child or infant is being treated as part of family-centered care is a necessary component of pediatric pain management.[54] Allowing the option of family presence and

Table 43-1. Techniques for Sedation and Analgesia in Pediatric Patients

Nonpharmacologic Techniques	Pharmacologic Agents for Analgesia and Sedation
Family-centered care	Nonopioids
Reassurance and explanation	Acetaminophen
Family presence	Aspirin
Inclusion of parents/caregivers as assistants	NSAIDs—oral
(when appropriate)	Ibuprofen
Music	Naproxen
Humor	NSAIDs—parenteral
Cognitive techniques	Ketorolac
Guided imagery	Opioids
Sensory focusing	Codeine
Controlled breathing	Morphine
Relaxation	Hydromorphone
Biofeedback	Meperidine
Yoga	Fentanyl
Psychotherapy	Sedative/hypnotics
Individual	Chloral hydrate
Family	Benzodiazepines
Hypnosis/hypnotherapy	Midazolam
Acupuncture	Diazepam
Massage therapy	Lorazepam
Physical therapy	Barbiturates
Transcutaneous electrical nerve stimulation (TENS)	Methohexital
Additional Techniques for Neonates/Infants	Pentobarbital
Oral sucrose	Thiopental
Breast feeding	Etomidate
Oral tactile stimulation (pacifier)	Propofol
Kangaroo care (KC) maternal skin-to-skin contact	Ketamine (dissociative agent)
Swaddling	Nitrous oxide (inhalation agent)
Parental holding	

giving the patient and family choices and control when possible will help allay anxiety and fear, and promote patient/family cooperation.[54]

Examples of nonpharmacologic approaches to pediatric pain management include the following:

- Family-centered care (giving information to patients/families, allowing choices when possible, family presence option for procedures, and so forth)
- Relaxation techniques
- Distraction
- Yoga
- Music
- Guided imagery
- Biofeedback
- Hypnotherapy
- Psychotherapy (for the patient and/or family)
- Physical therapy
- Massage therapy
- Hypnosis
- Acupuncture
- In infants, oral sucrose and pacifiers are additional nonpharmacologic modalities

Relaxation techniques decrease anxiety and foster muscle relaxation. The relaxation techniques of controlled breathing and stepwise muscle relaxation are appropriate for preschool and older children.

Distraction techniques can be used in patients of any age. Distraction techniques focus the child's attention away from pain onto activities that capture their attention. Examples of attention-sustaining activities in all ages of patients are conversation, music, and television. In toddlers and school age children, blowing bubbles and play activities can be attention sustainers. In older children and adolescents, video games and the telephone are other common activities used for distraction.

Yoga has been used for chronic pain. Yoga is based on the use of body poses, often accompanied by types of breathing, to enhance a feeling of well-being. Studies in adults indicate yoga may be of value.

Biofeedback utilizes a mechanical device to give *feedback* during relaxation, controlled breathing, or hypnotherapy activities. When the desired response occurs, positive visual and/or auditory feedback is given.

Individual and/or family psychotherapy has been valuable in dealing with issues that may accompany chronic or acute pain, such as anxiety, stress, depression, and school/work/ social/relationship problems.

Physical therapy and massage therapy have been especially helpful with chronic musculoskeletal pain. Benefits extend beyond improved function and decreased pain to improved mood and sleep.

Hypnotherapy and acupuncture have shown some success in treating patients with pain. Hypnotherapy is useful in children if school age or older.

In infants, nonpharmacologic techniques include oral sucrose, oral tactile stimulation (pacifiers), kangaroo care maternal to skin contact, and parental holding.

Pharmacologic Agents for Pediatric Sedation and Analgesia

Nonsystemic pharmacologic agents involving topical, local, and regional anesthetic techniques are valuable in the management of painful procedures and conditions. These are discussed in other chapters.

Systemic Pharmacologic Agents for Pediatric Pain Management

The two major classes of drugs used for pediatric systemic pharmacologic pain therapy are the nonopioids (primarily NSAIDs) and the opioids (Table 43-2).

NONOPIOIDS

Acetaminophen

Acetaminophen has both analgesic and antipyretic but little anti-inflammatory properties. It is generally a safe drug but toxicity can occur with an overdose or excessive cumulative doses over days. Acute liver failure can occur with an acetaminophen overdose. Acetaminophen lacks the gastrointestinal (GI) and antiplatelet effects of the NSAIDs and aspirin, which makes it useful in many patients such as those with a history of GI bleeding, ulcers, gastritis, platelet diseases, and bleeding disorders. An advantage of acetaminophen is that it can be given rectally as well as orally, making it useful in the patient that cannot take oral medications (e.g., vomiting patient). Acetaminophen undergoes liver metabolism mainly by conjugation with a minor amount metabolized by the P-450 enzyme system.

Nonsteroidal Anti-inflammatory Drugs (NSAIDs)

Acetaminophen and NSAIDs have supplanted aspirin as the most commonly used antipyretics and oral nonopioid analgesics in children.

In pediatric patients, the most commonly used NSAIDs are the oral drugs ibuprofen and naproxen, and the parenteral drug ketorolac.

Side effects of the NSAIDs are rare but GI bleeding, renal impairment, and platelet dysfunction/altered hemostasis can occur. Thus, NSAIDs should be used with caution or avoided in patients with impaired kidney function, those at risk for bleeding, or when surgical hemostasis is an issue (e.g., flap laceration repairs). Impairment of renal function secondary to short-term NSAID use is very rare in normovolemic pediatric patients, though the risk is increased in the face of hypovolemia or cardiac dysfunction.

Both NSAIDs and aspirin inhibit the cyclooxygenase (COX) enzyme that catalyses the formation of arachidonic acid from prostanoids. There are two COX enzymes: COX-1 and COX-2. COX-1 is found in gastric mucosa, platelets, liver, and kidneys. COX-2 resides in peripheral nerves, the spinal cord, and monocytes, and is also induced by inflammation and injury. Analgesia occurs with COX-2 inhibition, while COX-1 inhibition causes the GI side effects. The selective COX-2 inhibitors (e.g., celecoxib and rofecoxib) possess analgesic potency similar to other existing NSAIDs and have been touted to produce a lower incidence of gastric, renal, hematologic, and hepatic side effects. However, recent reports have identified an increased risk of serious heart disease (acute myocardial infarction and sudden death) and an increased risk of hospitalization for GI bleeding leading to warnings about these side effects and the removal of valdecoxib and rofecoxib from the market.[55,56] A recent meta-analysis of the COX-2 inhibitor valdecoxib (Bextra) has also found an increased risk of major cardiovascular events.[57] Whether the toxicity associated with the COX-2 inhibitors,

Table 43-2. Analgesics for Pediatric Sedation and Analgesia

Drug	Parenteral (IV/IM) Dose (mg/kg)	Enteral (PO) Dose (mg/kg)	Alternate Route Dose (mg/kg)	Maximum Dose Adult Dose	Precautions/Side Effects Contraindications/Toxicity		Comments
Nonopioids							
Acetaminophen*‡ (antipyretic, analgesic) No anti-inflammatory activity	NA	15 mg/kg PR	15 mg/kg PR	75 mg/kg qd 4 g qd Adult 325, 650, to 1000 mg q dose	G6PD deficiency	Liver failure with overdose (↑ risk if chronic alcohol use, other drugs)	Avoids GI/ platelet effects of NSAIDs/ aspirin Can use in patients with history of ulcer, GI bleeding, platelet dysfunction
Ibuprofen‡ (NSAID) (antipyretic, analgesic)	NA	10 q 6–8 h JRA 30–50 qd ÷ q 6 h inflammatory disease 400–800 mg q dose q 6–8 h	NA	40 mg/kg qd 800 mg per dose JRA 2.4 g qd Inflammatory disease 3.2 g qd Adults 3.2 g qd 400–800 mg q dose	Active GI bleeding Ulcers Renal failure	GI upset, (↓ with milk) Bleeding Platelet dysfunction Granulocyto- penia Anemia	Use cautiously if aspirin hypersensi- tivity, liver/renal insufficiency, on anticoa- gulants, severe dehydration
Aspirin*† (NSAID) (antiplatelet agent, analgesic)	NA	15 q 4–6 h PO/PR Anti-inflammatory 60–100 qd ÷ q 6 h Kawasaki disease 80–100 qd ÷ q 6 h	15 q 4 h PR	60–80 mg/ kg qd 4 g qd Adults 325, 650 mg q dose	Avoid if patient has chicken pox or flu- like illness and age <16 years With other NSAIDs Severe renal failure	GI upset Platelet dysfunction Gastritis Tinnitus Liver toxicity	Association with Reyes syndrome Use cautiously if bleeding disorder, renal disease, gastritis

(*Continued*)

Table 43-2. Analgesics for Pediatric Sedation and Analgesia (*Continued*)

Drug	Parenteral (IV/IM) Dose (mg/kg)	Enteral (PO) Dose (mg/kg)	Alternate Route Dose (mg/kg)	Maximum Dose Adult Dose	Precautions/Side Effects Contraindications/Toxicity		Comments
Naproxen[‡] (NSAID) (antiplatelet agent, analgesic)	NA	5–10 q 8–12 JRA 10–20 qd ÷ q 12 h	NA	*15 mg/kg 1.25 g qd* Adults 250–500 mg q dose	GI bleeding Platelet disorders	GI upset (↓ with milk) Thrombocytopenia GI bleeding Tinnitus Vertigo	Use cautiously if GI disease, renal or liver disease, heart disease, on anticoagulants
Ketorolac[‡] (NSAID) (antiplatelet agent, analgesic)	Child >50 kg and adults 0.5 q 6 h up to 30 mg	Child >50 kg and adults 10 mg q dose	NA	*10 mg PO q dose 40 mg PO qd 30 mg IV/IM q dose 120 mg qd IV/IM*	Renal/hepatic failure ↑ Bleeding risk	GI upset GI bleeding Thrombocytopenia Nephritis	Use in children supported by literature and practice but not yet recommended by manufacturer Use ≤5 days (↑ toxicity >5 days)
Opioids							
Codeine*,[§] (narcotic analgesic, antitussive)	1.0 IM/ PO/SC Adults 15–60 mg q 4–6 h	Onset 30–60 min Duration 3–4 h	IM/PO/SC same dose[‡]	*60 mg q dose 60–120 mg qd* Adults 15–60 mg q dose q 4–6 h	Contraindicated IV →histamine release, CV side effects	Nausea Vomiting Pruritus Constipation Hypotension CNS/respiratory depression	Synergistic effect with Acetominophen
Morphine*,[¶] (narcotic, analgesic)	0.1–0.2 IV/IM/SC q 2–4 h IV onset 5–10 min, IV duration 3–4 h	0.2–0.5 PO q 4–6 h Onset 30–60 min Duration 4–5 h	0.1–0.2 SC (same as IM/IV sustained PO release and transdermal patch forms available)	*15 mg q dose IV/IM/SC* Adults 10–30 mg PO 2–15 mg IV/IM/SC q dose	Hypotension Respiratory/ CNS depression (↑ risk if IV push)	Seizures in neonates Nausea Vomiting Pruritus Sedation	Infusions postop 0.01– 0.04 mg/kg/h Cancer, sickle cell

Drug	Route / Dose / Onset	Contraindications / Precautions	Side Effects	Comments
Hydromorphone*,¶ (narcotic, analgesic)	IM/SC onset 10–30 min, duration 4–5 h 0.015 IV/SC q 4–6 h; IV onset 5–10 min; IV duration 3–4h 0.03–0.1 PO; Onset 30 min; Adults 1–4 mg PO q dose SQ same as IV/IM 5 mg PO q dose; Adults 1–2 mg q dose IV/IM	Neonates; Use with caution infants/young child (↑CNS effects)	Biliary spasm constipation ↑ICP Nausea Pruritus Sedation Constipation	0.04–0.07 mg/kg/h; Adults 0.8–10 mg/h; ↓ incidence of side effects (compared to morphine)
Meperidine*,¶ (narcotic, analgesic)	1–2 IV/IM/SC/PO; IV onset 5 min; IV duration 3–4 h; IM/SQ onset 10–15 min NA 1.5–2.0 PO; PO onset 30–60 min; PO duration 2–4 h Do not use with MAO inhibitors 100–150 mg q dose; Adults 50–150 mg, q dose q 3–4 h.	Contraindicated MAO inhibitor ↑ICP Dysrhythmias Seizures from metabolite normeperidine (renal excretion) Wheezing from sodium bisulfite	Respiratory depression* Hypotension* *↑ risk if IV push Seizures Tachycardia Nausea/vomiting Pruritus, Seizures Caution renal disease	Greater euphoria than morphine; Use with caution in renal failure, sickle cell, seizures, asthma
Fentanyl*,¶ (narcotic, analgesic)	1–3 mcg/kg IV/IM q 30–60 min; IV onset 1–2 min.; IV duration 0.5–1 h Oralet 10–15 mcg q dose; Contraindicated <10 kg; Oralet max 400 mcg q dose Transdermal patch onset 6–8 h, duration 72 h peak 24 h Avoid rapid IV push ↑ risk of rigidity, respiratory depression	Bradycardia ↑ unbound drug in newborns ↑ICP Respiratory depression	Chest wall rigidity* Respiratory depression* *↑ risk if IV push or high dose (>mcg/kg)	Age <6 months ↓ dose by half to 0.5–1.5 mcg/kg (cytochrome P-450 metabolism)

(*Continued*)

Table 43-2. Analgesics for Pediatric Sedation and Analgesia (*Continued*)

Drug	Parenteral (IV/IM) Dose (mg/kg)	Enteral (PO) Dose (mg/kg)	Alternate Route Dose (mg/kg)	Maximum Dose Adult Dose	Precautions/Side Effects Contraindications/Toxicity	Comments
	Give IV over 2–3 min Infusion 1–3 mcg/kg/h	(up to 1600 meq has been used in adults)			Can occur with low dose High incidence Nausea/vomiting with oralet	Transdermal safety/efficacy in adults, not established in pediatrics

IV, intravenous; IM, intramuscular; JRA, juvenile rheumatoid arthritis; MAO, monoamine oxidase inhibitors; NA = not applicable (not available); NSAID = nonsteroidal anti-inflammatory drug; PO, oral; PR, rectal.

Note: The commonly used maximum dose is and adult dose listed. In some cases, doses may be lower or higher. Adolescents often receive the adult dose.

For maximum dose, when mg/kg or total dose is listed, generally use the lower of the two.
The parenteral (IV/IM) and enteral (PO) and alternate route (PR or SC) are given in mg/kg doses unless otherwise indicated.

Note: Fetanyl is in micrograms (mcg).

*Adjust dose in renal failure.

†Aspirin has fallen out of favor because of association with Reyes Syndrome so it is not generally used for its antipyretic or analgesic properties with acute illness. However, it is used as an analgesic for chronic pain with such diseases as Juvenile Rheumatoid Arthritis or Kawasaki's disease.

‡Recent concern regarding increased risk of serious heart disease (sudden death, heart attack) in adults on Cox-2 inhibitors.

§Often combined with acetaminophen.

¶Effects reversed by naloxone.

This table is not intended to imply a standard of care. Individual patients require individual tailored care and clinician judgment.

rofecoxib, and valdecoxib, will extend to other COX-2 inhibitors such as celecoxib (Celebrex) remains to be seen although caution has been advised.[58]

When used concomitantly with opioids, NSAIDs decrease the opioid requirements and side effects by as much as 35–40%. The GI upset secondary to the oral NSAIDs can be decreased if they are taken with milk or food. Ibuprofen should be used with caution in patients with aspirin hypersensitivity. All of the NSAIDs should be used cautiously in patients with renal or hepatic insufficiency or a bleeding diathesis.

Aspirin

Because of the association of aspirin with Reye's syndrome the use of aspirin in pediatric practice has fallen out of favor. However, there are still indications for the use of aspirin in the treatment of Kawasaki disease and for various rheumatologic disorders.

OPIOIDS

Opioids are indicated for the treatment of moderate-to-severe pain in pediatric patients including fractures, postoperative pain, patients with pain from sickle cell disease, and cancer pain.

The main side effects of the opioids are respiratory depression, hypotension, nausea, vomiting, pruritus, and urticaria/rashes.

In pediatrics, opioids are employed too infrequently and in inadequate doses for many reasons including concerns for side effects, such as respiratory depression and fears of addiction. The risk of apnea and respiratory depression that may occur with opioids, especially in neonates, can be minimized by adjusting the rate of administration, the dose, and the dosing interval along with appropriate monitoring. Infants, particularly neonates and premature infants, have an increased volume of distribution and decreased renal clearances. By 3 months of age, the kidney's clearance of opioids and opioid respiratory suppression approaches that of the adult.

The preferred antiemetics for opioid-induced nausea and vomiting in pediatric patients are the 5 HT-3 receptor antagonists. Compazine and other dopaminergic antiemetic drugs may cause dystonic reactions that can be especially disturbing in children.

Patient-controlled analgesia (PCA) has been used in patients as young as 6 years of age. Nurse-administered analgesia (NCA) or a continuous infusion of an analgesic drug may be appropriate for younger children and children with special health care needs.

Factors to be considered in the selection of a specific opioid include potency, efficacy, side effects, toxicity, onset, duration, and route of administration. In infants and children, morphine is often the initial choice for parenteral boluses and infusions. Patients with reactive airway disease may possibly demonstrate an increased sensitivity to morphine because it causes the release of histamine (i.e., wheezing) but this is rare, and overall morphine is well tolerated. Rash, nausea, and pruritus are other prominent side effects of morphine.

Meperidine has seen less use than other parenteral opioids because of the accumulation of its metabolite, normeperidine, which has excitatory effects on the heart and central nervous system (e.g., seizures and dysphoria) with repetitive dosing. Fentanyl has the advantages of a short half-life, useful for painful procedures, and minimal cardiac effects except for bradycardia making it a valuable option for infants/children with cardiac disease. However, a rare side effect, chest wall and glottic rigidity, can occur especially with high doses of fentanyl given by a rapid bolus. This can be treated with supplemental oxygen and assisted ventilation though neuromuscular blockade may be required.

Many oral opioids are available: codeine, morphine, oxycodone, methadone, fentanyl, hydromorphone, and meperidine. These are often available in combination with acetaminophen (e.g., acetaminophen with codeine and oxycodone with acetaminophen). Tramadol, a recently introduced oral opioid, has morphine-like u_1 receptor agonism but is incompletely antagonized by naloxone. It also blocks some reuptake of norepinephrine and serotonin at nerve terminals. Fentanyl lollipops, somewhat popular when first introduced, have seen less use recently because of the relatively high incidence of side effects, specifically nausea, vomiting, and pruritus.

Alternate routes of administration are available with some opioids. For example, fentanyl, morphine, and methadone are available in a sustained released form applied as a skin patch. Morphine and hydromorphone are available in rectal suppositories. They can be used in patients unable to tolerate oral medication, although rectal suppositories may be contraindicated in neutropenic or immunosuppressed patients.

PROCEDURAL SEDATION AND ANALGESIA FOR PEDIATRIC PATIENTS

The indications for, use of, and drugs for PSA for all age groups, especially pediatrics, has expanded greatly in recent years (Tables 43-3 and 43-4). The procedures for which pediatric procedural sedation is administered have a developmental and age predilection and generally belong to one of the three categories: (1) fracture reduction, (2) laceration repair, and (3) diagnostic imaging (most commonly for computed tomography).

Because infants (<1 years of age) have a disproportionately larger head than the body, they usually incur minor traumatic head injuries secondary to rolling off a bed or accidentally being dropped. Diagnostic radiology

Table 43-3. Indications for Procedural Sedation and Analgesia in Pediatric Patients

Airway Management
Rapid sequence intubation
Diagnostic: Bronchoscopy, laryngoscopy
Therapeutic: Chest tube placement, foreign body removal from airway (from oro/naso
  pharynx to larynx to bronchi) using laryngoscopy or bronchoscopy or other instruments

Diagnostic Procedures
Neurologic: Lumbar puncture, subdural puncture, ventricular puncture, ventriculostomy
Hematologic: Bone marrow aspiration
Orthopedic: Arthrocentesis
Ophthalmologic: Slit lamp examination
Gastrointestinal: Paracentesis, peritoneal lavage, gastric intubation, feeding tube replacement
Cardiothoracic: Thoracentesis, pericardiocentesis
Orthopedic: Arthrocentesis
Genitourinary: Suprapubic bladder aspiration

Therapeutic Procedures
Repair of lacerations
Dermatologic: Abscess incision and drainage, removal of foreign body, fishhook removal,
  removal of skin lesions/masses
Orthopedic: Fracture reduction, reduction of dislocation
Neurologic: Removal of excessive cerebrospinal fluid by lumbar or ventricular puncture
Hand surgery: Repair of fingernail/finger avulsion injuries, drainage of paronychia/ felon
Genitourinary: Reduction of inguinal hernia, detorsion of torsed testes, reduction of prolapsed
  rectum or uterus, examination of genitalia under anesthesia
Vascular: Central line placement, arterial line placement
Cardiac: Cardioversion
Dental: Incision and drainage of abscess, and so forth
Gastroenterology: EGD, sigmoidoscopy (treat bleeding, remove foreign body, and so forth)
Ophthalmic: Foreign body removal
Otolaryngology: Tympanocentesis, foreign body removal

Diagnostic Imaging (radiology)
Computerized tomography
Magnetic resonance imaging
Barium enemia
Upper GI
Ultrasonography

Procedures in Specific Patient Populations
Special needs children
Psychiatric patients
Mentally challenged patients

EGD: esophagogastroduodenoscopy.

Table 43-4. Sedatives for Pediatric Sedation and Analgesia

Sedatives	Anxiolytic	Analgesic	Sedative-Hypnotic	Reversal Agent	Parenteral (IV/IM) Dose (mg/kg)	Enteral (PO/PR) Dose (mg/kg)	Alternate Routes of Administration Dose (mg/kg)	Maximum Dose
Chloral hydrate	–	–	+	–	NA	low dose 25–50 may repeat in 30 min high dose 60–80 onset 30 min peak 30–60 min duration 60–90 min (often prolonged)	NA	100 mg/kg range 25–100 mg/kg 1 g infants 2–2.5 g children
Benzodiazepines Midazolam	+	–	+	+	0.05–0.1 over 2–3 min (may give 0.02–0.03 mg/kg then repeat) 0.1–0.3 for RSI IV onset 2–3 min IV duration 60 min IM onset 5–30 min IM duration 60–90 min	0.5–1.0 PO/PR onset 10–30 min duration 60–90 min adults 0.5–2.0 mg q dose IV maximum 20 mg q dose PO/PR	0.3–0.5 intranasal (IN) or sublingual IN onset 3–5 min IN duration 60 min IN can be uncomfortable IN maximum 7.5 mg	IV/IM 6 mg (age ≤5 years) IV/IM 10 mg (age >6 years and adults) ↓ IV/IM dose to 0.02mg/kg if giving with opioids or in at risk patients
Barbiturates Methohexital	–	–	+	–	1–3 IV titrated slowly usual 1–1.5 IV IV onset 1 min IV duration 10 min IM onset 10 min	25 PR onset 10–15 min duration 60 min	NA	3 mg/kg IV 1 g PR

(*Continued*)

Table 43-4. Sedatives for Pediatric Sedation and Analgesia (*Continued*)

Sedatives	Anxiolytic	Analgesic	Sedative-Hypnotic	Reversal Agent	Parenteral (IV/IM) Dose (mg/kg)	Enteral (PO/PR) Dose (mg/kg)	Alternate Routes of Administration Dose (mg/kg)	Maximum Dose
Barbiturates Thiopental	–	+	–		2–6 IV titrated slowly if low BP, ↓ dose to 1–2 IV onset 1 min duration 15 min	25 PR onset 10–15 min duration 60–120 min	NA	1 g PR
Barbiturates Pentobarbital	–	+	–		1–6 IV, 4–6 IM IV onset 3–5 min, IM 10 min duration IV 15–45 min, IM 1–2 h barbiturate coma loading dose 10–15 mg/kg/h over 1–2 h maintenance dose 1–3 mg/kg/h	2–6 PO/PR onset 15–60 min duration 120–240 min	NA	IV/PO 200 mg IM/PR 150 mg 6 mg/kg IV/IM/PO/PR
Ketamine (Dissociative anesthetic)	+	+	–		1–1.5 IV (repeat 0.5–1.0 IV for long procedures) titrate slowly IV onset < 1 min IV duration 10–20 min 5 IM IM onset 5–15 min	6–10 PO* 10–15 PR* PO/PR onset 20 min PO/PR duration 60–120 min *avoid PO/PR less efficacy more side effects	Avoid intranasal/ PO/PR Use IM if no IV access	May use with antisialogogue glycopyrrolate (preferred) or atropine

Etomidate	−	+	−	+	NA	IM duration 30–90 min 0.1–0.3 IV titrated slowly usual dose: PSA −0.3 RSI onset <1 min duration 3–10 min	NA	0.6 mg/kg
Propofol	+	−	−	+	NA	1–1.5 IV titrated slowly usual induction dose 1.5 (adult 100 mg bolus) onset <1 min duration 8 min infusion 50–150 mcg/kg/min	NA	3–3.5 mg/kg

(Continued)

Table 43-4. Sedatives for Pediatric Sedation and Analgesia (*Continued*)

Sedative	Cardiovascular Side Effects	Respiratory Side Effects	Neurologic Side Effects	GI/Other Side Effects	Contraindications	Precautions	Comments
Chloral hydrate	Cardiac depressant Hypotension Dysrhythmias	Apnea Respiratory depression Laryngospasm Bronchiolitis patients ↓ O₂ saturation	Paradoxical reaction Prolonged sedation Hangover effect	Gastritis Esophagitis Nausea Vomiting	Hepatic/Renal disease Age >3 year Use with caution preterm/term neonates (Hyperbilirubinemia)	↓ Side effects in special needs children Inadequate sedation up to 30–40% of time	Best to avoid: delayed onset/ offset, side effects, and high failure rate. Other better sedatives available
Benzodiazepines	No, unless hypovolemic or hypotensive then ↓ BP	Apnea Respiratory depression (↑ if coadminister opioids or barbiturates)	Paradoxical reaction Prolonged sedation Hangover effect	Vomiting Cough Hiccups	Glaucoma Shock Protease inhibitor drugs (Cytochrome P 450 metabolism)	Patients with respiratory depression (alcohol, COPD, BPD)	↓ dose in renal/hepatic disease, severe CHF/elderly, chronically ill. ↑ seizure threshold (used to treat seizures, ↓ CBF, ↓ ICP)
Barbiturates	Cardiac depressant Hypotension (vasodilatation, negative inotrope)	Apnea Respiratory depression (↑ if coadminister opioids or benzodiazepines) Laryngospasm	Paradoxical reaction Prolonged sedation Hangover effect	—	Porphyria Shock, Hypovolemia Severe liver disease Methohexital with seizure disorders	Patients with respiratory depression (alcohol COPD, BPD) IV infiltration can cause tissue necrosis, intra-arterial injection can cause vasospasm gangrene	Causes ↓ ICP, ↓ IOP (thiopental/ pentobarbital) used in head/eye injury patients. Avoid metho hexital for RSI Thiopental → histamine release (use cautiously if asthmatic)

Agent	Cardiovascular	Respiratory	CNS / Emergence	Emesis	Contraindications	Cautions	Comments
Ketamine (Dissociative anesthetic)	Sympathomimetic Effect ↑BP ↑HR	Laryngospasm (<1%) (↓ if use with antisalogue)	Emergence reaction (no ↓ with midazolam) ↑ICP, ↑IOP, ↑muscle tone	Emesis Salivation Give with antisialogue-glycopyrolate (preferred) or atropine	↑ICP ↑IOP	Thyroid disease Severe CV disease Age <3 month, Pneumonia (↑ risk laryngospasm)	Causes bronchodilation (asthma therapy) Excellent CV and respiratory stability
Etomidate	—	Minimal respiratory depressant	Myoclonic movements (↓ with opiate, benzodiazepine, paralytic) Seizures	Nausea Vomiting	Adrenal insufficiency	Seizure disorders High incidence of pain with injection Give with lidocaine to ↓ injection pain	Do not use as sole agent for RSI. (can cause facial myoclonus) Good choice if shock, CAD, trauma
Propofol	Cardiac depressant (↓ SVR, ↓ CO, ↓ baroreflex, ↓ HR response) Vasodilatation Bradydysrhythmias Negative inotrope	Apnea Respiratory depression (↑ if given with opioids or benzodiazepines)	Dysphoric reactions Myoclonic movements Posturing, seizure-like activity, seizures	No, (is mild antiemetic)	Egg/ Soybean/ EDTA allergy Shock Severe CV disease or hypotension	Hypotension/ volume depleted, if administer with drugs with negative chronotropic effect (fentanyl, succinylcholine)	↓ dose in elderly ↑ dose in pediatrics Propofol infusion syndrome

BP: blood pressure; HR: heart rate; ICP: intracranial pressure; IOP: intraocular pressure; COPD: chronic obstructive pulmonary disease; BPD bronchopulmonary dysplasia; CHF: congestive heart failure; CV: cardiovascular; CBF: cerebral blood flow; CAD: coronary artery disease; RSI: rapid sequence induction; CO: cardiac output; SVR: systemic vascular resistance. Reversal agent for benzodiazepines is flumazenil.

This table is not intended to imply a standard of care. Individual patients require individual tailored care and clinician judgment.

studies (e.g., CT scan) to rule head injury is the primary indication for PSA in this age group.

Toddlers are just beginning to ambulate and tend to collide with objects (especially furniture) resulting in facial and scalp lacerations. Older toddlers (age 18–36 months) are curious, beginning to explore their surroundings and using their hands reaching for objects and tend to incur hand injuries such as lacerations to the fingers and nail beds and fingertip avulsions. Preschool age (4 years and older) and school age children are involved in independent play and outdoor activities such as climbing, which can lead to falls with resultant fractures, especially of the forearm and wrist. In older school age children and adolescents, sports injuries are responsible for most of the minor traumatic injuries.

The types of clinical procedures requiring PSA are (1) airway management (specifically rapid sequence intubation), (2) therapeutic procedures (e.g., fracture reduction, laceration repair, and incision and drainage), (3) diagnostic procedures (e.g., lumbar puncture, arthrocentesis, and bone marrow aspiration), (4) access (e.g., central venous lines, arterial lines, and placement of various catheters/tubes), and (5) in *special health care needs* patients or patients with behavioral/psychiatric issues in whom cooperation is difficult or impossible to obtain (Table 43-3).

The pharmacologic agents used for analgesia and sedation can be categorized into (1) analgesics (2) sedative hypnotics, (3) dissociative agents, and (4) inhalational agents. The dissociative agent (ketamine) and the inhalational agent (e.g., nitrous oxide) generally have the same indications as the sedative/hypnotics, although they are pharmacologically very different drugs. Furthermore, drugs in the various groups may be coadministered to achieve the desired PSA. Examples of such combinations include fentanyl/midazolam. Many of the drugs employed for PSA can be given by multiple routes of administration.

With the advent of newer, more effective, and safer drugs, some of previous pharmacologic regimens used for PSA, specifically DPT and chloral hydrate, have seen a justifiable precipitous decline in usage and are not recommended.[31,33,59–67] The common PSA drugs are reviewed in other chapters. Table 43-3 summarizes key facts relevant to use of the PSA drugs.

SUMMARY

Patients of all ages, even preterm newborns, experience pain. Previous experiences with pain may affect later behavioral and physiologic responses to pain. Inadequate analgesia in the past may decrease analgesic effectiveness at a later time. Nonpharmacologic pain management techniques are safe, often effective, based on patients' age and development, may not work in all patients, and do not obviate the need for drug therapy.

There are many choices of drugs for sedation and the treatment of pain. The choice of drugs for PSA depends on many factors. These parameters include the patient (age, comorbidity, allergies, medications, special needs), whether the procedure is painless or painful, the procedure itself, the duration of the procedure, and facility specific (e.g., ED and hospital) factors.

Key considerations for safe and effective PSA for the pediatric patient include the selection of appropriate drugs, given in appropriate doses, on selected patients in the proper environment with adequate monitoring by physicians able to manage any untoward events that may occur.

REFERENCES

1. Anand KJ, Hickey PR. Pain and its effects in the human neonate and fetus. *N Engl J Med.* 1987;317(21):321–329.
2. American Academy of Pediatrics and Canadian Paediatric Society. Prevention and management of pain and stress in the neonate. *Pediatrics.* 2000;105 (2):454–461.
3. Greco CD, Aner MM, LeBel A. Acute pain management in infants and children. In: Warfield CA, Bajwa ZH (eds). Principles and Practice of Pain Medicine, New York: McGraw-Hill 2004:541–552.
4. Desparmet-Sheridan JP. Pediatric Pain. In: Raj PP (ed). Pain Medicine, A Comprehensive Review. St. Louis: Mosby 2003: 351–358.
5. Valman HB, Pearson JF. What the fetus feels. *Br Med J.* 1980;280:233–234.
6. Henderson-Smart DJ, Pettigrew HJ, Campbell DJ. Clinical apnea and brain neural function in preterm infants. *N Engl J Med.* 1983;308:353–357.
7. Bursch B, Zelter LK. Pediatric pain management. In: Behrman RE, Kliegman RM, Jenson HB. (eds). Nelson Textbook of Pediatrics. Philadelphia: WB Saunders 2004:358–366.
8. Berde C, Cairns B. Developmental pharmacology across species: promise and problems. *Anesth Analg.* 2000;91:1–5.
9. Fitzgerald M. The postnatal development of cutaneous afferent fibre input and receptive field organization in the rat dorsal horn. J Physiol (Lond) 1985;364:1–18.
10. Eland JM, Anderson JE. The experience of pain in children In: Jacox A., ed. Pain a source book for nurses and other health professionals. Boston: Little Brown. 1977.
11. Purcell-Jones G, Dormon F, Sumner E. Pediatric anesthetists' perception of neonatal and infant pain. *Pain.* 1988; 33:181–187.
12. Broome ME, Richtsmeirer A, Maikler V, et al. Pediatric pain practices: A national survey of health professionals. *J Pain Symptom Manage.* 1996;11:312–320.

13. Romsing J. Assessment of nurses judgment for analgesic requirements of postoperative pain. *J Clin Pharm Ther.* 1996;21:159–163.

14. Goddard JM, Pickup SE. Postoperative pain in children. *Anesthesia.* 1996;51:588–590.

15. De Lima J, Lloyd-Thomas AR, Howard RF, et al. Infant and neonatal pain; anaesthetists' perceptions and prescribing patterns. *Br Med J.* 1996;313:787.

16. Porter FL, Wolf CM, Gold J, et al. Pain and pain management in newborn infants: a survey of physicians and nurses. *Pediatrics.* 1997;100:626–632.

17. McGrath PA, Brigham MC. The assessment of pain in children and adolescents. In: Turk DC, Melzack R (eds). Handbook of Pain Assessment. New York: The Guilford Press; 1992:295–314.

18. Schechter NL, Berde CB, Yaster M. Pain in infants, children, and adolescents an overview. In: Schechter NL, Berde CB, Yaster M, eds. Pain in Infants, Children, and Adolscents. Baltimroe, MD: Williams & Wilkins; 1993:3–9.

19. American Academy of Pediatrics and American Pain Society. The assessment and management of acute pain in infants, children, and adolescents. *Pediatrics.* 2001;108(3):793–797.

20. Selbst SM, Clark M. Analgesic use in the emergency department. *Ann Emerg Med.* 1990;19:1010–1013.

21. Lewis LM, Lasater LC, Brooks CB. Are emergency physicians too stingy with analgesics? *South Med J.* 1994;87:7–9.

22. Petrack EM, Christopher NC, Kriwinsky J. Pain management in the emergency department: patterns of analgesic utilization. *Pediatrics.* 1997;99:711–714.

23. Ngai B, Duchame J. Documented use of analgesics in the emergency department and upon release of patients with extremity fractures (letter). *Acad Emerg Med.* 1997;4:1176–1178.

24. Alexander J, Manno M. Underuse of analgesia in very young pediatric patients with isolated painful injuries. *Ann Emerg Med.* 2003;41(5):617–622.

25. Hawk W, Crockett RK, Ochsenchlager DW, et al. Conscious sedation of the pediatric patient for suturing: a survey. *Pediatr Emerg Care.* 1992;6:84–88.

26. Cook BA, Bass JW, Nomizu, et al. Sedation for children for technical procedures: current standard of practice. *Clin Pediatr.* 1992;137–142.

27. Ilkanipour K, Jeuls CR, Langdorf MI. Pediatric pain control and conscious sedation. A survey of emergency medicine residencies. *Acad Emerg Med.* 1994;1:368–372.

28. Krauss B, Zurakowski D. Sedation patterns in pediatric and general community hospital emergency departments. *Pediatr Emerg Care.* 1998;14(2):99–103.

29. Cimpello LB, Khine H, Aoner JR. Practice patterns of pediatric versus general emergency physicians for pain management of fractures in pediatric patients. *Pediatr Emerg Care.* 2004;20(4):228–232.

30. Goldman RD, Balasubramanian S, Wales P, et al. Sedation and analgesia for incarcerated inguinal hernia in the pediatric emergency department. (submitted for publication).

31. Mace SE. Clinical policy on pediatric procedural sedation (letter to editor). *Ann Emerg Med.* 2005.

32. Zempsky WT, Cravero JP, Committee on Pediatric Emergency Medicine and Section on Anesthesiology and Pain Medicine. Relief of pain and anxiety in pediatric patients in emergency medical systems. *Pediatrics.* 2004;114(5):1348–1356.

33. Mace SE, Barata IA, Cravero JP, et al. Clinical policy: evidence-based approach to pharmacologic agents used in pediatric sedation and analgesia in the emergency department. *Ann Emerg Med.* Oct 2004;44(4)342–377.

34. American College of Emergency Physicians Clinical Policy: Procedural Sedation. Approved October 20, 2004 by ACEP Board of Directors, for publication. Annals of Emergency Medicine, 2005.

35. Reynolds M, Fitzgerald M. Long-term sensory hyperinnervation following neonatal skin wounds. *J Comp Neurol.* 1995;358:487.

36. Reynolds M, et al. Neonatally wounded skin induces NGF-independent sensory neurite outgrowth in vitro. *Brain Res.* 1997;102:275.

37. Anand KJ, Coskun V, Thrivikraman KV, et al. Long-term behavioral effects of repetitive pain in neonatal rat pups. *Physiol Behav.* 1999;66:627.

38. Johnston CC, Stevens BJ. Experience in a neonatal intensive care unit affects pain response. *Pediatrics.* 1996;98(5): 925–930.

39. Taddio A, Ipp M, et al. Effect of neonatal circumcision on pain responses during vaccination in boys. *Lancet.* 1995; 345:291–292.

40. Johnston CC, Stevens BJ, Franck LS, et al. Factors explaining lack of response to heelstick in preterm infant. *J Obstet Gynecol Neonatal Nurs.* 1999;28:587–594.

41. Grunau RVE, Whitfield MF, Petrie JH, et al. Early pain experience, child and family factors, as precursors of somatization: a prospective study of extremely premature and full term children. *Pain.* 1994;56:353–359.

42. Oberlander TF, Grunau RV, Whitfield MF. Behavioral responses in former extremely low-birthweight infants at 4 months corrected age. *Pediatrics.* 2000:105:E6–E18.

43. Grunau RV, Whitfield MF, Petrie JH. Pain sensitivity and temperament in extremely low-birth-weight premature toddlers with preterm and full-term controls. *Pain.* 1994;58:341.

44. Grunau RE, Whitfield MF, Petric J. Children's judgments about pain at age 8-years: do extremely low birthweight (≤1000 g) children differ from full birthweight peers? *J Child Psychol Psychiatry.* 1998;39:587–594.

45. Bushila D, Zmora E, Bolotin A. Pain sensitivity in prematurely born adolescents. *Arch Pediatr Adoles Med.* 2003; 157:1079–1082.

46. Taddio A, Katz JK, Ilersich AL, et al. Effect of neonatal circumcision on pain response during subsequent routine vaccination. *Lancet.* 1997;349:599–603.

47. Weisman SJ, Bernstein B, Schechter NL. Consequences of inadequate analgesia during painful procedures in children. *Arch Pediatr Adolesc Med.* 1998;152:147–149.

48. Anand KJS, McIntosh N, Lagercrantz H, et al. Analgesia and sedation in preterm neonate requiring ventilatory support. *Arch Pediatr Adolesc Med.* 1999;153:331–338.

49. Friis-Hansen B. Body composition during growth. In vivo measurements and biochemical data correlated to differential anatomical growth. *Pediatrics.* 1971;47:169–181.

50. Berde CB, Sethna NF. Analgesics for the treatment of pain in children. *N Engl J Med.* 2002;347(14):1094–1103.

51. Cote CJ. Pediatric Anesthesia. In: Miller RD (ed). Miller's Anesthesia. Philadelphia: Elsevier Churchill Livingstone; 2005:2367–2398.

52. Pang LM. Physiologic considerations. In: Kraus B, Brustowicz RM (eds). Pediatric Procedural Sedation and Analgesia Philadelphia. Lippincott, Williams and Wilkins 1999:47–54.

53. Nies AS. Principles of therapeutics. In: Hardman JG, Limbird LE, Goodman-Gilman A (eds). Goodman & Gilman's The Pharmacological Basis of Therapeutics. New York: McGraw-Hill, 2001:45–66.

54. Brown K, Chambain N, Dietrich A, et al. Family-centered care for the pediatric patient in the emergency department. *Ann Emerg Med.* in press.

55. Bombardier C, Laine L, Reicin A, et al. Comparison of upper gastrointestinal toxicity of rofecoxib and naprocoxib in patients with rheumatoid arthritis. *N Engl J Med.* 2000; 343:1520–1528. (VIGOR trial)

56. Memorandum from David J. Graham, MD, MPH, Associate Director for Science. Office of Drug Safety to Paul Seligman, MD, MPH, Acting Director, Office of Drug Safety entitled, "Risk of Acute Myocardial Infarction and Sudden Cardiac Death in Patients Treated with COX-2 Selective and Non-Selective NSAIDs." September 30, 2004.

57. Fitzgerald G, Furberg C, eds. Valdecoxib meta-analysis signals significant cardiovascular risk. Presented 11-10-04 at American Heart Association Scientific Sessions 2004; available American Heart Association Website. *http://www.theheart.org* (last accessed 1-11-05).

58. Mukherjee D, Nissen SE, Topol EJ. Risk of cardiovascular events associated with selective COX-2 inhibitors. *JAMA.* 2001;286(8):954–959.

59. Terndrup TE, Dire DJ, Madden CM, et al. A prospective analysis of intramuscular meperidine, promethazine, and chlorpromazine in pediatric emergency department patients. *Ann Emerg Med.* 1991;20:31–35.

60. Committee on drugs. American Academy of Pediatrics. *Pediatrics.* 1995;95(4):598–602.

61. Weir MR, Segapeli JH, Tremper LJ. Sedation for pediatric procedures. *Mil Med.* 1986;151:181–184.

62. Nathan JE, Stewart West M. Comparison of chloral hydrate-hydroxyzine with and without meperidine for management of the difficult pediatric patient. *J Dent Child.* 1987;437–444.

63. Gaulier JM, Merle G, Lacassie E, et al. Fatal intoxications with chloral hydrate. *J Forensic Sci.* 2001;46(6):1507–1509.

64. Cote CJ, Notterman DA, Karl HW, et al. Adverse sedation events in pediatrics: a critical incident analysis of contribution factors. *Pediatrics.* 2000;105:805–814.

65. Cote CJ, Karl HW, Notterman DA, et al. Adverse sedation events in pediatrics analysis of medications used for sedation. *Pediatrics.* 2000;106:633–644.

66. Englehart DA, Lovins ES, Hazenstab CB, et al. Unusual death attributed to the combined effects of chloral hydrate, lidocaine, and nitrous oxide. *J Anal Toxicol.* 1998;22:246–247.

67. Caksen H, Odabas D, Unerune A, et al. Respiratory arrest due to chloral hydrate in an infant. *J Emerg Med.* 342–343.

44

Geriatrics

Fredric M. Hustey
Jacques S. Lee

HIGH YIELD FACTS

- Older adults may have a tendency to underreport pain.
- Age and cognitive impairment are risk factors for inadequate pain management.
- A geriatric-specific approach, with attention to psychosocial issues, is particularly important when managing pain in older persons.
- Normal physiologic changes associated with aging can affect drug metabolism, drug clearance, and increase the risk of toxicity. These changes should be taken into account when prescribing analgesia and sedation for the older patient.
- A review of past medical history and medications should be done on every older patient prior to prescribing analgesia to avoid potentially dangerous interactions.
- Common analgesics such as indomethacin, propoxyphene, meperidine, and amitriptyline are potentially dangerous in older patients and should be avoided.

OVERVIEW

In 1996, the Society for Academic Emergency Medicine Geriatric Task Force proposed 11 principles to guide the approach to older patients in the emergency department (ED). These include key factors that should be considered when treating pain in the older patient: the patient's presentation is frequently complex or atypical, the effects of comorbid diseases must be considered, polypharmacy is common and may be a factor in management, the recognition of the possibility for cognitive impairment is important, the likelihood of decreased functional reserve must be anticipated, and social supports may be inadequate.

Older patients tend to have more comorbidities and take more medications than younger counterparts.

Preexisting conditions can be adversely affected by the addition of another drug. There is an increased potential for dangerous medication interactions. In addition, normal physiologic changes associated with aging can affect drug metabolism, drug clearance, and increase the risk of toxicity. All of these factors must be considered when developing a strategy for pain management and procedural sedation.

Psychosocial issues are especially important in this population. The rapid pace associated with ED care can make it difficult to explore issues beyond a well-defined single presenting complaint. However, good patient care demands the ability to rapidly explore a patient's psychosocial context, which may be particularly important when managing older patients with painful conditions.[1] Psychosocial factors may contribute to the ED visit. For example, did tripping hazards in the home cause the injury? Did caregivers' concerns regarding pain management precipitate the ED visit? Is there any evidence of elder abuse or neglect? Consideration should also be given to psychologic factors that may affect the patient's perception and expression of pain. Is fear of an underlying cause dreaded by the patient causing them to minimize their pain (e.g., denial of anginal symptoms) or conversely, to worsen pain severity (e.g., unexplained abdominal pain in a patient who recently lost a loved one due to cancer). Assessing home support is crucial for effective discharge planning. Is the patient sufficiently pain-free and mobile to accomplish the requisite activities of daily living without assistance? If not, home health aides or community agencies may be useful in providing additional support.

EPIDEMIOLOGY

While there are significant numbers of patients who seek care due to new onset pain (such as from a traumatic musculoskeletal injury) or worsening chronic pain (such as worsening osteoarthritis or spinal stenosis), the incidence and prevalence of these conditions in older ED patients is not well documented. However, pain is prevalent in the geriatric population. In the community setting, previous studies suggest that up to 50% of older people suffer from persistent pain. In addition, 80% of nursing home patients may suffer from significant pain that is undertreated.[2]

PHYSIOLOGY OF AGING

There are many physiologic changes associated with the aging process. Many of these changes can affect responses to pharmacotherapy, medication tolerance, and the threshold for toxicity. Both the pharmacokinetic and pharmacodynamic responses of drugs are affected. The result can be higher peak concentrations for given doses (such as with propofol), increased bioavailability, and prolonged clearance of medications. Older patients are also more likely to suffer from hypoalbuminemia due to comorbidities as well as protein-calorie malnutrition. This may increase the free fraction of protein-bound medications and further contribute to increased toxicity.

Cardiovascular changes considered a normal part of the aging process include an increase in peripheral vascular resistance, decrease in left ventricular compliance, reduced response of heart rate to catecholamines, and increased dependence of diastolic filling on atrial contraction. Pathologic changes may result in significant coronary artery disease, cardiomyopathy, congestive heart failure, and valvular dysfunction (such as aortic stenosis). While most of these changes are more likely to be problematic in the patient undergoing procedural sedation, in some instances they may also affect choices for home going analgesia.

There is a progressive loss of renal function associated with the aging process. The resultant reduction in the glomerular filtration rate, however, is not necessarily reflected by an elevation of the serum creatinine. What may be considered a normal creatinine in a 37-year-old man may signify renal insufficiency in a frail 87-year-old female. This decrease in renal reserve may leave older patients more susceptible to analgesics with nephrotoxic effects, such as long-acting nonsteroidal anti-inflammatory drugs (NSAIDs). In addition, medication doses may need to be adjusted. For those medications excreted by the kidneys, adjustments should be made based on creatinine clearance and *not* based solely on an abnormal lab value.

There is also a decline in pulmonary function. A decrease in the efficiency of gas exchange is signified clinically by a decrease in PaO_2 and less efficient elimination of CO_2. Impaired defense against inhaled matter as well as a less effective mucociliary reflex increases the risk for aspiration and pulmonary infection. There is also a marked decrease in chest wall compliance, requiring an increased muscular effort for adequate ventilation. These factors are important to consider in patients undergoing sedation and analgesia in the ED or those being placed on outpatient analgesics that may further impair respiratory function.

While some degree of cerebral atrophy is part of the normal aging process, in healthy patients cognition and behavior essentially remain normal; however, pathologic cognitive impairment (such as dementia) is common in older patients seeking emergency care.[3,4] These patients may have increased susceptibility to agents with potential central nervous system (CNS) side effects. Some potential complications include prolonged recovery time in patients undergoing procedural sedation, medication-induced delirium, and falls.

Age may also effect pain perception. The belief that normal aging results in reduced sensory acuity, including sensitivity to pain, was reported as early as 1931. Harkins coined the phrase *presbyalgos* to describe this phenomenon[5]; however, studies assessing the existence of presbyalgos have often yielded contradictory results. Gibson and Farrell recently summarized the literature in this area.[6] The number of myelinated and unmyelinated sensory fibers in the skin appears to decline with age. The bulk of evidence also supports a modest but reproducible increase in the pain threshold, particularly for brief, localized, peripheral, or visceral noxious stimuli; however, caution should be used in applying this information in the clinical setting. Rather than implying that older people are less likely to need analgesics, it may mean that they have less warning when a painful stimulus is becoming injurious. Older people also appear to be more prone to upregulation in the face of a persistent noxious stimuli, and prolongation of hyperalgesia after injury. Clinically, this may result in a propensity toward chronic pain and prolonged disability.

PAIN CONTROL IN THE EMERGENCY DEPARTMENT

There are several barriers that may make it harder to achieve adequate pain control in the older patient. The perception that older patients are frail, and cannot handle "stronger" analgesics may lead to the undertreatment of pain. This is supported by evidence that physicians are more hesitant to prescribe adequate analgesia for older patients, even those with metastatic disease.[7,8] Age and cognitive impairment have also been identified as factors associated with inadequate pain management.[9] In addition, older adults tend to underreport pain. These patients may be afraid of burdening caregivers, and may be reluctant to use the word pain to describe their discomfort.[10,11] Comorbidities, medications, and the physiology of aging should not prevent the clinician from striving to achieve adequate pain control.

PAIN MEASUREMENT

Failure to accurately assess pain intensity may be a barrier to adequate pain control.[12-15] This may be particularly true with older patients. While age itself does not appear to limit a patient's ability to use pain assessment tools, higher rates of cognitive, psychomotor, and visual disability found in older populations may complicate pain assessment.[16] This may explain why scales that require better hand-eye coordination and visual acuity, such as the visual analog scale (VAS), are more difficult for elderly patients to complete. Studies have shown that up to 19–25% of persons over 65 fail to correctly use the VAS in clinical and experimental pain settings.[16,17] Other scales of pain intensity, such as the verbal descriptor scale, numeric rating scale, or faces pain scale have significantly lower failure rates, with no significant difference between younger and older age groups.

Pain assessment in patients with severe cognitive deficits may be particularly challenging. While patients with mild-to-moderate cognitive impairment have been shown to provide reliable self-reports of pain intensity, memory deficits may limit the usefulness of recalled pain severity.[11,18] Observation of behavioral cues to pain (increased agitation and verbalization or reduced activity) as well as physical signs of increased sympathetic output (tachycardia, elevated blood pressure, and diaphoresis) may be the only clues to the presence of acute pain.[19]

Multidimensional pain assessments tools such as the McGill Pain Questionnaire offer the advantage of measuring the emotional impact, and perceived significance of the pain experience to the patient. Unfortunately, the McGill Pain scale required an average of 24 minutes to complete among older patients, limiting their clinical use in the emergency setting.[20]

In summary, the VAS may not be the ideal tool for measuring pain intensity among older patients. However, the decision to consistently assess pain severity among elderly ED patients is much more important than deciding which specific pain assessment tool to use.[21]

ACUTE PAIN CONTROL

Older persons with most types of acute, severe pain in the ED should be treated with titrated intravenous (IV) narcotics. Oral medications are unlikely to be sufficiently potent or rapid acting. Medications given via the intramuscular route are difficult to titrate, since peak absorption may be delayed by hours.

Parenteral meperidine has been shown to be an independent predictor of delirium, perhaps due to the psychoactive effects of its metabolite normeperidine, and should be avoided in older patients.

When titrating IV narcotics, it is best to follow the principle of "starting low and going slow." It is particularly important to calculate per kilogram doses for older patients. Starting at the lower end of recommended dose ranges may be appropriate for elders not used to narcotics; however, pain intensity should be reevaluated frequently and narcotics repeated until the patient's pain is adequately controlled.

SELECTED GERIATRIC PAIN SYNDROMES

Vertebral Compression Fractures

Lower back pain is the most common painful complaint among older persons in the community and nursing home settings.[22] Vertebral compression fractures are among the most common causes of acute back pain, affecting 40% of women 80 years and older.[23] The high potential for chronic pain, functional decline, and increased mortality after vertebral compression fractures is gaining recognition.[24] Discovery of a fragility fracture, such as a vertebral compression fracture arising spontaneously or after a trivial injury, should be a "red-flag." These patients should be referred to their primary care physician for investigation of osteoporosis, and consideration of bone-preserving bisphosphonate therapy, since they are at double the risk for a subsequent Colles' and hip fracture.[25] In addition to the use of traditional analgesics, salmon calcitonin may be beneficial. At a dose of 200 units by intranasal spray daily, salmon calcitonin reduces pain intensity within 1 week, reduces the total dose of analgesics required, and reduces the duration of bed rest.[26–28] The side effects profile of salmon calcitonin administered intranasally is similar to placebo, and it can also reduce chronic pain severity.

Hip Fractures

Poor pain control among older patients with hip fractures is well documented. Since many patients with hip fractures also suffer from cognitive decline, concern about inducing delirium may contribute to oligoanalgesia. However, when other risk factors for delirium are controlled for, cognitively-impaired patients given less than the equivalent of 10 mgs of morphine per day postoperatively were 4 times more likely to become delirious compared to patients given >30 mg equivalents per day. Cognitively intact patients given very low dose narcotics were 25 times more likely to become delirious, and patients with one episode of severe pain postoperatively were 9 times more likely to become delirious, clearly, inadequate analgesia is more of a threat for delirium than opioid use, even in cognitively impaired elders.[9]

Traction using a foam boot or skin tape has been advocated to reduce pain while awaiting surgery. Unfortunately, this can cause skin and neurovascular comprise, and recent studies have failed to demonstrate any analgesic effect.[29,30]

In contrast, several studies confirm that the "three-in-one" modified femoral nerve block reduces pain severity and narcotic analgesic requirements.[31] A recent study demonstrated that postgraduate physician-trainees could achieve a high rate of success with the technique after a 30-minute training session and one supervised procedure.[32]

The technique involves injecting long-acting local anesthetic proximally along the femoral nerve sheath, thus blocking the femoral, obturator, and lateral cutaneous nerves.[33]

Postherpetic Neuralgia

Postherpetic neuralgia (PHN) is a potentially devastating complication following reactivation of varicella-zoster infections. Persons over 65 develop zoster 8–10 times more frequently than those under 20, with a lifetime incidence of 23.8%.[34] Although definitions vary, pain that persists for more than 3 months after the rash has healed can be considered PHN. Elders are nearly twice as likely to have persistent PHN pain, affecting 10–15% of those over 65.[34] The burning, constant pain can be very distressing to patients, preventing sleep, and leading to loss of function and depression.[35] Early recognition of the unilateral, vesicular rash is critical, since early antiviral therapy reduces the incidence of PHN by half[36]; however, once chronic neuropathic pain is established, achieving effective analgesia may be difficult. While opioids have traditionally been considered ineffective in neuropathic pain,[37] two randomized trials have shown long-term oxycodone and morphine to have similar effectiveness and tolerability when compared to tricyclic antidepressants for the pain of PHN.[38,39] Topical 5% lidocaine gel applied under an occlusive dressing may also significantly relieve pain.[40] In contrast, topical capsaicin has shown only equivocal effectiveness and poor compliance due to the intense burning application.

Tricyclic antidepressants (TCAs) are effective in reducing pain severity in PHN and are considered first-line therapy; however anticholinergic side effects and postural hypotension significantly limit their use by older patients.[41] Rowbotham recently demonstrated the benefits of gabapentin among 229 patients with PHN (median age 72 years): 42% of patients randomized to gabapentin rated their pain as moderately or much improved, compared to 12% among the placebo group.[42] Since the initiation of TCAs and anticonvulsant therapies require dose titration and clinical monitoring for side effects, emergency physicians will not typically initiate these medications; however, the emergency physician can be instrumental in referring such patients for follow-up with a specialist who is aware of the expanding therapeutic options available for the treatment of PHN.

PHARMACOTHERAPY

Common Drug-Drug Interactions

It is especially important to review all concurrent medications of older patients prior to initiating outpatient analgesic therapy. They are unfortunately more likely to be prescribed multiple medications than younger patients, and may be more susceptible to drug-drug interactions. We will focus on the most commonly encountered interactions.

Acetaminophen—Warfarin

Clinical studies have since demonstrated a dose-dependent prolongation of international normalized ratio (INR) in patients on long-term warfarin who add acetaminophen to their medications. This seems to be particularly likely among older patients with congestive heart failure or chronic atrial fibrillation.[43] Patients needing regular acetaminophen during an episode of acute pain should be advised to have their INR followed weekly by their primary care physician.

NSAID—Antihypertensive Agents

Prostaglandins appear to be important in the regulation of blood pressure. NSAIDs, through their inhibition of cyclooxygenase-dependent prostaglandin synthesis, have been shown to interfere with the antihypertensive effects of diuretics, beta-blockers, and ACE inhibitors. Older patients, who are more likely to have low-renin essential hypertension, are thought to be more susceptible to NSAID antagonism of antihypertensive agents. The risks and benefits of adding NSAIDs should be assessed, and patients should be advised to have their blood pressure monitored while taking these medications. Recent reports of serious heart disease and an increased risk of hospitalization for gastrointestinal bleeding have raised concerns about the use of COX-2 inhibitors, especially in the elderly.

Morphine—Rifampin

Although rifampin is an uncommon drug, its ability to completely inhibit the analgesic effects of morphine warrants mention.[44,45]

Morphine—Ranitidine

Conversely, morphine-ranitidine interactions can compete with hepatic enzymes that metabolize morphine, prolonging clinical activity.[44]

DISCHARGE MEDICATIONS

Deciding on pharmacotherapy after discharge should involve many factors, including the degree of severity of pain, previous analgesics tried, type of condition, and comorbidities. In general, for mild-to-moderate pain, progression from non-opioid-analgesics such as acetaminophen to nonsteroidal anti-inflammatory drugs is appropriate.[2]

For patients who have not tried anything prior to their ED visit and have mild-to-moderate pain, acetaminophen is a reasonable and relatively safe option. It is the first-line therapy in patients with mild-to-moderate pain secondary to degenerative joint disease, and carries fewer risks than NSAIDs. For patients who require (and who do not have contraindications to) an NSAID, shorter-acting agents (such as ibuprofen) may be warranted. NSAIDs are also often an agent of choice for conditions in which the concomitant anti-inflammatory effect is desired to treat the disease process (such as in gout). The association of COX-2 inhibitors with heart disease raises concerns about their use.

For patients with more painful conditions, those who have already tried nonnarcotic agents without success, or those with contraindications to suitable alternatives, narcotics should be considered. There are several possible reasons why physicians may be reluctant to prescribe opioid analgesics in older patients. While older patients may be more susceptible to the side effects of opioid analgesics (for example, sedation, dizziness, and constipation), they also may be more sensitive to analgesic properties.[46] Fear of drug dependency or addiction may also result in a failure to treat pain; however, true narcotic addiction in older patients is probably rare, even in those with persistent pain syndromes.[2] Narcotics may be the optimal initial choice for many patients. In general, when narcotics are used, it is safer to start at lower doses and then increase slowly as needed.

Many analgesics considered safe in younger patients could have potentially serious consequences in an older age group. An expert consensus panel developed a comprehensive list of potentially inappropriate medications in older patients in 1997.[47] This was updated in 2003.[47] Unfortunately, many of the medications on this list have been commonly used in older ED patients.[48]

While narcotic analgesics are often appropriate for the management of acute pain in the elderly, there are several commonly prescribed narcotics that should be avoided. Propoxyphene and related products (such as Darvocet) offer few analgesic advantages over acetaminophen, but carry more side effects such as the risk of excessive drug accumulation, ataxia, and dizziness.[2] If narcotics are indicated, other combination agents such as hydrocodone/acetaminophen (Percocet) may be safer and more effective. Oral meperidine (Demerol) is sedating, may lower the seizure threshold,[47] and can induce hypotension and bradycardia. Pentazocine (Talwin) is a mixed narcotic agonist/antagonist that causes more CNS side effects than other narcotic drugs. Hallucinations and confusion are potential problems in patients taking this medication.

Certain NSAIDs may also be dangerous in older patients. Indomethacin, which is often prescribed for gout, produces more CNS side effects than any other NSAID.[47] Other choices, such as ibuprofen, may be preferable. Ketorolac (Toradol) should also be avoided due to the risk for gastrointestinal bleeding.[49] In addition, shorter-acting NSAIDS may be preferable to long-acting nonselective agents (such as naproxen and pyroxicam), and long-acting agents should be avoided entirely for long-term management of pain.

Muscle relaxants are poorly tolerated in older patients. They often lead to anticholinergic side effects, sedation, and weakness. Their effectiveness at doses tolerated in older patients is at best questionable, and they should generally be avoided.[47] For patients with chronic or neuropathic pain, amitriptyline should never be used. It has strong anticholinergic properties, is very sedating, and can lead to falls and urinary retention.[47] While not completely without risk, alternative agents such as gabapentin (Neurontin) are preferable.

Some medications may cause problems in patients with specific comorbidities. NSAIDs may exacerbate peptic ulcer disease and increase bleeding risk in patients taking anticoagulants. They may cause further impairment of renal function in patients with existing renal insufficiency. NSAIDs should be generally avoided in these patients. Muscle relaxants have anticholinergic side effects, and may cause urinary obstruction in patients with benign prostatic hypertrophy (BPH). Narcotic agents may also contribute to acute urinary retention in patients with BPH, as well as worsen constipation.

SEDATION

Geriatric patients require special consideration when preparing for procedural sedation. Many of these patients have significant comorbidities that may affect the response to sedation. False teeth should be removed. The increased risk of aspiration associated with age should be appreciated. Higher sensitivity to sedatives and analgesics may result in apnea or hypotension. Coronary artery disease or cardiomyopathy may predispose to arrhythmias or myocardial ischemia. For those patients who require bag-mask ventilation due to apnea or oxygen desaturation, increased age and loss of teeth are associated with higher failure rates. In order to avoid some of these potential complications, the principle of "starting low and going slow" should be followed when administering medications, and analgesia should be used in conjunction with sedation in most cases.

There are many agents to choose from when procedural sedation is indicated. Some of the more common agents used include narcotics, benzodiazepines, etomidate, propofol, and methohexital. Choices may be influenced by patient comorbidities, the reason for the procedure, and presenting condition.

There are many disadvantages to using narcotics with benzodiazepines alone in the older patient. Doses required for maintaining adequate sedation and analgesia for many procedures are limited by the risk of respiratory depression. Patients might develop apnea only to awake in distress as attempts are made to relocate a fracture or dislocated joint. Recovery times tend to be longer than that for other shorter-acting agents, and postprocedural delirium is a risk. This is especially problematic in the geriatric population, which is more sensitive to the effects of these agents, and is also more likely to have preexisting CNS abnormalities, such as dementia. For patients undergoing brief procedures that are commonly associated with severe pain (such as DC cardioversion), alternative sedative agents in combination with narcotic analgesics may be preferable.

Etomidate may be ideal in older patients with cardiovascular disease or hypotension due to a relative lack of cardiovascular side effects.[50] In usual doses, it has no significant effect on heart rate, blood pressure, cardiac output, or coronary perfusion pressure.[51] It may however induce myoclonus,[52] and should probably be avoided in older patients with this condition. It should also be used with caution in older patients with seizure disorder. As etomidate has no analgesic properties, concomitant administration of a narcotic analgesic for painful procedures should be strongly considered.

Propofol should be used with caution in older patients. These patients tend to have higher peak plasma concentrations for a given IV dose, and are more prone to the side effects of apnea, oxygen desaturation, airway obstruction, and hypotension. Lower doses are recommended for procedural sedation in older patients. In general, both the loading and maintenance doses should be started at 50% of that recommended for adults and titrated to effect.

The short duration of action of methohexital make it attractive for older patients undergoing brief procedures; however, side effects may limit its use in patients with cardiopulmonary disease. As with other barbiturates, methohexital may cause circulatory depression, apnea, and oxygen desaturation.[53] In addition, nausea and skeletal muscle hyperactivity can also occur. As older patients are more prone to aspiration, vomiting in this group may be particularly problematic.

REFERENCES

1. McNamara RM, Rousseau E, Sanders AB. Geriatric emergency medicine: a survey of practicing emergency physicians. *Ann Emerg Med.* 1992;21(7):796–801.
2. AGS Panel on Persistent Pain in Older Persons. The management of persistent pain in older persons [see comment]. *J Am Geriatr Soc.* 2002; 50(suppl 6):S205–S224.
3. Hustey FM, Meldon SW. The prevalence and documentation of impaired mental status in elderly emergency department patients [see comment]. *Ann Emerg Med.* 2002;39(3): 248–253.
4. Hustey FM, Meldon SW, Smith MD, et al. The effect of mental status screening on the care of elderly emergency department patients. *Ann Emerg Med.* 2003;41(5):678–684.
5. Harkins SW, Price DD, Martelli M. Effects of age on pain perception: thermo nociception. *J Gerontol.* 1986;41(1):58–63.
6. Gibson SJ, Farrell M. A review of age differences in the neurophysiology of nociception and the perceptual experience of pain. *Clin J Pain.* 2004;20(4):227–239.
7. Bernabei R, Gambassi G, Lapane K, et al. Management of pain in elderly patients with cancer. SAGE Study Group. Systematic Assessment of Geriatric Drug Use via Epidemiology [see comment] [erratum appears in JAMA 1999 Jan 13;281(2):136]. *JAMA.* 1998;279(23):1877–1882.
8. Cleeland CS, Gonin R, Hatfield AK, et al. Pain and its treatment in outpatients with metastatic cancer [see comment]. *N Engl J Med.* 1994;330(9):592–596.
9. Morrison RS, Siu AL. A comparison of pain and its treatment in advanced dementia and cognitively intact patients with hip fracture. *J Pain Symptom Manage* 2000; 19(4):240–248.
10. Weiner DK. Improving pain management for older adults: an urgent agenda for the educator, investigator, and practitioner [comment]. *Pain.* 2002;97(1–2):1–4.
11. Ferrell BA. Pain management. *Clin Geriatr Med.* 2000;16(4): 853–874.
12. Choiniere M, Melzack R, Girard N, et al. Comparisons between patients' and nurses' assessment of pain and medication efficacy in severe burn injuries. *Pain.* 1990;40(2): 143–152.
13. Harrison A. Comparing nurses' and patients' pain evaluations: a study of hospitalized patients in Kuwait. *Soc Sci Med.* 1993;36(5):683–692.
14. Drayer RA, Henderson J, Reidenberg M. Barriers to better pain control in hospitalized patients. *J Pain Symptom Manage.* 1999;17(6):434–440.
15. Rupp T, Delaney KA. Inadequate analgesia in emergency medicine. *Ann Emerg Med.* 2004;43(4):494–503.
16. Herr KA, Garand L. Assessment and measurement of pain in older adults. *Clin Geriatr Med.* 2001;17(3):457–478, vi.
17. Herr KA, Mobily PR. Comparison of selected pain assessment tools for use with the elderly. *Appl Nurs Res.* 1993;6(1):39–46.
18. Weiner DK, Peterson BL, Logue P, et al. Predictors of pain self-report in nursing home residents. *Aging* (Milano). 1998;10(5):411–420.

19. Frampton M. Experience assessment and management of pain in people with dementia. *Age Ageing*. 2003;32(3):248–251.

20. McGuire D. Assessment of pain in cancer inpatients using the McGill Pain Questionnaire. *Oncol Nurs Forum*. 1984; 11(6):32–37.

21. Lee JS. Pain measurement: understanding existing tools and their application in the emergency department. *Emerg Med* (Fremantle). 2001;13(3):279–287.

22. Ferrell BA. Pain management in elderly people. *J Am Geriatr Soc*. 1991;39(1):64–73.

23. Melton LJ III, Kan SH, Frye MA, et al. Epidemiology of vertebral fractures in women. *Am J Epidemiol*. 1989;129(5): 1000–1011.

24. Truumees E. Medical consequences of osteoporotic vertebral compression fractures. *Instr Course Lect*. 2003; 52:551–558.

25. Haentjens P, Autier P, Collins J, et al. Colles fracture, spine fracture, and subsequent risk of hip fracture in men and women. A meta-analysis. *J Bone Joint Surg Am*. 2003; 85-A(10):1936–1943.

26. Pun KK, Chan LW. Analgesic effect of intranasal salmon calcitonin in the treatment of osteoporotic vertebral fractures. *Clin Ther*. 1989;11(2):205–209.

27. Lyritis GP, Paspati I, Karachalios T, et al. Pain relief from nasal salmon calcitonin in osteoporotic vertebral crush fractures. A double blind, placebo-controlled clinical study. *Acta Orthop Scand Suppl*. 1997;275:112–114.

28. Silverman SL, Azria M. The analgesic role of calcitonin following osteoporotic fracture. *Osteoporos Int*. 2002;13(11): 858–867.

29. Rosen JE, Chen FS, Hiebert R, et al. Efficacy of preoperative skin traction in hip fracture patients: a prospective, randomized study. *J Orthop Trauma*. 2001;15(2):81–85.

30. Parker M. Pre-operative traction for fractures of the proximal femur. *Cochrane Database Syst Rev*. 2003;3: CD000168.

31. Parker MJ, Griffiths R, Appadu BN. Nerve blocks (subcostal, lateral cutaneous, femoral, triple, psoas) for hip fractures. *Cochrane Database Syst Rev*. 2001(2):CD001159.

32. Fletcher AK, Rigby AS, Heyes FL. Three-in-one femoral nerve block as analgesia for fractured neck of femur in the emergency department: a randomized, controlled trial. *Ann Emerg Med*. 2003;41(2):227–233.

33. Winnie AP, Ramamurthy S, Durrani Z. The inguinal paravascular technic of lumbar plexus anesthesia: the "3-in-1 block." *Anesth Analg*. 1973;52(6):989–996.

34. Bowsher D. The lifetime occurrence of Herpes zoster and prevalence of post-herpetic neuralgia: a retrospective survey in an elderly population. *Eur J Pain*. 1999;3(4):335–342.

35. Dworkin RH, Hartstein G, Rosner HL, et al. A high-risk method for studying psychosocial antecedents of chronic pain: the prospective investigation of herpes zoster. *J Abnorm Psychol*. 1992;101(1):200–205.

36. Jackson JL, Gibbons R, Meyer G, et al. The effect of treating herpes zoster with oral acyclovir in preventing postherpetic neuralgia. A meta-analysis. *Arch Intern Med*. 1997;157(8): 909–912.

37. Kost RG, Straus SE. Postherpetic neuralgia—pathogenesis, treatment, and prevention. *N Engl J Med*. 1996;335(1):32–42.

38. Watson CP, Babul N. Efficacy of oxycodone in neuropathic pain: a randomized trial in postherpetic neuralgia. *Neurology*. 1998;50(6):1837–1841.

39. Raja SN, Haythornthwaite JA, Pappagallo M, et al. Opioids versus antidepressants in postherpetic neuralgia: a randomized, placebo-controlled trial. *Neurology*. 2002;59(7):1015–1021.

40. Rowbotham MC, Davies PS, Fields HL. Topical lidocaine gel relieves postherpetic neuralgia. *Ann Neurol*. 1995;37(2): 246–253.

41. Kanazi GE, Johnson RW, Dworkin RH. Treatment of postherpetic neuralgia: an update. *Drugs*. 2000;59(5):1113–1126.

42. Rowbotham M, Harden N, Stacey B, et al. Gabapentin for the treatment of postherpetic neuralgia: a randomized controlled trial. *JAMA*. 1998;280(21):1837–1842.

43. Lehmann DE. Enzymatic shunting: resolving the acetaminophen-warfarin controversy. *Pharmacotherapy*. 2000; 20(12):1464–1468.

44. Lugo RA, Kern SE. Clinical pharmacokinetics of morphine. *J Pain Palliat Care Pharmacother*. 2002;16(4):5–18.

45. Fromm MF, Eckhardt K, Li S, et al. Loss of analgesic effect of morphine due to coadministration of rifampin. *Pain*. 1997;72(1–2):261–267.

46. Kaiko RF, Wallenstein SL, Rogers AG, et al. Narcotics in the elderly. *Med Clin North Am*. 1982;66(5):1079–1089.

47. Beers MH. Explicit criteria for determining potentially inappropriate medication use by the elderly. An update. *Arch Intern Med*. 1997;157(14):1531–1536.

48. Caterino JM, Emond JA, Camargo CA, Jr. Inappropriate medication administration to the acutely-ill elderly population: a nationwide emergency department study. *J Amer Geriatric Society*. 2004;52:1847–1855.

49. Fick DM, Cooper JW, Wade WE, et al. Updating the Beers criteria for potentially inappropriate medication use in older adults: results of a US consensus panel of experts [erratum appears in Arch Intern Med. 2004 Feb 9;164(3):298]. *Arch Inter Med*. 2003;163(22):2716–2724.

50. Gooding JM, Weng JT, Smith RA, et al. Cardiovascular and pulmonary responses following etomidate induction of anesthesia in patients with demonstrated cardiac disease. *Anesth Analg*. 1979;58(1):40–41.

51. Evers AS, Crowder CM. General anesthetics. In: Hardman JG, Limbird LE, Gilman AG, eds. *Goodman Gilman's the Pharmacological Basis of Therapeutics*. New York: McGraw-Hill; 2001:337–365.

52. Giese JL, Stanley TH. Etomidate: a new intravenous anesthetic induction agent. *Pharmacotherapy*. 1983;3(5):251–258.

53. Miner JR, Biros M, Krieg S, et al. Randomized clinical trial of propofol versus methohexital for procedural sedation during fracture and dislocation reduction in the emergency department. *Acad Emerg Med*. 2003;10(9):931–937.

45

Sedation and Analgesia in the Pregnant Patient

Scott Bailey
Pamela Dyne

HIGH YIELD FACTS

- Consider possible teratogenic and/or negative physiologic effects on the fetus from pharmacologic intervention but give drugs when indicated.
- Pregnancy causes ↑ sensitivity to diuretics, morphine, and aortocaval compression (use left lateral decubitus positioning).
- Pregnancy causes ↓ absorption of inhaled gases so preoxygenate prior to procedures.
- Pregnancy causes ↑ difficulty with intubations from weight gain, upper airway edema/hyperemia, and breast enlargement.
- Assume a full stomach and ↑ risk of aspiration in pregnant patients (use Sellick maneuver during intubation).
- ↑ hepatic metabolism, ↑ renal excretion occurs in pregnancy (give drugs more frequently).
- ↑ incidence of side effects to amide local anesthetics in pregnancy (monitor closely, consider ↓ initial dose).
- Know the differential diagnosis and treatment for the common complaints of headache and back/pelvic pain during pregnancy.

INTRODUCTION

The treatment of painful conditions in the pregnant patient presents challenges to the physician because of concern for teratogenic and/or negative physiologic effects on the fetus as a result of pharmacologic interventions. Every maternal organ system undergoes change during gestation, which alters drug absorption, metabolism, and elimination. This chapter will provide an understanding of the practical implications of these altered pharmacokinetics, along with useful nonpharmacologic adjunctive treatment modalities. This will facilitate the delivery of safe and efficacious care to the gravid patient.

PHYSIOLOGIC CHANGES OF PREGNANCY

The multiple, profound physiologic adaptations in pregnancy alter the disposition and effects of systemic analgesics, local anesthetics, sedatives, and hypnotics. Drugs given during pregnancy may negatively impact the embryo or fetus by (1) lethal or teratogenic effects, (2) placental vascular constriction impairing nutrient and gas exchange, (3) anoxic injury from uterine hypertonia, and (4) altered maternal biochemistry. The fetus is at the greatest risk for teratogenesis during the period of organogenesis from the 3rd to the 8th week. Drugs given before this period usually have a dichotomous impact: either no effect or causing abortion. Drugs given after 8 weeks may alter the growth of previously normally formed tissues (Table 45-1).[1]

Cardiovascular

In pregnancy, the circulation becomes hyperdynamic with the cardiac output increasing by up to 50%. This is accomplished by increases in left ventricular mass, stroke volume, and heart rate.[2] These physiologic changes make pregnant women very sensitive to drugs that decrease intravascular volume or preload (diuretics, morphine), or which cause negative inotropy and chronotropy (systemically absorbed lidocaine). The enlarging uterus also causes aortocaval compression giving rise to the *supine hypotensive syndrome*, which is usually most significant in the third trimester. This makes left lateral patient positioning critical during administration of drugs which might induce or exacerbate hypotension (morphine, fentanyl, propofol).

Respiratory Tract: Lungs

In pregnancy, respiratory tract changes occur as a result of progesterone and due to the mechanical impact of the enlarging uterus. The respiratory rate, minute ventilation, and plasma pH increase, while the lung vital capacity and functional reserve decrease. These changes impair the absorption of inhaled agents making the pregnant patient more prone to hypoxia during procedural sedation or intubation. However, the impact on the fetus is lessened by the fact that the fetus operates on a steeper part of the oxygen-Hgb dissociation curve, and considerable oxygen reserve may be created for the fetus by the preprocedural administration of high flow oxygen for 5 minutes.[2]

Table 45-1. Physiologic Changes of Pregnancy

Organ System	Physiologic Changes	Clinical Impact	Consequences/ Clinical Actions
Cardiovascular	↑ cardiac output by ↑ left ventricular mass ↑ stroke volume ↑ heart rate Aortocaval compression	↑ Sensitivity to drugs ↓ intravascular volume or ↓ preload or drugs with negative inotrope Supine hypotensive syndrome	↑ Sensitivity to diuretics, morphine ↓ intravascular volume, preload, negative inotrope: lidocaine (systemic) Left lateral decubitus positioning
Respiratory Lungs	↑ progesterone Mechanical pressure of gravid uterus	↑ Respiratory rate ↑ minute ventilation ↑ plasma pH ↓ lung vital capacity ↓ functional reserve capacity ↑ susceptibility to hypoxia (offset by fetus acts on steep part of oxygen—Hgb dissociation curve)	↓ absorption of inhaled gases/anesthetics (nitrous oxide) Preoxygenate patient with high flow oxygen for 5 minutes prior to intubation
Respiratory Upper airway	Hyperemia/edema of mouth/upper airway Weight gain Breast enlargement	Edematous hyperemic tissues in upper airway	↑ difficulty with intubations, nasopharyngeal procedures
Gastrointestinal	↓ lower esophageal sphincter tone Delayed gastric emptying (due to progesterone) Uterine compression of abdomen	In pregnant patients "assume a full stomach"	↑ risk of aspiration of gastric contents Use Sellick maneuver during intubation
Hepatic and renal	↑ hepatic metabolism and ↑ renal excretion of most drugs and their metabolites	↑ drug-dosing regimens for many drugs (exception: local anesthetics)	Give drugs more frequently (exception: local anesthetics)
Hepatic and renal: local anesthetics	↓ plasma protein binding ↑ fraction of free active drug	↓ threshold for aberrant reactions to amide local anesthetics Local reactions: allergic reactions, tissue necrosis from vasoconstrictors, intravascular infiltration (bradydysrhythmias, hypotension), CNS reactions: hallucinations and unresponsiveness	↑ incidence of side effects to amide local anesthetics Monitor for reactions Consider modest initial ↓ dose

Respiratory Tract: Upper Airway

Considerable hyperemia and edema occur in the mouth and upper airways, which, in conjunction with weight gain and breast enlargement make tracheal intubation or nasopharyngeal procedures potentially more difficult.

Gastrointestinal

Every late-term pregnant patient is "assumed to have a full stomach" because of progesterone-induced delayed gastric emptying, decreased lower esophageal sphincter tone, and uterine compression of abdominal contents.[3]

Because pregnant patients are at greater risk for aspiration of gastric contents, the Sellick maneuver (holding of cricoid pressure) is an imperative during intubation.

Hepatic and Renal Metabolism

In pregnancy, hepatic metabolism and renal excretion of most drugs and metabolites increases. This may necessitate increases in many drug-dosing regimens in pregnancy; however, local anesthetics are an exception. Pregnancy-related decreases in plasma protein binding contribute to increased local and systemic effects. A study of bupivacaine total and free fractions, and of albumin and alpha-1-glycoprotein concentrations through pregnancy found that the fraction of free, active drug increased and correlated strongly with concomitant decreases in concentrations of those proteins.[4] Thus, a lower threshold exists for maternal aberrant reaction to amide class local anesthetics. These reactions include local problems including allergic reactions and tissue necrosis from vasoconstriction because of epinephrine content, and intravascular infiltration leading to bradydysrhythmias and hypotension (particularly with bupivacaine). Central neurologic effects of auditory and visual hallucinations and decreased responsiveness may also result. Monitor carefully for these effects and consider a modest initial dose reduction when using this class of medications.

PROCEDURAL SEDATION AND ANALGESIA FOR THE PREGNANT PATIENT

- Provide both sedation and analgesia if sedation for a painful procedure is required.
- Consider the clinical effects of physiologic changes (Table 45-1).
- Consider the pregnancy class when administering drugs to pregnant patients but give drugs when needed (Table 45-2).
- Use a local anesthetic approach when possible.
  - Local infiltration of wound or a hematoma block.
  - Distal single nerve block.
  - Specialized regional blocks (consider anesthesiology consult): brachial plexus block (shoulder dislocation), Bier block.
  - Neuraxial approach (consider an anesthesiology consult): epidural anesthesia (hip dislocation, large lower extremity laceration, or fracture needing reduction).

Table 45-2. Pregnancy Class for Sedatives and Analgesics*

Drug	Pregnancy Class
Local anesthetics	
Lidocaine	B
Bupivacaine	C
Sedatives	
Barbiturates	
Pentobarbital	D
Benzodiazepines	
Diazepam	D
Lorazepam	D
Midazolam	D
Etomidate	C
Propofol	B
Ketamine	B
Narcotic analgesics	
Fentanyl	C
Morphine	C

*Pregnancy class may differ based on the reference used. See Chap. 20 for discussion.

SPECIAL CIRCUMSTANCES: PAINFUL CONDITIONS IN PREGNANCY HEADACHE

Headaches in pregnant patients may be the symptom of a serious neurologic or systemic process, the continuation of a previously known benign headache pattern, or the de novo occurrence of episodic benign headaches. Important causes of secondary headache in pregnancy include preeclampsia, eclampsia, hemolytic anemia, *e*levated *l*iver enzymes, and *l*ow *p*latelet-count (HELLP) syndrome, meningitis, subarachnoid hemorrhage, and aneurismal bleeding. Patients with potentially dangerous disease states *may* have focal neurologic deficits or systemic signs of toxicity or sepsis such as fever, cardiopulmonary abnormalities, hepatomegaly, petechiae, uterine tenderness, anemia, and thrombocytopenia. A complete physical examination including a detailed neurologic examination with retinal visualization and appropriate screening laboratory studies is indicated.

Dangerous conditions causing headaches are relatively rare compared to the more common type of headaches in pregnancy: migraine and tension-type headaches. Gender-specific differences in headache prevalence exist, and are believed to result from gender-specific steroid cycling. The lifetime prevalences of migraine is 25% in women and 8% in men, and of tension-type headache is 88%

Fig. 45-1. Age/gender demographics of migraine headache. Prior to the age of 12, incidence of migraine headache is equal among boys and girls. After age 12, migraine headache increases among females, reaching a peak at age 40, with a female to male ratio of 3:1. (Source: Lipton RB, Stewart WF. Migraine in the United States: a review of epidemiology and health care use. *Neurology.* 1993;43 (suppl 3):S6–S10. Copyright 2001 by AAN Enterprises, Inc. *Neurology*, online. *http://www.neurology.org/.* Used with permission.)

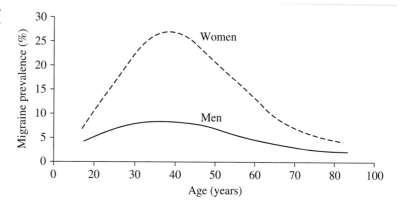

in women and 69% in men.[5] Before the age of 12, the prevalence of migraine in boys is equal to or slightly greater than that in girls, but after puberty the female predominance becomes evident. The ratios of migraine prevalence in women to men are 2:1 at age 20, 3:1 at 40, and 2.5:1 at 70[6] (Fig. 45-1).

The noncycling, high estrogen levels of pregnancy generally raise the threshold for the perception of pain.[7] Even so, many patients will still have new-onset headache, or new pain patterns compared to old headaches because of the complex interactions of pregnancy-induced changes in neural structure and physiology, and soft tissue and vascular tone.[8–10] Approximately 50% of pregnant women with migraines will experience a 50% reduction in headache severity by the end of the first trimester, and another 30% will experience some improvement later in pregnancy. Tension headache improves for only about 25% of patients during pregnancy.[11]

A "wait and see" approach to the treatment of headache during pregnancy with the hope of spontaneous remission will leave a large proportion of sufferers without treatment and is not recommended. Active and effective treatments with nonmedical and medical approaches are warranted.

NONPHARMACOLOGIC TREATMENTS FOR HEADACHES

- Effective in this usually highly motivated patient population because of the desire to avoid potential fetal toxins.
- Identification and control of headache *triggers.*
  - Regulate sleep patterns.
  - Stress management.

- Discontinue alcohol, nicotine, caffeine.
- Dietary irregularities—shown to be causal of headache more in women than men. Advise eating small, frequent meals, avoidance of restrictive diets except for nutrition-poor foods known to trigger headaches.

- Refer for physical therapy, relaxation training, and biofeedback. Primary and follow-up studies have shown a reduction in migraine and tension-type headache for 80% of patients so treated with a durable response rate of 65% of patients 1 year postpartum.[12,13]

- Two high-caliber resource organizations for patient information and self-help can be accessed at the following:
  - National Headache Foundation: *http://www. headaches.org/consumer/index.html*
  - American Council on Headache Education (ACHE) *http://www.achenet.org/*

PHARMCOLOGIC TREATMENTS FOR HEADACHES

Medical treatment of pain in pregnancy requires vigilant attention to potential adverse effects on mother and fetus, which are listed in Table 45-3. Some clinical "pearls" of medical pain management for headache in pregnancy include the following:

- Avoid nonsteroidal anti-inflammatory drugs (NSAIDs) around conception and near term.

- Avoid prolonged use (i.e., >3 days per week) of any analgesic to avoid rebound daily headaches in the case of NSAIDs, and of dependence on opioids.

Table 45-3. Pharmacologic Therapy for Headache in Pregnancy

Medications Feeding	Periconceptual and First Trimester	Second > Third Trimester	Breast
Acute Abortive Treatment			
Simple analgesics			
Aspirin	C	C > D	Caution: fetal bleeding risk
Acetaminophen	B	D	Compatible
Caffeine	B	B	Compatible
Narcotics*			
Morphine	C	B	Compatible
Hydromorphone	C	B	Compatible
Methadone	C	B	Compatible
Butorphanol	C	B	Compatible
Codeine	C	C	Compatible
Meperidine	C	C	Compatible
Propoxyphene	C	C	Compatible
NSAIDs†‡			
Ibuprofen	B	B > D	Compatible
Naproxen	B	B > D	Compatible
Indomethacin	B	B > D	Compatible
Barbiturates			
Butalbitol	C	C	Caution: sedation
Phenobarbital	C	C	Caution: sedation
Benzodiazepines			
Diazepam	D	D	Unknown effects
Lorazepam	D	D	Unknown effects
Antihistamines			
Meclizine	B	B	Unknown
Dimenhydrinate	B	B	Unknown
Cyproheptadine	B	B	Contraindicated: neonatal sedation
Antiemetics/Neuroleptics			
Emetrol	B	B	Compatible
Metoclopramide	B	B	Concern
Promethazine	C	C	Concern
Trimethobenzamide	C	C	Unknown
Prochlorperazine	C	C	Compatible
Tryptans‖ and Ergots§			
Naratriptan	C	C	Pump and dump
Rizatriptan	C	C	For 4 hours after dosing
Sumatriptan	C	C	For 4 hours after dosing
Zolmitriptan	C	C	For 4 hours after dosing
Ergotamine	X-placental vasoconstriction	X	Vomiting, diarrhea, convulsions
Dihydroergotamine	X-placental vasoconstriction	X	Vomiting, diarrhea, convulsions

Table 45-3. Pharmacologic Therapy for Headache in Pregnancy (*Continued*)

Medications Feeding	Periconceptual and First Trimester	Second > Third Trimester	Breast
Prophylactic Treatment			
Antihypertensives			
Metoprolol	C	C	Compatible
Atenolol	D: low birth weight	D	Concern for neonatal bradycardia
Diltiazem	C	C	Compatible
Nifedipine	C	C	Compatible
Verapamil	C	C	Compatible
Antidepressants			
Bupropion	B	B	Concern
Fluoxetine	B	B	Concern
Nefazodone	C	C	Concern
Sertraline	C	C	Concern
Paroxetine	C	C	Concern
Amitriptyline	D	D	Concern
Anticonvulsants			
Neurontin	C	C	Unknown
Carbamazepine	C	C	Compatible
Phenobarbital	D	D	Compatible
Phenytoin	D	D	Compatible
Valproate	D	D	Compatible
Corticosteroids			
Prednisone	B	B	Compatible
Dexamethasone	C	C	Compatible
Cortisone	D	D	Compatible

*All are elevated to class D if use is prolonged or near term (fetal withdrawal risk).
†Early effect: impaired embryo implantation—avoid if trying to conceive.
‡Late effect: fetal pulmonary hypertension and labor difficulties—class B before 32 weeks and class D after 32 weeks EGA.
¶Selective serotonin agonists.
§Nonselective serotonin agonists.

Source: Adapted from Spierings ELH. *Headache.* Butterworth-Heinemann; 1998:153–185; and American Council for Headache Education, Planning Pregnancy While Managing Migraine, Web publication, Nov. 20, 2001.

- Reassure a pregnant patient if she inadvertently takes a dose of a triptan drug. A postmarketing patient registry documenting the usage experience of 220 patients has shown no ill effects from isolated exposures to triptans.[14]

- If an enteral route of administration is used for treatment of headache and nausea, administer the antiemetic or prokinetic agent 15 minutes prior to the analgesic. GI peristalsis and absorption is frequently impaired during migraines.

BACK AND PELVIC PAIN

Back and pelvic pain in a pregnant patient often represents a benign musculoskeletal disorder, but it is important to consider the onset of labor and genitourinary disorders such as vaginitis, cystitis, pyelonephritis, and nephrolithiasis. The evaluation of low back pain requires a history including the chronicity of the pain and the character of the pain, assessment for fever and costovertebral angle tenderness, and laboratory tests: urinalysis, blood urea nitrogen (BUN)/creatinine, and complete blood count. Assessment of fetal heart tones

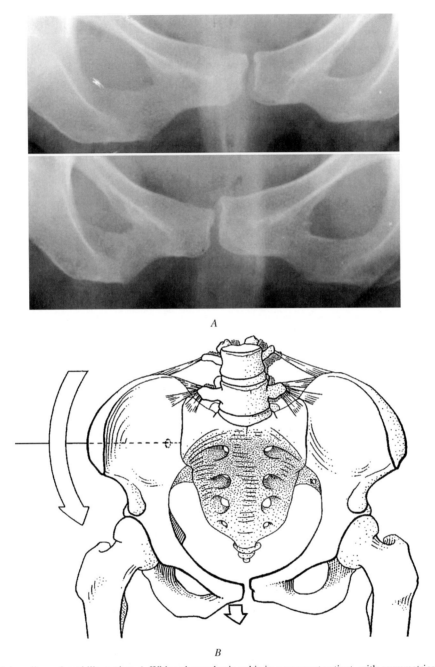

A

B

Fig. 45-2. Pelvic radiograph and illustration. *A.* Widened symphysis pubis in a pregnant patient, with asymmetrically, anteriorly rotated right hemi-pelvis. *B.* Schematic of rotary forces on sacroiliac (SI) pain, giving rise to SI microtrauma and regional pain. (Source: X-ray and schematic diagram adapted from Mens JMA, Vleeming A, Snijders C, et al. The active straight leg raise test and mobility of the pelvic joints. *Eur Spin J.* 1999;8:468–473. Used with permission.)

by Doppler is appropriate for patients greater than 10–12 weeks EGA when fetal heart tones become detectable.

The incidence of musculoskeletal back pain in pregnancy is estimated at 30–50% becoming most common in the 6th month and lasting until 6 months postpartum. Risk factors for back pain in pregnancy include preexisting back pain and multiparity.[15,16] It is hypothesized that changes in spinal loading and in the hormonal milieu make the pregnant woman more prone to back pain. Growth of the fetus causes abdominal wall distention, which results in loss of abdominal wall muscular tone and leaves the lumbar paraspinus musculature unbalanced and prone to strain. The center of gravity shifts backward in the pelvis and abdomen as pregnancy progresses. This along with minimal change in lumbar lordosis results in posterior displacement of the spinal column.[17] The hormone relaxin rises 10-fold during pregnancy, reaching a zenith at 38–42 weeks of pregnancy.[18] This allows the ligamentous laxity necessary for pelvic expansion during gestation and parturition, but also destabilizes multiple joints. The symphysis pubis widens from 0.5 mm to as much as 12 mm. This allows rotary stress at the sacroiliac (SI) joint and causes SI microtrauma and pain[19] (Fig. 45-2). In the spinal column, support from the anterior and posterior spinal ligaments weakens, making associated structures more susceptible to anterior shearing forces and increasing discogenic and facetogenic symptoms.

The three common types of back pain during pregnancy are in order of frequency: SI pain, lumbar pain, and nocturnal back pain.[20] Sacroiliac pain associated with pregnancy is much more common and is distinct from true sciatica, which has a prevalence of only 1% in pregnancy.[21] SI pain is a posterior pelvic pain, with discomfort spreading across the upper buttocks and sacrum, either unilaterally or bilaterally, and typically starting in the second trimester and persisting or progressively worsening through the pregnancy as the relaxin levels peak.[22] Pain in the anterior pelvis is termed *symphiolysis pubis*, and pain in all three joints, *pelvic girdle syndrome*.[23,24]

Nocturnal back pain occurs alone or in conjunction with lumbar or SI pain. Putative mechanisms for this include end-of-day cumulative muscle fatigue, and tissue edema redistribution causing retroperitoneal venous plexus engorgement.[25,26]

Several bedside examinations aid in the clinical diagnosis of low back pain and help distinguish SI pain from the other types of back and pelvic pain in pregnant patients:

Gower's Maneuver

As the patient attempts to rise from a chair or squatting position, she will need to turn toward one side, and lift the trunk by supporting her weight on her arms and pushing upward if she has SI pain.

Posterior Pelvic Provocation Test

Place the patient in a supine position with the hip of the affected side in 90° of flexion. Apply gentle downward pressure on the flexed femur while stabilizing the other side of pelvis. This test is positive for SI pain if the pain is reproduced by the pressure (81% sensitivity, 80% specificity).

Fabere Test

*F*lexion *ab*duction *e*xternal *r*otation *e*xternal side:
Place the patient in a supine position with the hip of the affected side flexed, abducted, externally rotated, and the external side of the ankle resting over the other extended leg.

Ventral Gapping Test

Place the patient in a supine position. Manual distraction of the sides of the pelvis reproduces SI pain.

Dorsal Gapping Test

Place the patient in a supine position. Manual compression of the sides of the pelvis reproduces SI pain.

TREATMENT OF LOW BACK PAIN

The treatment of pregnancy-related musculoskeletal pelvic and low back pain is primarily nonpharmacologic in nature. Moderately strong clinical research data and expert physical medicine opinion support such an approach.[27–29] Physical therapy seems to be most effective if the treatment is specialized for a patient's particular needs, and if a regular program of stabilizing exercises is followed. Evidence suggests that at least 50% of patients show significant improvement.[30] Emergency department (ED) physicians can and should initiate treatment immediately by providing simple instructions on posture, footwear, leg elevation, and by making a referral to a competent physical therapy provider.[31] Table 45-4 summarizes the clinical features and management options for musculoskeletal pelvic and back pain in pregnancy.

SUMMARY

Analgesia and sedation in the pregnant patient is a challenge because of concern for the teratogenic and/or negative physiologic effects on the fetus as a result of

Table 45-4. Back Pain in Pregnancy

Pain Entity	Characteristic Symptoms	Physical Examination	Treatment
Sacroiliac pain	Pain distal and lateral to lumbar spine and deep gluteal Exacerbated by prolonged positions and weight bearing, standing, walking	No hip pathology or neurologic deficits (+) Posterior pelvic provocation test (+) Gapping tests, dorsal and ventral (+) Fabere test	Cold or hot packs Refer for nonelastic trochanteric belt Refer for physical therapy, customized treatment and exercise regimen
Lumbar pain	Pain in lumbar area only ± Radiation to lower extremity Exacerbated by prolonged weight bearing and sitting More persistent in nature, including postpartum	No hip pathology or neurologic deficits Discogenic pain: pain increases with waist flexion and standing Facetogenic pain: pain increases with waist extension and rotation to affected side	Avoid high heeled shoes While sitting, elevate leg of affected side While standing, place leg on a stool Refer for physical therapy, customized treatment, and exercise regimen Refer for TENS placement Whirlpools are contraindicated
Nocturnal pain	Pain that occurs at night, alone or with the above	No specific signs	Cold or hot packs Refer for physical therapy

TENS: transcutaneous electric nerve stimulation.

Source: Adapted from Colliton J. Managing backache pain during pregnancy. *Medscape Gen Med.* 1999;1(2).

pharmacologic treatment. Many profound physiologic changes occur during pregnancy that alter a drug's metabolism and effects. Local and regional anesthesia employing local infiltration, hematoma block, nerve blocks, regional blocks, or a neuraxial approach can be valuable in treating pregnant patients with painful injuries/conditions. Nonpharmacologic techniques can also be useful in treating painful disorders such as headaches. It is important for the physician to be familiar with the differential diagnosis and treatment options for back/pelvic pain and headaches, two commonly encountered disorders in pregnant patients.

REFERENCES

1. Dilts PV, Jr. Normal pregnancy, labor and delivery. Chap. 248. In: Beers MH, Berkow R, eds. The Merck Manual of Diagnosis and Therapy. Whitehouse Station, NJ: Merck Research Laboratories, 1999, pp. 2016–2031.
2. Lapinsky SE, Kruczynski K, Slutsky AS. Critical care in the pregnant patient. *Am J Respir Crit Care Med.* 1995;152 (2):427–455.
3. Penning D. Trauma in pregnancy. *Can J Anesth.* 2001;6(48): R1–R4.
4. Faure EA. Anesthesia for the pregnant patient, University of Chicago Obstetrical Anesthesia. http://daccx.bsd.uchicago. edu/manuals/obstetric/obanesthesia.html
5. Lawrence CT, et al. Measurements of Maternal Protein Binding of bupivacaine throughout pregnancy, *Anesth Analg.* 1999;89:965.
6. Rasmussen BK, Jensen R, Schroll M, et al. Epidemiology of headache in a general population prevalence study. *J Clin Epidemiol.* 1991;44:1147–1157.
7. Lipton RB, Stewart WF. Migraine in the United States: a review of epidemiology and health care use. *Neurology.* 1993;43(suppl 3):S6–S10.
8. Watanabe S, Otsubo Y, Araki T. The current perception thresholds in pregnancy. *J Nippon Med Sch.* 2002;69(4): 342–346.
9. Oshima M, Ogawa R, Menkes DL. Current perception threshold increases during pregnancy but does not change across menstrual cycle. *J Nippon Med Sch.* 2002;69(1): 19–23.
10. Marcus, D. Management of headache in women, *J Gend Specif Med.* 1999;2(4):47–50.
11. Aloisi AM. Gonadal Hormones and sex differences in pain reactivity, *Clin J Pain.* 2003;19:168–174.
12. Chancellor AM, Wroe SJ, Cull RE. Migraine occurring for the first time in pregnancy. *Headache.* 1990;30:224–227.
13. Scharff L, Marcus D, Turk D. Maintenance of effects in the nonmedical treatment of headaches during pregnancy. *Headache.* 1996;36:285–290.
14. Marcus D, Scharf L, Turk D. Nonpharmacologic management of headaches during pregnancy. *Psychosom Med.* 1995;6(57):527–535.

15. Baker B. Triptans Not Advised for Migraines in Pregnancy, *Fam Pract News*. March 5, 2000.

16. Mantle MJ, Greenwood RM, Corey HL. Backache in pregnancy. *Rheumatol Rehabil*. 1977;16:95–101.

17. To WW, Wong MWN. Factors associated with back pain symptoms in pregnancy and the persistence of pain 2 years after pregnancy. *Acta Obstet Gynecol Scand*. 2003;82:1086–1091.

18. Hummel P. Changes in posture during pregnancy. Philadelphia, PA: W.B. Saunders; 1987.

19. Calguneri M, Bird HA, Wright V. Changes in joint laxity during pregnancy. *Ann Rheum Dis*. 1982;41:126–128.

20. Colliton J. Managing back pain during pregnancy. *Medscape Gen Med*. 1999;1(2). www.medscape.com

21. Albert H, Godskesen M, Westergaard J. Prognosis in four syndromes of pregnancy-related pelvic pain, *Acta Obstet Gynecol Scand*. 2001;80:505–510.

22. Ostgaard HC, Anderson GB, Karlson K. Prevalence of back pain in pregnancy. *Spine*. 1991;16(5):549–552.

23. To WWK, Wong MWN. Factors associated with back pain symptoms in pregnancy and the persistence of pain 2 years after pregnancy, *Acta Obstet Gynecol Scand*. 2003;82: 086–1091.

24. Albert H, Godskesen M, Westergaard J. Prognosis in four syndromes of pregnancy related pelvic pain. *Acta Obstet Gynecol Scand*. 2001;80:505–510.

25. Damen L, Buyruk HM, Guler-Uysal F, et al. Pelvic pain during pregnancy is associated with asymmetric laxity of the sacroiliac joints, *Acta Obstet Gynecol Scand*. 2001;80: 1019–1024.

26. Fast A, Weiss L, Parikh S, et al. Night backache in pregnancy: Hypothetical pathophysiological mechanisms. *Am J Phys Med Rehabil*. 1989;68:227–229.

27. Stuge B, Laerum E, Kirkesola G, et al. The efficacy of a treatment program focusing on specific stabilizing exercises for pelvic girdle pain after pregnancy—a randomized controlled trial. *Spine*. 2004;29(4):351–359.

28. Stuge B, Hilde G, Vollestad N. Physical therapy for pregnancy-related low back and pelvic pain: a systematic review. *Acta Obstet Gynecol Scand*. 2003;82:983–990.

29. Mantel MJ, Greenwood RM, Currey HL. Backache in pregnancy. *Rheumatol Rehabil*. 1977;16(2):95–101.

30. Mens J M A, Vleeming A, Snijders C, et alStam H J, Ginai, A. The active straight leg raise test and mobility of the pelvic joints, *Eur Spin J*. (1999);8:468–473;468–473.

31. Stuge B, Laerum E, Kirkesola G, et al. The efficacy of a treatment program focusing on specific stabilizing exercises for pelvic girdle pain after pregnancy. *Spine*. 2004;29(4): 351–359.

46

The Palliative Approach to Pain Management in the Emergency Department

Tammie E. Quest
Robert J. Zalenski

HIGH YIELD FACTS

- Palliative care meets the physical, psychologic, social, and spiritual needs of patients/families with chronic progressive life-threatening illness.
- Untreated pain is physically, emotionally, psychologically, and spiritually devastating for patients/families.
- The balance of curative and palliative therapies needs to be individualized for each specific patient/family.
- It is unethical for physicians to provide inadequate treatment of pain and other symptoms at the end-of-life for fear of hastening death.
- Double effect is the provision of adequate medication by a physician that is intended to relieve suffering but *unintentionally* hastens death.
- Double effect is sanctioned by the U.S. Supreme Court and should be differentiated from physician-assisted suicide (illegal in most states).
- Pain is multidimensional with physical, emotional, and spiritual aspects.
- In patients on opiates, determination of morphine equivalents can help guide therapy.
- Develop a stepwise plan utilizing opiates plus adjuvant drugs plus nonpharmacologic therapy as needed.

INTRODUCTION: DEFINITIONS AND PRINCIPLES

Palliative care is provided to patients to aggressively meet the physical, psychologic, social, and spiritual care needs of patients and families across the continuum of diagnosis to death or cure in patients living with chronic, progressive, life-threatening illness such as cancer, progressive neurologic, pulmonary, or cardiovascular conditions.[1] Palliative care is best initiated early in the disease and should continue till cure or death in an effort to alleviate suffering (Fig. 46-1).[2]

Moderate-to-severe hospital pain is predictive of persistent pain in patients with serious illness. Of over 5000 patients with serious illness needing hospitalization, 50% of patients reported pain, with over 15% in extremely or moderately severe pain half of the time.[3] Of those patients who had experienced moderate-to-severe pain nearly half the time, at follow-up of survivors, 40% had persistent, severe pain.[4] Pain is a predominant physical symptom that left untreated makes the experience of living and dying with serious illness physically, emotionally, psychologically, and spiritually devastating for patients and families. In patients who eventually die of their disease, chronic unremitted pain can lead to poor quality of life, depression, anxiety, and isolation. The treatment of pain within the palliative care model can be best illustrated within the context of care for the patient with cancer, a relatively common pain emergency.

Every patient needs the right individualized balance of a curative and palliative approach. Every physician, and especially the emergency physician (EP), needs to have curative and palliative maneuvers in his or her portfolio. The ideal EP needs to be able to extend a patient's time, restore function, relieve pain, and provide comfort. Time extension (i.e., "saving lives") and function restoration are not always possible. Even when possible, they are sometimes not wanted or are too burdensome for the patient.

The EP must be sufficiently knowledgeable about prognosis, to assess realistic possibilities, and be able to share them with the patient or their surrogate to determine whether they are desirable.[5–7] For the patient who arrives with death imminent, the doctor must be able to speak to the patient and/or family about the death that is about to happen, and to recommend an appropriate code status, such as to allow natural death rather than resuscitate—and then protect the patient by writing a do not attempt resuscitation (DNAR) order. If extending time/restoring function is neither doable nor desirable, the EP must know how to relieve suffering and provide comfort. Fortunately both these gifts are always possible and desirable. No place

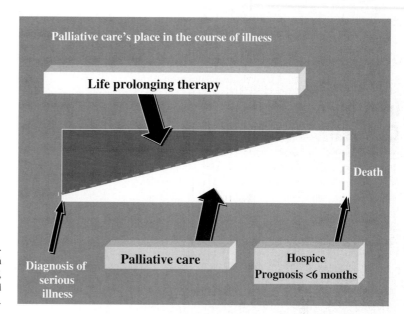

Fig. 46-1. Continuum of care model. (Reproduced with permission from Emanuel LL, Von Guten C, Ferris F, eds. The Education in Palliative and End-of-Life Care (EPEC) Curriculum).

is better equipped for titrating powerful drugs to provide the relief of pain, breathlessness, or anxiety. One must be reminded that patients do not say: "I know you cannot cure me, so just make me as comfortable as possible," though fortunately physicians often end up knowing and doing just that.

BARRIERS TO PAIN TREATMENT IN THE PALLIATIVE CARE SETTING: OLIGOANALGESIA AND DOUBLE EFFECT

Attitudes, knowledge, beliefs, and cultural norms all create barriers to optimal pain management in the emergency department (ED) setting[8] and include some of the following: (1) insufficient time in emergency medicine curricula for pain assessment and management—the Model of Clinical Practice of Emergency Medicine at the present time does not explicitly require training in chronic pain management or palliative medicine principles and practice, (2) paucity of continuous quality improvement programs for patients with malignant and nonmalignant pain, (3) a negligible research and evidence base for treatment of patients' pain crises in the ED, (4) opioid phobia among ED physicians manifest as inappropriate concern about addiction, and (5) misunderstanding of the concept of *double effect*. Double effect is the provision of adequate medication by a physician that *unintentionally* hastens death but is provided with the *intent* to relieve of suffering. This is different from provision of medication that is intentionally

administered to cause a patient's death (physician-assisted suicide).[9] Double effect is sanctioned by the U.S. Supreme Court whereas physician-assisted suicide is illegal in most states. As a result of the above barriers, patients suffer from *oligoanalgesia*, the undertreatment of pain.[10–12] All barriers not withstanding, there is widespread consensus that it is unethical for physicians to provide inadequate treatment of pain and other symptoms at the end-of-life for fear of unintentionally hastening death.

THE EMERGENCY PHYSICIAN AS MANAGER OF ACUTE PAIN

With significant barriers to effective pain management encompassing knowledge, attitudes, and beliefs regarding pain treatment, one key to excellent pain control in the ED is a team approach to the detection, assessment, treatment, and monitoring of painful conditions such as acute cancer pain. There must be constant communication between the ED care team (e.g., nurse, physician, social worker, and chaplain) and patient/family to create an environment for pain relief in which members of the health care team embrace the spirit and practice of pain relief as the principal goal.

As has been emphasized in previous chapters, the gold standard for pain control is what the patient reports as his or her level of pain. Pain must indeed become the fifth vital sign, and be recorded for each patient entering the ED.[13] Severe pain using a numerical rating scale then triggers early assessment and treatment. The new model of medicine requires ongoing efforts to diagnose and palliate, to provide time extension and comfort. It must be reemphasized that many chronic pain patients and patients suffering from pain in the setting of chronic life-threatening illness such as cancer may report very high pain scores in the face of severe uncontrolled pain, but appear calm and outwardly undisturbed by his or her pain. Thus the patient needs to be adequately assessed for pain (see further), and to have further diagnostic approaches either formulated or foreclosed. He or she should then be started on a stepwise approach to the treatment, reassessment, and titration of medications to the painful condition at hand. Notably, significant barriers still exist in the assessment and treatment of pain in the cognitively impaired and nonverbal patient.[14,15]

PAIN CLASSIFICATION AND THE MULTIDIMENSIONAL PALLIATIVE APPROACH TO PAIN TREATMENT MODEL

In palliative medicine, physicians use a multidimensional model of pain where there is a physical, emotional, and spiritual aspect of the pain.[16] Optimally, all three aspects need to be at least briefly addressed in order to provide adequate pain relief. Physical pain needs to be classified correctly so that appropriate drugs or other therapies can be used effectively. Pain here will be classified as nociceptive (somatic or visceral) and neuropathic. The first two are likely to be responsive to opiates; neuropathic pain has a variable response to opiates.

- *Nociceptive* pain is produced by damaged tissue or organs.
- *Somatic nociceptive* pain is produced if the body part is musculoskeletal or cutaneous.
- *Visceral nociceptive* pain is produced if the body part is an internal organ, such as the liver, pancreas, or stomach.
- *Neuropathic* pain is produced if the sensory afferent nerve itself is damaged or destroyed by the cancer or disease process.

Apart from the report of physical pain sensation itself, there is the patient's emotional response to the pain. The patient can be fearful, angry, anxious, depressed, or withdrawn. In the case of malignancy, the patient who believes his or her pain indicates a recurrence is likely to be filled with fear. The patient who thought that he or she had been cured may well be angry or very sad at the diagnosis of recurrence or metastasis. In any case, the patient may well become depressed or withdrawn due to persistent unrelenting pain. Although such emotional states cannot be definitely treated in the ED, a start toward healing can be taken by the recognition or validation of the emotion (you seem very afraid of the pain you are having) and an explanation of likely causes of the pain "I'm afraid the cancer has spread to another part of your body" or "I do not believe that the pain you are having today is caused by the regrowth of your cancer," or "I am uncertain as to what is causing your pain today, but let's get you feeling better and don't necessarily think the worst—that it is your cancer again." Think of severe depression, which can be induced by pain or the cancer itself, as a stab wound to the soul, and consider referral to the doctor of such traumatic illness, the psychiatrist.

Finally, there is oftentimes a spiritual component of pain. This refers to how a pain can be exacerbated by a spiritual belief or context into which the pain is inserted or nested. A patient who blames himself or herself for causing cancer will often suffer more deeply from the pain; a patient who believes he or she deserves eternal punishment for his or her deeds on earth, will feel a pain that threatens his or her physical existence more deeply. Most often these are matters for the chaplain or minister, but any clues or hints dropped by the patient should be briefly explored and the patient advised to seek spiritual guidance.

Just as these dimensions may deepen the pain crisis, and may make it more intense, some patient predilections may make him or her more resistant to usual remedies. One such patient characteristic is the use of chemical coping. By this are meant patients who use alcohol, recreational drugs, or abuse prescription drugs to get through life's difficulties and their own inadequacies. Screening for alcohol or drug abuse is an important step in the assessment of treatment options for pain management. Chemical coping is both a risk factor for inadequate response to opiate analgesia and a marker of likely opiate escalation and even possible diversion.

THE PALLIATIVE APPROACH: CANCER PAIN AS A MODEL

The EP will be called on to assess and treat patients with pain associated with malignancy, an unambiguously serious, chronic, life-threatening disease. It is estimated that pain occurs in approximately 50% of all cancer patients and in 74% of advanced cancer. While not all pain in palliative medicine is associated with malignancy, the principles and practice of pain management associated with malignancy is well studied and serves as a useful backdrop to discuss optimal pain management of patients with severe, progressive, and potentially life-limiting disease. Not surprisingly, metastatic cancers have a higher prevalence of pain than do nonmetastatic disease. Different tumor sites have varying prevalences of pain, with multiple myeloma (100%), advanced sarcoma (100%), head and neck (80%), genitourinary (77%), esophageal (74%), and prostate (74%) cancers with the highest pain prevalences. This contrasts with the lower rates for hematologic malignancies, such as leukemia (5%).[17] While the number of patients who present with uncontrolled pain and new or established diagnoses of cancer is not currently known, a search of the topics of cancer pain and emergency management revealed no relevant citations. It is clear, however, that in case series of malignancies requiring emergency hospitalization, pain is the most frequent presenting symptoms. In the coming two decades, the number of elderly patients will markedly increase, which will result in even higher numbers of patients with cancer.

Notably, over 34 million people without progressive life-threatening illness suffer from nonmalignant chronic pain that lasts 6 months or more.[18] Common conditions that cause chronic nonmalignant pain include musculoskeletal or neurodegenerative structural lesions. Other common causes include arachnoiditis, reflex sympathetic dystrophy, adhesions, systemic lupus, headaches, degenerative arthritis, fibromyalgia, and neuropathies. The principles used, particularly when titrating opiates, are also useful in the care of patients with chronic and nonmalignant pain.

MANAGING CANCER PAIN IN THE ED: THE CASE OF JR

J.R. is a 72-year-old woman with metastatic breast cancer with widespread bone metastasis who presents at 8 a.m. Her son accompanies her. She has refused any further chemotherapy or surgery. She has now developed back pain that she rates 10/10 increasing over the last 2 weeks and has been taking her medications that include morphine sustained release tablets 100 mg every 12 hours with morphine immediate release at 30 mg every 2 hours, she has taken five doses in the last 24 hours. On further questioning, she took in addition two Percocet (5 mg oxycodone/ 325 mg acetaminophen) every 4 hours for six doses without relief. She is alert, awake, and has no neurologic deficits. She has not taken her medication that morning. Her vitals: BP 100/60, HR 110, RR 14, oxygen saturation 95% on room air. How should we manage her pain?

Step 1: Classify the Type of Pain and Devise a General Pain Management Strategy

Except for treatment of pathologic fractures, the pain stimulus associated with cancer is not likely to be rapidly removed as with a previously healthy patient with new fracture or a patient with sickle cell disease with vasoocclusive crisis that will resolve over days with potential recurrence. A good history, physical examination, and strategic management of pain yields optimum success in the ED.[19] There are a great many cancer pain syndromes,[20] and the EP should be expected to be familiar with only a selected few of these, since this subset is more likely to present in the ED and to be responsive to available therapeutic regimens. The main entities are tumor-related somatic or visceral pain syndromes. These include (1) bone pain from metastatic disease or pathologic fractures, (2) headache or facial pain from intracerebral tumor or base of skull metastases, and (3) visceral abdominal pain from pancreatic tumors or peritoneal carcinomatosis. Two other categories are tumor-related neuropathic pain: neuralgias such as trigeminal neuralgia and plexopathies from the neck, brachial plexus, or lumbosacral nerve roots. Some cancer patients will present with pain that arises from damaged nerves rather than damaged tissue, which is identified as neuropathic pain. In review, such pain usually is along a nerve distribution, is described as lancinating or burning. Advanced neuropathic pain can be reproduced by light touch (allodynia). Occasionally a patient might experience an exacerbation of a chronic pain from cancer therapy—such as postthoracotomy or postbreast surgery pain presentations. Patients who have had radical neck dissection can have severe neck pain with neuropathic components. Head and neck cancer has the highest associated pain prevalence.

Somatic and visceral pain syndromes in general tend to be remarkably responsive to opiates with neuropathic pain being less responsive but in many cases still useful. However, when the clinician suspects a single bone lesion causing pain that is not in the setting of pathologic fracture, he or she can initiate consultation with the radiation oncologist for localized, limited, treatment as well as start opiates for the immediate relief of pain. Importantly, in the case of headache from cerebral metastasis where resection is not an option or not wanted, the initiation of corticosteroids such as dexamethasone (start at 4 mg tid) as well as consultation with radiation oncology for palliative whole-brain radiation might be of use.

Because her pain is 10/10, and generalized to the bones, we can assume that her pain is somatic in nature, not likely to be responsive to focal radiation, so we will initiate opiates. The World Health Organization suggests that patients who have a pain level greater than 5/10 should have opiates initiated regardless of prior use. In patients who are opiate naïve, lower doses may be used compared to those that are opiate tolerant.

Step 2: Clarify Goals of Treatment with the Patient, Family, and ED Team

The palliative approach is centered on achieving the goals of the patient in keeping with modalities acceptable to the pain. The clinician must not forget that pain in these patients sits within a complex disease entity. Communication between patient, family, and the ED team is critical in the successful management of the patient's pain.[21]

When intervening in the treatment of physical pain, it is not reasonable to insist on complete pain relief in the ED setting. Titration of pain medications takes time and fine-tuning can be performed on an outpatient or inpatient basis. A good rule of thumb is to expect at least 50% reduction in the pain as an initial goal. Just as no patient should be admitted to the floor that has any instability of traditional vital signs, so a patient with an unstable fifth (pain $\geq 7/10$) vital sign should not be discharged from the ED. No patient with severe uncontrolled pain should be transferred to a lower level of care, e.g., the medical ward. Such practices only serve to guarantee poor care and dissatisfied or even psychologically traumatized patients and/or families.

A discussion with the patient and family should include the following: (1) affirmation that pain relief at 50% is an initial reasonable goal with a goal to relieve pain to its lowest level either in the ED or by admission, (2) that the intent of the administration of pain medications is the relief of suffering and (3) that continual communication between the patient, family regarding pain relief, goals, or concerns and the ED team is paramount. It must be realized that some patients and families may be concerned with addiction or euthanasia regarding the use of opiates and these concerns should be addressed honestly and openly. It is worthwhile to assure the never-addicted but fearful patient or family that "He/you cannot become addicted to morphine as long as he/you is using it to treat the cancer pain."

Work-up that includes labs, radiographs, and other diagnostic tests should be discussed with the patient and family to make sure that they are consistent with the goals of care for that patient. Patients should be given the option to not undergo work-up beyond pain management if it is determined by the patient/family and clinician that this is not be consistent with the goals of care (e.g., the detection of renal failure on routine labs that the patient or family would not want further treatment even if discovered when

"comfort only" is the focus). The emergency practitioner should discuss goals of care whenever a possible poor quality of life raises the question of whether time should be extended or when the disease course itself is likely to be incompatible with extending the patient's time.

Step 3: If Opiates will be Used—Determine how much Opiates the Patient is Taking and Use as a Guide

After discussion with patient and family regarding the goal of pain treatment, the clinician must rationally begin treatment. In patients who are currently taking opiates, the clinician should first consult an equianalgesic dosing table[22,23] (Table 46-1) as a guide to convert opiates to *morphine equivalents*.[24] *Morphine equivalents* are the universal language to covert easily between types of medications. Morphine equivalents are the milligrams of total morphine used in a 24-hour period when all opiates are converted to morphine. For example in JR:

1. Morphine sustained release: 100 mg/12 h × 2 = 200 mg for 24 h.
2. Morphine IR: 30 mg × 5 in 24 h = 150 mg in 24 h.
3. Percocet: 2 tabs = 10 mg × 6 dose in 24 h = 60 mg oxycodone.

$$10 \text{ mg oxycodone} = 15 \text{ mg morphine oral}$$
$$60 \text{ mg oxycodone} = X \text{ morphine oral}$$
$$X = 90 \text{ mg morphine oral}$$

Total morphine in 24 hours used by JR (1, 2, and 3) = 440 mg in 24 hours.

Table 46-1. Equianalgesic Dosing

Equianalgesic Doses of Opioid Analgesics		
Oral/Rectal Dose (mg)	**Analgesic**	**Parenteral Dose (mg)**
100	Codeine	60
—	Fentanyl	0.1
15	Hydrocodone	—
5	Hydromorphone	1.5
2	Levorphanol	1
150	Meperidine	50
15	Morphine	5
10	Oxycodone	—

(Reproduced with permission from Emanuel LL, Von Guten C, Ferris F, eds. The Education in Palliative and End-of-Life Care (EPEC) Curriculum).

Step 4: Determine the Route of Administration

The route of administration must be determined and will determine the time of onset of expected pain relief since the pharmacokinetics differ depending on the preparation. In the ED, the intravenous (IV) route is the most convenient route of administration for pain medication. However, patients with severe, chronic, life-limiting disease, especially at the end-of-life may have difficult IV access or not want an IV. The EP should be familiar with how to dose opiates by multiple routes. Opiates may be dosed intravenously or subcutaneously, orally, enterally (through a gastric or duodenal feeding tube), transmucosal/buccal, rectally, and transdermally. The subcutaneous route is equally effective with the same risk of complications as the standard peripheral IV. Subcutaneous administration is particularly useful if an IV will be established with delay (e.g., central line placement). Subcutaneous boluses or infusions should be done with 25 or 27-gauge needles to minimize patient discomfort.

Intramuscular injections are *not* recommended since subcutaneous infusion is less painful and just as effective. Transdermal medications cannot be titrated in the ED setting since their onset of action is slow and may not reach steady state for 24 hours.

In this case, JR agrees to have an IV peripheral line initiated, which is done with no complication.

Step 5: Initiate a Rapid Titration Protocol

Rapid parenteral titration protocols allow for rapid relief of pain and are preferable to oral routes when pain is severe and uncontrolled. In choosing an opiate for rapid titration, a priori there is little to no difference in side effects. There may be special considerations because of the metabolism and excretions of opiates by the liver and kidney, respectively, in patients with severe renal insufficiency or failure with oliguria or anuria the use of morphine should be used with caution. Because one of the two metabolites, morphine-6-glucoronide, has a longer half-life than morphine, opiate dosing should be given as needed. Hydromorphone or fentanyl do not have this metabolite and can be safely given in long-acting form. Only patients with severe liver dysfunction need adjustment dosing. Patients with liver metastasis without failure do not need dosing adjustments.

Several dosing strategies for cancer pain have been described.[25] Few focus specifically on the emergency setting. Three published protocols in the emergency setting include the following:

- Rapid titration with IV morphine[26] and without immediate oral conversion[27] (Fig. 46-2)
- Fentanyl fast titration[28] (Fig. 46-3)

In acute pain exacerbation it is useful to recognize that the patient's total daily dose may be increased by

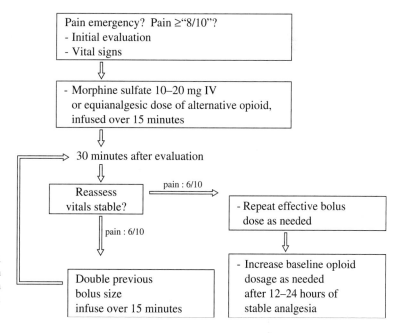

Fig. 46-2. Rapid titration with morphine. (Reprinted with permission from Hagen NA, Elwood T, Ernst S. Cancer pain emergencies: a protocol for management. *J Pain symptom Manage* 2003;26:46).

Pain emergency? Pain ≥"8/10"?
- Initial evaluation
- Vital signs

⇩

- Morphine sulfate 10–20 mg IV
  or equianalgesic dose of alternative opioid,
  infused over 15 minutes

⇩

30 minutes after evaluation

⇩

Reassess vitals stable?   → pain : 6/10 →   - Repeat effective bolus dose as needed

pain : 6/10 ⇩   ⇩

Double previous bolus size infuse over 15 minutes   - Increase baseline opioid dosage as needed after 12–24 hours of stable analgesia

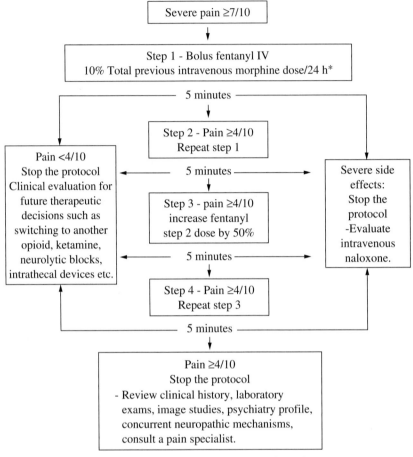

Fig. 46-3. Rapid titration with fentanyl. (Reproduced with permission from Guilherme L, Soares L, Martins M, et al. Intravenous fentanyl for cancer pain: a "fast titration protocol for the emergency room. *J Pain Symptom Manage* 2001;21:878.)

50–100% or more. In the case of JR, we have determined that we will be using the opiate by IV route. She is currently using 440 mg a day of oral morphine equivalents or 18 mg/h of oral morphine. With a potency ratio of 3:1 oral:IV we can calculate the amount of IV equivalents per day JR is using and then the hourly rate if we divide by 24:

$$\frac{440 \text{ mg oral morphine/24 h} = X \text{ mg IV/24 h}}{15 \text{ mg oral morphine} = 5 \text{ mg IV}}$$

$$X = 146 \text{ mg IV/24 h}$$

$$X = 6 \text{ mg/h IV morphine}$$

Knowing what JR is currently taking per hour that is not providing pain relief is useful in gauging where the

patient may respond. That said, these protocols could be initiated when the baseline opiate usage is unknown as well as understanding that the effective dose may be 50–100% more than the patient is currently taking.

Clinicians should be familiar with the concept of cross-tolerance. Cross-tolerance refers to the subtle way in which a different opiate reacts in a given patient when applying equianalgesic dosing principles. When switching opioids in a patient who has controlled pain, the dose may be reduced by 25–50% (that is give 50–75% of the equianalgesic dose). In a patient with uncontrolled pain, opiate dosing should not be reduced significantly. Notably, there is no ceiling effect (dose at which the medication is no longer effective) when using pure opiates and that there is no theoretical dose that is too high for a patient.

Step 6: Write and Order Opiates and Discuss this with Your ED Team

As noted previously, many barriers exist to the administration of opiates. Many nurses may be fearful to give more than a certain amount of opiate during a certain interval and may be unfamiliar with the principle of double effect. The clinician prescriber should have an explicit conversation regarding the pain management plan, and the need for rapid titration to achieve pain relief.

Most clinicians at some point in their career fear respiratory depression and death in a patient as a result of opiate administration. Systematic literature review reveals that the rate of respiratory depression in opiate-tolerant patients is almost negligible when appropriate equianalgesic dosing principles are used.[25] Patients on chronic opioids have pharmacologic tolerance to respiratory depression. As opioid doses increase, respiratory depression does not occur in the setting of overdose. Somnolence always occurs before respiratory depression. For patients on opioids in the outpatient setting, somnolence is predictive of overdose as the patient will not be awake enough to take the next dose.

Respiratory depression with a respiratory rate of 6–8 is typically tolerated. In the event that respiratory depression occurs, patients should not receive the usual dose of naloxone used in patients with intentional narcotic overdose:

- Dilute 0.4 mg of naloxone in 10 mL of sterile water (0.04 mg/mL) and give 0.1–0.2 mg IV q 1–2 minute until patient is alert. If repeat drowsiness occurs, repeat.

This method succeeds in reversing the respiratory depression without reversing the analgesic effect of the opiate.[2]

Step 7: Anticipate and Treat the Common Side Effects of Opiates

Medication allergy, urticaria, nausea, vomiting, and sedation are the most common side effects seen with opioid analgesia in the ED setting. Medication allergy should be treated as usual. Should the patient have had a previous allergic reaction or adverse event from morphine sulphate, than either IV hydromorphone (Dilaudid) or fentanyl can be used. Urticaria and pruritus can be managed with antihistamines. Nausea and acute vomiting is most easily treated with dopaminergic agents such as prochlorperazine (10 mg), metochlorpramide (10 mg), or haldoperidol (1 mg). Some patients may experience drowsiness 30–60 minutes after bolus of opiates as plasma levels peaks. Sedation should be distinguished from exhaustion due to sleep deprivation from pain. Constipation is universal with opiates and if the patient is discharged, must be attended to. Bowel stimulants such as senna, 17 mg bid should be started on day 1 rather than waiting for the patient to develop painful constipation on day 3. The clinician must be aware that the source of pain in patients with acute exacerbation of pain might be due to constipation.

Step 8: Initiate the Use of an Adjuvant Medication if Indicated

The use of nonsteroidal anti-inflammatory drugs (NSAIDs) is an important adjunct for the pain of bony metastases, and all patients without contraindication should be started or continued on NSAIDS. Steroids also interrupt the cyclooxygenase pathway, and can be considered for bony pain flares, particularly if the patient has been steroid responsive in the past. This should be discussed with the patient's oncologist or palliative care physician. In general, the patient should have one medication adjusted at a time, so that the effects of changes can be tracked and anticipated.

In patients with neuropathic pain, although opioids may be partly effective in treating such pain, adjunctive agents are more effective. For lancinating pains, the patient can be safely started on gabapentin (Neurontin) at a dose of 300 mg three times a day, which has been proven to be effective. Neurontin also has the advantage of a low incidence of side effects, lack of hepatic metabolism, and drug interactions, and is well tolerated. Tegretol is an alternative agent, but needs monitoring of plasma concentrations and close follow-up. Noripramine can be started for burning pain at a dose of 100 mg per day. However, although such secondary amines are safer than tricyclic antidepressants, they should not be used in elderly patients, those with severe heart disease, glaucoma, symptomatic prostatic hypertrophy or neurogenic bladder, or organic brain syndrome, and so are unlikely to be initiated in the ED.

It is important to understand that radiation therapy is excellent treatment for painful cancer infiltration, and should be used whenever possible. In conjunction with the patient's attending physician, radiation therapy should be initiated at the earliest possible time. Consideration can be given to sending the patient to radiation oncology for a single treatment fraction, which may produce the beginning of therapeutic effect within a few days. Most often pain relief is well underway within 2 weeks of starting radiation therapy, usually requiring that opiates be tapered at that time.

Step 9: Multiple Reassessments and Attend to Other Aspects of Pain

Patients undergoing a rapid titration protocol should be reassessed every 15–30 minutes for pain relief. As the patient's physical pain is treated she may become more responsive to other therapies. If the pain cannot be managed successfully (pain <4) in the ED within a reasonable amount of time (4–6 hours) then the patient should be admitted for further management. When ED chaplain services are available, a referral can be made for a spiritual assessment. While ED clinicians may not feel this should be a routine part of care, studies have shown repeatedly that this can be a very important part of the chronic illness experience.

Indicators of poor response to pharmacotherapy include incident pain (pain with movement), neuropathic pain, tolerance to opioids, a history of alcohol or drug abuse, and psychologic distress. Opioid dose and the presence of confusion have not been predictive of a poor response.[29,30]

Step 10: Determine the Appropriate Disposition of the Patient

JR is treated in the ED with 50 mg IV total of morphine over 4 hours with good relief of pain—the pain is now 3/10. She is requesting to be discharged. What should we do?

No explicit guidelines exist for the ED disposition on oral therapy following parenteral therapy for severe cancer pain in the emergency setting. As stated previously, patients with severe uncontrolled pain that is unable to be remitted below an acceptable level for the patient, should be admitted for continued pain management in the hospital as well as in cases where it is anticipated that the patient will not be able to receive the appropriate medication as an outpatient. Many hospitals in the United States and Canada have palliative care hospital-based consultation services that are experts in pain management—particularly in the setting of chronic life-threatening conditions. These services should be consulted if there are any questions or concerns. Typically, patients need to be followed for 12–24 hours to determine a good estimate of opiate need with conversion of IV to oral dosing using equianalgesic tables as a guide. With many EDs increasingly having observational units this may be the best place to establish a new baseline dose of opiates. That said, in keeping with the goals of care of the patient and family, the patient may want to be discharged from the ED.

If discharged, patients should not drive home or operate machinery within 5 days of dose escalation. In opiate-tolerant patients, they should be sent home with an increase in their long-acting medication, with an appropriate increase in their breakthrough dose. If the EP were to discharge the patient, the following should be considered:

- In severe pain, the total daily opiate dose may be increased by 50–100%. When titrated without close monitoring, patients may experience potentially unwanted side effects such as drowsiness. Careful attention should be paid to the route of administration for outpatient care that will be most effective.

- All patients should be discharged with adequate medication to treat opiate side effects such as nausea and constipation.

- When available: consult with the palliative care or pain service while the patient is in the ED to discuss discharge recommendations.

- Follow-up (phone or in person) and communication is essential between the EP, the patient/family, and primary care clinician responsible for outpatient pain control.

- A pain diary after leaving the ED is essential—to record the effects of the new medication regimen and the quantity and frequency of use of breakthrough medications. This can be given to the patients' primary care doctor to adjust doses as needed.

SUMMARY

In summary, nociceptive somatic (soft tissue, muscle, bones) or visceral tumor expansion in the abdominal cavity from the liver, pancreas, or gastric, or pelvic carcinomas, are highly responsive to opioid therapy. Patients can be rapidly titrated to comfort levels, which usually require single or multiple boluses of 5 mg IV morphine or equivalent for opiate naïve and 10 mg boluses for opiate-tolerant patients. Opiate naïve patients should be started on a short-acting opiate as guided by the therapy needed to reduce pain in the ED by 50%. Patients on opiates typically need doses increased from 50 to 100% for severe exacerbations and 25–50% for moderate ones. Follow-up should be arranged with oncology, the pain service, or palliative care.

Not all pain will be opiate responsive. When a patient is found to be nonresponsive to repetitive dosing, particularly when sedation limits dose escalation, alternative components of the pain should be considered. Eventual involvement of other members of an interdisciplinary team, such as psychologist, chaplain, or social worker, would be helpful, and such referrals should be encouraged.

For pain management in the ED, educational interventions have been shown to result in beneficial changes in pain management by physicians. It is clear that a widespread, intense effort will be needed over the coming decade especially with the growth of the elderly population and the increase in numbers of patients with cancer.

REFERENCES

1. World Health Organization. *Definition of Palliative Care.* 2004.

2. Emanuel LL, von Guten C, Ferris F, eds. *The Education in Palliative and End-of-Life Care (EPEC) Curriculum.* EPEC Project Feinberg School of Medicine, Chicago, IL: Northwestern University; 2003.

3. Desbiens NA, Wu AW, Broste SK, et al. Pain and satisfaction with pain control in seriously ill hospitalized adults: findings from the SUPPORT research investigations. For the SUPPORT investigators. Study to Understand Prognoses and Preferences for Outcomes and Risks of Treatment. *Crit Care Med.* 1996;24:1953–1961.

4. Desbiens NA, Wu AW, Alzola C, et al. Pain during hospitalization is associated with continued pain six months later in survivors of serious illness. The SUPPORT Investigators. Study to Understand Prognoses and Preferences for Outcomes and Risks of Treatments. *Am J Med* 1997;102(3):269–276.

5. Lamont EB, Christakis NA. Some elements of prognosis in terminal cancer. *Oncology* (Huntington). 1999;13(8):1165–1170; discussion 1172–1174, 1179–1180.

6. Lamont EB, Christakis NA. Complexities in prognostication in advanced cancer: "to help them live their lives the way they want to." *JAMA.* 2003;290(1):98–104.

7. Takayesu JK, Hutson HR. Communicating life-threatening diagnoses to patients in the emergency department. *Ann Emerg Med.* 2004;43(6):749–755.

8. Rupp T, Delaney KA. Inadequate analgesia in emergency medicine. *Ann Emerg Med.* 2004;43(4):494–503.

9. Hawryluck LA, Harvey WR. Analgesia, virtue, and the principle of double effect. *Palliat Care.* 2000;16(suppl): S24–S30.

10. Todd KH, Samaroo N, Hoffman JR. Ethnicity as a risk factor for inadequate emergency department analgesia. *JAMA.* 1993;269(12):1537–1539.

11. Sobel RM, Todd KH. Risk factors in oligoanalgesia. *Am J Emerg Med.* 2002;20(2):126.

12. Tamayo-Sarver JH, Dawson NV, Cydulka RK, et al. Variability in emergency physician decision making about prescribing opioid analgesics. *Ann Emerg Med.* 2004;43(4): 483–493.

13. Davis MP, Walsh D. Cancer pain: how to measure the fifth vital sign. *Clev Clin J Med.* 2004;71(8):625–632.

14. Horgas AL, Elliott AF. Pain assessment and management in persons with dementia. *Nurs Clin North Am.* 2004;39(3): 593–606.

15. Frampton M. Experience assessment and management of pain in people with dementia. *Age Ageing.* 2003;32(3):248–251.

16. Bruera E, Michaud M, Vigano A, et al. Multidisciplinary symptom control clinic in a cancer center: a retrospective study. *Support Care Cancer.* 2001;9(3):162–168.

17. Bruera ED, Portenoy RK, eds. *Cancer Pain: Assessment and Management.* Cambridge, England: Cambridge University Press; 2003.

18. Bruera E, Neumann CM, Gagnon B, et al. Edmonton Regional Palliative Care Program: impact on patterns of terminal cancer care. *CMAJ.* 1999;161(3):290–293.

19. Bruera E, Lawlor P. Cancer pain management. *Acta Anaesth Scand.* 1997;41(1 pt 2):146–153.

20. Portenoy RK, Lesage P. Management of cancer pain. *Lancet.* 1999;353(9165):1695–1700.

21. Berry DL, Wilkie DJ, Thomas CR Jr, et al. Clinicians communicating with patients experiencing cancer pain. *Cancer Invest.* 2003;21(3):374–381.

22. Pereira J, Lawlor P, Vigano A, et al. Equianalgesic dose ratios for opioids. A critical review and proposals for long-term dosing. *Pain Symptom Manage.* 2001;22(2):672–687.

23. Levy MH. Pharmacologic treatment of cancer pain. *N Engl J Med.* 1996;335(15):1124–1132.

24. Arnold R, Weissman DE. Calculating opioid dose conversions #36. *Palliat Med.* 2003;6(4):619–620.

25. Davis MP, Weissman DE, Arnold RM. Opioid dose titration for severe cancer pain: a systematic evidence-based review. *Palliat Med.* 2004;7(3):462–468.

26. Mercadante S, Villari P, Ferrera P, et al. Rapid titration with intravenous morphine for severe cancer pain and immediate oral conversion. *Cancer.* 2002;95(1):203–208.

27. Hagen NA, Elwood T, Ernst S. Cancer pain emergencies: a protocol for management [see comment]. *J Pain Symptom Manage.* 1997;14(1):45–50.

28. Soares, LG, Martins M, Uchoa R. Intravenous fentanyl for cancer pain: a "fast titration" protocol for the emergency room. *J Pain Symptom Manage* 2003;26(3):876–881.

29. Mercadante, S, Portenoy RK. Opioid poorly-responsive cancer pain. Part 1: clinical considerations. *J Pain Symptom Manage* 2001;21(2):144–150.

30. Caraceni A, Martini C, Zecca E, et al. Breakthrough pain characteristics and syndromes in patients with cancer pain. An international survey. *Palliat Med.* 2004;18(3):177–183.

47

Alternate Routes for the Systemic Delivery of Analgesics and Sedatives

Sharon E. Mace

HIGH YIELD FACTS

- Many drugs can be given for local and systemic effects by "nontraditional" routes of administration: transdermal and transmucosal (respiratory tract, nasal, oral [PO], rectal).
- Advantages of alternate routes of drug delivery are painless, easy to administer, needleless (no risk of needlestick exposure), cost-effective, no first-pass metabolism.
- Alternative methods of drug administration avoid the problems inherent with the "traditional" parenteral and oral administration of drugs.
- Problems with the traditional routes for giving drugs include for IV: painful, takes time/equipment/personnel to administer, cost, risk of needlestick, and for PO: decreased bioavailability if the patient is vomiting, has gastrointestinal (GI) disease, and from first-pass metabolism and destruction by hostile environment of GI tract.
- Side effects and toxicity are often less with alternate routes but can occur with any route of drug administration whether a traditional or alternate method.

OVERVIEW

The use of alternate routes of drug administration has seen an increase in the past decade.[1] This trend is likely to continue in the future.[2] There are several reasons for this including problems with the traditional routes of drug administration, the unique advantages of the nontraditional techniques, and perhaps, more importantly, pharmacologic advances including new drug formulations and drug delivery systems (Tables 47-1 and 47-2).[2–6]

Alternate routes of drug administration, transdermal and transmucosal, were once considered novel techniques of drug delivery but now are commonplace.[1,6] Many different types of drugs can be given via alternative routes of drug delivery for their local or systemic effects (Table 47-3).

Although the oral (PO) route followed by the parenteral route are the traditional and the most common methods for giving drugs, there are several other alternative routes with their own advantages and disadvantages (Table 47-2).[1,6] There are many factors to consider when selecting a route for delivering a pharmacologic agent. Some of these parameters are efficacy, reliability, rapid onset, duration, ease of administration, patient comfort, side effects or toxicity, patient/family acceptance, need for equipment and personnel for administration, and cost-effectiveness (Table 47-4).

ADVANTAGES AND DISADVANTAGES OF ALTERNATE ROUTES OF DRUG ADMINISTRATION

Advantages of these alternative techniques of drug administration include painless, patient acceptance, needleless (avoids the risk of needlestick injuries), immediate availability, ease of administration, large absorptive surface, rapid drug absorption/availability/onset, fewer systemic side effects, eliminates the gastrointestinal (GI) destruction of a drug, and avoids hepatic first-pass metabolism (Table 47-2).[1–9]

The use of alternative methods of drug delivery also avoids some of the problems inherent with the more traditional intravenous and PO routes. Such problems are related either to pharmacologic issues or to patient considerations. Medications given orally may undergo destruction in the GI tract with loss of pharmacologic activity.[7,8] Drugs given via the oral route may undergo hepatic first-pass metabolism resulting in decreased drug availability.[7,8] Drugs administered orally need to be absorbed from the GI tract and pass into the systemic bloodstream then travel to exert their effect on various organs. Thus, there is a delay in the drug's onset of action. For most oral sedatives and/or analgesics, the onset is about 20–30 minutes with a peak at 1 hour and an effect lasting several hours. If rapid onset (e.g., within seconds to a few minutes) is desired then avoid PO or rectal (PR) administration. For almost all emergency department procedures a quick onset and offset are preferred so a drug's effect that has a slow onset and lasts hours is not desirable as occurs with many PO medications.

Intravenous (IV) administration gives a faster onset but necessitates the time consuming labor-intensive painful procedure of starting an IV line, which may be

Table 47-1. Disadvantages of Traditional Routes of Drug Administration

Parenteral (IV/IM)
Painful
Need to secure a line (IV route)
Time consuming (IV route)
Risk of needlestick
Need for equipment/devices (IV setup, IV infusion pump)
Cost (expense of equipment for administering and personnel to administer and set up the IV equipment)

Enteral (PO/PR)
↓ absorption with emesis, abnormal gut motility, GI diseases
May be rejected if poor taste
First-pass metabolism (↓ drug availability)
Destruction by hostile environment of stomach (highly acidic—low pH)

IM, intramuscular; IV, intravenous; PO, oral; PR, rectal.

Table 47-2. Advantages and Disadvantages of Alternate Routes of Drug Administration*

Advantages: Alternate Routes of Drug Administration
Patient factors
  Painless
  Patient acceptance
  Needless: avoids risk of needlestick injuries
  May not require sterile technique
  Route is immediately available
  Ease of administration
  No need for equipment for administration
  No need for personnel to administer
  Cost-effective
Pharmacologic factors
  Large absorptive surface with significant blood flow
  Rapid drug absorption/availability → rapid onset
  ↓ systemic side effects (e.g., inhaled vs. parental beta-agonists or inhaled vs. oral steroids)
  Direct medication absorption
  Avoids GI destruction
  Avoids hepatic first-pass metabolism → more drug available more quickly than PO
  Absorption rate/plasma concentration often equivalent to IV administration
  Often greater CSF/plasma concentration for intranasal administration than for IV or PO
  Greater bioavailability than PO (drains into systemic not portal system)

Disadvantages: Alternate Routes of Drug Administration
  Patient acceptance (e.g., rectal)
  Patient discomfort (e.g., intranasal or rectal may be uncomfortable)
  Variable absorption (especially rectal)
  Local irritation: rashes, skin irritation, itching (transdermal route)

CSF: cerebrospinal fluid.

*Advantages may vary somewhat depending on the specific transdermal or transmucosal route.

Table 47-3. Medications Administered by Alternate Routes of Drug Administration*

Transdermal
Topical anesthetics: EMLA, LMX-4, lidocaine, tetracaine, LET, TAC
Narcotics: fentanyl patches, morphine patches, duragesic patches
Cardiac: nitroglycerin, clonidine
Dermatologic: cortisone cream, mupriocin cream
Hormones: estradiol, testosterone, birth control pill
Miscellaneous: scopolamine, nicotine

Transmucosal
Respiratory tract mucosa: inhalation route
   Administered via nebulization, aerosol, powder, vapor
   Inhalation anesthetics: nitrous oxide
   Pulmonary medications: β-agonists (e.g., albuterol, atrovent, and epinephrine), antivirals,
      antifungal, surfactant, hormones
Respiratory tract mucosa: direct installation
   Topical anesthetics: lidocaine, cetacaine for procedures such as bronchoscopy, laryngoscopy
   Resuscitation drugs: narcon, atropine, lidocaine, epinephrine
Nasal mucosa
   Sedatives: benzodiazepine (midazolam), ketamine (not recommended because of erratic
      absorption)
   Nasal sprays/drops: decongestants
   Topical anesthetics: lidocaine, tetracaine (prior to procedures)
   Illegal drugs: cocaine (also for ENT procedures)
Oral mucosa (sublingual, buccal)
   Sedatives: fentanyl *lollipops*
   Cardiac: nitroglycerin, clonidine
   Topical anesthetics: lidocaine, tetracaine, cetacaine
   Psychiatric: olanzapine
   Miscellaneous: nicotine gum
Rectal mucosa
   Sedatives: benzodiazepines (midazolam), barbiturates (methohexital, pentobarbital, thiopental),
      ketamine (not recommended because of erratic absorption)
   Anticonvulsants: benzodiazepines, diazepam, paraldehyde
   Analgesic/antipyretic: acetaminophen

EMLA: eutectic mixture of local anesthetic; LET: lidocaine epinephrine tetracaine; TAC: tetracaine
adrenaline cocaine.
*This is not an all-inclusive list but gives some examples.

quite difficult in certain patient populations: the infant, young child, intravenous drug users, patients with fragile veins including patients on steroids, and chronically ill patients with sclerosed and/or fragile veins. There is also the risk of a needlestick injury with securing an IV line. Other routes such as transmucosal, e.g., respiratory or intranasal, have a rapid onset and offset, avoid a painful IV, and the possibility of a needlestick injury.[9]

Oral drug administration may not be possible in a patient with persistent vomiting. Patient factors associated with oral drug administration also include palatability.

Will the patient or child take the medicine or reject it if the drug has a poor or bitter taste? Individual variability in GI absorption is common and may affect the bioavailability of an individual drug.[10] Patients with bowel obstruction, hypermotility, short gut syndrome, malabsorption, celiac disease, sprue, colitis, and other GI disorders may have an even greater variability and unpredictable drug absorption/bioavailability.

In general, only 5–10% bioavailability occurs with oral medications because of GI and hepatic destruction, while intranasal drug delivery yields bioavailability from

Table 47-4. Parameters for Selection of a Route of Drug Administration

Parameters
Efficacy
Reliability
Rapid onset
Duration
Ease of administration
Patient comfort
Side effects
Toxicity
Patient/family acceptance
Need for technology (e.g., IV devices and pumps) and personnel for administration
Cost–effectiveness

Routes of Administration

Traditional
Parenteral
    Intravenous
    Intramuscular
Oral

Alternate or Nontraditional
Transdermal
Transmucosal
    Respiratory tract mucosa
        Inhalation or direct installation
    Nasal mucosa
    Oral (sublingual, buccal) mucosa
    Rectal mucosa
    Vaginal mucosa

negligible (nearly 0%) to almost 100%, and IV medication has nearly 100% bioavailability.[9]

There are some disadvantages and potential problems or risks associated with alternate routes of drug administration. While patient acceptance is usually positive for most alternate routes such as transdermal or via the oral transmucosa, rectal administration may be acceptable in an infant but is aesthetically unpleasant and rejected by an adolescent. Intranasal or rectal drug administration may be uncomfortable for some drugs and in some patients. Local irritation at the site can occur with transdermal or transmucosal drug administration.

In addition to these patient variables, a major pharmacologic problem is variable absorption leading to an inadequate effect or toxicity. Rectal administration has resulted in erratic absorption for some drugs.[6,10]

Nasal delivery of drugs ranges from minimal to nearly 100%.[9] Because of anatomy, nasal administration of drugs may yield a greater ratio of cerebrospinal fluid (CSF) to plasma drug concentration than IV or oral administration.[11,12] Absorption of pharmacologic agents via the dermis can vary depending on factors such as thickness of the patient's skin and local blood flow, creating the potential for toxicity or undermedicating.[13,14]

PATHOPHYSIOLOGY AND PHARMACOLOGY OF TRANSMUCOSAL AND TRANSDERMAL DRUG ADMINISTRATION

Transmucosal drug administration at any of the various mucosal surfaces; whether skin, respiratory tract, nose, oral cavity, vagina, or the rectum involves passage or transport across a cell membrane.[7,10] There are four transport mechanisms across this cellular barrier: (1) transcellular, (2) transcytosis, (3) carrier-mediated, and (4) paracellular transport (Fig. 47-1).

Transcellular is diffusion across the cell membrane through the cell and out the other side passing through the cell membrane on the opposite side. Only small molecules such as oxygen or carbon dioxide can pass through cells by diffusion. Transcytosis involves the interaction of the molecule with the cell membrane to form a vesicle or lipid bilayer around the molecule. The vesicle can travel to the other side of the cell and be released, or be digested and destroyed within the cell.

Carrier-mediated transport also involves interaction of the molecule with the cell membrane. Instead of forming a vesicle as with transcytosis, the molecule reversibly binds to complexes in the lipid bilayer of the cell membrane. This allows the molecule to enter the inside of the cell. Once inside the cell, the molecule complex disassociates. Next the molecule moves across to the other side of the cell, where it again forms this reversible complex in the cell's lipid bilayer. Then the drug molecule can break the reversible bond to be released outside the cell. Paracellular transport occurs when the molecule can pass between cells, thus, enabling it to cross the cellular barrier (Fig. 47-2).

Additional obstacles to the passage of drugs across the mucosa also occur. For example, proteolytic enzymes in the GI tract or in the oral cavity can breakdown and destroy peptides and proteins.[7,8,10] The mucus in the lungs, the nose, and in the GI tract also impedes the transport of molecules. The highly acidic very low pH of the stomach leads to the denaturation and the destruction of proteins.[7,8,10]

Drug absorption across the mucosa; whether the skin, oral, nasal, or respiratory mucosa; depends on many factors.[8,15]

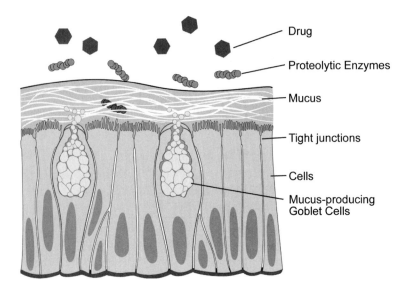

Fig. 47-1. Barriers to drug absorption: the cell membrane, proteolytic enzymes, and mucosa layers serve as a barrier to drug absorption. (Reprinted with permission from Department of Medical Illustration-Cleveland Clinic Foundation.)

Absorption is inversely related to the thickness of the mucosa.[8,15] Absorption decreases as the thickness (H) of the skin or other mucosal layer increases. Absorption increases when there is a higher concentration of drug in the delivery vehicle (C), a greater surface area of the delivery site on the skin or other mucosa (S), and a longer time or duration the drug is in contact with the skin or other mucosa (T). Absorption (A) varies directly with the permeability coefficient (P) times the drug concentration (C) times the surface area (S) times the time of contact (duration) (T) or $A = P \times C \times S \times T$.

If P equals the drug's diffusion coefficient (D) times the partition coefficient of the drug between the delivery medium and the skin or mucosa (K_p) divided by H then $P = D\frac{K_p}{H}$. Therefore, $A = P \times C \times S \times T$ or $A = \frac{DK_pCST}{H}$.

SPECIFIC ROUTES OF DRUG ADMINISTRATION

What are the advantages/disadvantages, clinical uses, practical considerations, and pathophysiology/pharmacology of the various routes of drug administration?

Transdermal Drug Administration

Variables affecting the absorption of a drug via the skin can be divided into pharmacologic and patient factors

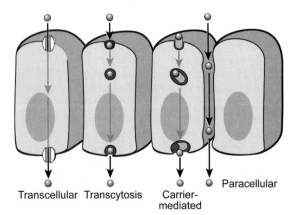

Transcellular Transcytosis Carrier-mediated Paracellular

Fig. 47-2. Transport mechanisms across cellular barrier: the mechanisms for transport across the cell membrane: transcellular, transcytosis, carrier-mediated, paracellular. (Reprinted with permission from Department of Medical Illustration-Cleveland Clinic Foundation.)

Table 47-5. Factors Affecting Drug Absorption

Pharmacologic (drug) Factors
Type of molecule (e.g., proteins/peptides are subject to enzymatic hydrolysis/destruction)
Lipid solubility
Molecular size
pH of drug (affects ionization)
Concentration of drug
Local barriers (pH, mucous, enzymes)
Additives to drug
Drug delivery vehicle
Particle size (especially for respiratory tract mucosa)
Drug solubility

Patient Factors
Transdermal drug administration
  General health
  Age: skin thickness, blood flow
  Skin thickness
  Skin temperature
  Application site on skin
  Time (duration) of contact with skin
  Hydration of skin
  Skin microbial flora (affects drug metabolism)
  Integrity of stratum corneum (intact or broken skin)
  Blood flow to skin (affected by overall health, vascular disease, skin temperature)
  Skin disease present (e.g., psoriasis and eczema)
Respiratory transmucosal absorption
  General health
  Surface area
  Respiratory disorders: ↓ absorption with pneumonia (↑ mucous), pulmonary edema (↑ fluid), COPD/pulmonary
    fibrosis (↓ surface area 2° to alveolar destruction), pulmonary emboli or vasculitis (↓ blood flow)
Nasal transmucosal absorption
  General health
  Nasal mucosal health: ↓ absorption with nasal discharge, epistaxis, nasal mucosal disease, or destruction
Oral transmucosal
  General health
  Oral disease: ↑ absorption: stomatitis, mucositis, blisters, gingivitis
Rectal transmucosal absorption
  General health
  Site where drug is delivered (length of rectal catheter)
  Drainage via superior rectal veins to liver (hepatic metabolism) or via inferior and middle rectal veins to
    systemic circulation
  Presence or absence of stool
  pH of rectal contents (affects drug ionization)
  How long drug is in rectum or is it expelled?

COPD: chronic obstructive pulmonary disease.

(Table 47-5) (Fig. 47-3). Pharmacologic parameters that can affect drug absorption and kinetics are lipid solubility, molecular size, the pH of the drug, drug concentration, the membrane permeability of the transdermal drug delivery system, the drug vehicle formulation, and the depot of drug in the skin.[7,10,15] Individual factors include skin thickness, application site on skin, time in contact with the skin, skin's hydration, integrity of the

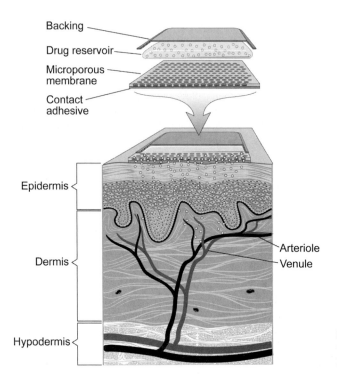

Fig. 47-3. Transdermal drug absorption. (Reprinted with permission from Department of Medical Illustration-Cleveland Clinic Foundation.)

stratum corneum (Is the skin broken or intact?), healthy or diseased skin (Is eczema or another skin disorder present?), the skin's microbial flora (affects drug metabolism), and blood flow to the skin.[6] Dermal blood flow is a function of many variables including the patient's overall health (Is hypotension, shock, or a low blood flow state present?), vascular disorders (Is vascular disease present such as a vasculitis, Raynaud's disease or peripheral vascular disease?), the skin temperature, and by *additives* applied to the skin or in the drug.[6,7,15]

The age of the patient is a consideration in transdermal drug administration since skin blood flow and skin thickness vary with age.[6,15] The geriatric patient with peripheral vascular disease and a decreased dermal blood flow may be undermedicated, while a pediatric patient especially an infant with a thinner skin and a rich dermal blood flow could be toxic with the same transdermal medication patch. An example of such toxicity resulted when newborns were washed with hexachlorophene.[16–18] Central nervous system toxicity including seizures occurred from the toxic systemic blood levels due to the high absorption because of the neonate's large body surface area and very thin skin.[16–18]

Absorption via the dermal route is known to be increased by skin disease, accidental application across a mucous membrane, and by pulling off a superficial layer of skin.[19] Psoriasis causes a thickened epidermis with decreased absorption, while eczema allows increased absorption because of broken skin.

The main barrier to the dermal absorption of exogenous substances including drugs through the skin is the stratum corneum (the top layer of the skin). Passage through the stratum corneum is the rate-limiting step for percutaneous absorption. The establishment of a concentration gradient creates a driving force for drug movement across the skin. Other factors affecting absorption include the following:

The release of drug from the vehicle = Kp

Drug diffusion across the skin layers = diffusion coefficient = D

The thickness of the stratum corneum = H

The concentration of drug in the vehicle = C

Therefore,

$$\text{absorption } (A) = P \times C \times S \times T = A = \frac{K_p DCST}{H}.$$

The practical implication is that drug absorption can be increased by such maneuvers as applying an occlusive dressing. An occlusive dressing decreases water loss from the transepidermal layer of skin, thereby increasing hydration by increasing the water content of the stratum corneum. This is why topical anesthetics such as LMX-4 and EMLA cream are applied using a bioclusive dressing. There are also substances which increase drug penetration through the skin: propylene glycol, urea, and dimethyl sulfoxide; substances commonly used in skin ointments or creams. [6] Where the medication is applied can affect absorption since some anatomic regions have thinner or thicker skin. Patient age is also a factor since the skin thickness (*H*) is thinner in infants especially preterm infants and in the elderly which allows for greater skin permeability.

A problem with transdermal drug administration is achieving consistent therapeutic drug levels in different patients and in the same patient across time under different physiologic conditions. Blood levels of drugs given transdermally can match that achieved with parenteral administration and thus, be equally effective. The downside with transdermal drug administration is the long onset and offset. There is a significant delay before therapeutic blood levels are attained. With transdermal fentanyl, for example, uptake starts in 1 hour, low therapeutic levels occur in 6–8 hours, and peak blood levels occur 24 hours after administration.[1,6] Similarly, blood concentrations fall slowly after removal of the patch. The slow onset and variable absorption from transdermal administration generally eliminates the ability to use the narcotic patch (morphine or fentanyl) for acute pain relief, although the use for chronic pain relief is well established. Use of the patch does not eliminate side effects (such as nausea or vomiting) or toxicity including respiratory depression.

Occasionally, local irritation, redness, pruritus, or a rash may occur at the site of drug application. However, transdermal drug administration has significant advantages: painless application, ready availability in all patients without needing time and equipment (such as IVs) for application, and avoids the risk of a needlestick. Transdermal drug administration generally has negligible systemic absorption and few side effects, although toxicity and even deaths have been reported usually secondary to accidental increased absorption through mucous membranes or when an excessive dose was given.[20,21]

Transdermal drug administration has widespread clinical usage. The use of topical anesthetics (see Chap. 26) is only one of many applications of transdermal drug administration. Other uses include narcotic administration for patients with chronic pain such as cancer patients (examples: morphine and fentanyl patches), cardiac medication delivery (nitroglycerin and clonidine), hormone delivery, birth control, nicotine, and miscellaneous drugs such as scopolamine patches for treatment of motion sickness as well as the dermatology pharmacopeia[13–15, 22–25] (Table 47-3).

Key considerations for the safe and efficacious use of transdermal drug delivery include: use recommended dosages (do not exceed the maximum dose), do not use on (or near) mucous membranes, and do not apply over broken or diseased skin (e.g., eczematous skin), since this will increase drug absorption and blood levels of the drug.

Transmucosal Drug Administration

Transmucosal drug administration is the delivery of medications through a mucosal surface. Since the mucosa has an abundant vascular supply without a layer of stratum corneum epidermidis, drug absorption is rapid and efficient with quick drug delivery to the systemic circulation.

Medications are frequently applied to the mucous membranes for their local effects. Such topical applications often involve the mucous membranes of the ocular conjunctiva, the nasopharynx, the oropharynx, the colon, the bladder, the urethra, and the vagina.[1] The use of topical ophthalmic medications, topical otolaryngologic drugs, and inhaled pulmonary medications is well established.[1] In addition, medications are given locally with systemic absorption resulting in the desired systemic therapeutic effect. Examples include the use of rectal diazepam to treat seizures and the application of synthetic antidiuretic hormone to the nasal mucosa for its systemic effect[10,26] (Table 47-3).

A major advantage of transmucosal drug administration is that it averts the problems of oral drug administration, which includes degradation by first-pass hepatic metabolism, degradation by enzymes throughout the GI tract, and destruction by the hostile environment of the acidic stomach with its low pH[7] (Tables 47-1 and 47-2).

Factors determining transmucosal drug absorption can be divided into pharmacologic and patient factors (Table 47-5). Pharmacologic parameters are lipid solubility, molecular size, the pH and ionization of the drug, the drug delivery vehicle, and the drug concentration (these are essentially the same factors as for transdermal drug administration).[10] Patient factors involve duration of contact with the mucosa and the blood flow to the mucosa (especially venous drainage) (again similar factors to that for transdermal drug delivery).[6]

Transmucosal drug absorption further depends on the specific site and is subdivided into mucosa of the respiratory tract and GI tract; specifically, nasal, oral (sublingual or buccal), and rectal mucosa.

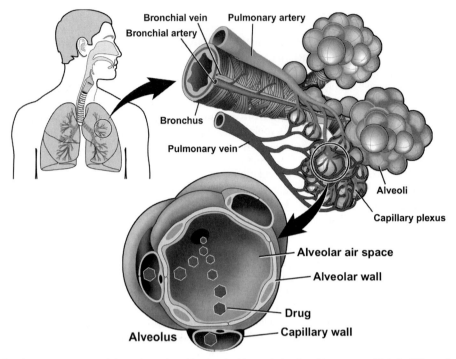

Fig. 47-4. Respiratory tract mucosal drug absorption. (Reprinted with permission from Department of Medical Illustration-Cleveland Clinic Foundation.)

Respiratory Tract Mucosal Drug Administration

The large surface area of the lung allows rapid access to the circulation (Fig. 47-4). Advantages of the pulmonary route are the rapid nearly instantaneous absorption into the blood and elimination of the hepatic first-pass loss of drug. When treating pulmonary disorders, delivery of the drug at the local desired site of action minimizes or eliminates many drug side effects and toxicity.[27] Past problems with this route of administration have involved control of the drug dosage and bulky unwieldy devices for drug administration. Such problems have disappeared with various technological improvements.[10] There is a greater bioavailability with respiratory tract mucosal drug administration because drainage is into the systemic circulation unlike oral drug administration which drains into the portal circulation.[10] Many drugs can be given via this route including solutions of drugs which can be atomized, aerosolized, and inhaled.

Inhalation is the most common method for respiratory tract mucosal drug administration, although direct installation is also used.[6] In general, inhaled drugs are deposited on the upper airway mucosa but this is a function of particle size, and drug solubility, as well as the delivery vehicle and the patient's respiratory pattern. Fat-soluble medications gravitate toward the distal airways and are more quickly absorbed than water-soluble drugs that tend to stay in the upper airway. The particle size is also a determining factor with intermediate size (1–5 μm) particles reaching the distal airways and large (>5 μm) particles depositing in the nasopharynx.[28,29]

There is a vast array of medications that are given via inhalation into the respiratory tract mucosa: inhalational anesthetics including nitrous oxide, bronchodilators (albuterol, ipratropium, epinephrine), corticosteroids, antibiotics, antifungals, antiviral agents, surfactant, hormones, and sedatives.[6,27]

Direct installation into the respiratory tract mucosa has generally been used for topical anesthesia prior to airway procedures and during resuscitation. The key to attaining higher systemic blood levels by direct instillation is to dilute the drug in sufficient volume to be propelled into the distal airway with positive pressure ventilation or to deposit the drug beyond the tip of the endotracheal tube.[30] Typically, lidocaine, atropine, epinephrine, naloxone (and previously valium) can be administered by this route.

Nasal Mucosal (Intranasal) Drug Administration

As with other transmucosal routes, intranasal drug delivery has unique advantages. It is painless, needleless, avoids needlestick injuries, does not require sterile technique, has a large absorptive highly vascular surface resulting in rapid drug absorption and systemic drug levels (in blood and CSF), and avoids first-pass metabolism yielding a greater bioavailability than with oral medications.[9]

As with other transmucosal routes, factors influencing drug absorption involve pharmacologic and patient factors including the patient's general and nasal mucosal health. Decreased drug absorption occurs when there is copious nasal discharge, bloody secretions, epistaxis, and nasal mucosal damage/destruction.[9]

Techniques for increasing absorption are to administer half of the drug dose into each nostril, which effectively doubles the available absorptive area.[9] Use the most concentrated form of drug available to limit the volume of solution administered. Large drug volumes (e.g., greater than 0.5–1.0 cc per nostril) may drain out of the nose, thereby decreasing absorption and effectiveness. Drug delivery vehicles using atomization versus drops or sprays also increase absorption.

There are multiple techniques for the administration of intranasal medications: nasal sprays, inhalers, atomizers, dipping a cotton swab into the medicated solution and applying it to the nasal mucosa, or injecting with a needleless syringe.

Clinical uses of intranasal medications involve not just over the counter nasal sprays (for example, decongestants) but also topical anesthetics (e.g., 4% lidocaine) for nasal procedures from nasal packing for epistaxis to nasogastric tube placement, and intranasal corticosteroids for allergic rhinitis.[31–33] Intranasal medications administered for their systemic effects include naloxone for opiate overdose, the benzodiazepine midazolam to control of seizures, fentanyl or sufentanil for analgesia,

midazolam, ketamine or sufentanil for sedation, vasopressin for antidiuretic hormone replacement, and butorphanol for treatment of migraine headaches.[1,6,9,34–41] The intranasal route is also a popular avenue for various illegal drugs, e.g., cocaine.

Unlike other transmucosal routes of drug administration, intranasal drug administration has some unique considerations (Fig. 47-5). Pharmacologic agents applied to the nasal mucosa are absorbed via three pathways: into the systemic circulation via the capillary bed (as with other transmucosal locations), but also by the olfactory neurons, and directly into the CSF.[6] For some pharmacologic agents, nasal administration yields a higher CSF/plasma ratio than oral or even intravenous administration.[6] It is likely that drugs can diffuse through the perineural space surrounding the olfactory nerves into the subarachnoid space.[6]

Intranasal drug absorption and effect generally has a rapid onset and offset but there is a possibility of continued absorption. Potential mechanisms for continued drug absorption are from absorption of swallowed medication after nasal administration or differential neuronal and/or CSF drug transfer or transport.[6]

Oral (Sublingual, Buccal) Drug Administration

Considering that nitroglycerin has been administered sublingually for over 100 years, oral mucosal drug delivery is clinically well established and may be the oldest medical transmucosal alternative route of systemic drug delivery.[8]

The surface area of the oral mucosa is much less than that of the GI tract (1750 times greater surface area) or the skin (100 times greater surface area).[8] But the oral mucosa is highly vascularized and pharmacologic agents

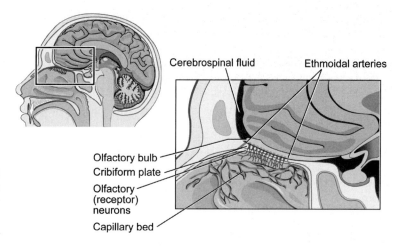

Fig. 47-5. Nasal transmucosal drug absorption. (Reprinted with permission from Department of Medical Illustration-Cleveland Clinic Foundation.)

Cerebrospinal fluid

Ethmoidal arteries

Olfactory bulb

Cribiform plate

Olfactory (receptor) neurons

Capillary bed

Sublingual administration   Buccal administration

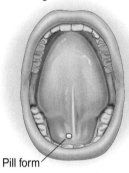 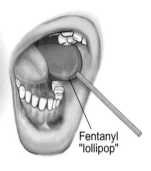

Pill form   Fentanyl "lollipop"

Fig. 47-6. Oral (sublingual, buccal) transmucosal drug absorption. (Reprinted with permission from Department of Medical Illustration-Cleveland Clinic Foundation.)

absorbed via the oral mucosa directly enter the systemic circulation. This has the advantage of bypassing the GI tract and the first-pass metabolism of the liver.[42–45]

The anatomic structures of the oral cavity are the tongue, the floor of the mouth, cheeks, hard palate, soft palate, and the lips (Fig. 47-6). The oral mucosa is the lining of the oral cavity and consists of the sublingual, buccal, gingival, palatal, and labial mucosa. The ventral surface of the tongue, the floor of the mouth (sublingual), and the cheeks (buccal) make up approximately 60% of the oral mucosal surface area. The sublingual and buccal tissues have a greater permeability than other tissues in the mouth.[8] These facts explain the various methods for giving oral transmucosal drugs: usually by placing the drug under the tongue (e.g., sublingual nitroglycerin) or sucking on a fentanyl lollipop. There are many vehicles for administering drugs: sprays, tablets, lozenges, solutions, patches, adhesive films, and even chewing gum (e.g., nicotine gum).

There is an additional barrier to drug absorption in the oral cavity: the enzymes in the mouth which rapidly degrade and destroy any protein or peptide molecules.[8] This is why the bioavailability of proteins or peptides (but not all pharmacologic agents) given via the oral transmucosal route is generally <5%.[8] As with the enteral route, absorption can be variable. Furthermore, a drug's penetration through the oral mucosa can be affected by disorders that affect the integrity of the oral mucosa such as stomatitis, mucositis, blisters, or glossitis.[6]

Various drugs have been administered via the oral transmucosal route. Some pharmacologic agents administered via the oral transmucosal route include sedatives (midazolam), analgesics (fentanyl, morphine, buprenorphine), cardiovascular (nitroglycerin, clonidine), psychiatric (olanzapine), and nicotine. There is also promising research on oral transmucosal administration of the sedatives

(midazolam and etomidate) and the opioid analgesics (morphine).[46–50] When compared with nasal and/or rectal midazolam, the sublingual route was effective, had better patient acceptance, and higher plasma concentration.[8,48,49] Oral mucosal delivery of etomidate was effective in producing sedation and detectable blood levels.[50]

The oral transmucosal delivery of the opioid fentanyl is via a sugar-based lozenge on a handle, the fentanyl lollipop. The fentanyl *Oralet* has been used to treat breakthrough cancer pain and pain in pediatric patients.[1,51–53] Oral transmucosal fentanyl citrate (OTFC) is contraindicated in children <10 kg, has an onset in 15 minutes, and is given in a 10–15 μg/kg dose up to 400 mg in pediatric patients and up to 1600 mg in adults in one study. Its use has been somewhat limited by the side effects of nausea, vomiting, and facial pruritus.[1]

Rectal Drug Administration

The rectal transmucosa allows for the absorption of many drugs.[54,56] Clinical examples of rectal drug administration include acetaminophen for its antipyretic and analgesic effect, diazepam or midazolam for the treatment of seizures, and numerous sedatives: midazolam, ketamine, methohexital, thiopental, and pentobarbital (Table 47-3).[57–63]

Rectal administration can be used in vomiting patients, is easy to administer, a painless alternative to parenteral medication, and in infants/young children is comparable to taking a rectal temperature. One contraindication to rectal drug administration is an immunosuppressed patient with the potential for an abscess with even minimal trauma.

There are several considerations when administering medications via the rectal transmucosa. There can be much variation in drug absorption due to anatomy, drug factors, the administration of the drug, and patient

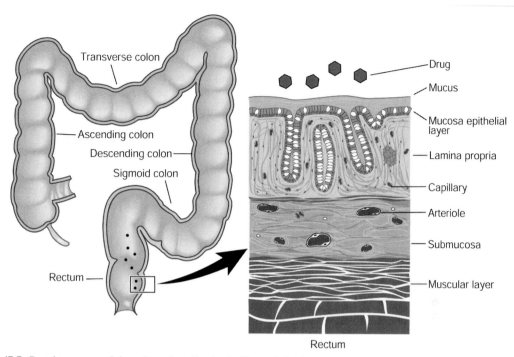

Fig. 47-7. Rectal transmucosal drug absorption. (Reprinted with permission from Department of Medical Illustration-Cleveland Clinic Foundation.)

factors (Fig. 47-7). Drug parameters include the concentration of the drug, drug diluent volume, and drug formulation (time to liquefaction of suppositories).[64] For example, a 2% methohexital solution yielded higher blood levels for a longer duration than a 10% methohexital solution at the same 25 mg/kg dose.[65] Local parameters affecting drug absorption are drug location in rectum (site in rectum where drug is delivered depends on the length of the rectal catheter), absence or presence of stool in rectum, pH of the rectal contents (affects drug ionization), and how long the drug is retained in the rectum or if is it expelled.[66,67] The superior aspect of the rectum is drained by the superior rectal veins which drain into the liver, therefore, drugs given high up in the rectum undergo hepatic metabolism. The inferior part of the rectum first drains into the inferior and middle rectal veins and then into the systemic venous system. It is possible that drugs given higher up in the rectum will undergo greater hepatic first-pass metabolism.

The main disadvantage of rectal transmucosal administration is the variable absorption. Generally, the onset takes minutes and the effects last for hours, although rapid nearly complete absorption can occur and result in toxicity.

PRACTICAL CONSIDERATIONS AND THE FUTURE

Because of the disadvantages associated with the "conventional" routes of drug administration, unique routes and/or methods for giving pharmacologic agents especially analgesics and sedatives are being developed and there is much promising research.

However, there should be a word of caution. Use of a "local" site for transmucosal drug administration often decreases systemic side effects or toxicity but not always. In fact, serious complications such as seizures and even fatal toxicity have been associated with transdermal or transmucosal drug administration especially in infants and young children.[16–18,20,21,68,69] Such fatal toxic effects have generally occurred after an accidental ingestion or when an individual mistakenly received an excessive dose of medication(s) and was not properly monitored. Therefore, no matter what the route or technique of drug administration, procedural sedation and analgesia requires careful pre and postprocedure evaluation on selected patients using appropriate drugs in recommended doses given in the proper environment with adequate monitoring by trained and qualified physicians.

Advances in transdermal drug delivery involve chemical, physical, technological, and even computer microprocessing research. Various chemical enhancers or additives can be applied to the skin or other mucosal layer or incorporated into the vehicle used for delivery of the drugs.[19] Such enhancers are "safe" and increase drug transport and absorption across the skin or other mucosal barriers, or limit degradation of the drug (as by lessening the effect of enzymes, a layer of mucous, or the acidic pH of the stomach). Microstructured arrays, dubbed *microneedles*, create microscopic pores that can penetrate the skin's stratum corneum allowing the drug to bypass the body's layer of cells that acts as a barrier.

Another way of delivering medication, the use of drug implants, has had a variety of clinical uses from birth control to delivering chemotherapy at localized sites of action, or in coronary artery stents. Expansion of drug implants for systemic as well as local delivery of pharmacological agents is another area of active research.

Emerging technologies from iontophoresis, phonophoresis, or electroporation (which creates transient permeable pores in the stratum corneum) may increase drug absorption across the body's cellular barrier. Use of magnetic energy (magnetophoresis), radio waves, microlasers, thermal patches (the temperature affects absorption), high-speed particles, or liquids may develop into a practical commercial technology for drug delivery in the future.

Active delivery devices are already utilized to deliver subcutaneous insulin. Use of a microprocessor-controlled feedback system when combined with a noninvasive continuous monitoring system will allow automatic modulation of drug delivery. This will allow temporal real-time control over drug transport.

Improvements in the vehicles for drug delivery from gels to patches that use existing passive delivery technology are already being tested.[2] Research in "active delivery devices" is ongoing. [2] Undoubtedly, new devices and technologies and additional pharmacologic agents will be available for transdermal and transmucosal drug delivery in the near future.

SUMMARY

The use of nontraditional routes of drug administration is likely to undergo rapid expansion in the future. Such alternative methods of drug delivery avoid the problems inherent with the traditional methods of drug administration including the pain of an IV stick or IM shot, and the risks of a needlestick injury; or the decreased bioavailability that can occur if the patient is vomiting, has GI disease, and from hepatic first-pass metabolism.

There are numerous benefits of such nontraditional routes of administering drugs including painless, needleless (no risk of needlestick injuries), no need for equipment or personnel for administration, cost-effective, and avoids hepatic first-pass metabolism and destruction in the GI tract. Variable drug absorption can be a disadvantage of the alternate routes of drug administration. There are some unique considerations for the various alternative routes of administration, transdermal and transmucosal (respiratory tract, nasal, oral, or rectal). The use of alternative routes of drug administration is an area of active research that holds promise for the development of many new pharmacologic agents with continuing improvements in the drug delivery vehicles.

REFERENCES

1. Gaukroger PB. Novel techniques of analgesic delivery. In: Malviya S, Naughton NN, Tremper KK, eds. *Sedation and Analgesia for Diagnostic and Therapeutic Procedures.* Totowa, NJ: Humana Press; 2003:195–201.
2. Meidan VM, Michniak BB. Emerging technologies in transdermal therapeutics. *Am J Ther.* 2004;11:312–316.
3. Stanley TH. New routes of administration and new delivery systems of anesthetics. *Anesthesiology.* 1988;68:665–668.
4. McQuay HJ. The logic of alternative routes (Editorial). *J Pain Symptom Manage.* 1990;5:75–77.
5. Mather LE. Novel methods of drug delivery (abstract). Pain 1990;(suppl 5):5250.
6. Committee on drugs—American Academy of Pediatrics. Alternate routes of drug administration-advantages and disadvantages. *Pediatrics.* 1997;100(1):143–152.
7. Blanchette J, Kavimandan N, Peppas NA. Principles of transmucosal drug delivery of therapeutic agents. *Biomed Pharmacol.* 2004;142–151.
8. Zhang H, Zhang J, Streisant JB. Oral mucosal drug delivery—clinical pharmacokinetics and therapeutic applications. *Clin Pharmacokinet.* 2002;41(9):661–680.
9. Wolfe TR, Bernstone T. Intranasal delivery: an alternative to intravenous administration in selected emergency cases. *J Emerg Nurs.* 2004;30(2):141–146.
10. Wilkinson GR. Pharmacokinetics. The dynamics of drug absorption, distribution, and elimination. In: Hardman JG, Limbird LE, Goodman Gilman A, eds. *Goodman and Gilman's The Pharmacological Basis of Therapeutics.* New York: McGraw-Hill; 2001:3–31.
11. Sakane T, Akizuki M, Yoahida MK, et al. Transport of cephalexin to the cerebrospinal fluid directly from the nasal cavity. *J Pharm Pharmacol.* 1991;43:449–451.
12. Binhammer RT. CSF anatomy with emphasis on relations to nasal cavity and labyrinthine fluids. *Ear Nose Throat J.* 1992; 71:292–294.
13. Roy SD, Flynn GL. Transdermal delivery of narcotic analgesics: pH, anatomical, and subject influences on cutaneous

permeability of fentanyl and sufentanil. *Pharm Res*. 1990;7: 842–847.

14. Biddle C, Gilliland C. Transdermal and transmucosal administration of pain-relieving and anxiolytic drugs: a primer for the critical care practitioner. *Heart Lung*. 1992;21:115–124.

15. Wyatt EL, Sutter SH, Drake LA. Dermatological pharmacology. In: Hardman JG, Limbird LE, Goodman-Gilman A, eds. *Goodman and Gilman's The Pharmacological Basis of Therapeutics*. New York: McGraw-Hill; 2001:1795–1818.

16. Bressler K, Walson PD, Fulginitti VA. Hexachlorophene in the newborn nursery: a risk benefit analysis and review. *Clin Pediatr*. 1977;16:342–351.

17. Marquardt ED. Hexachlorophene toxicity in a pediatric burn patient. *Drug Intell Clin Pharm*. 1986;20:624.

18. Tyrala EE, Hillman LS, Hillman RE, et al. Clinical pharmacology of hexachlorophene in newborn infants. *J Pediatr*. 1977;91:481–486.

19. Lerner EV, Bucalo BD, Kist DA, et al. Topical anesthetic agents in dermatologic surgery. *Dermatol Surg*. 1997;23:673–683.

20. Daya MR, Burton BT, Schleiss MR, et al. Recurrent seizures following mucosal applications of TAC. *Ann Emerg Med*. 1988;17:646–648.

21. Dailey RH. Fatality secondary to misuse of TAC solution. *Ann Emerg Med*. 1988;17:159–160.

22. Miser AW, Narung PK, Dothage JA, et al. Transdermal fentanyl for pain control in patients with cancer. *Pain*. 1989;37:15–21.

23. Horimoto Y, Tomie H, Hanzawa K, et al. Scopolamine patch reduces postoperative emesis in paediatric patients following strabismus surgery. *Can J Anaesth*. 1991;38:441–444.

24. Gora ML. Nicotine transdermal systems. *Ann Pharmacother*. 1993;27:742–750.

25. Sorenson JC, Crook D, Godsland IF, et al. Oral versus transdermal hormone replacement therapy. *Int I Fertil Menopausal Stud*. 1993;38(suppl 7):30–35.

26. Scott RC, Basag FM, Neville BGR. Buccal midazolam and rectal diazepam for treatment of prolonged seizures in childhood and adolescence: a randomized trial. *Lancet*. 1999;353:623–626.

27. Undem BJ, Lichtenstein LM. Drugs used in the treatment of asthma. In: Hardman JG, Limbird LE, Goodman-Gilman A, eds. *Goodman and Gilman's The Pharmacological Basis of Therapeutics*. New York: McGraw-Hill; 2001:733–754.

28. Scheuch G, Stahlofen W. Deposition and dispersion of aerosols in the airways of the human respiratory tract: the effect of particle size. *Exp Lung Res*. 1992;18:343–358.

29. Everend ML, Hardy JG, Milner AD. Comparison of nebulized aerosol deposition in the lungs of healthy adults following oral and nasal inhalation. *Thorax*. 1993;48:1045–1046.

30. Mace SE. The effect of technique of administration on the endotracheal absorption of medication. *Ann Emerg Med*. 1986;15(5):552–556.

31. Wolfe TR, Fosnocht DE, Linscott MS. Atomized lidocaine as topical anesthesia for nasogastric tube placement: a randomized, double-blind, placebo-controlled trial. *Ann Emerg Med*. 2000;35:421–425.

32. Singer AJ, Konia N. Comparison of topical anesthetics and vasoconstrictors vs lubricants prior to nasogastric intubation: a randomized, controlled trial. *Acad Emerg Med*. 1999;6: 184–190.

33. Mabry RL. Corticosteroids in the management of upper respiratory allergy: the emerging role of steroid nasal sprays. *Otolaryngol Head Neck Surg*. 1992;107:855–860.

34. Barron ED, Ramos J, Colwell C, et al. Intranasal administration of naloxone by paramedics. *Prehosp Emerg Care*. 2002;6:54–58.

35. Borland ML, Jacobs I, Geelhoed G. Intranasal fentanyl reduces acute pain in children in the emergency department: a safety and efficacy study. *Emerg Med* (Fremantle). 2002;14:275–280.

36. Bates BA, Schutzman SA, Fleisher GR. A comparison of intranasal sufentanil and midazolam to intramuscular meperidine, promethazine, and chlorpromazine, and chlorpromazine for conscious sedation in children. *Ann Emerg Med*. 1994;24:646–651.

37. Wermeling DP, Miller JL, Archer SM, et al. Bioavailability and pharmacokinetics of lorazepam after intranasal, intravenous, and intramuscular administration. *J Clin Pharmacol*. 2001;41: 1225–1231.

38. Theroux MC, West DW, Corddry DH, et al. Efficacy of intranasal midazolam in facilitating suturing of lacerations in preschool children in the emergency department. *Pediatrics*. 1993;91:624–627.

39. McGlone RG, Renasinghe S, Durham S. An alternative to "brutaine": a comparison of low dose intramuscular ketamine with intranasal midazolam in children before suturing. *J Accid Emerg Med*. 1998;15:231–238.

40. Yealy DM, Fillis JH, Hobbs GD, et al. Intranasal midazolam as a sedative for children during laceration repair. *Am J Emerg Med*. 1992;10:584–587.

41. Abrams R, Morrison JE, Villasenor A, et al. Safety and effectiveness of intranasal administration of sedative medications (ketamine, midazolam, or sufentanil) for urgent brief pediatric dental procedures. *Anesth Prog*. 1993;40:63–66.

42. Administration of drugs by the buccal route. *Lancet*. 1987;1:666–667.

43. de Vries ME, Bodde HE, Verboef JC, et al. Developments in buccal drug delivery. *Crit Rev Ther Drug Carrier Syst*. 1991;8:271–303.

44. Motwani JG, Lipworth BJ. Clinical pharmacokinetics of drugs administered buccally and sublingually. *Clin Pharmacokinet*. 1991;21:83–94.

45. Harris D, Robinson JR. Drug delivery via the mucous membranes of the oral cavity. *J Pharm Sci*. 1992;81:1–10.

46. Gong L, Middleton RK. Sublingual administration of opioids. *Ann Pharmacother*. 1992;26:1525–1527.

47. Manara AR, Bodenham AR, Park CR. Analgesic efficacy of perioperative buccal morphine. *Br J Anaesth*. 1990;64: 551–555.

48. Karl HW, Rosenberger JL, Laruch MG, et al. Transmucosal administration of midazolam for premedication of pediatric patients: comparison of the nasal and sublingual routes. *Anesthesiology*. 1993;78:885–891.

49. Geldner G, Hubmann M, Knoll R, et al. Comparison between three transmucosal routes of administration of midazolam in children. *Paediatr Anaesth.* 1997;7:103–109.

50. Streisand JB, Jaarsma RL, Gay MA, et al. Oral transmucosal etomidate in volunteers. *Anesthesiology.* 1998;88(1):89–95.

51. Lind GH, Marcus MA, Mears SL, et al. Oral transmucosal fentanyl citrate for analgesia and sedation in the emergency department. *Ann Emerg Med.* 1991;20:1117–1120.

52. Schechter NL, Weisman SJ, Roswenblulm M, et al. The use of oral transmucosal fentanyl citrate for painful procedures in children. *Pediatrics.* 1995;95:335–339.

53. Schutzman SA, Burg J, Liebelt E, et al. Oral transmucosal fentanyl citrate for premedication of children undergoing laceration repair. *Ann Emerg Med.* 1994;24:1059–1064.

54. van Hoogdalem E, Lebauer AG, Bremmer DD. Pharmacokinetics of rectal drug administration. Part I: general considerations and clinical applications of centrally acting drugs. *Clin Pharmacokinet.* 1991;21:11–26.

55. Choonara LA. Giving drugs per rectum for systemic effect. *Arch Dis Child.* 1987;62:771–772.

56. Van Hoogdalem EJ, de Boer AG, Breimer DD. Pharmacokinetics of rectal drug administration: Part II: clinical applications of peripherally acting drugs and conclusions. *Clin Pharmacokinet.* 1991;21:110–128.

57. Gaudreault P, Guay J, Nicol O, et al. Pharmacokinetics and clinical efficacy of intrarectal solution of acetaminophen. *Can J Anaesth.* 1988;35:149–152.

58. Fisgin T, Gurer Y, Tezic T, et al. Effects of intranasal midazolam and rectal diazepam on acute convulsions in children: prospective randomized study. *J Child Neurol.* 2002;17:123–126.

59. Malinovsky JM, Lejus C, Servin F, et al. Plasma concentrations of midazolam after i.v. nasal or rectal administration in children. *Br J Anaesth.* 1993;70:617–620.

60. Tsai SK, Mok MS, Lippmann M. Rectal ketamine vs intranasal ketamine as premedicants in children, *Anesthesiology.* 1990; 73:A1094.

61. Beebe DS, Belani KG, Chang PN, et al. Effectiveness of preoperative sedation with rectal midazolam, ketamine, or their combination in younger children. *Anesth Analg.* 1992; 75:880–884.

62. Roelfee JA, van der Bijil P, Stegmann DH, et al. Preanesthetic medication with rectal midazolalm in children undergoing dental extractions. *Oral Maxillofac Surg.* 1990; 48:791–797.

63. Pomeranz ES, Chudnofsky CR, Deegan TJ, et al. Rectal methohexital sedation for computed tomography imaging of stable pediatric emergency department patients. *Pediatrics.* 2000;105:1110–1114.

64. Laishley RS, O'Callaghan AC, Lerman J. Effects of dose and concentration of rectal methohexitone for induction of anaesthesia in children. *Can Anesth Soc J.* 1986;33: 427–432.

65. Forbes RB, Vandewalker GE. Comparison of two and ten percental rectal methohexitone for induction of anaesthesia in children. *Can J Anesth.* 1988;35:345–349.

66. Khalil SN, Florence FB, Van den Nieuwenhuyzen MC, et al. Rectal methohexital; concentration and length of the rectal catheters. *Anesth Analg.* 1990;70:645–649.

67. Jantzen JP, Erdmann K, Witton PK, et al. The effect of rectal pH values on the absorption of methohexital. *Anesthetist.* 1986;35:496–499.

68. Gourlay GK, Boss RA. Fetal outcome with use of rectal morphine for postoperative pain control in an infant. *Br Med J.* 1992;304:766–767.

69. Safety of novel fentanyl dosage forms questioned: several deaths attributed to misuse of patch. *Am J Hosp Pharm.* 1994;51:870.

48

Devices
Intravenous Opioid Patient-Controlled Analgesia (PCA) and Transcutaneous Electrical Nerve Stimulation (TENS)

Sharon E. Mace
Michael F. Murphy

HIGH YIELD FACTS

- Patient-controlled analgesia (PCA) is the self-administration of analgesia, generally opioids.

- PCA has many indications including postoperative analgesia, treatment of cancer pain, and sickle cell crisis.

- Nurse-controlled analgesia (NCA) or family-controlled analgesia (FCA) can be used in patients without the motor and cognitive skills to operate a PCA device.

- NCA or FCA can be used in young children (<4–6 years), special needs patients, cognitively impaired (e.g., some geriatric patients).

- Transcutaneous electrical nerve stimulation (TENS) is a type of electroanalgesia.

- Electroanalgesia uses electrical stimulation to treat pain and includes deep brain stimulation, dorsal column stimulation, and TENS.

- TENS is noninvasive, inexpensive, safe, and can be used in all ages of patients for selected types of pain.

PATIENT-CONTROLLED ANALGESIA

Background and Technique

The pain associated with major surgery, acute medical conditions, major trauma, and invasive medical procedures is generally given the rubric *acute pain*. It is ordinarily abrupt in onset, peaks in minutes to hours, and is anticipated to be severe for no more than 1–2 days. It is distinct from *chronic pain*.

Over the past 15 years, the emphasis given to acute pain management by government agencies, accrediting bodies, professional organizations, practitioners, and individuals in pain has driven the implementation of acute pain management services and techniques. This has led to the development of new drugs, new medication delivery systems, and new protocols to improve the way we manage pain in general, and acute pain in particular.

A substantial component of this emerging patient care discipline is education:

- Of health care professionals with respect to the importance of prompt evaluation and management of pain.

- Of patients to ensure that they demand and receive appropriate pain management.

Along with this shift in thinking, there has been a change in philosophy and perspective: from the caregiver deciding how much pain the patient has, how much analgesic medication to administer and how often, to patients deciding how much pain they have and how much medication they take. Transferring this "control" to patient-controlled analgesia (PCA) has had a tremendously positive influence on patient satisfaction and comfort. In addition, patient control compensates for the fact that pain intensity is rarely constant. For example, it may be exacerbated by patient movement or coughing. One may effectively take advantage of this feature of pain and PCA by advising the patient to demand a dose from the PCA prior to moving or coughing.

The devices employed as intravenous (IV) PCA pumps are programmable, medication dose controllers with a patient-activated demand feature. They are capable of administering a continuous background infusion of a medication while at the same time permitting intermittent fixed bolus dose supplementation. Ordinarily a loading dose of an opioid is administered to lower the pain score to an acceptable level for the patient, followed by patient-controlled intermittent bolus dosing, continuous infusion, or both.

Morphine is the most commonly used agent. The total *titrated* loading dose is typically in the 0.1–0.2-mg/kg range, and the bolus 0.5–1.5 mg/dose with a lockout of 5–10 minutes. Some set a 4-hour maximum dose limit of 20–30 mg in an average adult. A 4-hour limit is useful in that it triggers an increase in dose or a decrease in dose lockout interval in the event the patient has inadequate pain control for any reason (e.g., acute tolerance). The only other agent used with any regularity is hydromorphone (Dilaudid). The bolus dose is 0.1–0.3 mg with a lockout of 5–10 minutes.

It is of utmost importance that it be appreciated by family and staff that PCA systems *must* only be operated by the patients themselves. The inherent safety of this system is related to the fact that analgesia occurs before respiratory depression and drowsiness. If the latter occurs it will do so slowly permitting intervention, and will preclude additional self-dosing. Well-meaning family members, friends, and health care providers activating the devices have produced overdoses and fatalities.

Patients are ordinarily switched from IV PCA to equivalent oral dosing regimens at days 2–4, or when oral medications are tolerated.

Clinical Applications

IV PCA is typically employed in the inpatient setting, for postsurgical patients where pain management is a significant issue. Common examples include orthopedic surgery, abdominal and pelvic surgery, and some types of thoracic surgery. It is particularly valuable in the opioid-habituated patient. The pain from major truncal surgical procedures such as pelvic exenterations, radical urologic surgery, and thoracic surgery is typically managed post-operatively by epidural opioid analgesia with or without a patient-controlled option.

Some other specific subsets of patients with acute pain may be particularly amenable to management with IV PCA:

- Sickle cell crisis.[1–4]
- Acute pain in children as young as 4 years old, though particularly in older children.[5–9]
- Burn patients.[10–12]
- Emergency department patients suffering from trauma.[13]

Advantages and Disadvantages of Patient-Controlled Analgesia (PCA)

Studies of PCA have documented wide variations in individual patient analgesic requirements. Furthermore, with PCA, patients could titrate their own analgesic needs better than the health care staff, and patients did not abuse the setup. Indeed, frequently patients' dosage requirements by PCA were less than with standard parenteral orders.[14]

The advantages of PCA include (1) automatic adjustments to the needs of the individual patient, (2) less nursing staff time needed, (3) cost-effectiveness, (4) decreased medication error (pump can be set up once with a premixed bag from pharmacy vs. medications drawn up and given episodically by different staff members), (5) more immediate response to patient needs/requests, (6) potential for decreased drug requirement (less side effects such as sedation and emesis) and perhaps earlier weaning off drugs and earlier mobilization, and (7) more even level drug administration with less peak and trough drug levels.[14–18] The patient can also "premedicate" prior to a painful procedure (such as a dressing change in a burn patient) (Table 48-1).

There are disadvantages to be considered. The patient needs to have some hand motor skills and cognition to be able to operate the bedside device when in pain. Equipment problems and machine malfunction can occur but are rare. Further-more, use of the device does not eliminate side effects from the drugs. There is also an initial capital equipment expense.

The primary concern with opioid administration by any technique is respiratory depression. PCA is considered safer than bolus doses of opioids given by a nurse at set intervals. As the patient's serum opioid level starts to rise, he or she falls asleep and no longer pushes the button to self-administer the drug.[19] Somnolence generally occurs before respiratory depression. However, there is an incidence of significant respiratory depression of 1.7%, so close patient monitoring is still needed. Other side effects from the opioids can occur including nausea, emesis, sedation, and pruritus.

Another concern with PCA is that when the patient is sleeping or is pain free, no drug is given. This lets the drug's therapeutic level to drop to a level where constant pain control is forfeited. A solution to this problem is to infuse a constant "background" level of opioid. However, baseline infusions of any opioid have the potential to defeat the *patient control* safety feature inherent in the technique. A baseline infusion may be of particular use in the patient who is opioid-habituated to replace the patient's baseline requirement.

Use of Patient-Controlled Analgesia in Pediatric Patients

PCA has been used in patients as young as 4 years old.[14,15] However, not all children aged 4–6 years are able to master the use of the PCA equipment. The use of PCA in pediatric patients does provide another benefit. It allows children to exercise some control over their

Table 48-1. Advantages and Disadvantages of Patient-Controlled Analgesia (PCA)

Advantages of PCA

Allows individual dosing to accommodate wide patient variability

"Immediate" drug administration/response to patient needs (no wait for nurse to respond, go to obtain and draw up medication, and so forth)

Decreased nursing staff time

Cost-effective

Increased patient safety (somnolence occurs before respiratory depression, patient falls asleep, and does not get more drug)

Often, ↓ drug requirement (↓ side effects, ↓ sedation → earlier mobilization)

More "even" therapeutic drug levels (↓ variation in peak/trough drug levels)

↓ Chance of medication error (preset/premixed drug in a pump vs. drug drawn up by different personnel every few hours and then given)

Can use for all types of acute pain (postop, cancer) in all types of setting (OR, recovery room, ICU, ward, ED, and so forth)

↑ Patient/family satisfaction

Patient can have some control over their situation

Patient can ↑ dose prior to painful event (e.g., dressing change)

Disadvantages of PCA

Need motor/cognitive skills to use (cannot use in children ≤4 years of age, special needs patients, patients unable to use hands [e.g., stroke patients and s/p hand surgery] [use nurse or family-controlled PCA])

May ↓ side effects/toxicity but still can occur

Initial capital expenditure for equipment

↓ Therapeutic drug level when patient is asleep or pain free (use background or baseline dose)

Equipment problems/machine malfunction can occur although it is rare

---

situation and make choices.[14,19] In general, PCA has the same advantages and disadvantages as with adult patients with the exception of the more frequent use of a background infusion in pediatric patients.[15,20] Unlike adults, in pediatric patients, the use of a baseline or basal opioid infusion may improve the sleep pattern when compared with no baseline infusion.

Nurse- or Family-Controlled Analgesia

PCA does require some motor and cognitive abilities. So what options are there for patients <4 years of age, the "special needs" patient, or the patient with limited motor function of the hand (as with a patient status posthand surgery)? Nurse- or family (parent)-controlled analgesia can be used.[21–23] With nurse-controlled analgesia (NCA), the bedside nurse activates the PCA device. With family (parent)-controlled analgesia (FCA), the parent can work the PCA pump for the child. One study of adolescents on postoperative day 1 showed a strong agreement between parents and adolescents.[24] However, in other studies, parents and health care workers underestimated the child's pain.[25–27] When FCA is used, one family member is designated the "primary pain manager" who is the only person who can activate the pump. A "secondary pain manager" may also be designated and he (or she) is allowed to activate the PCA pump only when the "primary pain manager" is not present. Such "pain managers" have been instructed in the use of PCA and a pain manager(s) is required to be present 24 hours a day. Generally, with FCA a baseline infusion is not used (or is used at a lower rate) and the lockout intervals are longer than for PCA.

Summary—Intravenous Opioid Patient-Controlled Analgesia

PCA is a valuable technique of pain management in adult and pediatric patients. It has an established record of efficacy and safety. PCA was designed to treat postoperative pain but it's use has been expanded to treat many different types of patients from cancer patients to those with sickle cell disease to burn patients. PCA has several built-in safety features including lockout periods and maximum (or ceiling) levels of drugs. PCA has many advantages, and side effects/problems tend to be rare but can occur. NCA or FCA is an option in patients unable to operate the PCA devices (e.g., very young, cognitively impaired [Alzheimer's patients], special needs patients, or those without hand motor function).

ELECTROANALGESIA

Definitions and Types of Electroanalgesia

Transcutaneous electrical nerve stimulation (TENS) is a nonpharmacologic electroanalgesic technique or the use of electrical stimulation for the treatment of pain.[28] Electroanalgesia has also been described as an *interventional* method (as compared to a *pharmacologic* method) of pain therapy, a nonpharmacologic technique, and as a "physical intervention" for pain management.[29] Such techniques are a way to augment the *usual* or *conventional* analgesic modalities.[30] The side effects/toxicity of pharmacologic agents has given impetus to the development of such electroanalgesia.

Electrical stimulation or neurostimulation for the treatment of pain includes (1) implanted central devices: spinal cord stimulation (SCS), deep brain stimulation, and motor cortex stimulation, (2) implanted peripheral devices: facial stimulation and peripheral nerve stimulation, and (3) TENS.[31–34] The implanted electroanalgesic devices tend to be used more for severe intractable pain, while TENS has been used for both acute and chronic pain (Table 48-2).[34]

Some experts have described the various electroanalgesic techniques as a spectrum from TENS to percutaneous neuromodulation therapy (PNT) to SCS.[35] TENS is considered noninvasive, inexpensive, and without complications.[32] PNT is intermediate because it is minimally invasive, has few complications, and an intermediate cost, while SCS is highly invasive, costly, and can have serious complications.

Invasive Electroanalgesia

There are invasive neurosurgical procedures involving spinal cord or intracerebral locations used to provide analgesia.[31–34] SCS or dorsal column stimulation (DCS) involves the implantation of electrodes percutaneously into the dorsal epidural space. Epidural stimulation involves an open surgical procedure with electrodes sewn onto the dura. Deep brain stimulation involves intracerebral techniques using electrical stimulation of the periventricular and periaqueductal grey matter (*periaqueductal grey stimulation*) or *thalamic stimulation* with electrodes implanted in various thalamic sensory nuclei.[32–34]

Peripheral Electrical Nerve Stimulation

TENS should be distinguished from similar types of peripheral electrical nerve stimulation including percutaneous electrical nerve stimulations (PENS) or

Table 48-2. Types of Pain in Adults Treated with TENS

Musculoskeletal pain
    Head/neck pain, low back pain, cervical spine pain, fractured ribs, joint (knee pain, arthritis)
    Traumatic injuries: fractures, sprains
    Other: bone healing
Postoperative pain
Cancer pain
Neuropathic pain
    Phantom limb, diabetic neuropathy, posttherapeutic neuralgia
Neurologic disorders:
    Multiple sclerosis, peripheral nerve injuries, root/plexus injuries, spinal cord injury, stroke
Obstetrics/gynecologic
    Pregnancy, labor and delivery, pelvic pain/dysmenorrhea
Gastrointestinal diseases
    Pancreatitis, postop ileus
Vascular diseases
    Raynaud's phenomenon, thrombophlebitis
Cardiac pain (angina)
Other
    Dental pain, bladder pain, pruritus

---

precutaneous neuromodulation therapy (PNT).[28] PENS involves insertion of ultrafine acupuncture needle probes into soft tissues or muscles to stimulate peripheral nerve fibers in the dermatonal distribution of the patient's pain symptoms. PENS combines the principles of TENS by placing electrodes in the patient's symptomatic dermatones and Chinese acupuncture by placing 32–37-gauge acupuncture needles at the Chinese accupoints. It has been theorized that PENS can "overcome" the resistance of the skin, thereby delivering the electrical stimulus nearer the peripheral nerve endings, which may be an advantage. PENS has also been termed PNT.

Transcutaneous Electrical Nerve Stimulation (TENS)

A TENS unit delivers small amounts of electrical energy through the skin via 2–4 cutaneous electrodes attached via a set of wires to a small plastic box (about 2 in. × 1 in. × 3 in.).[35] TENS devices deliver energy from the external stimulator via wires to electrodes placed on the skin using conductive electrode gel pads. Similar to a pacemaker, TENS units can be programmed to vary the electrical energy delivered by modifying the rate, amplitude, pulse width, wave form, and so forth.

Multiple *modes* of TENS for pain management have been developed.[35,36] Conventional (*high rate* or *high frequency*) uses a high frequency (10–100 Hz) and a low to medium intensity. *Strong low rate* (*acupuncture like*) has a frequency <10 Hz with a high intensity. *Brief-intense* uses a high intensity with a 60–150 Hz. *Pulse-train* or *burst* employs a high frequency of 60–100 Hz modulated by low carrier (0.5–4 Hz) and a low to high intensity. *Modulated* uses a low to high intensity while modulating the frequency, pulse, duration, and amplitude.[36] *Hyperstimulation* uses a frequency of 1–100 Hz and a high intensity (based on current density).[36] High rate conventional TENS is the most widely used type of TENS.[35]

In addition to the variable output from the TENS unit itself, there is also variability in the type of electrodes and more importantly, placement of the electrodes.[37] Parameters that may affect TENS stimulation include (1) site of electrode placement, (2) application technique, (3) the mode used (e.g., frequency and intensity), and (4) treatment duration.[38,39] Patient variables, such as subcutaneous fat or obesity and skin resistance, which is affected by weight, size, age, skin thickness, and so forth, also exist.[35] With the tremendous heterogeneity of devices, patients, acute versus chronic pain, and the underlying etiology or disease causing the pain, it is understandable that large numbers of blinded randomized-controlled trials (RCT) are nonexistent and that

research based on defined clinical end points or outcomes is difficult at best. The need for high quality RCT involving TENS has been cited by many.[40–42] Furthermore, there has been very little research or clinical practice data regarding TENS in pediatric patients.[35]

The Clinical Use of TENS

Given this background, what can be said about TENS and how can it be related to clinical practice? In adults, TENS has been used to treat acute and chronic pain including postoperative pain, cancer pain, musculoskeletal pain, obstetric/gynecologic pain, neuropathic pain, and even cardiac (anginal) pain (Table 48-2).[28,34,35,41,43]

What are the success rates with TENS therapy? The likelihood of benefit (e.g., pain reduction) is extremely variable. Estimates of the percent of patients improving (e.g. decreased pain) with short-term TENS therapy is 50–80% and with long-term therapy 6–44%.[44] Others report the clinical effectiveness of TENS for chronic pain in the 12–60% range. For chronic pain secondary to musculoskeletal disorders, only a "small percentage" of patients' experience long-lasting benefits.[45] Another study, however, found a 55% decrease in pain medications and a 69% decrease in the use of physical/occupational therapy for chronic pain patients with TENS use.[46] Others have reported improved quality of life (return to work, increased social activities, decrease in other therapies) for chronic pain patients with long-term TENS use.[47] Most studies report a 15–30% decrease in the need for narcotic pain medications in postoperative patients with the use of TENS.

With chronic pain, the response to TENS therapy is gradual with a slow onset of analgesic effect.[28] Again, the marked differences in results have been related to TENS parameters (electrode site, electrode placement, mode, frequency, intensity, and duration of electrical stimulation) plus patient variables including psychologic factors. There is also difficulty in eliminating the placebo effect of therapy, or in devising a "blinded" study with sham stimulation devices; additional factors that confound research and study results.[30,40]

Systematic Reviews of TENS

With the use of TENS for chronic pain, the Cochrane collaboration found "inconclusive" results and concluded that "large multicenter RCTs of TENS in chronic pain are urgently needed."[40] In another report, the Cochrane collaboration found "no evidence to support the use of the TENS device in the treatment of chronic low back pain" and noted that "clinicians and researchers should consistently report the characteristics of the TENS device and the application techniques used."[38] The meta-analysis lacked data on how TENS effectiveness is affected by four important factors: type of application, site of application, treatment duration of TENS, optimal frequencies and intensities.[38]

The Philadelphia panel used the methods of the Cochrane Collaboration to evaluate RCTs and observational studies on the use of TENS in adults. Their conclusions were that TENS is of benefit for the knee pain of osteoarthritis but not for chronic neck pain and there were insufficient studies to evaluate chronic back pain.[48–50]

A systematic literature review using a modified Chalmers rating system by Reeve et al. considered studies dealing with the efficacy of TENS for low back pain. They concluded there was "moderate but contradictory evidence that TENS would benefit workers with chronic low back pain."[51,52] Gadsby et al. using the Cochrane rating system identified studies using TENS and ALTENS (acupuncture-like TENS). Their findings were: "There is evidence from the limited data available that TENS/ALTENS reduces pain and improves range of motion in chronic back pain patients, at least in the short term. A large trial of ALTENS and TENS is needed to confirm these findings."[53]

Clinical Uses—Summary

TENS is more effective in patients who have a peripheral nociceptive source for their pain, such as patients with peripheral nerve injuries, stump pain, and musculoskeletal pain. TENS is not as efficacious in patients who lack a peripheral nociceptive source for their pain, for example, central pain states, psychosocial pain, and those with drug dependence.[43] According to a review of long-term studies, TENS was most effective with well localized pain, pain due to deafferentation, if the treatment can be applied in close proximity to the nervous structure supplying the painful area, and if there were adequate lemniscal fibers remaining in order to transmit the stimulation from the device.[33]

Advantages and Contraindications/Side Effects of TENS

The major advantages of TENS are noninvasive, inexpensive, very safe, and with few side effects or complications (Table 48-3).[34] TENS is contraindicated in patients with a pacemaker or AICD because of concerns it may interfere with the device.[34] In pregnant women, TENS should not be applied to the abdominal muscles because it may precipitate labor although it may be placed on other parts of the body.[35] TENS should not be placed over the region of

---

Table 48-3. Advantages and Contraindications/Side Effects of TENS

Advantages of TENS
Noninvasive
Inexpensive
Few, if any, side effects or complications
Simple, can be used at home
No age restrictions (can be used in geriatric or pediatric patients)
Does not require a formal therapist or physical therapy treatment session (may be cost-effective)
No systemic side effects
Does not interfere with other therapy
Patient controlled (can be individualized)
Can be used with acute or chronic pain
May relieve reflex muscle spasm (which allows for movement, physical therapy)

Contraindications/Side Effects of TENS
Contraindicated in patients with pacemakers, AICD
Should not be applied to abdominal muscles in pregnant women (can apply to other parts of body)
Should not be applied over carotid sinus
Local irritation: dermatitis, itching, redness, skin necrosis
Variable efficacy

AICD: automatic implantable cardioverter defibrillator.

the carotid sinus because of concern that carotid stimulation could precipitate a vasovagal reflex and cause asystole.[35]

Local irritation (dermatitis, redness, itching) is not uncommon but usually just necessitates a change in the type of electrode or its placement.[37] Changing the electrode sites on a regular basis helps prevent skin breakdown. Additional electrode gel may decrease skin irritation and decrease skin impedance.

Pediatric Considerations with TENS

Experience with TENS use in children has been limited, although case reports indicate its successful use in pediatric patients.[35,54] Low-rate acupuncture-like TENS can cause visible muscle twitching and can be uncomfortable so young children will not use the TENS device.[35] Therefore, it is probably best not to use the acupuncture-like mode in young children. The conventional (high rate or high frequency) mode is preferred.[35]

As with adults, improper electrode placement may be ineffective or even cause more pain. Proper electrode placement may be even more critical in children because if a bad initial experience occurs, both the child and the parent will probably not allow a second trial. Some clinicians have developed pediatric protocols for TENS, which allow the children along with their parents to make the "detailed" adjustments after letting the child become familiar and comfortable with the device.[35]

Mechanism of Action of TENS

There are several theories that have been proposed to explain the mechanism of actions of TENS: peripheral, spinal, supraspinal, and endogenous opioid theories.[55] The spinal theory is based on Melzack and Wall's gate control theory and involves a frequency-dependent blockade. Uses of the TENS unit causes electrical nerve stimulation and excitation of the large mechanofibers in the periphery. These mechanofibers then stimulate the enkephalin-containing interneurons in the dorsal horn of the spinal cord, which produces analgesia. The supraspinal theories involve the release of endogenous opioids (e.g., endorphins, enkephalins, and dynorphins) within the central nervous system (CNS), which suppresses the transmission and perception of noxious stimuli from the periphery.

The nociceptive impulses are transmitted by the unmyelinated C-fibers while the large myelinated fibers inhibit or moderate the nociceptive impulses carried by the unmyelinated C-fibers. The impulses created by the TENS unit are transmitted by the large myelinated fibers which inhibit the nociceptive impulses carried by the unmyelinated C-fibers. By the gate theory of Melzack and Wall, when the various impulses (from the nociceptors via the unmyelinated C-fibers or from the large myelinated inhibitory fibers) arrive in the dorsal horn of the spinal cord, modification or modulation occurs. Currently, evidence suggests that such modulation occurs not only in the dorsal horn of the spinal cord but also at the dorsal root ganglion level and more centrally in the midbrain.

TENS has been shown to cause an increase in the local cutaneous blood flow, suggesting a direct peripheral effect.[56] Research has documented an increase in endorphins from TENS or electroacupuncture use.[57–60] One study used naloxone to abolish the effect of TENS which implicates a neurochemical role.[61] Another study documented an increase in levels of epinephrine, serotonin, and dopamine.[62]

Electroanalgesia may increase the plasma opioids[63] or the number of opioid receptors.[64] In a murine study, high frequency TENS acted via delta opioid receptors while low frequency TENS worked via mu opioid receptors.[65] Another study found that TENS had an effect at both the dorsal horn and at suprasegmental levels.[66] A study in humans found that TENS use resulted in an increase in the mechanical and tactile pain thresholds and increased the latency of the peripheral action potential.[67] Research has also shown a decrease in the action potential of the A-delta fiber nerves, which carry the transmission of pain from the nociceptors.

Indeed, it is possible that the analgesic effect of TENS may involve more than one mechanism. There may be different mechanisms based on the TENS frequency. High-rate conventional TENS is intended to stimulate the large densely myelinated inhibitory nerve fibers while low-rate acupuncture-like TENS is designed to increase the release of endorphins.

SUMMARY—TRANSCUTANEOUS ELECTRICAL NERVE STIMULATION (TENS)

TENS is an electroanalgesic technique using electrical stimulation via skin electrodes to treat pain. TENS is non-invasive, inexpensive, and safe. It is contraindicated in patients with pacemakers or automatic implantable cardioverter defibrillators (AICDs). Unfortunately, there has been a relative lack of large randomized clinical trials regarding TENS therapy. TENS may be effective in decreasing pain and improving the quality of life in selected patients, especially those patients with a peripheral nociceptive source for their pain who are not opioid dependent. TENS has been used successfully in both adult and pediatric patients. The actual mechanism for the action of TENS is unknown. It may involve an increase in endorphins and/or an increase in opioids and be mediated by various neurotransmitters with changes in the periphery modified by input from the dorsal root ganglion, dorsal horn of the spinal cord, and the CNS.

REFERENCES

1. Stinson J, Naser B. Pain management in children with sickle cell disease. *Paediatr Drugs.* 2003;5(4):229–241.
2. Johnson L. Sickle cell disease patients and patient-controlled analgesia. *Br J Nurs.* 2003;12(3):144–153.
3. Ballas SK. Management of sickle pain. *Curr Opin Hematol.* 1997;4(2):104 111.
4. Ackerman WE III, Juneja M. Patient-controlled analgesia for management of pain associated with acute sickle cell crisis. *South Med J.* 1993;86(2):254.
5. Pounder DR, Steward DJ. Postoperative analgesia: opioid infusions in infants and children. *Can J Anaesth.* 1992;39(9): 969–974.
6. Birmingham PK, Wheeler M, Suresh S, et al. Patient-controlled epidural analgesia in children: can they do it? *Anesth Analg.* 2003;96(3):686–691, table of contents.
7. Bhatt-Mehta V, Rosen DA. Management of acute pain in children. *Clin Pharm.* 1991;10(9):667–685.
8. Litman RS. Recent trends in the management of acute pain in children. *J Am Osteopath Assoc.* 1996;96(5):290–296.
9. Marchetti G, Calbi G, Villani A. PCA in the control of acute and chronic pain in children. *Pediatr Med Chir.* 2000;22(1): 9–13.
10. Gallagher G, Rae CP, Kinsella J. Treatment of pain in severe burns. *Am J Clin Dermatol.* 2000;1(6):329–335.
11. Kinsella J, Glavin R, Reid WH. Patient-controlled analgesia for burn patients: a preliminary report. *Burns Incl Therm Inj.* 1988;14(6):500–503.
12. Rovers J, Knighton J, Neligan P, et al. Patient-controlled analgesia in burn patients: a critical review of the literature and case report. *Hosp Pharm.* 1994;29(2):106, 8–11.
13. Flemming A, Adams HA. Analgesia, sedation and anaesthesia in emergency service. *Anaesthesiol Reanim.* 2004;29(2): 40–48.
14. Gaukroger PB. Patient controlled analgesia in children. In: Schecter WL, Berde CB, Yaster M, eds. *Pain Control in Infants, Children, and Adolescents.* Baltimore, MD: Williams & Wilkins; 1993:203–212.
15. Wu CL. Acute postoperative pain. In: Miller RD, ed. *Miller's Anesthesia.* Philadelphia, PA: Elsevier Churchill Livingstone; 2005:2229–2762.
16. Lloyd-Thomas AR. Modern concepts of paediatric analgesia. *Pharmacol Ther.* 1999;83:1–20.
17. Specialized pharmacologic approaches to pain: continuous intravenous opioids. In: DiGregorio GJ, Barbieri EJ, Sterling GH, et al. *Handbook of Pain Management.* West Chester, PA: Medical Surveillance; 1991:74–75.
18. Benzion HT. Surgery. In: Raj PP, ed. *Pain Medicine A Comprehensive Review.* St. Louis, MO: Mosby; 1996:43–48.
19. Tobias JD. Postoperative pain management. *Pediatr Ann.* 1997;26:490–499.
20. Feldman D, Reich N, Foster JMT. Pediatric anesthesia and postoperative analgesia. *Pediatr Clin North Am.* 1998;45: 1525–1537.
21. Lehr VT, BeVier P. Patient controlled analgesia for the pediatric patient. *Orthop Nurs.* 2003;22:298–306.
22. Kanagasundaram SA, Cooper MG, Lane LJ. Nurse-controlled analgesia using a patient-controlled analgesia device: an alternative strategy in the management of severe cancer pain in children. *J Paediatr Child Health.* 1997;33: 352–355.
23. Kotzer AM, Coy J, LeClaire AD. The effectiveness of a standardized educational program for children using patient-controlled analgesia. *J Soc Pediatr Nurs.* 1999;3(3): 117–126.
24. Gil KM, Ginsberg B, Muir M, et al. Patient controlled analgesia: the relation of psychological factors to pain and analgesic use in adolescents with postoperative pain. *Clin J Pain.* 1992;8:215–221.
25. Singer AJ, Richman PB, Kowalska A, et al. Comparison of patient and practitioner assessments from commonly performed emergency department procedures. *Ann Emerg Med.* 1999;33:652–658.
26. Romsing J. Assessment of nurses judgment for analgesic requirements of postoperative children. *J Clin Pharm Ther.* 1996;21:159.
27. St-Laurent-Gagnon T, Bernard-Bonnin AC, Villeneuve E. Pain evaluation in preschool children and their parents. *Acta Paediatr.* 1999;88:422–427.
28. White PF, Shitong L, Chiu JW. Electroanalgesia: its role in acute and chronic pain management. *Anesth Analg.* 2001; 92:505–513.
29. Chen H, Lamer TJ, Rho RH, et al. Contemporary management of neuropathic pain for the primary care physician. *Mayo Clin Proc.* 2004;79:1533–1545.
30. White PF. The role of non-opioid analgesic techniques in the management of pain after ambulatory surgery. *Anesth Analg.* 2002;94:577–585.
31. Muir A, Molloy AR. Neuraxial implants for pain control. *Int Anesthesiol Clin.* 1997;35:171–196.
32. Neurosurgical approaches to pain. In: DiGregorio GJ, Barbieri EJ, Sterling GH, et al. *Handbook of Pain Management.* West Chester, PA: Medical Surveillance; 1991:76–79.
33. Manning DC, Loar CM, Raj PP, et al. Neuropathic pain. In: Raj PP, ed. *Pain Medicine A Comprehensive Review.* St. Louis, MO: Mosby; 2003:77–93.
34. Rushton DN. Electrical stimulation in the treatment of pain. *Disabil Rehabil.* 2002;24:407–415.
35. Eland J. The use of TENS with children. In: Schecter NL, Berde CB, Yaster M, eds. *Pain in Infants, Children, and Adolescents.* Baltimore, MD: Williams & Wilkins; 1993331–340.
36. Rakel B, Barr JO. Physical modalities in chronic pain management. *Nurs Clin North Am.* 2003;38:477–494.
37. Titler MG, Rakel BA. Nonpharmacologic treatment of pain. *Crit Care Nurs Clin North Am.* 2001;12:221–232.

38. Milne S, Welch V, Brosseau L, et al. Transcutaneous electrical nerve stimulation (TENS) for chronic low back pain. *Cochrane Database Syst Rev.* 2005;1.

39. Chesterton LS, Foster NE, Wright CC, et al. Effect of TENS frequency, intensity, and stimulation site parameter manipulation on pressure pain thresholds in healthy human subjects. *Pain.* 2003;106:73–80.

40. Carroll D, Moore RA, McQuay HJ, et al. Transcutaneous electrical nerve stimulation (TENS) for chronic pain. *Cochrane Database Syst Rev.* 2005;1.

41. Longhurst JC. Alternative approaches to the medical management of cardiovascular disease: acupuncture, electric nerve, and spinal cord stimulation. *Heart Dis.* 2001;3:215.

42. Casimiro L, Brosseau L, Milne S, et al. Acupuncture and electropuncture for the treatment of RA. *Cochrane Database Syst Rev.* 2005;1.

43. Rowlingson JC. Chronic pain. In: Miller RD, ed. *Miller's Anesthesia*. Philadelphia, PA: Elsevier Churchill Livingstone; 2005:2763–2786.

44. Lampl C, Kreczi T, Klingler D. Transcutaneous electrical nerve stimulation in the treatment of chronic pain: predictive factors and evaluation of the method. *Clin J Pain.* 1998;14:134–142.

45. Robinson AJ. Transcutaneous electrical nerve stimulation (TENS) for the control of pain in musculoskeletal disorders. *J Orthop Sports Phys Ther.* 1996;24:108–116.

46. Chabal C, Fishbain DA, Weaver M, et al. Long-term transcutaneous electrical nerve stimulation (TENS) use: impact on medication, utilization, and physical therapy costs. *Clin J Pain.* 1998;14:66–73.

47. Fishbain DA, Chabal C, Abbott A, et al. Transcutaneous electrical nerve stimulation (TENS) treatment outcome in long-term users. *Clin J Pain.* 1996;12:201–214.

48. Philadelphia P. Philadelphia Panel evidence-based clinical practice guidelines on selected rehabilitation interventions for knee pain. *Phys Ther.* 2001;81:1675–1700.

49. Philadelphia P. Philadelphia Panel evidence-based clinical practice guidelines on selected rehabilitation interventions for neck pain. *Phys Ther.* 2002;81(10):1701–1717.

50. Philadelphia P. Philadelphia Panel evidence-based clinical practice guidelines on selected rehabilitation interventions for low back pain. *Phys Ther.* 2002;81(10):641–674.

51. Reeve J, Corabian P. *Transcutaneous Electric Nerve Stimulation (TENS) and Pain Management*. Report prepared for the Canadian Coordinating Office for Health Technology Assessment. 1995.

52. Reeve J, Menon D, Corabian P. Transcutaneous electrical nerve stimulation (TENS): a technology assessment. *Int J Technol Assess Health Care.* 1996;12:299–324.

53. Gadsby JG, Flowerdew MW. The effectiveness of transcutaneous electrical nerve stimulation (TENS) and acupuncture- like transcutaneous electrical nerve stimulations (ALTENS) in the treatment of patients with chronic low back pan. In: Bombardier C, Nachemson A, Deyo R, et al, eds. *CMSG Back Module of the Cochrane Database of Systematic Reviews*. Oxford: The Cochrane; 1996.

54. Merkel SI, Gutstein HB, Malviya S. Use of transcutaneous electrical nerve stimulation in a young child with pain from open perineal lesions. *J Pain Symptom Manage.* 1999;18:376–381.

55. Sluka KA, Walsh D. Transcutaneous electrical nerve stimulation: basic science mechanisms and clinical effectiveness. *J Pain.* 2003;4:109–121.

56. Cramp AF, Gilsenan C, Lowe AS, et al. The effect of high and low frequency transcutaneous electrical nerve stimulation upon cutaneous blood flow and skin temperature in healthy subjects. *Clin Physiol.* 2000;20:150–157.

57. Sjolund B, Terenius L, Eriksson M. Increased cerebrospinal fluid levels of endorphins after electroacupuncture. *Acta Physiol Scand.* 1977;100:382–384.

58. Abbate D, Santanaria A, Brambilla, et al. β-endorphin and electroacupuncture. *Lancet.* 1980;2:1309.

59. Hans JS, Chen XH, Sun SL, et al. Effect of low and high frequency TENS on Met-enkephalin-Arg-Phe and dynorphin. A immunoreactivity in human lumbar CSF. *Pain.* 1991;47:295–298.

60. Salar G, Job I, Mingrino S. Effect of transcutaneous electrotherapy on CSF B-endorphin content in patients without pain problems. *Pain.* 1981;10:169–172.

61. Sjolund BH, Eriksson MBE. The influence of naloxone on analgesia produced by peripheral conditioning stimulation. *Brain Res.* 1979;173:295–301.

62. Akil H, Liebeskind JC. Monaminergic mechanisms of stimulation produced analgesia. *Brain Res.* 1975;94:279–296.

63. Facchinetti F, Sandrini G, Petraglia F, et al. Concomitant increase in nociceptive flexion reflex threshold and plasma opioids following transcutaneous nerve stimulation. *Pain.* 1984;19:295–303.

64. Gao M, He LF. Increase of mu opioid receptor density in rat central nervous system following formalin nociception and its enhancement by electroacupuncture. *Acta Physiologica Sinica.* 1996;48:125–131.

65. Sluka KA, Deacon M, Stibal A, et al. Spinal blockade of opioid receptors prevents the analgesia produced by TENS. *J Pharmacol Exp Ther.* 1999;289:840–846.

66. Urasaki E, Wada S, Yasukouchi H, et al. Effects of TENS on central nervous system amplification of somatosensory input. *J Neurol.* 1998;245:143–148.

67. Walsh DM, Lowe AS, McCormack K, et al. TENS: Effect on peripheral nerve conduction, mechanical pain threshold, and tactile threshold in humans. *Arch Phys Med Rehabil.* 1998;79:1051–1058.

49

Hypnosis as Treatment for Pain

Alex L. Rogovik
Ran D. Goldman

HIGH YIELD FACTS

- Hypnosis is an effective method of pain and anxiety control.
- Hypnosis is accepted by the American Medical Association (AMA) as a medical therapy.
- Hypnotic techniques include induction of analgesia, suggestions, cognitive reframing, metaphors, imagery, and posthypnotic suggestions.
- Hypnosis is reimbursable.
- Hypnotherapy is used for acute pain and chronic pain.
- Hypnosis may be more effective in children than in adults.

THE EVOLUTION OF A NEW ANALGESIC METHOD

Franz Anton Mesmer (1734–1815) was the "father" of hypnosis, which gained popular recognition in the late eighteenth century in Paris. He believed that humans, like iron and minerals, possess magnetic forces and that uneven distribution of these forces in the body may result in illness. Mesmer wanted to redistribute magnetic forces to prevent transferring from one person to another. He was well-known as a hypnotic showman, but his performances ended in 1784, when a commission judged that animal magnetism does not exist.[1]

James Esdaile (1850) was one of the first physicians who documented the use of hypnosis for pain. He practiced hypnosis in India as the only form of anesthesia for amputations and tumor resections. During World War II, some hypnosis clinicians provided pain relief to injured soldiers when field hospitals ran short of drugs. In 1958, hypnosis was accepted by the American Medical Association (AMA) as a medical treatment, when administered by an appropriately trained practitioner.[2] According to the current procedural terminology (CPT) 2005 professional edition under the psychiatry codes, hypnotherapy is listed as CPT code 90880.

The definition of hypnosis has been a matter of debate. While some patients describe their hypnotic experience as an altered state of consciousness, others see it as focused attention in a normal state. According to Barber,[3] hypnosis is an "altered condition or state of consciousness characterized by a markedly increased receptivity to suggestion, the capacity for modification of perception and memory, and the potential for systematic control of a variety of usually involuntary physiological functions." The altered state of consciousness, or dissociation, is the basis for hypnotic analgesia. Recent positron emission tomography cerebral blood flow scans showed that hypnosis modulates activity in the anterior midcingulate cortex and enhances the interaction between the midcingulate cortex and a large cortical and subcortical neural network of bilateral insula, pregenual anterior cingulate cortex, presupplementary motor area, right prefrontal cortex and striatum, and thalamus and brainstem.[5,6]

Hypnotic susceptibility predicts the degree of analgesia.[7–9] As many as 10–15% of the population is highly responsive to hypnosis, 70–80% are moderately responsive, and 10–15% are minimally responsive or unresponsive. Training does not increase suggestibility score nor does it enhance the effects of hypnosis for analgesia.[10] One meta-analysis found correlation ($r = 0.44$) between hypnotic suggestibility and therapeutic outcome, but the small number of studies providing correlation coefficients (6/57) was not sufficient to confirm this relationship.[11]

The ability to get hypnotized depends on genetic and environmental variables. Women have high hypnotizability scores,[12] similar hypnotizability was found among twins[13] and language used was also a determining factor.[14] Hypnotic ability does not seem to reduce the effects of other analgesic medications, acupuncture, relaxation, distraction, or the placebo effect.[15]

Hypnotic techniques for pain relief include induction of analgesia, suggestions, cognitive reframing, metaphors, imagery, posthypnotic suggestions, and other methods.[4,7,16]

There are multiple hypnotic techniques for analgesia[4,7,16] and the four main steps include (1) assessment of hypnotizability, (2) induction of analgesia and development of individual strategies for the treatment of pain, (3) direct suggestions, cognitive reframing, metaphors, and imagery, and (4) psychodynamic reprocessing of emotional factors in chronic pain.[17]

Previous induction techniques such as swinging pendulums, whirling disks, or upward straining eyes are used much less than previously. Today, increased emphasis is put on self-hypnosis, and more permissive (Ericksonian) hypnotists have become more popular than authoritarians. Pain itself can be used as the initial focus, with simultaneous relaxation and calmness suggestions.

CLINICAL STUDIES

In the last two decades hypnosis was found to be effective as an analgesic for both acute and chronic pain conditions. Contraindications to hypnosis include severe psychiatric illness or developmental delay, undiagnosed and untreated illness presenting with pain, and conflict with religious beliefs.[18,19]

Hypnosis for Acute Pain

Burn Wound Debridement and Dressing Change

Hypnosis has been successfully employed as a nonpharmacologic treatment of pain in patients with burns.[20,21] In a patient with severe burn injury who was hypnotized using a three-dimensional computer virtual reality world, a 40% decrease in pain was noted immediately and the next day, but returned to the previous level when the intervention stopped.[22] Anxiety decreased significantly before and during dressing change in 30 hypnotized patients with intramuscular analgesia compared to stress reduction strategy with medications. There was no significant difference between the groups in the level of pain reduction.[23] Similarly, self-reported pain, anxiety, and use of analgesic drugs between treatment sessions significantly decreased during and after rapid induction hypnotic analgesia for dressing changes in 15 burn patients compared to 15 controls.[24] Another study found hypnotized patients and their nurses to report significant pain reduction compared to prewound debridement baseline, using a visual analogue scale. Hypnosis was better than attention, information, or no treatment.[25]

Even for severe burns, hypnosis was beneficial.[26,27] Among 61 severely burned patients with a high level of baseline pain, randomized to either hypnosis or a relaxation control group, patients reported reduced posttreatment pain compared to controls.[26] In 32 patients given opioids and randomized for hypnosis, lorazepam, hypnosis with lorazepam, or placebo groups; no significant differences in pain were found,[27] possibly due to a low baseline pain level measured during dressing changes.

Invasive Medical Procedures

Hypnosis and self-hypnosis have been used extensively in invasive medical procedures and surgery with a moderate-to-large hypnoanalgesic effect in both clinical and experimental settings.[28]

Thirty hypnotized patients undergoing interventional radiologic procedures reported reduced pain and use of patient-controlled analgesia (P <0.01) compared to controls.[29] During percutaneous vascular and renal procedures much less analgesia was used by 241 patients using self-hypnosis and attention when compared to the control patients.[30] When 49 patients with cystic fibrosis were taught self-hypnosis, they reported pain relief for headache and medical procedures 86% of the time.[31] Hypnosis was also found as an effective analgesic and anxiolytic for dermatologic[32] and dental procedures.[33]

Operative Surgery

The analgesic effects of hypnosis were investigated in the preoperative period, during an operation (as an adjunct to analgesics), and in facilitating postoperative pain relief. A meta-analysis of 20 studies on the effectiveness of adjunctive hypnosis with 1624 surgical patients demonstrated that almost 90% of surgical hypnotized patients had a better outcome compared to patients in control groups, and there were no differences in the induction methods used.[34]

Preoperative Hypnosis

Presurgical hypnosis reduced postsurgical pain and distress in a randomized controlled trial of 20 women undergoing excisional breast biopsies.[35] In one study, tape-recorded hypnosis instructions administered before molar teeth surgery did not reduce pain, increased the incidence of vomiting, but significantly reduced anxiety.[36] However, in a larger trial on 337 patients undergoing plastic surgical procedures under hypnosis, postoperative nausea and vomiting were reported by only 1% of patients in the hypnosis group, 13% in the relaxation group, and 27% in the intravenous sedation (midazolam and fentanyl) group. Adjunct hypnosis provided better pain and anxiety relief, allowed for a significant reduction in anesthetics needed, and improved patient satisfaction.[37]

Intraoperative Hypnosis

Successful intraoperative routine use of hypnosis (revivication of pleasant life experiences) in combination with procedural intravenous sedation was reported in more than 1650 procedures in plastic and endocrine surgery.[38] Almost 200 thyroidectomies and 21 cervical explorations for hyperparathyroidism, performed under hypnoanesthesia using Erickson's method, revealed that hypnosis is effective in providing intraoperative and post-operative pain relief and can be used in most patients.[39] In a prospective randomized study of patients undergoing parathyroid surgery, hypnoanesthesia (hypnosis plus local anesthesia and minimal sedation) significantly reduced postoperative pain and was associated with better hemo-dynamic parameters than conventional anesthesia.[40]

When tape-recorded positive intraoperative suggestion was used in another group undergoing total abdominal hysterectomy, postoperative pain or use of morphine were similar to placebo.[41] However, patients undergoing hysterectomy required less rescue analgesics compared with a control group, with no increase in adverse events.[42] Fewer narcotics were also used by hypnotized patients during angioplasty, and the cardiologist was able to keep the balloon inflated 25% longer compared to controls.[43]

Postoperative Hypnosis

Postoperative hypnosis significantly decreased pain intensity and anxiety after orthopedic surgery pro-cedures.[44] Tape-recorded therapeutic suggestions with music significantly decreased pain intensity compared with the control blank tape ($P < 0.002$) in the immediate postoperative period in patients undergoing varicose vein or inguinal hernia repair under general anesthesia.[45]

Obstetrics

Since hypnosis is a method with no known adverse effects, it has been suggested as a safe alternative to analgesia in labor. Women are found to be confident, in control, and actively involved with the provider team[46] and infants are calm and alert.[19] The best time to learn self-hypnosis for childbirth pain relief is the antepartum period[47] and group methods consisting of training sessions in the third trimester have been recommended.[7] As few as four hypnotic sessions were found to be superior to supportive counseling in the preparation of pregnant adolescents for labor and delivery, when medication use and complications were measured.[48]

One trial with self-hypnotized women found no dif-ference in pain relief or analgesic intake during labor in 65 women.[49] This was in contrast to two other studies that documented reduced anxiety[50] and pain, shorter stage 1 labor, reduced drug use, and more spontaneous deliveries.[51] A meta-analysis of three trials of hypnosis

for pain management in labor ($n = 189$) found hypnosis to increase patient satisfaction. This was in contrast to music, audio analgesia, and aromatherapy.[52]

Hypnosis for Chronic Pain

Hypnosis is a valuable and frequently neglected resource of pain relief for patients with chronic and terminal illness.[53] Patients with chronic pain are usually receptive to the idea as part of a pain management program and patients with chronic pain bring to the office a "sur-prisingly sophisticated knowledge" of clinical hypnosis.[54]

Hypnosis is a useful complementary treatment for phantom limb pain[55,56] and was significantly more effective than "minimal treatment" in patients with myofascial pain.[57] Hypnosis treatment significantly decreases ($P < 0.001$) pain frequency, duration, and intensity in patients with tem-poromandibular disorders, and the effect is maintained for at least 6 months.[58] Osteoarthritis subjective pain was significantly lower with eight-session hypnosis and patients required fewer analgesics compared to a relaxation technique.[59] Chronic pain intensity was significantly decreased in the hypnotized patient compared to attention technique as control, and the change was sustained on a 1-month follow-up.[60] Even in patients with sickle cell disease, self-hypnosis was reported to be associated with a significant reduction in the number of "pain days," nights of "bad sleep" and the use of analgesics.[61]

Headache

Hypnotherapy is an effective intervention in the treatment of migraine[62] and chronic tension-type headaches.[63] Headache ratings and medication use decreased in all four treatment groups (hypnosis and other techniques) compared to the waiting for treatment group in 66 patients with migraines.[64] The effectiveness of hypnotherapy in the treatment of chronic tension-type headache was evaluated in several studies. Melis et al.[65] observed significant decreases in headache intensity, headache hours, and headache days in the hypnosis group in contrast with a waiting for treatment control group ($P < 0.05$). When patients with chronic headache used cognitive self-hypnosis and relaxation training, a significant reduction in the headache index scores[66] and psychologic distress[67] were noted. In both studies, the improvement was maintained during the follow-up period.

Zitman et al.[68] compared hypnotic imagery, which was explicitly presented as hypnosis or not presented as hypnosis, to an abbreviated form of autogenic training (a self-relaxation procedure popular in Europe) in the treatment of tension headache and found that all three treatments were equally effective. After a 6-month follow-up period, the group to which hypnosis was presented was superior to autogenic training. When 144 patients with chronic headache were randomly allocated to cognitive self-hypnosis or autogenic training treatment groups for 7 weeks, their pain appraisals and coping strategies significantly improved.[69] In a study of the efficacy of hypnosis and acupuncture in 25 patients with various head and neck pain syndromes both treatments were effective, with hypnosis reducing pain by a mean of 4.8 units, compared to 3.7 for acupuncture ($P = 0.26$).[70] Hypnosis was more beneficial for patients with psychogenic pain.

Irritable Bowel Syndrome

Hypnosis is effective for treatment of irritable bowel syndrome dominated by pain. One survey reported reduced abdominal pain ($P < 0.0001$) and back pain ($P < 0.05$) compared to a control group, and quality of life and well-being also improved.[71] Hypnosis also increased mean pain sensory threshold ($P < 0.05$) in patients with elevated intestinal sensitivity measured using a barostat distension technique leaving normal sensory perception unchanged.[72] Of 27 patients, hypnotherapy decreased or eliminated pain and flatulence in 24, two stopped the treatment prematurely, and one patient remained symptomatic.[73]

Another study found that rectal pain thresholds were unaffected by treatment with hypnosis audiotapes.[74] However, when a self-hypnosis audiotape was compared with individual hypnotherapy in a randomized controlled trial, symptoms improved in 76% of the hypnotherapy patients and 59% of the tape group. Self-hypnosis audiotape can be recommended as a second-line treatment for irritable bowel syndrome, reserving individual hypnosis for failures.[75]

Cancer-Related Pain

Evidence from randomized trials supports the value of hypnosis for cancer-induced pain,[76–79] and oncology professionals are interested in knowing more about hypnosis.[80] In 67 patients undergoing bone marrow transplantation randomly assigned to hypnosis training, cognitive behavioral coping skills training, therapist contact control or no intervention control groups, hypnotherapy did not reduce the use of opioids but was effective in reducing reported oral pain.[81] Hypnosis is also effective for pain and anxiety alleviation in pediatric cancer patients undergoing lumbar punctures[82] and bone marrow aspirations.[83]

Hypnosis and Analgesia in Children

Hypnotic ability in children is limited below the age of 3, appears at 5–6 years, raises to a peak at 7–14 years, and then gradually diminishes. Unlike adults, differences between boys and girls are insignificant.[13,14,84] Hypnosis was used in the treatment of anxiety, phobias, post-traumatic stress, sleepwalking, behavioral disorders, conversion reactions, anorexia nervosa, enuresis, soiling, intractable cough, speech and voice problems, tics, learning disabilities, drug abuse, dermatologic problems, diabetes, juvenile rheumatoid arthritis, and pain control.[13] Children usually respond better than adults to hypnotherapy for control of both acute and chronic pain[85] and could be assessed using Children's Hypnotic Susceptibility Scale or the Stanford Hypnotic Clinical Scale for Children.[86]

Adults are usually cataleptic while under hypnosis, but children often appear restless or fidget during the procedure.[13] They require different approaches than adults for hypnosis,[87] and highly hypnotizable children often need no induction.

Painful Medical Procedures in Children

Hypnosis was successfully used for alleviating pain during bone marrow aspirations and lumbar punctures in pediatric cancer patients. A randomized controlled trial in 30 children aged 5–15 undergoing bone marrow aspirations demonstrated that children receiving hypnosis reported reduced pain compared to their own baseline and compared to a control group.[83] Children with lymphoblastic leukemia undergoing bone marrow aspirations reported similar pain on the graphic 1–100 rating scale and fear on a faces scale with hypnosis or indirected play, although fear and pain decreased in both groups relatively to the baseline.[88] When 3–6-year-old patients with leukemia underwent bone marrow aspirations under hypnosis, external observers reported an immediate decrease in pain, anxiety, and distress in the hypnotic imaging group in comparison with the distraction and control groups, although no effect was found in the patient self-reports.[89] Similarly, hypnosis significantly reduced pain and anxiety during bone marrow aspirations[90] and lumbar punctures in children and adolescents with cancer.[82,90]

Monitoring of children during dental procedures showed that hypnotic suggestions of a favorite and pleasant place can be used successfully before and during the administration of local anesthesia to mitigate pain-related stress.[91] Hypnosis was also used successfully to diminish pain and anxiety for angulated forearm fracture reduction in four emergency pediatric patients who had no access to other analgesia.[92] Similarly, postoperative pain and anxiety were significantly lower in the hypnosis/guided imagery group in a randomized controlled trial of 52 children during surgery.[93]

Chronic Pediatric Pain

Hypnotherapy and self-hypnosis have been demonstrated to be effective in the treatment of chronic pain in children. Among 303 patients presenting to a pediatric pulmonology center with chronic chest pain who received hypnotherapy, improvement was reported in 80%. No symptoms worsened and no new symptoms appeared following the treatment.[94] Combined hypnosis and acupuncture for chronic pediatric pain was highly acceptable, not associated with adverse effects and resulted in significant alleviation of both child- and parent-rated pain and anticipatory anxiety.[95]

Most children can learn self-hypnosis, which is an efficacious treatment for recurrent pediatric headache.[96] Intensity and number of chronic and episodic headaches in hypnosis or self-hypnotized children were lower than in behavior therapy and "talks to the doctor" groups.[97] Self-hypnotherapy for functional abdominal pain in five children was associated with resolution of pain in four of them within 3 weeks.[98]

Although child hypnosis does not currently qualify as "efficacious" according to criteria for empirically supported therapies because of the lack of treatment specification,[99] the results of controlled studies demonstrated that clinical hypnosis and self-hypnosis for children and adults in pain are beneficial.

SUMMARY

Hypnosis has a long and rich history, and has been accepted by the AMA as a medical treatment when administered by an appropriately trained practitioner. Hypnotic susceptibility is the most important factor for analgesic effect and highly hypnotizable patients benefit the most. Numerous studies have shown adjunctive hypnosis and self-hypnosis to be effective in the treatment of acute pain caused by burn wound debridement and dressing change, invasive medical procedures, operative surgery, and labor. Clinical evidence suggests the benefit of hypnosis and self-hypnosis for chronic pain, such as chronic tension headache and migraine, irritable bowel syndrome dominated by pain, and pain caused by cancer therapy.

Controlled studies found hypnosis effective in children, who are more hypnotizable than adults, for painful medical procedures; such as bone marrow aspirations and lumbar punctures, in cancer treatment, headache, and chronic pain conditions.

REFERENCES

1. Sapp M. *Hypnosis, Dissociation, and Absorption: Theories, Assessment, and Treatment.* Springfield, IL: Charles C Thomas; 2000.
2. Simon EP, James LC. Clinical applications of hypnotherapy in a medical setting. *Hawaii Med J.* 1999;58:344–347.
3. Barber J. Hypnosis and suggestion in the treatment of pain: a clinical guide. New York: Norton; 1996.
4. Evans FJ. Hypnosis: an introduction. In: Fredericks LE, ed. The use of hypnosis in surgery and anesthesiology: psychological preparation of the surgical patient. Springfield, IL: Charles C Thomas; 2001:3–30.
5. Faymonville ME, Laureys S, Degueldre C, et al. Neural mechanisms of antinociceptive effects of hypnosis. *Anesthesiology.* 2000;92:1257–1267.
6. Faymonville ME, Roediger L, Del Fiore G, et al. Increased cerebral functional connectivity underlying the antinociceptive effects of hypnosis. *Brain Res Cogn Brain Res.* 2003;17: 255–262.
7. Hilgard ER, Hilgard JR. *Hypnosis in the Relief of Pain.* New York: Brunner Mazel; 1994.
8. Sandrini G, Milanov I, Malaguti S, et al. Effects of hypnosis on diffuse noxious inhibitory controls. *Physiol Behav.* 2000; 69:295–300.
9. Ray WJ, Tucker DM. Evolutionary approaches to understanding the hypnotic experience. *Int J Clin Exp Hypn.* 2003;51:256–281.
10. Milling LS, Kirsch I, Burgess CA. Brief modification of suggestibility and hypnotic analgesia: too good to be true? *Int J Clin Exp Hypn.* 1999;47:91–103.
11. Flammer E, Bongartz W. On the efficacy of hypnosis: a meta-analytic study. *Contemp Hypn.* 2003;179–197.
12. De Pascalis V, Russo P, Marucci FS. Italian norms for the Harvard Group Scale of Hypnotic Susceptibility, Form A. *Int J Clin Exp Hypn.* 2000;48:44–55.
13. Olness K, Kohen D. Hypnosis and hypnotherapy with children. New York: Guilford; 1996.
14. Yapko MD. Trancework: an introduction to the practice of clinical hypnosis. New York: Brunner-Routledge; 2003.
15. Evans FJ. Hypnosis and the management of chronic pain. In: Fredericks LE, ed. The use of hypnosis in surgery and anesthesiology: psychological preparation of the surgical patient. Springfield, IL: Charles C Thomas; 2001:31–56.
16. Gafner G, Benson S. Hypnotic techniques: for standard psychotherapy and formal hypnosis. New York: Norton; 2003.
17. Eimer BN. Clinical applications of hypnosis for brief and efficient pain management psychotherapy. *Am J Clin Hypn.* 2000;43:17–40.
18. Eimer BN, Freeman A. Pain management psychotherapy: a practical guide. New York: Wiley; 1998.

19. Ketterhagen D, VandeVusse L, Berner MA. Self-hypnosis: alternative anesthesia for childbirth. *MCN Am J Matern Child Nurs.* 2002;27:335–341.

20. Patterson DR, Jensen MP. Hypnosis and clinical pain. *Psychol Bull.* 2003;129:495–521.

21. Gallagher G, Rae CP, Kinsella J. Treatment of pain in severe burns. *Am J Clin Dermatol.* 2000;1:329–335.

22. Patterson DR, Tininenko JR, Schmidt AE, et al. Virtual reality hypnosis: a case report. *Int J Clin Exp Hypn.* 2004;52:27–38.

23. Frenay MC, Faymonville ME, Devlieger S, et al. Psychological approaches during dressing changes of burned patients: a prospective randomized study comparing hypnosis against stress reducing strategy. *Burns.* 2001;27:793–799.

24. Wright BR, Drummond PD. Rapid induction analgesia for the alleviation of procedural pain during burn care. *Burns.* 2000;26:275–282.

25. Patterson DR, Everett JJ, Burns GL, et al. Hypnosis for the treatment of burn pain. *J Consult Clin Psychol.* 1992;60: 713–717.

26. Patterson DR, Ptacek JT. Baseline pain as a moderator of hypnotic analgesia for burn injury treatment. *J Consult Clin Psychol.* 1997;65:60–67.

27. Everett JJ, Patterson DR, Burns GL, et al. Adjunctive interventions for burn pain control: comparison of hypnosis and ativan: the 1993 Clinical Research Award. *J Burn Care Rehabil.* 1993;14:676–683.

28. Montgomery GH, DuHamel KN, Redd WH. A meta-analysis of hypnotically induced analgesia: how effective is hypnosis? *Int J Clin Exp Hypn.* 2000;48:138–153.

29. Lang EV, Joyce JS, Spiegel D, et al. Self-hypnotic relaxation during interventional radiological procedures: effects on pain perception and intravenous drug use. *Int J Clin Exp Hypn.* 1996;44:106–119.

30. Lang EV, Benotsch EG, Fick LJ, et al. Adjunctive non-pharmacological analgesia for invasive medical procedures: a randomised trial. *Lancet.* 2000;355:1486–1490.

31. Anbar RD. Self-hypnosis for patients with cystic fibrosis. *Pediatr Pulmonol.* 2000;30:461–465.

32. Shenefelt PD. Biofeedback, cognitive-behavioral methods, and hypnosis in dermatology: is it all in your mind? *Dermatol Ther.* 2003;16:114–122.

33. Schaerlaekens M. Hypnosis and dentistry: water and fire? *Rev Belge Med Dent.* 2003;58:118–125.

34. Montgomery GH, David D, Winkel G, et al. The effectiveness of adjunctive hypnosis with surgical patients: a meta-analysis. *Anesth Analg.* 2002;94:1639–1645.

35. Montgomery GH, Weltz CR, Seltz M, et al. Brief presurgery hypnosis reduces distress and pain in excisional breast biopsy patients. *Int J Clin Exp Hypn.* 2002;50:17–32.

36. Ghoneim MM, Block RI, Sarasin DS, et al. Tape-recorded hypnosis instructions as adjuvant in the care of patients scheduled for third molar surgery. *Anesth Analg.* 2000;90: 64–68.

37. Faymonville ME, Fissette J, Mambourg PH, et al. Hypnosis as adjunct therapy in conscious sedation for plastic surgery. *Reg Anesth.* 1995;20:145–151.

38. Faymonville ME, Meurisse M, Fissette J. Hypnosedation: a valuable alternative to traditional anaesthetic techniques. *Acta Chir Belg.* 1999;99:141–146.

39. Defechereux T, Meurisse M, Hamoir E, et al. Hypnoanesthesia for endocrine cervical surgery: a statement of practice. *J Altern Complement Med.* 1999;5:509–520.

40. Defechereux T, Degauque C, Fumal I, et al. Hypnosedation, a new method of anesthesia for cervical endocrine surgery. Prospective randomized trial study. *Ann Chir.* 2000;125:539–546.

41. Dawson P, Van Hamel C, Wilkinson D, et al. Patient-controlled analgesia and intra-operative suggestion. *Anaesthesia.* 2001; 56:65–69.

42. Nilsson U, Rawal N, Unestahl LE, et al. Improved recovery after music and therapeutic suggestions during general anaesthesia: a double-blind randomized controlled trial. *Acta Anaesthesiol Scand.* 2001;45:812–817.

43. Weinstein EJ, Au PK. Use of hypnosis before and during angioplasty. *Am J Clin Hypn.* 1991;34:29–37.

44. Mauer MH, Burnett KF, Ouellette EA, et al. Medical hypnosis and orthopedic hand surgery: pain perception, postoperative recovery, and therapeutic comfort. *Int J Clin Exp Hypn.* 1999;47:144–161.

45. Nilsson U, Rawal N, Enqvist B, et al. Analgesia following music and therapeutic suggestions in the PACU in ambulatory surgery; a randomized controlled trial. *Acta Anaesthesiol Scand.* 2003;47:278–283.

46. Schauble PG, Werner WEF, Rai SH, et al. Childbirth preparation through hypnosis: the hypnoreflexogenous protocol. *Am J Clin Hypn.* 1998;40:273–283.

47. Goldman L. The use of hypnosis in obstetrics. *Psychiatr Med.* 1992;10:59–67.

48. Martin AA, Schauble PG, Rai SH, et al. The effects of hypnosis on the labor processes and birth outcomes of pregnant adolescents. *J Fam Pract.* 2001;50:441–443.

49. Freeman RM, Macaulay AJ, Eve L, et al. Randomized trial of self hypnosis for analgesia in labour. *Br Med J* (Clin Res Ed). 1986;292:657–658.

50. Mairs DAE. Hypnosis and pain in childbirth. *Contemp Hypn.* 1995;12:111–118.

51. Harmon TM, Hynan MT, Tyre TE. Improved obstetric outcomes using hypnotic analgesia and skill mastery combined with childbirth education. *J Consult Clin Psychol.* 1990;58: 525–530.

52. Smith CA, Collins CT, Cyna AM, et al. Complementary and alternative therapies for pain management in labour. *Cochrane Database Syst Rev.* 2003(2):CD003521.

53. Douglas DB. Hypnosis: useful, neglected, available. *Am J Hosp Palliat Care.* 1999;16:665–670.

54. Lynch DF Jr. Empowering the patient: hypnosis in the management of cancer, surgical disease and chronic pain. *Am J Clin Hypn.* 1999;42:122–130.

55. Rosen G, Willoch F, Bartenstein P, et al. Neurophysiological processes underlying the phantom limb pain experience and the use of hypnosis in its clinical management: an intensive examination of two patients. *Int J Clin Exp Hypn.* 2001;49: 38–55.

56. Oakley DA, Whitman LG, Halligan PW. Hypnotic imagery as a treatment for phantom limb pain: two case reports and a review. *Clin Rehabil.* 2002;16:368–377.

57. Winocur E, Gavish A, Emodi-Perlman A, et al. Hypnorelaxation as treatment for myofascial pain disorder: a comparative study. *Oral Surg Oral Med Oral Pathol Oral Radiol Endod.* 2002;93:429–434.

58. Simon EP, Lewis DM. Medical hypnosis for temporomandibular disorders: treatment efficacy and medical utilization outcome. *Oral Surg Oral Med Oral Pathol Oral Radiol Endod.* 2000;90:54–63.

59. Gay MC, Philippot P, Luminet O. Differential effectiveness of psychological interventions for reducing osteoarthritis pain: a comparison of Erikson [correction of Erickson] hypnosis and Jacobson relaxation. *Eur J Pain.* 2002;6:1–16.

60. Edelson J, Fitzpatrick JL. A comparison of cognitive-behavioral and hypnotic treatments of chronic pain. *J Clin Psychol.* 1989;45:316–323.

61. Dinges DF, Whitehouse WG, Orne EC, et al. Self-hypnosis training as an adjunctive treatment in the management of pain associated with sickle cell disease. *Int J Clin Exp Hypn.* 1997;45:417–432.

62. Matthews M, Flatt S. The efficacy of hypnotherapy in the treatment of migraine. *Nurs Stand.* 1999;14:33–36.

63. Spinhoven P, ter Kuile MM. Treatment outcome expectancies and hypnotic susceptibility as moderators of pain reduction in patients with chronic tension-type headache. *Int J Clin Exp Hypn.* 2000;48:290–305.

64. Friedman H, Taub HA. Brief psychological training procedures in migraine treatment. *Am J Clin Hypn.* 1984;26:187–200.

65. Melis PM, Rooimans W, Spierings EL, et al. Treatment of chronic tension-type headache with hypnotherapy: a single-blind time controlled study. *Headache.* 1991;31:686–689.

66. ter Kuile MM, Spinhoven P, Linssen AC, et al. Autogenic training and cognitive self-hypnosis for the treatment of recurrent headaches in three different subject groups. *Pain.* 1994;58:331–340.

67. Spinhoven P, Linssen AC, Van Dyck R, et al. Autogenic training and self-hypnosis in the control of tension headache. *Gen Hosp Psychiatry.* 1992;14:408–415.

68. Zitman FG, van Dyck R, Spinhoven P, et al. Hypnosis and autogenic training in the treatment of tension headaches: a two-phase constructive design study with follow-up. *J Psychosom Res.* 1992;36:219–228.

69. ter Kuile MM, Spinhoven P, Linssen AC, et al. Cognitive coping and appraisal processes in the treatment of chronic headaches. *Pain.* 1996;64:257–264.

70. Lu DP, Lu GP, Kleinman L. Acupuncture and clinical hypnosis for facial and head and neck pain: a single crossover comparison. *Am J Clin Hypn.* 2001;44:141–148.

71. Houghton LA, Heyman DJ, Whorwell PJ. Symptomatology, quality of life and economic features of irritable bowel syndrome—the effect of hypnotherapy. *Aliment Pharmacol Ther.* 1996;10:91–95.

72. Lea R, Houghton LA, Calvert EL, et al. Gut-focused hypnotherapy normalizes disordered rectal sensitivity in patients with irritable bowel syndrome. *Aliment Pharmacol Ther.* 2003;17:635–642.

73. Vidakovic-Vukic M. Hypnotherapy in the treatment of irritable bowel syndrome: methods and results in Amsterdam. *Scand J Gastroenterol Suppl.* 1999;230:49–51.

74. Palsson OS, Turner MJ, Johnson DA, et al. Hypnosis treatment for severe irritable bowel syndrome: investigation of mechanism and effects on symptoms. *Dig Dis Sci.* 2002;47:2605–2614.

75. Forbes A, MacAuley S, Chiotakakou-Faliakou E. Hypnotherapy and therapeutic audiotape: effective in previously unsuccessfully treated irritable bowel syndrome? *Int J Colorectal Dis.* 2000;15:328–324.

76. Pan CX, Morrison RS, Ness J, et al. Complementary and alternative medicine in the management of pain, dyspnea, and nausea and vomiting near the end of life. A systematic review. *J Pain Symptom Manage.* 2000;20:374–387.

77. Vickers AJ, Cassileth BR. Unconventional therapies for cancer and cancer-related symptoms. *Lancet Oncol.* 2001;2(4):226–232.

78. Shukla Y, Pal SK. Complementary and alternative cancer therapies: past, present and the future scenario. *Asian Pac J Cancer Prev.* 2004;5:3–14.

79. Sellick SM, Zaza C. Critical review of 5 nonpharmacologic strategies for managing cancer pain. *Cancer Prev Control.* 1998;2:7–14.

80. Zaza C, Sellick SM, Willan A, et al. Health care professionals' familiarity with non-pharmacological strategies for managing cancer pain. *Psychooncology.* 1999;8:99–111.

81. Syrjala KL, Cummings C, Donaldson GW. Hypnosis or cognitive behavioral training for the reduction of pain and nausea during cancer treatment: a controlled clinical trial. *Pain.* 1992;48:137–146.

82. Liossi C, Hatira P. Clinical hypnosis in the alleviation of procedure-related pain in pediatric oncology patients. *Int J Clin Exp Hypn.* 2003;51:4–28.

83. Liossi C, Hatira P. Clinical hypnosis versus cognitive behavioral training for pain management with pediatric cancer patients undergoing bone marrow aspirations. *Int J Clin Exp Hypn.* 1999;47:104–116.

84. Plotnick AB, O'Grady GJ. Hypnotic responsiveness in children. In: Wester WC, O'Grady DJ, eds. *Clinical Hypnosis with Children.* New York: Brunner/Mazel; 1991:19–33.

85. O'Grady DJ. Hypnosis and pain management in children. In: Wester WC, O'Grady DJ, eds. *Clinical Hypnosis with Children.* New York: Brunner/Mazel; 1991:213–229.

86. Council JR. Measures of hypnotic responding. In: Kirsch I, Capafons A, Gardena-Buelna E, Amigo S, eds. *Clinical Hypnosis and Self-Regulation: Cognitive-Behavioral Perspectives.* Washington, DC: American Psychological Association; 1999:119–140.

87. Vandelberg B. Hypnotic responsivity from a developmental perspective: insights from young children. *Int J Clin Exp Hypn.* 2002;50:229–247.

88. Katz ER, Kellerman J, Ellenberg L. Hypnosis in the reduction of acute pain and distress in children with cancer. *J Pediatr Psychol.* 1987;12:379–394.

89. Kuttner L. Favorite stories: a hypnotic pain-reduction technique for children in acute pain. *Am J Clin Hypn.* 1988; 30:289–295.

90. Zeltzer L, LeBaron S. Hypnosis and nonhypnotic techniques for reduction of pain and anxiety during painful procedures in children and adolescents with cancer. *J Pediatr.* 1982; 101:1032–1035.

91. Peretz B, Bimstein E. The use of imagery suggestions during administration of local anesthetic in pediatric dental patients. *ASDC J Dent Child.* 2000;67:263–267.

92. Iserson KV. Hypnosis for pediatric fracture reduction. *J Emerg Med.* 1999;17(1):53–56.

93. Lambert SA. The effects of hypnosis/guided imagery on the postoperative course of children. *J Dev Behav Pediatr.* 1996; 17;307–310.

94. Anbar RD. Hypnosis in pediatrics: applications at a pediatric pulmonary center. *BMC Pediatr.* 2002;2:11.

95. Zeltzer LK, Tsao JC, Stelling C, et al. A phase I study on the feasibility and acceptability of an acupuncture/hypnosis intervention for chronic pediatric pain. *J Pain Symptom Manage.* 2002;24:437–446.

96. Holden EW, Deichmann MM, Levy JD. Empirically supported treatments in pediatric psychology: recurrent pediatric headache. *J Pediatr Psychol.* 1999;24:91–109.

97. Gysin T. Clinical hypnotherapy/self-hypnosis for unspecified, chronic and episodic headache without migraine and other defined headaches in children and adolescents. *Forsch Komplementarmed;*6(suppl 1):44–46.

98. Anbar RD. Self-hypnosis for the treatment of functional abdominal pain in childhood. *Clin Pediatr* (Phila). 2001;40: 444–451.

99. Milling LS, Costantino CA. Clinical hypnosis with children: first steps toward empirical support. *Int J Clin Exp Hypn.* 2000;48:113–137.

50

Nonpharmacologic Interventions
Psychologic Techniques

Lance Brown
Lilit Minasyan

HIGH YIELD FACTS

- Psychologic techniques are used to provide pain relief to emergency department (ED) patients and in settings similar to the ED.
- Ideal psychologic techniques comply with relevant policies/regulations/laws, and are culturally acceptable for all involved.
- Psychologic techniques include humor, music, controlled breathing, guided imagery, sensory focusing, low-tech and high-tech distractions, and acupuncture/acupressure.
- Future techniques may make use of virtual reality technology.

INTRODUCTION

In many ways, psychologic techniques for the control of pain and anxiety in the emergency department (ED) have not been utilized or studied to the same extent that pharmacologic agents for sedation and anxiolysis have. There are several possible reasons for this. First, the human response to a given pharmacologic sedative is much more uniform than the response to psychologic techniques. Although the effective dose may very somewhat, if given a sufficient dose, patients will uniformly enter deep sedation when given intravenous propofol in the ED. The same cannot be said of humor, for example. By simply providing more material from the same comedian, some patients may laugh more and more hysterically while others remain insulted, bewildered, or uninterested. A video game that may effectively distract an adolescent during a procedure, may fail to capture the interest of an elderly patient. Second, because of this variable response, study results

may be difficult to interpret. Guided imagery where the patient imagines her pain to be shrinking away may work very well for a school-aged child, but not for an uptight adult who sees the exercises as silly and does not "buy in" to the process. Third, there may be reluctance on the part of physicians to clinically employ and scientifically study psychologic techniques because they do not seem "medical." Although effective, having a decrease in pain and anxiety by watching an interesting movie may seem too "common" or "simple" to constitute "medical treatment." Fourth, there seems to be a financial disincentive to employ psychologic techniques. We are not aware of an appropriate billing code for physicians when they provide handheld video games during laceration repair, for example.

Even given these difficulties, there is a small but growing body of literature regarding psychologic care and acute pain management. There are now efforts to improve the quality of the methodology for this kind of research.[1] In this chapter, we will explore the qualities of an ideal ED psychologic technique and review the available evidence regarding psychologic techniques for pain and anxiety control as it relates to ED care.

THE IDEAL PSYCHOLOGIC TECHNIQUE

When considering employing psychologic techniques in the ED, it is helpful to list highly desirable characteristics. Although it is unlikely that any single psychologic technique will exhibit all of these desirable characteristics for all patients, the identification of highly desirable features is a useful exercise. Various psychologic techniques can be held up to this theoretical standard for comparison and assessment. This may help clinicians in their selection of psychologic techniques for a particular patient and situation.

There are several features we have identified that should be present in the ideal psychologic technique (Table 50-1). The ideal psychologic technique would be age appropriate. This is especially true when the patients are infants and children. The rapid changes in developmental behavior, including the ability for abstract thinking and pretend play, make the selection of age-appropriate psychologic techniques paramount. Effective strategies for one age group will fail miserably for others. The ideal psychologic technique would comply with relevant policies, regulations, and laws and be culturally acceptable for all involved. Although possibly effective, an illegal technique would obviously wreak regulatory and administrative havoc on a medical facility. A vivid example of a culturally unacceptable psychologic technique would be the use of pornography. It is highly likely that many patients would be quite distracted (positively or negatively) by

Table 50-1. Characteristics of the Ideal Psychologic Technique

Age appropriate
Complies with relevant policies, regulations, and laws
Culturally acceptable for the patient, family, and staff
Does not interfere with clinical care
Does not require prior patient experience with the
    technique
Easy to teach and learn
Evidence-based effectiveness has been documented
High success rate
Inexpensive
Minimal preparation time needed
Pleasant for patient and staff
Poses no risk to the patient or staff
Requires little or no staff training
Requires no special skills from staff or patient

viewing erotic materials while undergoing procedures. However, it is highly doubtful that many families or staff members would find this technique to be culturally or socially acceptable. Although possibly effective, a psychologic technique that is not culturally acceptable to all involved will ultimately fail. The ideal psychologic technique should not interfere with clinical care. If the activity involves large, sweeping movements by the patient at a time when movement would be unsafe or if the activity is annoying to the individuals performing the procedure, this psychologic technique will not be effective. The ideal psychologic technique cannot require prior experience. Since the ED visit is a single encounter, the technique cannot require multiple practice sessions. The ideal psychologic technique will be easy to teach, easy to learn, require minimal preparation time, and require little or no staff training. Because there are multiple ED staff members working various shifts—typically with substantial time pressure to move quickly from one activity to another— selected techniques should require minimal preparation time and be brought to the bedside immediately prior to the procedure. The ideal psychologic technique should require no special skills from the staff or patient. Although juggling may be an effective distraction technique when performed by either the staff member or the patient, it would be unrealistic to expect many patients to juggle or to always have a staff member on duty who could juggle.

Although no currently available psychologic technique has all of these characteristics, there are some techniques that have some appealing features. Each of these techniques has some ideal qualities. It is clear that there are often no distinct boundaries between these psychologic techniques. Although the intent of a particular intervention may be to invoke humor, there are features to humorous activities that also induce relaxation and distraction. Regardless of the underlying neurobiology or psychology, techniques that are successful are worth considering for use in the ED. Available evidence, although typically scarce, will be presented for each technique discussed.

HUMOR

Humor has been advocated as a psychologic technique for acute pain management.[2] It is also clear that humor has widespread appeal, given the popularity of humorous movies and situational comedies on television. Given this, however, we were only able to identify four studies examining the role of humor that we considered potentially applicable to care in the ED.[3–6] The earliest study we could identify is by Cogan and colleagues and was published in 1987. These researchers examined the effects of listening to 20-minute long "laughter-inducing" audiotapes and compared the effects of these humorous tapes on pressure-induced pain thresholds to the effects of listening to other types of audiotapes (e.g., "relaxation inducing" and "dull narrative"). These researchers found that pain thresholds were higher in the laugher-inducing audiotape group than in other groups. In the early 1990s, Hudak and colleagues found similar results when transcutaneous electrical nerve stimulation (TENS) was used as the painful stimulus.[4] More recently, Weisenberg and colleagues assessed cold-pressor-induced pain thresholds for groups of subjects after viewing different kinds of movies for 15, 30, or 45 minutes.[5] These researchers found that subjects who had viewed the longest and most humorous movies had increased pain thresholds compared to the other groups (holocaust movie, neutral movie, and no movie).[5] Most recently, in 2001, Mahony and colleagues reported on the effects of humorous videos on acute pain thresholds.[6] Inflating a blood pressure cuff on the upper dominant arm of study subjects to induce pain, these researchers noted increased pain thresholds when the subjects were watching humorous videos. Groups of study subjects were given a specific expectation that the video would either increase or decrease their sensitivity to pain. These expectations also affected the pain threshold by adjusting it in the direction that the patient was told to expect.

We did not identify any studies that directly examined the effects of humor on pain experiences for patients in the ED. It is conceivable that properly using humor in the ED may increase patient pain thresholds. If future studies support the therapeutic uses of humor in the ED, this would support the use of (properly secured) televisions and DVD players in the ED for patients experiencing pain and during painful procedures.

COGNITIVE TECHNIQUES

Guided Imagery

Guided imagery is a technique that relies on the imagination of the patient. Guided imagery employs a voice (recorded or spoken) guiding the patient through a pleasant, imaginary scenario including sites, sounds, smells, tastes, and feelings. An example of this technique would be to have a staff member talk to a patient during a procedure about being at the beach, smelling the fresh sea air, and feeling the sand beneath her feet. The patient would then try to imagine herself at the beach.[7] Active involvement and acceptance of the process by the patient are requisite for this psychologic technique to be effective. We could not identify any studies that have evaluated the effectiveness of this technique in the ED. Guided imagery has also been called "leaving the pain behind" and "replacing pain with a familiar activity."[8]

Sensory Focusing

Unlike guided imagery during which the patient avoids thinking about the painful experience and instead focuses on something else, sensory focusing involves actively thinking about the ongoing pain.[8] When sensory focusing is employed, the patient is asked to focus on their experience of pain and to imagine that the pain is a physical object that can be manipulated by the patient. In this way, the patient is supposed to imagine the pain getting smaller or more distant and therefore more manageable. Like guided imagery, active involvement and acceptance of the process by the patient are required for this technique to be effective. We could not identify any studies that have evaluated the effectiveness of this technique in the ED. Sensory focusing has also been called "shrinking the pain" and "painting the pain."[8]

MUSIC

Listening to music has been recommended as a means of providing pain relief during procedures.[8] Lullabies for infants, fun "child-friendly" music for older children, and self-selected music for adolescents and adults can provide a sense of well-being and relaxation making painful procedures more tolerable. There is some very recent work that has explored the biologic basis for the soothing effects of music.[9] With regard to clinical care relevant to the ED setting, we have identified three applicable studies.

Berlin and colleagues published a qualitative review of their experience using music therapy in their ED for children undergoing invasive procedures.[10] They reported that their experience was generally positive and they recommend music therapy for use in the ED. Haythornthwaite and colleagues reported that for burn patients undergoing dressing changes, music was less effective than sensory focusing.[11] It is conceivable that the active participation needed for sensory focusing was the key difference in the effectiveness of the two techniques. In the only randomized, controlled trials of the use of music in the ED, Manegazzi and colleagues evaluated the effectiveness of music to relieve pain and anxiety during laceration repair in adults.[12] In this study, 19 patients listened to music and 19 control subjects did not. These researchers found a statistically significant decrease in perceived pain in the music group, but no statistically significant difference in anxiety between the groups.

CONTROLLED BREATHING

Using controlled breathing has been recommended as a way to increase patient relaxation and improve pain tolerance.[8] There appear to be two main forms of controlled breathing based on age. For children 4–12 years of age, the primary technique has been described as "blowing away the pain."[8,13] To use this technique, children are instructed to repeatedly blow out during the period of greatest pain intensity.[13] This process can be facilitated by the use of bubble wands, pinwheels, other similar objects, or imaginary candles.[8] For adults, the process seems to be quite different. Rather than a vigorous active blowing, adults seem to do better with slow, deep breathing. We were unable to identify any literature describing the use of controlled breathing in the ED setting.

DISTRACTION

Distraction is probably the most effective and best studied of the psychologic techniques.[14–18] We feel that it is important to acknowledge that other psychologic techniques could also be considered forms of distraction. This may cause some confusion when reading the literature regarding psychologic techniques. The classification of a humorous movie as "humor" or blowing bubbles as "controlled breathing" rather than "distraction" is necessarily arbitrary as these classifications clearly overlap.[19] Benefits and limitations of other psychologic techniques may apply to those techniques designated as "distraction." When considering using distraction techniques in the ED, classifying them as *low tech* or *high tech* may have some use in terms of cost and feasibility.

Low-Tech Distractions

Many inexpensive distraction techniques can be imagined including reading books, telling stories, playing with noisy objects, playing cards, or watching bubbles float through the air. In children's hospitals, these techniques are often associated with child life specialists.[20] Unfortunately, there have been few studies that have evaluated the effectiveness of these low-tech techniques in the setting of acute pain in the ED. We identified a single study that described the use of child life specialists during ED suturing.[20] In this study, children who received low-tech distractions provided by child life specialists during ED suturing expressed fewer fears than the control group who received standard care. We were also able to identify two studies that directly addressed inexpensive and simple distraction. Both studies examined the effectiveness of kaleidoscopes. In 1994, Vessey and colleagues reported on the successful use of a kaleidoscope as a distraction technique during phlebotomy in children 3–12 years of age.[16] Similarly, in 1997, Cason and colleagues reported on the use of kaleidoscopes as a distraction technique for 96 adults undergoing phlebotomy.[21] The authors reported a statistically significant difference in the pain perception in the kaleidoscope group compared to the control group. At this point there is reasonable evidence to suggest that kaleidoscopes are an effective low-tech distraction technique for phlebotomy and possibly for similar procedures.

High-Tech Distractions

Distraction techniques that involve relatively expensive electronic equipment can be considered high tech. We have had personal experience observing older school-aged children using handheld computer games and noticed the intense concentration these children seem to exhibit. We have observed that even though a wound repair is done and discharge is imminent, these children appear to have substantial reluctance in putting the game away. Similar phenomena are observed when it appears that a particular television show has captured a child's interest. We were unable to identify medical literature that discusses these handheld devices or television directly, but other forms of electronic entertainment have been studied. Lembo and colleagues studied the effects of audio stimulation, audio plus visual stimulation, and a control group who received neither form of stimulation.[22] In this study, the investigators evaluated the effects of these forms of distraction for 37 adults undergoing flexible sigmoidoscopy. Audio and visual stimulation was the most effective form of distraction in this study. Bentsen and colleagues took this idea a step further and studied the

effects of three-dimensional video glasses on cold pressor pain.[23] Perceived pain was lower in the three-dimensional video group than in the control group. The most extreme form of high-tech distraction, virtual reality, has also been studied recently. Recent work by Hoffman and colleagues has suggested that virtual reality may be a very effective form of distraction for pain reduction during acute painful events.[24–26] If further work in this area of study supports these positive findings, virtual reality may turn out to be quite useful in the ED. Virtual reality has the advantages of actively engaging the patient with minimal effort from her, involving multiple sensory inputs (at least sight and sound), providing individualized content, and wide applicability to a variety of patient groups and procedural indications. As the cost of this technology falls, we may see the use of computer-aided distraction become commonplace in the EDs of the future.[27]

ACUPUNCTURE AND ACUPRESSURE

Although acupuncturists may disagree with the categorization of acupuncture and acupressure as psychologic in nature, the current allopathic model of health and disease has yet to explain adequately any anatomic or physiologic reason for acupuncture to work. The traditional models of explaining how acupuncture works are bewildering to an allopath. Explaining acupuncture in traditional terms involves talking about imbalanced Qi (vital energy) and the flow of Qi through anatomically mysterious meridians. The explanation essentially involves the unblocking of the flow of Qi to one part of the body by inserting a hair-thin needle into a distant part of the body at an acupuncture point along the right meridian.[28,29] On the surface, this seems like quackery when evaluated using the current allopathic model of health and disease. However, many individuals seek out acupuncture care for a fairly large number of conditions and insurance companies have begun covering acupuncture.[29] In the allopathic model of health and disease, acupuncture, if it works, works by impacting the psychology of the patient. There may be a change in brain chemicals during acupuncture, but this has yet to be fully elucidated.

We identified two peer-reviewed articles in the medical literature that addressed acupressure in the emergency setting. Kober and colleagues performed a prospective, randomized, double-blind trial of using true acupressure points (Di4, KS9, KS6, BL60, and LG20), sham acupressure points (all over bony areas), and a control group that received no acupressure. There were 60 subjects in the study and the authors suggest that acupressure was helpful in relieving perceived anxiety, decreasing pain, and slowing the heart rate.[30] Members of the same research group also studied the effect of auricular acupressure on anxiety and pain in patients being transported by ambulance. The outcome was similarly positive in this study.[31]

We could not identify any studies of acupuncture in the ED setting. There are case reports of complications of acupuncture leading to ED visits, however. These include a case of a retroperitoneal abscess[32] and pneumothoraces.[33] There are reports for acupuncture being used in a variety of settings other than the ED, however.[34–36] The applicability of these studies to contemporary emergency medicine practice has yet to be explored and is unclear.

CONCLUSION

Psychologic techniques are currently being employed to provide pain relief to patients in the ED and in settings similar to that of the ED. We are at an early developmental stage in our understanding of these techniques. There are multiple psychologic techniques for the practitioner to consider. The best studied psychologic technique and the one for which there is the best supporting evidence is distraction. Computer generated distractions including virtual reality technology may have the greatest promise for effective distraction techniques of the future.

REFERENCES

1. Davidson KW, Goldstein M, Kaplan RM, et al. Evidence-based behavioral medicine: what is it and how do we achieve it? *Ann Behav Med.* 2003;26:161–171.
2. Stevensen C. Non-pharmacological aspects of acute pain management. *Complement Ther Nurs Midwifery.* 1995;1:77–84.
3. Cogan R, Cogan D, Waltz W, et al. Effects of laughter and relaxation on discomfort thresholds. *J Behav Med.* 1987;10:139–144.
4. Hudak DA, Dale JA, Hudak MA, et al. Effects of humorous stimuli and sense of humor on discomfort. *Psychol Rep.* 1991;69:779–786.
5. Weisenberg M, Raz T, Hener T. The influence of film-induced mood on pain perception. *Pain.* 1998;76:365–375.
6. Mahony DL, Burroughs WJ, Hieatt AC. The effects of laughter on discomfort thresholds: does expectation become reality? *J Gen Psychol.* 2001;128:217–226.
7. Halter CW. Using guided imagery in the emergency department. *J Emerg Nurs.* 1998;24:518–522.
8. Kuttner L. *A Child in Pain: How to Help, What to Do.* Vancouver, BC: Hartley & Marks; 1996.
9. Stefano GB, Zhu W, Cadet P, et al. Music alters constitutively expressed opiate and cytokine processes in listeners. *Med Sci Monit* 2004;10:MS18–27 (available at *http://www.MedSciMonit.com/pub/vol_10/no_6/5351.pdf*, last accessed July 15, 2004).
10. Berlin BK, Avondale BA. Music therapy with children during invasive procedures: our emergency department's experience. *J Emerg Nurs.* 1998;24:607–608.
11. Haythornthwaite JA, Lawrence JW, Fauerback JA. Brief cognitive interventions for burn pain. *Ann Behav Med.* 2001;23:42–49.
12. Menegazzi JJ, Paris PM, Kersteen CH, et al. A randomized, controlled trial of the use of music during laceration repair. *Ann Emerg Med.* 1991;20:348–350.
13. French GM, Painter EC, Coury DL. Blowing away shot pain: a technique for pain management during immunization. *Pediatrics.* 1994;93:384–388.
14. Kleiber C, Harper DC. Effects of distraction on children's pain and distress during medical procedures: a meta-analysis. *Nurs Res.* 1999;48:44–49.
15. Christenfeld N. Memory for pain and the delayed effects of distraction. *Health Psychol.* 1997;16:327–330.
16. Vessey JA, Carlson KL, Mcgill J. Use of distraction with children during an acute pain experience. *Nurs Res.* 1994;43:369–372.
17. Tanabe P, Ferket K, Thomas R, et al. The effect of standard care, ibuprofen, and distraction on pain relief and patient satisfaction in children with musculoskeletal trauma. *J Emerg Nurs.* 2002;28:118–125.
18. Fanurik D, Koh JL, Schmitz ML. Distraction techniques combined with EMLA: effects on IV insertion pain and distress in children. *Child Health Care.* 2000;29:87–101.
19. Sparks L. Taking the "ouch" out of injections for children. Using distraction to decrease pain. *MCN Am J Matern Child Nurs.* 2001;26:772–787.
20. Alcock DS, Feldman W, Goodman JT el al. Evaluation of child life intervention in emergency department suturing. *Pediatr Emerg Care.* 1985;1:111–115.
21. Cason CL, Grissom NL. Ameliorating adults' acute pain during phlebotomy with a distraction intervention. *Appl Nurs Res.* 1997;10:168–173.
22. Lembo T, Fitzgerald L, Matin K, et al. Audio and visual stimulation reduces patient discomfort during screening flexible sigmoidoscopy. *Am J Gastroenterol.* 1998;93:1113–1116.
23. Bentsen B, Svensson P, Wenzel A. The hypoalgesic effect of 3-D video glasses on cold pressor pain: reproducibility and importance of information. *Anesth Prog.* 2000;47:67–71.
24. Hoffman HG, Doctor JN, Patterson DR, et al. Use of virtual reality for adjunctive treatment of adolescent burn pain during wound care: a case report. *Pain.* 2000;85:305–309.
25. Hoffman HG, Patterson DR, Carrougher GJ. Use of virtual reality for adjunctive treatment of adult burn pain during physical therapy: a controlled study. *Clin J Pain.* 2000;16:244–250.
26. Hoffman HG, Garcia-Palacios A, Kapa V, et al. Immersive virtual reality for reducing experimental ischemic pain. *Int J Hum Comput Interact.* 2003;15:469–486,.
27. Reducing acute pain through computer-generated distraction in children. *http://www2.healthcare.ucla.edu/pedspain/rp7_comp.htm* (last accessed July 15, 2004).

28. *www.holisticonline.com/Acupuncture/acp_meridians.htm* (last accessed December 19, 2004).

29. *www.acupuncturebydrlee.com* (last accessed December 19, 2004).

30. Kober A, Scheck T, Greher M, et al. Prehospital analgesia with acupressure in victims of minor trauma: a prospective, randomized, double-blinded trial. *Anesth Analg.* 2002;95: 723–727.

31. Kober A, Scheck T, Schubert B, et al. Auricular acupressure as a treatment for anxiety in prehospital transport settings. *Anesthesiology.* 2003;98:1328–1332.

32. Cho YP, Jang HJ, Kim JS, et al. Retroperitoneal abscess complicated by acupuncture: case report. *J Korean Med Sci.* 2003;18:756–757.

33. Vilke GM, Wulfert EA. Case reports of two patients with pneumothorax following acupuncture. *J Emerg Med.* 1997;15: 155–157.

34. Brent R. Medical, social, and legal implications of treating nausea and vomiting of pregnancy. *Am J Obstet Gynecol.* 2002;186(5 suppl understanding):S262–S266.

35. Bielory L, Russin J, Zuckerman GB. Clinical efficacy, mechanisms of action, and adverse effects of complementary and alternative medicine therapies for asthma. *Allergy Asthma Proc.* 2004;25:283–291.

36. Rogenhofer S, Wimmer K, Blana A, et al. Acupuncture for pain in extracorporeal shockwave lithotripsy. *J Endourol.* 2004;18:634–637.

51

Future of Pain Management and Sedation in Emergency Medicine

James Ducharme

> *Pain, friends, is from the devil . . . Think now, I ask you . . . of your greatest suffering. Remember how each and every one of you, in your torment, would have exchanged your skin with the most wretched in the kingdom, just but you might have a minute, nay, a half-minute's relief.*
>
> D Miller, *Ingenious Pain*

INTRODUCTION

In his seminal book *Future Shock*, Alvin Toffler quoted the ironic Chinese proverb, "To prophesy is extremely difficult—especially with respect to the future."[1] In this final chapter, I will comment on future directions of pain management in emergency medicine. These are not "predictions" (which are best left to oracles and astrologers), but important advances that will probably occur (or are already occurring) over the next decade and will change how patients with pain are treated in the emergency department (ED).

THE MOVE TO MECHANISM-BASED PAIN CONTROL

Genomic research is revealing the multiple complex pathways that provide us with the sensation of pain and our reaction to it—either negative or positive. As a result, the approach to pain is increasingly a mechanism-based one that is rapidly replacing the symptom-based approach of the past. This will require a much better understanding of pain neurobiology by clinicians to ensure optimal matching of medication with the pain process. While morphine, normally considered the gold standard analgesic,

may be a poor analgesic for neuropathic pain, an agent that suppresses sodium channels—thereby diminishing neural discharge—may be very effective. Ultimately, as an individual's genomic code becomes available on a "smart card," medications will be chosen that not only fit the pain mechanism but are optimized for that person's genetic makeup. Such smart cards, as well as tools able to scan patients to identify precise pain mechanisms, remain at least a decade away. Without a definitive "pain-o-meter" we will have to continue to rely on physician-patient interaction and physician attitudes and knowledge to optimally assess and treat pain. This latter process is flawed as it exists and requires improvement.

THE GREATEST CHALLENGE—WILL WE CHANGE OUR ATTITUDES ABOUT PAIN CONTROL?

Each of us enters the medical domain with our own experience, cultural upbringing, and ethical viewpoints. During training, students are asked to integrate new knowledge and attitudes with little consideration of each individual's attitudes. It is not understood how individual values may impact this learning process. It is equally unknown to what degree various attitudes and values are modified by medical school. How are attitudes toward pain affected? Most students receive little training about either the neurobiology of pain or about pain management during training in medical school. This absence of a priority toward teaching about pain is in itself a powerful lesson. As Weinstein showed so well, we leave training with almost no change in our approach or in our attitudes toward pain and pain management from when we entered.[2] Psychologic characteristics associated with reluctance to prescribe opioids, and fears of patient addiction and drug regulatory agency sanctions are present before entering training. Cultural and religious values often stress the character and valor that results from enduring pain and hiding suffering. These attitudinal forces combined with inadequate education readily explain the prevailing misunderstanding of pain, opiophobia and oligoanalgesia among physicians.

An increasing amount of clinical pain research is being published in the emergency medicine literature. To varying degrees we have tried to make up for the lack of medical school pain education through CME. Opioid use in the management of pain has increased worldwide. Sensitivity to the need to better manage pain also appears to have waxed. Why is it, therefore, that Todd et al. were able to demonstrate almost no change in oligoanalgesic patterns of practice in 2002 from that demonstrated a decade earlier?[3]

The origins of opiophobia and societal attitudes about drug use and addiction are complex. In his book, *The American Disease—Origins of Narcotic Control*, David Musto noted that the United States has oscillated between periods of drug tolerance and drug intolerance.[4] The nineteenth century saw the advent of morphine, which was cheap, compact, and had a standard strength, the hypodermic needle, and unregulated patent medicines. Morphine, according to Sir William Osler, was "God's own medicine." Unfortunately, by 1900, America had developed a comparatively large addict population *and* a fear of addiction and addicting drugs. The Harrison Act, the first major American antinarcotic law was passed in 1914. It rapidly became clear that the actual enforcement of the Harrison Act would affect professionals and lead to indictments against physicians. The remainder of the twentieth century would see the attitudes of both clinicians and the public fluctuate with respect to potentially addictive drugs. Alcohol, despite being banned during prohibition, associated annually with thousands of deaths from motor vehicle collisions, and costing health care billions of dollars due to illness arising from its consumption, remained—and remains today—socially acceptable while opioid (and cocaine) use has not. This history, though fascinating, is too complex and nuanced to recount in this chapter. Nevertheless, readers should be aware that attitudes about drugs including analgesics have been shaped by two centuries of history.

Opiophobia is so powerful among medical professionals that clinicians either refuse to treat pain or opt for less effective analgesics with more adverse effects. In the SUPPORT trial, physicians did not increase analgesic use or better control severe pain even when specifically requested by patients with terminal cancer to do so.[5] Nonsteroidal anti-inflammatory drugs (NSAIDs) have been chosen as substitute analgesics despite high adverse effect rates. Industry has repeatedly stressed the benefits of their "opioid sparing effects" as if opioids were an undesired option. Gastrointestinal bleeding, congestive heart failure, and renal failure from NSAID use will result in untold numbers of deaths and hospitalizations, yet clinicians fear opioids more. Risk of addiction is often cited, despite rates as low as 0.03% when prescribed appropriately for acute pain.

Adding further to the emotional turmoil and stress physicians face when contemplating the use of opioids to manage pain is the potential malingerer, who seeks to obtain opioids for resale. The frequency with which emergency physicians might have to face such turmoil is considerable: according to at least two epidemiologic studies, more than 60% of patients registering in EDs across North America have pain as part of their complaint.[6,7] But even in inner city EDs, malingerers represent less than 2% of visits. Ever fearful of malingerers—1/30 as frequent as sufferers—physicians often avoid prescribing opioids to those in pain. Worse, patients may be unable to obtain opioids when prescribed due to their unavailability in many pharmacies.[8] Such attitudes lead to distortion of perception: 53% of emergency physicians believe 20% of those with sickle cell disease are addicted, 25% believe 50% are addicted. Large scale studies in fact place the rate of addiction in those suffering vasooc-clusive crises much lower, at 2% or less.[9] Such a viewpoint inevitably leads to skepticism and distrust of patient reporting.

Pain management cannot improve significantly until an approach to deal with attitudes and lack of education about pain in medical school is developed. This is a problem that needs to be addressed by all fields of medicine. Of patients admitted to the hospital with non-painful conditions, a large percentage are suffering from severe pain, often unrecognized. Teachers with better understanding of pain and medications must be identified, otherwise students will continue to learn the "old" biases from the traditional medical school training of "master-to-student" at the bedside. A revamping of medical school curricula that structures learning in such a way as to take into account the influences of individual cultural backgrounds is required. Pain education must become a priority in our training: it is, after all, the most frequent symptom of patients, yet the one we treat perhaps least well.

Education and ongoing assessment of attitudes cannot stop with completion of training. Reinforcement and ongoing education are essential. Marquie et al. demonstrated that the greater the clinical experience, the greater the risk of "systemic miscalibration".[10] They described that with increasing years of practice, physicians demonstrate increasing discordance in pain scoring when compared to patient self-reporting. Physicians score pain based on having witnessing thousands of patients in pain, not on an individual patient's experience. Without ongoing education, senior physicians risk providing less, not more, pain control. When a patient reports pain levels higher than that assessed by the physician (or nurse), the most frequent immediate reaction is to disbelieve the patient.

At present there is no standardized formal ongoing education with respect to pain, though some tentative efforts are being made. The State of California now requires all licensed physicians to undergo 12 hours of CME on pain-related topics to maintain licensure. Joint Commission on Accreditation of Healthcare Organizations (JCAHO) has mandated (with respect to pain in the ED) that health care workers carry out pain assessment and treat pain as a priority. Such a top-down approach does not ensure proper understanding and learning, however.[11] For optimal results clinicians must comprehend the extent of the problem and subsequently discover workable solutions, or change will never truly occur.

Caring for all Patients who are in Pain

In this book we have attempted to review all of the key areas of pain and pain management for the clinician. We have attempted to provide physiology based explanations for the various causes of pain and for the medications employed to treat them. Though many may consider chronic pain to be outside our area of practice or the expertise of emergency physicians it ought to be recognized that more than 40% of the patients in pain seen in the ED suffer from chronic pain.[7] It is imperative that emergency practitioners understand the nature of this pain, and recognize what can and cannot be offered to these patients in the ED, and if nothing else, how to properly educate and refer them. It serves little purpose, for example, to offer a patient with fibromyalgia an opioid when analgesics offer little if any benefit. Emergency practitioners need to somehow find the time in the midst of a busy shift to assess them properly. For many the ED is the only resource available, and often the default provider for others that were unable or unwilling to provide adequate pain relief or adequate explanations. ED physicians cannot affirm that patients with chronic pain are not *emergency* patients when data show that they are.

Recognizing the need for education and improvement in our approach to pain, let us explore where the future of pain management may lie.

FROM LABORATORY TO BEDSIDE

Knowledge about pain pathways and the neurobiology of pain is growing exponentially. The translation of laboratory animal study results and genomic research into clinical applications lags well behind this burgeoning knowledge. This is not due to lack of funding or interest, but rather the recognition of a pain system that is increasingly complex. Wang et al. studying rats with neuropathic pain

identified 148 genes in the dorsal root ganglion (DRG) that were up-regulated more than twofold, suggesting a heretofore unrecognized complexity of understanding required to successfully control pain.[12]

Though often normal practice, it ought to be recognized as simplistic thinking for many conditions to expect that a single agent can suppress the sensation of pain, particularly as multiple processes are occurring simultaneously. Consider the following example: a crush type injury produces local tissue hypoxia leading to peripheral nociceptor stimulation and the stimulation of acid sensing ion channels (ASIC) in afferent fibers. Reflex efferents lead to the release of calcitonin gene-related peptide (CGRP) and nitric oxide stimulating vasodilation, and the recruitment of additional nociceptors. Shortly thereafter, local inflammation leads to the release of kinins, prostaglandins, and potassium further stimulating the afferent nociceptive traffic, increasing the pain intensity. The release of cytokines into the circulation induces Cox-2 receptors in the spinal cord. It can be readily appreciated that a tactic aimed at blocking only one of these processes or products is unlikely to adequately control this patient's pain.

Research on analgesics with peripheral action has been frustrating as a result. Attempts to produce such agents have met with problems: dextromethorphan (an oral *N*-methyl-D-aspartate [NMDA] antagonist) causes excessive sedation before providing sufficient analgesia, and Cox-2 agents have recently been associated with an increased risk of death from ischemic heart disease. Since these same processes are essential aspects of normal physiology and have widespread effects, it may be difficult at times to foresee what adverse events may arise when one of these processes is interrupted with a therapeutic intent. It is anticipated that current genomic research will produce data that can be integrated into the clinical arena permitting a more effective risk:benefit tradeoff. It ought to be recognized that patient and care giver biases will still ultimately determine the success or failure of any pain control strategy.[13]

Delivery of Medication

It seems that novel methods of medication delivery are being developed almost daily. Some, such as liposomal encapsulated medications can be delivered by nebulization, providing rapid relief without requiring intravenous (IV) access.

Nanotechnology—allowing micromachines with a single function before destruction to be injected—may permit the targeted delivery of pain process interrupting medication, or the microscopic repair of damaged tissues removing the cause of pain. Altering the genome of targeted cells with modified viruses or by the injection of allogenic tissue into the subarachnoid space, may well allow control of chronic pain.[14]

Analgesic Medications

Perhaps more important than *how* medication is given, is ensuring that *the right* treatment *is* given.

Opioids

Patients suffering repetitive episodes of vasoocclusive crises have taught us that the metabolism of morphine may vary as much as tenfold among individuals. Genomic research has identified at least 15 different variants of the mu receptor. Thus, individuals may thus not only metabolize at a different rate, but respond differently to a given opioid. It may well be that certain patients receive no benefit from certain opioids, or benefit only transiently. For example, it is well known that up to 10% of Caucasians are unable to metabolize codeine to morphine to render it an effective analgesic.[15] Patients may well be providing important information when they state that a certain opioid has not "worked" in the past, though many clinicians may incorrectly interpret this as a marker of "drug seeking."

Finally, opioid specificity is such that an individual being treated with a nonspecific opioid (thereby occupying most mu receptors) may be unable to obtain rapid pain control should the dose of this same opioid be increased to manage an acute increase in their pain. Such variation mandates that physicians understand opioid physiology, and titrate opioids without preconceived notions of what an effective dose might be for the individual patient. ("One size does not fit all.") As an example, opioids such as fentanyl are often effective in achieving rapid control of pain in patients already receiving another opioid. Considerations such as these are even more important in averting suboptimal pain control for the discharged patient, who typically receives a fixed dose opioid combination that allows for little individual variation.

The appropriate and effective use of opioids in the management of severe pain leads us to address our fears of addiction and misuse. This is a long-term goal that probably will not be achieved quickly. Fortunately, research centered on the combination of cannabinoid antagonists with opioids may bear fruit in this regard. Studies in laboratory animals have demonstrated the successful prevention of addictive behavior of such combinations.[16,17] Such combination agents are speculated to prevent misuse by eliminating any positive reinforcement other than analgesia.

Cannabinoids

Cannabinoids act at CB_1 and CB_2 receptors both peripherally and centrally. They modulate release of neuropeptides from primary afferent receptors and inhibit the release of CGRP from sensory neurons, minimizing the local inflammatory response.[18] Clinical use of cannabinoids as analgesics has been slowed by legal issues, its adverse psychotropic effect profile, and a narrow therapeutic index (difficult to titrate to analgesia without inducing intoxication). In addition, many patients resist the notion of smoking cannabis to achieve analgesia. Alternative approaches to cannabinoid administration are forthcoming, including standardized oral formats that will decrease resistance to their use. Their mechanism of action suggests they could perform an important role in chronic pain control, especially in combination with other analgesics, each "attacking" different parts of the pain system.

Nonanalgesic Analgesics

The past decade has demonstrated an 'analgesic effect' for multiple medications not previously considered to be analgesics, particularly in patients with severe or poorly controlled pain. Dopamine antagonists such as prochlorperazine and metoclopramide are used routinely to treat acute migraine headaches.[19] Sodium channel blockers such as tricyclic antidepressants and carbamazepine, and calcium current inhibitors such as gabapentin are now considered staples in the management of neuropathic pain.[20]

Some agents were found to be effective even before we understood their mechanism of action (gabapentin). It is anticipated that genomic research will make this less likely in the future, as specific channels are targeted. Such a mechanistic approach to pain is supplanting the existing symptom- based approach. Current areas of high interest include tetrodotoxin (the neurotoxic agent from puffer fish) for neuropathic pain, calcitonin for the complex regional pain syndrome (CRPS), and agents affecting tumor necrosis factor and nerve growth factor for pain of inflammatory origin.[21–24]

Each of these approaches will permit more precision in targeting pain relief and perhaps decrease our reluctance to adequately treat pain.

All of this means that in the future pain will be controlled very differently than it is now. It will also require that physicians remain open to novel routes of administration, medications, and combinations of medications.

RELIEVING PROCEDURAL PAIN

Several chapters in this book have addressed methods that might be employed to minimize the pain patients suffer during the performance of medical procedures.

Some are more effective than others in eliminating procedural pain, and most are procedure and patient condition specific. *The objective ought to be to eliminate procedural pain altogether.* However, that would mean that many patients undergoing painful procedures in the ED would have to receive a general anesthetic, and that is not practical. Rather, one is left to determine the risk: benefit tradeoff inherent in the medications used to attenuate pain, and do so to the extent that it does not threaten the life or safety of the patient.

It was not that long ago that children requiring suturing of minor lacerations were bundled and simply expected to *endure* the procedure. Unfortunately this still occurs, albeit to a much lesser degree.

The failure to attenuate procedural pain for whatever reason (e.g., lack of knowledge about medications and how to use them) is not acceptable. Perhaps the most egregious transgression is for a health care provider to judge procedural analgesia as 'unnecessary' because:

- This will not take long.
- This does not hurt that much.
- I do not have time to do all that sedation stuff.

It should be the patient's decision that the procedure is not painful enough to warrant pain control, not the clinician's.

Recent work by Singer et al. demonstrated that even routine interventions can be very uncomfortable.[25] Very simple topical anesthesia for NG tubes or catheters can markedly decrease insertion pain, yet most centers have not established policies to make this routine and mandatory.[26,27] Similar apparent indifference is seen with IV starts and arterial punctures, despite evidence demonstrating no change in success rates and high levels of patient satisfaction.[28] It has to be asked: why the reluctance to prevent pain? Perhaps because patients are reluctant to insist on pain control related to the incorrect expectation they will have to endure pain in the hospital. Physicians as patient advocates need to be at the forefront of change rather than leaving themselves in the position of responding to patient frustration.

There has, however, been considerable progress toward a humane approach to the management of procedural pain, with a variety of national specialty societies establishing standards for procedural sedation in many countries. Issues of safety continue to be defined. For instance, it is not unusual to read publications in the emergency medicine literature touting the safety of a medication (and the dosing regime used) while at the same time reporting cases of apnea.[29] Inherent in the concept of safety is the ability to determine the depth of sedation

with some precision. Monitoring of the degree of sedation has gained popularity in the ICU and the OR, using bispectral (e.g., bispectral index [BIS]) and multichannel continuous electroencephalogram (EEG) monitoring.)[29,30] As discussed in Chapter (8), such monitoring is not yet sufficiently reliable to guide procedural sedation in the ED and remains a focus of research. The goal is to be able to determine if the patient is "deep enough: or "too deep," particularly in response to stimulation and with respect to the maintenance of protective airway reflexes and vital organ function.

As with analgesia, selection of an agent for procedural sedation will vary depending on the circumstances. No one drug will fit all scenarios. Hemodynamics, pain control, oxygenation, and maintenance of protective reflexes all must be considered. For example, while ketamine may the best agent in terms of pain relief and "sedation," the thalamus continues to receive afferent pain input during a procedure when ketamine is used, impacting postprocedural pain and analgesic requirements. The degree of thalamic stimulation is much greater when sedative hypnotic agents such as propofol, midazolam or etomidate are employed for painful procedures—the diencephalon remembers the experience even if the patient does not. This worsens the phenomenon known as *windup.* Analgesics and local long-acting anesthetics such as bupivacaine in addition to sedation are essential in the prevention of wind-up and in minimizing postprocedural pain.

Each agent has its own indications and contraindications and adverse effects. The best way to effectively employ these agents safely is to better understand each drug's limitations, improve monitoring, and establish standardized methods of reaching optimal end points without overshooting and placing the patient at risk.

ASSESSING PAIN

Great strides have already occurred in the development of standardized pain assessment tools. As Dr. Lee pointed out in Chapter 11, further inroads are required.

Prior to the development of patient-generated standardized pain reporting tools clinicians were left to guess how much pain the patient was experiencing relying for the most part on past experience with a diverse population of patients. This method has been shown to often lead to insufficient analgesia. The judgment of clinicians is colored by past experience rather than *this* patient; and by stereotyping, e.g., procedure 'A' requires IV opioids while procedure 'B' does not. In other words, the status quo is physician driven; the future will be patient driven.

Fundamental to the transition is the identification of barriers such as a lack of trust in patient reporting.

No practical multidimensional pain assessment tool currently exists for acute pain as seen in the ED. It should not be assumed that a scale used for chronic pain is valid in the acute setting. Such tools are essential in distinguishing between pain and suffering. As an example, with acute postoperative pain, an emotional component may predominate artificially decreasing a unidimensional self-reported pain severity score. Similarly, but in an opposite way, a perceived loss of control, or secondary gain, may markedly increase self-reported pain severity. The development and validation of a multidimensional pain severity assessment tool is fundamental to the growth of pain research in emergency medicine. Such research will allow clinicians to learn about the aspects of pain other than intensity that contribute to suffering, ultimately allowing better understanding and management of acute pain as it has with chronic pain.

For now, unidimensional pain scales should be used routinely, and not just on patients presenting with a chief complaint of a painful condition. No scale works for all patients, so that at least three or four should be available: an infant behavioral scale, a FACES scale, and a numerical rating scale are the minimum. Such assessment should become routine at triage, ensuring that those with more severe pain are seen more rapidly. Subsequent scoring during the ED stay has uncertain value in decreasing pain, despite the JCAHO mandate for such scoring. Caregivers need to recognize that many patients will not request medication due to their own perceptions and barriers. It is important that patients feel empowered to ask for analgesic medication and and that we ensure they receive it when requested.

Finally, we must continually evaluate our performance with respect to how adequately we relieve pain in our day-to-day practice. Satisfaction surveys do not determine the adequacy of pain management. Instead physicians should be surveying patients to determine how well their pain was relieved while under the department's care.

REFERENCES

1. Toffler A. *Future Shock*. New York: Random House; 1970.
2. Weinstein SM, Laux LF, Thornby JI, et al. Medical students' attitudes toward pain and the use of opioid analgesics: implications for changing medical school curriculum. *South Med J*. 2000;93(5):472–478.
3. Todd KH, Sloan EP, Chen C, et al. Survey of pain etiology, management practices and patient satisfaction in two urban emergency departments. *Can J Emerg Med*. 2002;4(4): 252–256.
4. Musto DF. *The American Disease—Origins of Narcotic Control*. 3rd ed. Oxford: Oxford University Press; 1999.
5. Desbiens NA, Mueller-Rizner N, Hamel MB, et al. Preference for comfort care does not affect the pain experience of seriously ill patients. The SUPPORT Investigators. Study to Understand Prognoses and Preferences for Outcomes and Risks of Treatment. *J Pain Symptom Manage*. 1998;16(5):281–289.
6. Cordell WH, Keene KK, Giles BK, et al. The high prevalence of pain in emergency medical care. *Am J Emerg Med*. 2002;20(3):165–169.
7. Todd KH, Ducharme J, Choiniere M, et al. Pain and pain-related functional interference among discharged emergency department patients. *Ann Emerg Med*. 2004;44 (suppl 4):s86.
8. Morrison RS, Wallenstein S, Natale DK, et al. "We don't carry that"—failure of pharmacies in predominantly nonwhite neighborhoods to stock opioid analgesics. *N Engl J Med*. 2000;342(14):1023–1026.
9. Shapiro BS, Benjamin LJ, Payne R, et al. Sickle cell-related pain: perceptions of medical practitioners. *J Pain Symptom Manage*. 1997;14(3):168–174.
10. Marquie L, Raufaste E, Lauque D, et al. Pain rating by patients and physicians: evidence of systematic pain miscalibration. *Pain*. 2003;102(3):289–296.
11. Gallagher RM. Physician variability in pain management: are the JCAHO standards enough? *Pain Med*. 2003;4(1):1–3.
12. Wang H, Sun H, Della PK, et al. Chronic neuropathic pain is accompanied by global changes in gene expression and shares pathobiology with neurodegenerative diseases. *Neuroscience*. 2002;114(3):529–546.
13. Ducharme J. The future of pain management in emergency medicine. *Emerg Clin North Am*. 2005;23:467–476.
14. Yeomans DC, Mannes A, Saitoh Y. Gene therapy for pain: different approaches toward a common goal. In: Dostrovsky JO, Carr DB, Koltzenburg M, eds. *Proceedings on the 10th World Congress on Pain: Progress in Pain Research and Management*. Seattle, WA: IASP Press; 2003:521–537.
15. Dresser GK, Bailey DG. A basic conceptual and practical overview of interactions with highly prescribed drugs. *Can J Clin Pharmacol*. 2002;9(4):191–198.
16. De Vries TJ, Homberg JR, Binnekade R, et al. Cannabinoid modulation of the reinforcing and motivational properties of heroin and heroin-associated cues in rats. *Psychopharmacology* (Berl). 2003;168(1–2):164–169.
17. Navarro M, Carrera MR, Fratta W, et al. Functional interaction between opioid and cannabinoid receptors in drug self-administration. *J Neurosci*. 2001;21(14):5344–5350.
18. Rice ASC, Farquhar-Smith WP, Bridges D, et al. Cannabinoids and pain. In: Dostrovsky JO, Carr DB, Koltzenburg M, eds. *Proceedings of the 10th World Congress on Pain: Progress in Pain Research and Management*. Seattle, WA: IASP Press; 2003:437–468.
19. Coppola M, Yealy DM, Leibold RA. Randomized, placebo-controlled evaluation of prochlorperazine versus

metoclopramide for emergency department treatment of migraine headache. *Ann Emerg Med.* 1995;26(5):541–546.

20. Rowbotham M, Harden N, Stacey B, et al. Gabapentin for the treatment of postherpetic neuralgia: a randomized controlled trial. *JAMA.* 1998;280(21):1837–1842.

21. Akopian AN, Souslova V, England S, et al. The tetrodotoxin-resistant sodium channel SNS has a specialized function in pain pathways. *Nat Neurosci.* 1999;2(6):541–548.

22. Appelboom T. Calcitonin in reflex sympathetic dystrophy syndrome and other painful conditions. *Bone.* 2002;30 (5 suppl 1):84–86.

23. Moreland LW. Inhibitors of tumor necrosis factor for rheumatoid arthritis. *J Rheumatol.* 1999;26(suppl 57):7–15.

24. Snider WD, McMahon SB. Tackling pain at the source: new ideas about nociceptors. *Neuron.* 1998;20(4):629–632.

25. Singer AJ, Richman PB, Kowalska A, et al. Comparison of patient and practitioner assessments of pain from commonly performed emergency department procedures. *Ann Emerg Med.* 1999;33(6):652–658.

26. Singer AJ, Konia N. Comparison of topical anesthetics and vasoconstrictors vs lubricants prior to nasogastric intubation: a randomized, controlled trial. *Acad Emerg Med.* 1999;6(3): 184–190.

27. Tanabe P, Steinmann R, Anderson J, et al. Factors affecting pain scores during female urethral catheterization. *Acad Emerg Med.* 2004;11(6):699–702.

28. Sacchetti AD, Carraccio C. Subcutaneous lidocaine does not affect the success rate of intravenous access in children less than 24 months of age. *Acad Emerg Med.* 1996;3(11): 1016–1019.

29. Strachan AN, Edwards ND. Randomized placebo-controlled trial to assess the effect of remifentanil and propofol on bispectral index and sedation. *Br J Anaesth.* 2000;84(4): 489–490.

30. Hans P, Bonhomme V, Born JD, et al. Target-controlled infusion of propofol and remifentanil combined with bispectral index monitoring for awake craniotomy. *Anaesthesia.* 2000;55(3):255–259.

INDEX

Page numbers followed by italic *f* or *t* denote figures or tables, respectively.